Mastering Clinical Embryology

Clinical scientists, embryologists, and reproductive technologists, at all levels, as well as trainees and students interested in assisted reproductive technology and reproductive medicine, will find here a clear synopsis of the best laboratory practice, clinical biology, assisted reproduction techniques, and advanced practical skills they will need to know as clinical practitioners. Expert embryologists and trainers contributed to the essential material as well as a number of advanced topics.

Mastering Clinical Embryology

Good Practice, Clinical Biology, Assisted Reproductive Technologies, and Advanced Laboratory Skills

Edited by

Alison Campbell, PhD

Chief Scientific Officer for Care Fertility Group

Honorary Professor at University of Kent

Walid E. Maalouf, MMedSci, PhD

Senior Scientific Advisor for Vitrolife Group

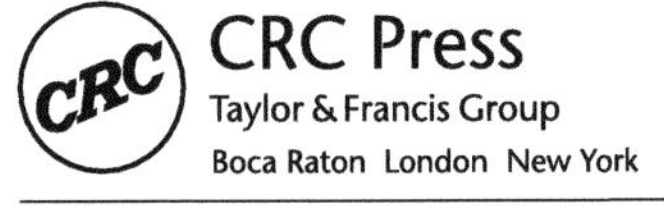

CRC Press is an imprint of the
Taylor & Francis Group, an **informa** business

Designed cover image: Shutterstock

First edition published 2024
by CRC Press
2385 NW Executive Center Drive, Suite 320, Boca Raton FL 33431

and by CRC Press
4 Park Square, Milton Park, Abingdon, Oxon, OX14 4RN

CRC Press is an imprint of Taylor & Francis Group, LLC

ISBN: 978-1-032-21674-4 (hbk)
ISBN: 978-1-032-21657-7 (pbk)
ISBN: 978-1-003-26950-2 (ebk)

DOI: 10.1201/9781003269502

Typeset in Times LT Std
by Apex CoVantage, LLC

Access the Support Material: www.routledge.com/9781032216577

Contents

Videos

Videos are accessible to readers of the book at www.routledge.com/9781032216577

Foreword

I was honoured and delighted to be invited to provide a foreword for this timely, focused, and important book. The book is 'focused' because it derives from the practice of teaching the importance of IVF as a medical science to students hoping to accomplish a career in or associated with clinical embryology. It is important because IVF has for the last four decades been a continuously changing landscape of innovation, improvement, evolution, and modification. The debunking of myths, jettisoning of irrelevant practice, and the teaching of important novel procedures, as well as how to pay close attention to detail and quality control all matter when delivering the highest service standards and live birth opportunity for patients. Clinical embryologists are generally – and should be – curious about *why* they do what they do, interested in opportunities to improve on what is current practice and, as such, are scientists dedicated to maximising the opportunity for gametes to fertilise and become viable embryos.

The practice of clinical embryology as a profession has evolved from its non-existence only four decades ago to a global discipline. Since the birth of the first IVF baby in 1978, following a preceding decade of failure upon failure, IVF has changed from simply not understanding what ingredients were needed in culture media, how to prepare spermatozoa for culture, using, literally, warming boxes (not even standard incubators) with test tubes gassed with a mixture of 5% CO_2 in air, not understanding that 'normal semen samples' may be incapable of fertilisation, that male infertility was as prevalent as female infertility, how best to introduce the embryo to the uterus, that ultrasound could be used for collecting eggs rather than laparoscopy, believing it would not be possible to freeze oocytes, and how to use and evolve gonadotrophins for ovarian stimulation – and these are just a few examples of how far the field has come! In those pioneering days live birth rates rarely exceeded 15%! Indeed, it was even then believed that most causes of infertility were female, and most gynaecological infertility specialists promulgated IVF as an option for couples *only* if the female had tubal occlusion!

One can rightly be amazed at how the dedicated, resourceful, and at times, courageous practitioners have changed the practice of IVF to its current level: expecting a live birth rate of ~50% in the best centres, the introduction of ICSI, which revolutionised the opportunity for infertile men to have their own genetic child, to gamete donation, surrogacy, embryo biopsy and preimplantation genetics, vitrification of oocytes, constant undisturbed incubation and the use of sophisticated time-lapse imaging incubators with algorithms based on the analysis of morphokinetics to aid in selecting the most viable embryos; all of which, and more, enabling for almost all infertile couples the chance of a healthy live birth. But it must also be recognised that by traversing the choreography of medical-science and engaging a corpus of ethical and moral discourse globally, IVF has been instrumental in redefining family life.

When I began in this field, over 40 years ago, many of the developments were not even envisaged, or were a kind of science fiction, or simply only a dream! It was for this reason, as well as the ignorance abounding in IVF practice, that I began my own journey to establish the world's first IVF degree. Some 30 years later one of my first star students – Professor Alison Campbell – and her proficient and dedicated team have picked up the mantle; and with the Liverpool John Moores University/CARE Fertility partnership, they will imbue the current generation of hopeful clinical embryologists with discovery and understanding of this magical medical science. A field of medicine and science integrated not only to help patients become parents through the vigorous, dedicated, and highly experienced practitioner/teachers, but to enlighten young minds on how best they can serve the patients who, in the future, will seek their help in bringing into the world the ultimate of all products of reproduction – a human baby.

But the joy of this profession only begins with the understanding of the highest standards of IVF practice; its continuing scientific research to develop new procedures and technologies will venture beyond the lifetime career of the current students, as it has mine; and I have little doubt that the quality, range, and breadth of subjects taught during this course, and delineated in the excellent chapters of this book, will provide the very best foundations for a vocation in IVF and its research. The IVF practitioner must, amongst many disciplines, be familiar with cell biology, genetics, cryobiology, cell and gamete manipulation, intelligent algorithms, and normal and abnormal embryonic cleavage. Beyond the science, they must be cognizant of regulation, ethics, the law and their variances across geographies and cultures. Involvement in the onerous discipline of human reproduction – and its many modes of manipulation – requires the utmost responsibility; after all, its meticulous practice will be accountable for a new human, and its lifespan!

All such disciplines are here in this timely, focused, and important book. I use this prerogative to wish the consumers of these pages the inspiration I was fortunate to embrace throughout a professional career. And, to the writers and teachers of these subjects, I wish you very many years of your continued dedication, which shall be of great benefit to future generations of students and their patients.

In the words of Theodore Roszak, "Nature composes some of her loveliest poems for the microscope and the telescope" (*Where the Wasteland Ends*, 1972).

Simon Fishel FRSB, 2023

Contributors

Ruth Arnesen
CARE Fertility, Daresbury, UK

Tom Bamford
CARE Fertility and University of Birmingham, UK

Amy Barrie
CARE Fertility, Nottingham, UK

Vipul Batra
Lifespan and Population Health, School of Medicine
University of Nottingham, UK

Marianna Belmpa
Hygeia IVF Embryogenesis, IVF Lab
Athens, Greece

Kathryn Berrisford
CARE Fertility Group, Nottingham, UK

Louise Best
CARE Fertility Group, London, UK

Debra Bloor
Care Fertility, Manchester, UK

Yealin Chung
CARE Fertility, Birmingham, UK

Natalie Davis
CARE Fertility, Northampton, UK

Nader Eid
Lifespan and Population Health, School of Medicine
University of Nottingham, UK

Juan Hernandez-Medrano
Faculty of Veterinary Medicine, University of Calgary
Calgary, AB, Canada

Kimberly Higgins
Centre for Reproduction and Gynaecology
Wales, UK

Kanna Jayaprakasan
Care Fertility, Nottingham
University Hospitals of Derby and Burton NHS Foundation Trust, Department of Gynaecology
Royal Derby Hospital, UK

Lucy Jenner
CARE Fertility, Nottingham, UK

Louise Kellam
CARE Fertility, Nottingham, UK

Gillian Lockwood
CARE Fertility, Tamworth, UK

Colleen Lynch
CARE Fertility, UK

Pedro Melo
University of Birmingham, UK

Lyndon Miles
Centre for Reproduction and Gynaecology
Wales, UK

Ishita Mishra
CARE Fertility, Birmingham, UK
Institute of Metabolism and Systems Research
University of Birmingham, UK

Sue Montgomery
Care Fertility, Manchester, UK

Hannah L. Morgan
Lifespan and Population Health, School of Medicine
University of Nottingham, UK

Rebecca Oakley
CARE Fertility, London, UK

Charlotte Palmer
CARE Fertility, Cheshire, UK

Claudia Passaro
CARE Fertility, Sheffield, UK

Catherine Pretty
CARE Fertility, UK

Alison Richardson
Care Fertility
Northampton, UK

Karen Sage
CARE Fertility, London & Nottingham, UK

Lessly Pilar Sepulveda-Rincon
Imperial College London, London, UK

Valerie Shaikly
Fertility Genetics, London, UK

Charmian Short
CARE Fertility, Northampton, UK

Rachel Smith
CARE Fertility, Sheffield, UK

Bryony Swift
CARE Fertility
Nottingham, UK

Tyl Taylor
Laboratory Services, North Carolina Fertility
Charlotte, NC, USA

Andrew Thomson
Centre for Reproduction and Gynaecology
Wales, UK

Mathew Tomlinson
Andrology Consulting, Nottinghamshire, UK

Alicia Urrutia
LifeAire Systems
Philadelphia, PA, USA

Adam J. Watkins
Lifespan and Population Health, School of Medicine
University of Nottingham, UK

Giles Watts
Liverpool John Moores University, Liverpool, UK

Selina Wilkinson
CARE Fertility, Manchester, UK

Kathryn C. Worrilow
LifeAire Systems
Pennsylvania, USA

1

Laboratory Design

Tyl Taylor and Alison Campbell

In-vitro fertilization (IVF) laboratory design encompasses many different aspects, all in an attempt to optimize conditions to allow for growth of human embryos outside of the reproductive tract, and thus optimizing patient outcomes. The IVF lab is responsible for sperm and oocyte collection, insemination/embryo creation, embryo culture, embryo storage and a multitude of other procedures that require the utmost care. An important priority of the IVF laboratory is to minimize stress and fatigue of embryologists and technicians and therefore limiting the probability of a mistake occurring. It is crucial to the success of the IVF lab and fertility team that the IVF lab be set up correctly. Laboratory setup involves many aspects, but at a minimum should include detailed consideration and optimization of the following: location, equipment, construction materials, secondary systems such as electrical and air handling systems, workflow, changing area, storage area, gas storage and supply to equipment and cryopreservation storage.

Space for administration is important to minimize paper, computers, clutter and distractions within the IVF lab, thus, the administrative offices should be kept separate from the IVF lab. Administrative duties include quality management, shipping and receiving embryos, and patient charting; all require a large amount of desk space and multiple network points to complete.

The IVF laboratory suite may consist of several areas, each with specific functions and requirements. The key areas are the main IVF laboratory (where oocyte and embryo preparation and culture take place, the cryolaboratory (where gamete and embryos cryostorage takes place) and the andrology laboratory (which is ideally separated into diagnostic and clinical andrology). This chapter will focus on the main IVF laboratory.

Figure 1.1 shows a sample layout of an effective IVF laboratory with specific areas: The main laboratory, Cryogenic laboratory and Andrology laboratory, and associated IVF clinic rooms.

1.1 Planning the IVF Laboratory

Perhaps the most critical stage in the whole process of establishing an IVF clinic is the planning of the IVF Lab. It should be noted that different areas have different building, regulatory and safety requirements, but an IVF lab needs to have special consideration for air quality, layout and present and future space requirements.

Air flow, positive pressure and the control of volatile organic compounds (VOCs) is of great importance to maintain air quality within the laboratory environment where procurement and processing of gametes and embryos occurs. VOCs are discussed in Chapter 2 but positive pressure minimises unwanted air and particles from reaching the IVF lab. This is accomplished by a specialized air handling unit, which includes filtration and air treatment, and through minimizing openings within the boundaries of IVF lab. For example, building a lab with a solid surface ceiling as opposed to drop down tiles, provides minimal area for air to escape and will help maintain positive pressure within the lab. The downside to having a solid ceiling is that access above the ceiling if an emergency arises, or for housing pipe work or cables, can be restricted. However, it is also possible to put access hatches into the ceiling so that areas can be reached. Although this does increase air loss and reduce positive pressure, it will also possibly prevent challenges later on, and, on balance, is generally part of an IVF lab specification. Another consideration relating to positive pressure within the IVF laboratory that is often overlooked, is the size of the space. The larger the space, the more air is needed to maintain the required positive pressure. Thus, the goal of building an IVF lab is to have a lab small enough to allow for proper movement of embryologists and large enough that it does not inhibit positive air flow. When designing an IVF laboratory, there is usually a specific area pre-allocated for the laboratory areas; which should include embryology, andrology and a cryolaboratory. Making the best use of the allocated space is important, and it should be flagged if the space provided is considered insufficient.

Electricity is also an important aspect to consider within the IVF lab. The IVF lab has a high electrical need due to the hoods, microscopes, lights, filters, and incubators, all of which must be usable at all times, even during a power outage. Careful planning of circuits, electrical loads, uninterrupted and backup power must be considered and drawn out by an electrician. The laboratory manager may be required to provide a detailed inventory of all equipment requiring power, to calculate total power requirement. At a minimum, all the critical equipment, such as incubators, should be on their own individual critical circuit and each of those circuits should have immediate back up/generator power should a power outage occur. Figure 1.2 shows a sample layout with power and network requirements for an andrology laboratory.

Water, although not an important aspect in the IVF lab *per se*, still must be taken into consideration. Briefly, sinks,

DOI: 10.1201/9781003269502-1

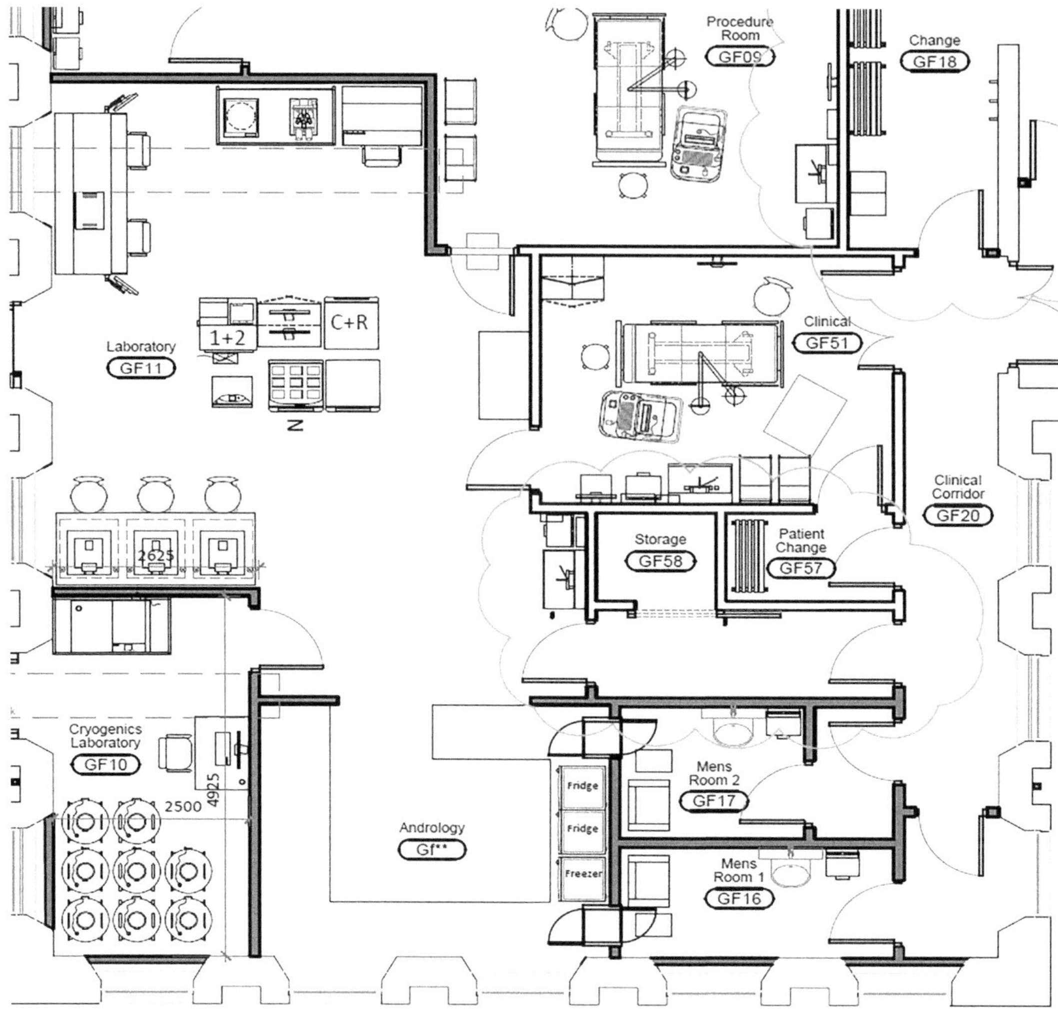

FIGURE 1.1 Sample layout of effective laboratory areas (main laboratory, cryogenic laboratory, and andrology) and associated IVF clinic rooms (by courtesy of CARE Fertility).

for hand washing, and eye wash stations, must be available within a designated distance from the laboratory entrance and work areas. Attention should be given to the placement of water pipes behind or above the walls. There are instances where pipes have burst and labs have been flooded, so if at all possible, minimizing laboratory exposure to excess piping is advisable. Additionally, the placement of pipes and electrical wiring can influence where shelving is put up or how case work is performed, so these must be thought out prior to building.

1.2 Equipment

Setting up an IVF laboratory from scratch requires detailed consideration of the treatments and services to be offered by that laboratory/clinic and the equipment required to deliver it. A budget is important to ensure procurement spending is managed and that the laboratory is suitably equipped to provide safe and effective gamete and embryo preparation, culture, and cryopreservation. User requirement specifications are essential to document what is required from each item of equipment and that the model or type of equipment selected meets those needs. For an incubator, for example, the following should be considered, as a minimum: footprint, gas and power requirements (e.g. does it mix gas or require ready-mixed gas?), recovery times after door opening, time lapse or standard, accuracy of gas and temperature controls, ease of use, servicing requirements and cost.

Electronic witnessing is common and well established in the UK, and less so in other countries and jurisdictions, although a few still utilize manual methods. Several systems are available which utilize different technologies and offer different working models. When designing the IVF laboratory, a decision on which witnessing system will be used is needed early on as some equipment can be provided with integrated witnessing plates and readers. Close working with manufacturers is important.

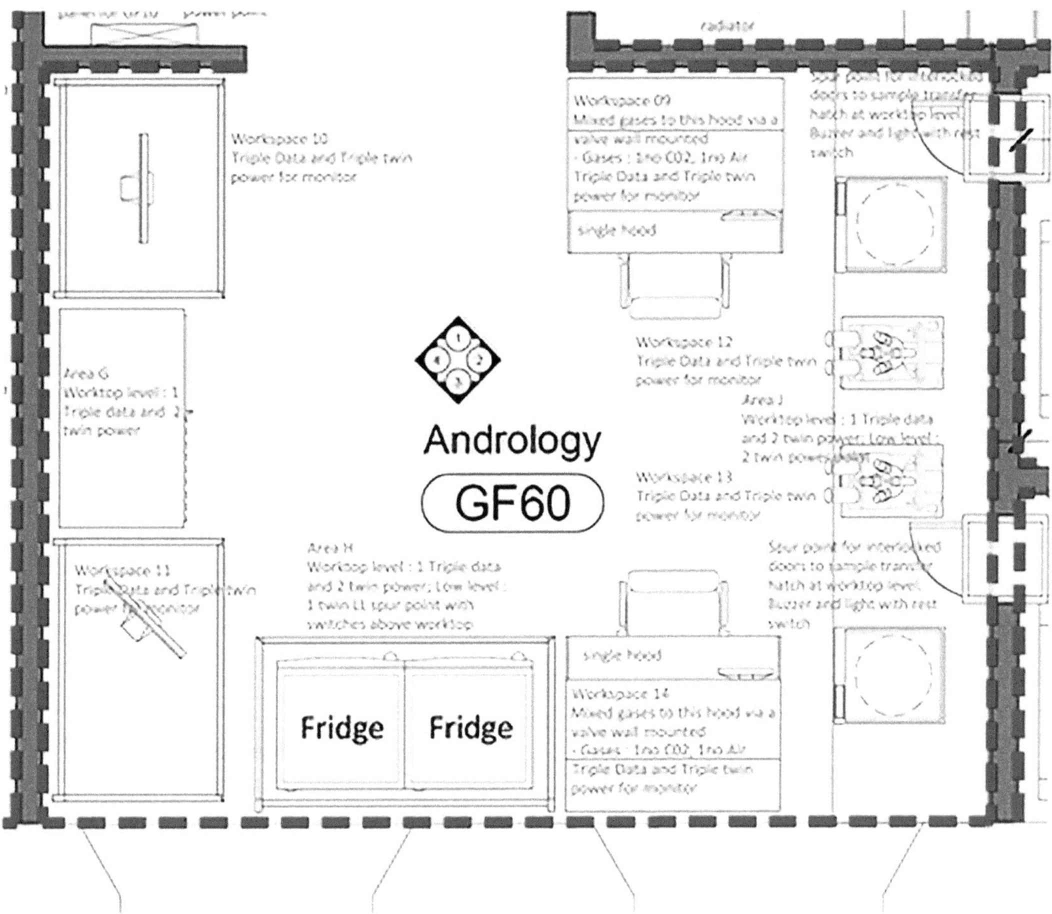

FIGURE 1.2 Example of andrology laboratory design (by courtesy of CARE Fertility).

Typically, for a new IVF laboratory, aiming for up to 500 oocyte recoveries per year, the following equipment are required, as a minimum:

- Incubators
- Class I and Class II workstations
- Stereo (andrology), dissecting and inverted microscopes
- Centrifuge
- Fridges
- Hand basin
- Benching
- Cryostorage tanks
- Ergonomic seating
- Micromanipulator (with laser if offering embryo biopsy for PGT)

1.3 Cryolaboratory

Since the advent of IVF, small vacuum tanks, or Dewars, have been used to store cryopreserved specimens. These Dewars can generally fit under laboratory benches and are easily moved, on wheeled bases. However, due to increasing demand for cryostorage space, in part due to the increase of freeze-all cycles and preimplantation genetic testing, freezing has become much more common and thus increasing the number of specimens within the IVF lab. It is not uncommon for large established IVF labs to have 30–50 Dewars, all within a dedicated room. These Dewars can have a circular footprint of approximately 50cm, so large spaces need to be planned out. Of note, an oxygen depletion monitor should be placed within the area to detect and alert to the displacement of oxygen by nitrogen, associated with a low-level air extraction system to make the area safe. Alarm repeaters should be cited outside of the cryostore, so that staff are alerted to low oxygen levels in advance of entering the affected area.

Gas storage is also an important consideration. IVF labs utilize large amounts of nitrogen, carbon dioxide, mixed gas, and liquid nitrogen. These tanks are often dirty and should not be brought into the IVF lab. The gases should be piped into the lab through specialty regulators to provide the optimum pressure for the devices they supply. An externally located tank storage room is advisable with access from the outside to minimize disturbance and contamination.

1.4 Future-Proofing

Future-proofing and scalability of the laboratory, in terms of electrical supply, network points and gases, is important. The cost of doing this is relatively small. Ensuring additional network and power sockets and peripheral gas supply is helpful in the long term and allows flexibility when the lab needs to expand to accommodate more equipment, staff and patient treatments. When planning a new lab, consideration must be given to the expected treatment cycles for the next few years but also aspirational targets for the further 5–10 years. Purchasing equipment and particularly laboratory benching, which is mobile, will offer flexibility to reorganize workflow and lab layout.

1.5 Location of the Laboratory

Before construction can begin the ideal location within the building should be determined. Ideally, IVF labs should be on the ground floor and not in a high-rise facility. The ground floor will minimize vibrations which can influence micromanipulation techniques. If high off the ground, the vibrations/disturbances could be more impactful during these techniques. Although the introduction of equipment such as antivibration tables does dampen the impact of vibrations, anything that can be done initially to limit disturbances should be taken.

Due to the delicate nature of embryology, minimizing personnel and unnecessary interactions with patients and visitors should be taken into account when building a facility. Thus, placing the embryology lab in the back of the facility, away from the waiting room and entrances will provide enough isolation for the procedures. One also needs to take into account the non-IVF areas that will be consistently accessed:

Operating Room (OR)
Changing Room
Storage
Cryopreservation storage

The operating/procedure room is where the patient and medical practitioner perform the oocyte retrieval and transfer and its location to the IVF lab is important to control for multiple variables. Ideally, there should be a small passthrough, or door, by which tubes for the oocyte retrieval and the embryo catheter during the embryo transfer can be passed through. Some facilities have full doors between the OR and the IVF lab but this is sometimes discouraged to prevent air contamination, increase positive pressure, and decrease unwanted employees into the IVF lab. A small passthrough allows the for the proper airflow and minimizes distractions but means that the embryologist is not responsible for the release of the embryo, which they have precisely loaded into the catheter. Regardless, the IVF lab should be as close as possible to the procedure rooms.

A changing room provides an area where embryologists, nurses, and doctors can change into theatre clothes, or scrubs. This area needs to be included during the initial planning phase. Typical changing rooms provide a bathroom and personal lockers. Some facilities provide showers as well; however, these are not mandatory. Regardless this should be a place where employees can wear their regular clothes to work and have room to change into proper scrub attire. Additional space is also needed for storage of supplies. The IVF Lab requires sufficient supplies of materials such as dishes, tubes, media, catheters, etc., and all supplies, apart from those in use, need to be stored outside the lab. Labs typically have shelving or storage whereby all these supplies can be unpacked, the cardboard discarded, and the supplies placed on shelving for easy access.

The vestibule is also an important feature to the IVF lab. Instead of having the IVF lab open up directly to the main area or hallway, the use of an auxiliary room or vestibule is often utilized. A vestibule can act as a storage room, but its main purpose is to add another layer of protection from the untreated air within the main clinic space. The embryologists can enter the auxiliary room and wait for the door behind to shut and then proceed into the IVF lab.

1.6 Materials

Reproductive material is extremely sensitive to outside sources of contamination so minimizing sources of contamination starts at the construction phase. Primarily, care should be taken to minimize VOCs. VOCs are expelled from a wide range of products including adhesives, plastics, paints, and resins. This means that everything from the floor to the walls to the equipment has some degree of VOC and minimizing this can only improve IVF outcomes. To minimize VOC, non-VOC material should be utilized whenever possible. Almost everything can be purchased, although more expensive, as non-VOC. If no VOC material cannot be utilized, then a low VOC may suffice however care should be taken and the material allowed to "off-gas" for an extended period of time to reduce the overall VOCs. Stainless steel, and no VOC resins and epoxies, make for great building materials for any IVF lab.

All flooring, walls and ceiling should have non-porous materials for easy cleaning and disinfecting. In regard to benching, there are multiple choices, and each has its own advantages and disadvantages. The key consideration is avoidance of VOCs and possible contamination. With that in mind the following substrates offer low VOC and are non-porous, allowing for easy cleaning: phenolic resin, epoxy resin, stainless steel and laminate. Additionally, cabinetry should be made out of stainless steel. All countertops, cabinetry, equipment, should have ample time to off-gas, lowering possible contamination. Additionally, a burn in time should be implemented, whereby the temperature is turned up in the lab for a few days.

1.7 Other Considerations

Another consideration that can be overlooked is access and the size of doorways. IVF equipment can be very large and heavy, especially the laminar flow hoods. All this equipment must be brought in from a truck into the lab. If the doorway is not wide or tall enough or the hallways are too tight for a turn, then the optimal equipment may not be able to be utilized.

Also often overlooked is the heat output from all the electrical equipment. If the space is crowded with electric equipment, the heat generated by this equipment can impact the temperature in the air. For this reason, it is important to discuss with the proper contractors the impact on the air handling system, power requirements and temperature in the IVF lab.

1.8 Final Word

Safety of gametes and embryos, and the provision of optimal conditions for their manipulation and culture, are paramount in the IVF laboratory. When establishing an IVF laboratory, careful planning is required; involving expert advisors, to ensure efficacy and success. In addition, the working conditions and ergonomics for the laboratory staff should not be underestimated. The laboratory should be laid out with short distances between critical equipment (working triangles) and with comfortable, adjustable, and supportive seating so that the staff can work at their best level at all times and always maximize patient chances of becoming pregnant.

REFERENCES

Cairo Consensus Guidelines on IVF Culture Conditions. There is only one thing that is truly important in an IVF laboratory: everything. *Reproductive BioMedicine Online*. 2020 Jan 1;40(1):33–60.

Cohen J, Alikani M, Gilligan A, Schimmel T. Setting up an ART laboratory. In Gardner D, et al., eds, *Textbook of assisted reproductive techniques*. CRC Press, Boca Raton, 2012, pp. 41–48.

ESHRE Guideline Group on Good Practice in IVF Labs, et al. Revised guidelines for good practice in IVF laboratories (2015). *Human Reproduction*. 2016 Apr 1;31(4):685–686.

2

IVF Cell Culture: VOCs and Air Quality

Alicia Urrutia and Kathryn C. Worrilow

2.1 What Are VOCs?

Volatile organic compounds (VOCs) are carbon containing compounds that can be found in all living organisms. These chemicals are easily vaporized, allowing them to serve as hazardous air pollutants. VOCs contain not only carbon but are also comprised of other elements including hydrogen, oxygen, chlorine, bromine, sulphur, or nitrogen (**1**). VOCs are released from a number of common activities such as the burning of fuel, construction, and the use of solvents, paints, glues, and other household products (**1–4**). They can be found in paint thinners, lacquer thinners, insect repellents, air fresheners, wood preservatives, aerosol sprays, degreasers, automotive products, and dry-cleaning fluids (**1, 3, 5**). Some of the most common VOCs include benzene, formaldehyde, toluene, xylene, phenol, formaldehyde, and acetaldehyde (**6**).

VOCs are classified based on their biochemical structures and can be separated into over 300 biochemical groups (**6**). Some of these groups include polar, nonpolar, low molecular weight, high molecular weight, fungal, microbial, and biogenic. Some classification groups denote the chemical structure of the VOC and other groups refer to their origin. For example, fungal VOCs are produced by viable and proliferating fungi. Over 300 unique fungal VOCs have been identified and they comprise a vast array of compounds such as acids, alcohols, aldehydes, aromatics, esters, ketones, terpenes and thiols (**7**). Microbial VOCs are released by microorganisms and these compounds have been identified as belonging to the alkane, alkene, alcohol, ester, ketone, terpenoid and sulphur families (**8**). Terpenes and isoprenes are among the biogenic VOCs that are released by plants, trees, shrubs and vegetation (**9**).

2.2 Methods of Measuring VOCs

There are a number of methods available to measure airborne VOCs. Certain methods, such as the use of photoionization detectors (PID), quantify the total concentration in parts per million (ppm) or parts per billion (ppb) of VOCs present (**10, 11**). Other methods, such as canister testing, provide speciation and concentration of the specific VOCs present in a sample using gas chromatography-mass spectrometry (GC-MS) (**12**). Other sensor technology is commercially available, but PID and canister testing are the most widely used to measure VOC levels in in vitro fertilization (IVF) laboratories (**13**).

2.2.1 PID Sensors

PID sensors consist of a pump that pulls ambient air into a small chamber. Inside the chamber, there is a short-wave-length ultraviolet (UV) lamp that produces photons. These photons interact with the VOCs in the sample by ionizing the molecules. The ionization process excites the molecules and causes them to lose an electron and become positively charged ions. There are two polarized electrodes on either side of the chamber and the positively charged ions move towards the electrodes. This process creates a measurable electric current that is converted into a voltage signal. The voltage signal is proportional to the concentration of the VOCs in the sample and is reported in ppb or ppm (**10, 11, 14**). Due to the nature of PIDs and the manner in which they operate, they are unable to distinguish between specific compounds and are only able to report total VOC levels (**10, 11**). Isobutylene is a stable calibration gas that is commonly used for the calibration of PID units (**11**).

Since all VOCs have unique biochemical properties, the ease of ionization differs depending on the specific VOC. The ability of a compound to be ionized is known as its ionization energy (IE) or ionization potential (IP). The IE is measured for individual compounds on an energy scale in units of electron-volts (eV). The higher the eV value, the more difficult the VOC is to ionize (**10**). Due to the different eVs of various VOCs, it is important to select a PID that contains a UV lamp that can ionize a wide range of VOCs. Each UV lamp used in a PID is filled with an inert gas that dictates the energy produced by the specific lamp (**11**). The specific lamps are able to ionize compounds with IEs lower than their specified voltage rating (**10, 11**). Lamps are most often filled with krypton, xenon, or radon (**14**). PID lamp energies range from 8.4 eV to 11.7 eV with the most common being 10.6 eV. Lamps with energies of 10.6 eV are capable of detecting benzene, aromatic compounds, amines, ammonia, ethanol, acetone among other compounds. The standard constituents of air that are not considered to be contaminants such as carbon dioxide, water vapor, nitrogen, oxygen, and helium have IEs that are higher than 11.7 eV. For this reason, they cannot be ionized or detected by PIDs (**11**).

2.2.2 Canister-Based Sampling

Canister-based sampling for VOCs has been in use since the 1980s with the original techniques being developed by the Environmental Protection Agency's (EPA) Air Monitoring Center in Research Triangle Park, North Carolina. The initial

DOI: 10.1201/9781003269502-2

method was described in the *EPA Compendium of Methods for the Determination of Toxic Organic Compounds in Ambient Air* and was referred to as TO-14 (**12, 15**). In 1999, Method TO-15 was introduced in the second edition of the *EPA Compendium of Methods for the Determination of Toxic Organic Compounds in Ambient Air* (**15, 16**). The TO-15 method was authorized to be revised in 2014, with the final revisions being published in 2019. This guidance provides individuals with canister sampling and analysis information based on the technology currently available and best practices within the field (**16**).

Canister sampling under the TO-15 method utilizes stainless-steel canisters that have been cleaned and evacuated to collect samples of ambient air (**16**). There are two types of samples that can be collected using the canisters, grab samples or time-integrated samples. For a time-integrated sample, the canister is fitted with a regulator to pull ambient air into the canister over a set period of time. The period of time for the sample to be taken ranges from hours to several days. For a grab sample, the canister is opened to the ambient air and the canister is quickly filled without the use of a regulator. A grab sample is generally completed within a few minutes (**15, 16**). The volume of gas collected utilizing this method can be up to 1 litre of air. After the samples are collected, they are sent to a certified laboratory for analysis. Once at the analysis laboratory, the canister is emptied into a preconcentrator that separates VOCs from the other components of air such as nitrogen, oxygen, argon, and carbon dioxide. The laboratory then utilizes a GC-MS to determine the speciation and concentration of the VOCs present in the sample. This method focuses on 97 specific VOCs and the minimum concentration that can be measured by this method is 0.5–0.020 ppb (**16**).

Both PID monitors and canister testing can be integrated into VOC monitoring protocols within IVF laboratories. PID monitors can be purchased commercially and installed within a laboratory to provide real-time, live monitoring of VOCs. Though such monitors are unable to give an indication of exactly which VOCs are present, they can be beneficial in understanding overall VOC levels and how the levels change depending on the activities of the lab or surrounding areas. Canister testing requires the use of a third-party laboratory and does not provide instantaneous feedback on VOC levels. Though it cannot provide live VOC data, canister testing can be used to identify the species and concentration of VOCs. Used in conjunction, PID monitors and canister testing can help IVF laboratories develop a clear understanding of their VOC load during various aspects of live operations. This critical environmental data can be used to adjust standard operating procedures, identify sources of VOCs, and implement VOC remediation tools. The environmental data can also be used to evaluate the effectiveness of any VOC remediation techniques that have been installed or used.

2.3 VOCs and IVF

The typical IVF facility has many sources of VOCs including but not limited to tissue culture plastic-ware, equipment off gassing, compressed medical gases, building materials, and cleaning protocols (**17, 18**). One study that obtained measurements of the VOCs released by laboratory plastic-ware determined that culture dishes commonly used in IVF release styrene, toluene, and acetone. The same study also determined that compressed gases contain benzene, freon, isopropanol, *n*-pentane, and acetaldehyde (**19**). Building materials, such as carpets, paints, particle board, and adhesives are known to release VOCs to indoor spaces. Among the compounds released by these materials are formaldehyde, acetaldehyde, toluene, xylenes, and acetone (**20, 21**).

Studies have been performed to better understand the mechanisms by which VOCs interact with mammalian cell culture processes and why these contaminants are detrimental to cell growth and often result in cell death. These studies utilized many different types of mammalian cells and common airborne VOCs to classify the mechanisms of action involved in cytotoxicity. The cells studied included bronchial epithelial cells, HepG2 liver cells, Jurkat T cells, fibroblast cells and human keratinocytes and the VOCs of interest were toluene, n-hexane, methyl ethyl ketone, xylene, benzene, formaldehyde, acetaldehyde, and acetone. The findings of these studies determined multiple cellular responses to the airborne VOCs that contribute to cytotoxicity. Among these responses were perturbed cellular membranes with leakage and disturbed homeostasis, increased intracellular calcium ions which leads to cell injury and death, impaired mitochondrial function, increased oxidative damage to DNA, reactive oxygen species (ROS) overproduction, increased fragmentation of DNA, interference with the replication of DNA and RNA within the cells, and proteasome inactivation leading to apoptosis, oxidized proteins and damage to DNA (**22–25**). Though the studies did not directly focus on embryos or the IVF process, they did focus on cultured mammalian cells and VOCs that are common to IVF facilities. It is reasonable to infer that similar cytotoxic mechanisms are occurring when VOCs are exposed to human gametes and embryos during the IVF cell culture process.

VOCs can exert embryotoxic effects during the growth of human embryos. VOCs can attach to the DNA during the growth of the embryo resulting in DNA fragmentation and reduced or arrested embryo growth (**26**). The presence of airborne VOCs has also been linked to increased DNA fragmentation in human sperm, without causing any other measurable differences in semen quality (**27**). The interference with the DNA has detrimental effects on pregnancy and implantation rates, even if the VOCs are present in very small concentrations (**28, 29, 30**). The presence of environmental pollutants during IVF procedures has been linked to low birth weight and prematurity (**31**). It has been reported that VOC levels of 0.5 ppm will allow blastocyst development and acceptable pregnancy rates but are associated with an increase in miscarriages (**26**). One study analyzed the impact of styrene, a VOC commonly found in plasticware, on day-3 human embryos and found that styrene has a negative impact on embryo growth and development resulting in reduced inner cell mass and trophectoderm scores as well as increases in aneuploidies (**32**).

Clinical pregnancy rates have been shown to decrease from 35% to 16% after exposure to VOCs released during building remodeling. This decrease can be attributed to the release of VOCs during the remodeling and construction process. In the same facility, pregnancy rates were reported to increase from 16% to 20% after cleanrooms were installed and then again to 59% as specific air purification units were installed and used. Additionally, after the implementation of the cleanroom, increases in fertilization rates and embryo quality were noted for transferable embryos. Improvements in air quality directly led to improvements in cleavage rates and can also be linked to improvements in clinical pregnancy (**28**). Another study retrospectively analyzed fertilization, cleavage and blastocyst conversion rates in the presence and absence of carbon filtration designed to remove VOCs from the air. The study results noted a significant decrease in fertilization, cleavage and blastocyst conversion rates during time periods without the use of carbon filters (**33**). High performance laboratories with VOC levels at less than or equal to 400 ppb demonstrated statistically significant increases in blastocyst conversion, implantation, and clinical pregnancy rates (**34, 35**). These studies indicate a clear association between air quality, cellular, and clinical outcomes in IVF facilities.

Though the specific embryotoxic mechanisms by which VOCs interact with embryos growing in culture are not fully understood, efforts have been made to provide a theoretical model to understand how airborne VOCs can partition from the air phase into the oil overlay, from the oil overlay into the cell culture media phase, and finally from the cell culture media phase into the cellular phase. The partitioning of the VOCs is governed by Henry's Law, the air-hexadecane partitioning constant and the octanol-water partitioning coefficient. The model uses thermodynamic principles to provide an understanding of the mass-transfer sequence followed by airborne VOCs as they migrate from the air to the embryo. This modeling identified seven VOCs (acrolein, formaldehyde, phenol, toluene, acetaldehyde, ethanol, isopropanol) that are prevalent within the typical IVF facility that should be of highest concern due to their high air-phase concentrations and embryotoxic levels within the media and embryos (**36**).

An international meeting was held in Cairo, Egypt in 2017 at the Upper Egypt Assisted Reproductive Symposium (UEARS) conference. The goal of the meeting was to come to an agreement on the technical and operational air quality recommendations within modern IVF facilities. The experts hailed from across the world with the majority of the participants coming from the United States, Canada, and the United Kingdom (**13**). Their recommendations and conclusions have become known as the "Cairo Consensus" and are well respected within the IVF community as best practices.

The participants agreed that clean air is critical for IVF laboratories. Based on a review of the specific needs of the IVF environment, they recommended target particulate levels of ISO Class7/GMP Grade B when the laboratory is in operation and Grade C when it is at rest. Their recommendation is to utilize high efficiency particulate air (HEPA) filtration and 10 to 15 air changes per hour (ACH) to achieve these targets. They also recognized the various sources of VOCs and recommended that the IVF laboratory be located away from sources of chemical and particulate contaminants such as parking garages and dry cleaners. Additionally, they recommended that VOC measurements be taken at all potential lab locations prior to commencing construction to best understand what chemical contaminants are present (**13**).

The Cairo Consensus report outlines basic design criteria for new construction IVF laboratories. These criteria provide a framework of targets that should be kept in mind when constructing a new IVF facility. Within these criteria, they made specific recommendations on air quality. These recommendations included less than 352,000 particles larger than 0.5 microns to 10 microns per cubic meter (ISO Class 7/GMP Grade B 'in operation' and Grade C 'at rest'), less than 10 colony forming units (cfu) per cubic meter, less than 2 spores per cubic meter and less than 500 μg per cubic meter of VOCs. This is equivalent to approximately 400–800 ppb total and less than 5 μg per square meter of aldehydes. They further recommended 15 total ACH with 3 fresh ACH and positive pressure between +38 to +50 pascals (Pa) in the laboratory. The recommendations outline the need for a dedicated air handling unit (AHU), set to run continuously, for the IVF suite with no recirculated air from adjacent spaces. VOC remediation technology is recommended to be implemented downstream of the AHU and prior to the HEPA filter. Additional measures to prevent high levels of VOCs within the laboratory are also suggested including the capability of the heating, ventilation, and air conditioning (HVAC) system to run isolated from the outside air in the event of an emergency. Construction materials to minimize VOCs are recommended for the ceilings, light fittings, doors, walls floors, countertops, windows, cabinets, and wood products to minimize the level of VOCs generated by the building materials. Once construction is complete it is recommended that a burn-in period of at least 2–3 weeks be observed to allow time for all construction materials to off-gas. Final recommendations are made on properly off gassing plasticware, avoiding scented personal hygiene and cosmetic products, and being cognizant to minimize activities and products that could introduce unwanted embryotoxic VOCs into the IVF laboratory environment (**13**).

2.4 Other Airborne Contaminants

Though VOCs are cytotoxic to the IVF process, they are not the only type of airborne contamination to consider. Airborne contamination can be broken into three different groups: chemical contamination, viable particulates, and nonviable particulates. VOCs are classified as chemical contamination. Viable particulates are biologicals that include viruses, bacteria, and fungi. Nonviable particulates are any non-living contaminants such as particulate matter or dust particles. It is critical that all types of airborne contamination be addressed and remediated within the IVF facility.

Nonviable particulates are often controlled using HEPA filters. These filters are mechanical air filters that are designed to remove 99.97% of particulates that have a size of 0.3 microns (**37**). This particle size was targeted as the design parameter because it is known as the most penetrating particle size (MPPS) and the most difficult size of particles to capture (**38**). The use of HEPA filters within IVF labs is a recommended best practice and cannot be ignored during the design process (**13**)

HEPA filters have also been traditionally employed to remove viable particulates from the airstream since many viable particulates fall within the size range that is captured by HEPA filters. Multiple studies have reported successful results in controlling viable particulates through the use of HEPA filters (**39, 40**). Since HEPA filters operate by capturing the particulates, the viable particulates that are captured are contained within the matrix of the filter and are able to continue to proliferate within the filter. The contained growth of fungal microorganisms provides an additional source of cytotoxic fungal VOCs. If bypass is present, some biologicals can become dislodged due to the high airflow passing through the filter and are able to reenter the airstream (**41**). Once these particulates are back in the airstream, they can circulate into the areas the filter was installed to protect.

Though HEPA filtration is effective in remediating nonviable particulates, it is not ideal for viable particulates. The use of ultraviolet germicidal irradiation (UVGI) has been used since the 1940s for air disinfection. The UVC band of ultraviolet (UV) light produces wavelengths between 200 and 280 nm and is the band that is traditionally used for air, surface, and water disinfection (**38, 42, 43**). The most effective wavelength for germicidal irradiation is 265 nm and most commercially available germicidal UV lamps emit up to 95% of their energy at 253.7 nm. The mechanisms of action of the UV light on microorganisms is well documented. The UV light penetrates the microorganism and causes molecular, DNA and RNA damage to the organism, thereby inactivating it. This inactivation prevents the organism from infecting individuals or reproducing (**38, 42, 43**). The susceptibility of various organisms to UV inactivation and the equations required to model the UV dose needed for inactivation are well defined. This information can be used to model and design airborne pathogen remediation systems located within the facility's ductwork (**38**). The use of UVGI can be extremely effective in eliminating airborne viable contaminants when applied correctly. It is critical that anyone designing a UVGI disinfection system must have been properly trained in UV dosing requirements and how to utilize the characteristics of the HVAC system and ductwork to properly design the airborne disinfection system.

2.5 VOC Remediation Methods

There are over 90,000 unique VOCs and each contain a unique biochemical structure. This provides a significant challenge to comprehensive remediation. HEPA filers are only effective on particulates 0.3 microns and larger and are unable to capture VOCs as they exist in the gas phase and are significantly smaller (**44**). Since mechanical filters are unable to capture and remove VOCs from the airstream, alternative methods of remediation exist. Some of the most common methods used in IVF facilities include potassium permanganate-impregnated activated carbon, photocatalytic oxidation and a novel and purposed multi-staged air purification technology, the LifeAire System.

2.5.1 Potassium Permanganate-Impregnated Activated Carbon

The use of potassium permanganate-impregnated activated carbon has been used successfully in IVF facilities for years (**13, 44**). Activated carbon remediates VOCs through a process called physical adsorption. During this spontaneous process, the VOCs are held to the surface of the activated carbon. One important characteristic of the activated carbon is that it contains many pores of different sizes that allow the gaseous VOCs to permeate and be adsorbed through the activated carbon (**45**). Adsorption is most successful for compounds with molecular weights above 45 g/mol. Low molecular weight compounds are not well adsorbed, due to their high volatility, and are not well remediated by activated carbon (**46**). The success of the adsorption also depends greatly on the pore structure and air temperature (**45**). Potassium permanganate has the ability to oxidize certain compounds, such as alcohols and ketones, that are not adsorbed by activated carbon (**44**). The oxidation process converts the VOCs into harmless oxidation products of carbon dioxide and water (**47**). Though potassium permanganate and activated carbon work well to complement each other on the groups of VOCs they remediate, they are not successful in comprehensively remediating all embryotoxic VOCs that may exist within the IVF laboratory.

2.5.2 Photocatalytic Oxidation (PCO)

Photocatalytic oxidation (PCO) is a technology that is commonly used to remediate VOCs. These devices use a honeycomb shaped reactor coated with titanium dioxide which acts as the photo-oxidative catalyst. The monolith is irradiated with UV light in the range of 254 or 365 nanometres, which are within the UVC and UVA band of UV radiation respectively. As air passes through the honeycomb shaped reactor, VOCs are adsorbed onto the catalyst where they are oxidized. In the presence of water vapor and oxygen, both of which exist in ambient air, the UV light interacts with the titanium dioxide catalyst and generates hydroxyl radicals. These hydroxyl radicals react with the adsorbed VOCs to break them down. This process creates carbon dioxide and water as byproducts (**48**). Though this technology can be effective in remediating VOCs, it is also known to produce embryotoxic byproducts. For example, incomplete oxidation of certain VOCs can lead to the production of formaldehyde, acetaldehyde, and acetone. The removal rate of these secondary pollutants is slower than their overall production rate and multiple studies have documented increases in these VOCs associated with the use of PCO technology (**48–52**). Another limitation of this technology is the fact that catalysts degrade over time and need to be replaced to continue to be effective. Several limitations specific to the PCO technology have been studied and published.

2.5.3 IVF-Purposed Air Purification: LifeAire System

The genesis of the LifeAire System occurred from within the IVF laboratory. An IVF lab director, after years of data collection, identified the airborne metrics necessary for successful embryogenesis. In the absence of a commercial solution available to deliver these metrics, a purposed air purification system was designed to deliver these aggressive metrics of airborne contaminants specific to IVF. It is a novel air purification system that targets the three families of airborne contaminants; VOCs, viable particulates, and nonviable particulates. This induct air purification system is integrated into the building's HVAC system downstream of the AHU. The system contains five stages of air purification technology. The first two stages consist of proprietary filter media that is specially formulated to remediate all airborne VOCs. The third stage is a high dose UV chamber that has been mathematically and genomically modelled to kill all airborne viable particulates in a single pass. The fourth stage is a polishing VOC filter, and the fifth stage is a final HEPA filer for all nonviable particulates. Multiple studies involving a large number of independent IVF facilities reported statistically significant increases in blastocyst conversion, implantation, clinical pregnancy, and ongoing pregnancy rates and statistically significant decreases in loss rate concomitant with the installation of the LifeAire System (**34, 35**). The extensive amount of efficacy data has allowed continued learnings and ongoing technological developments to the unique air purification system.

2.6 Summary

VOCs are easily vaporized carbon containing compounds that are found in all living organisms. They can be generated from many different activities including cleaning procedures, construction materials, burning fuel, the use of household products and equipment off gassing. Two common methods of measuring VOC concentrations are through the use of PID sensors and canister-based sampling. PID sensors utilize photons to excite the VOCs present and convert the electric current generated into a voltage signal that is proportional to the total VOC concentration. PID sensors are unable to differentiate between the different species of VOCs present and if the speciation and concentration of the specific VOCs is desired, canister-based testing can be used. In canister-based testing, a sample of air is collected according to EPA method TO-15 and sent to a certified laboratory for analysis.

VOCs are known to negatively impact mammalian cell culture processes resulting in detrimental cell growth and cell death. The presence of airborne VOCs in IVF laboratories have been reported to have detrimental effects on critical metrics of embryogenesis and clinical outcomes. The Cairo Consensus published technical and operational air quality recommendations for IVF facilities following an expert meeting held in Egypt in 2017. The report outlines design criteria and air quality targets for the construction of new IVF laboratories.

Airborne contamination is not limited to VOCs alone and includes viable and nonviable particulates. Nonviable particulates include any non-living contaminants such as dust. Viable particulates include all living airborne contamination such as viruses, bacteria, and fungi. Nonviable particulates are traditionally controlled through the use of HEPA filters, but such filtration methods are not ideal for viable particulates. Viable particulates are best remediated by destroying the DNA and RNA of the pathogen, thereby rendering them noninfectious. This can be achieved through the use of UVGI.

As there are so many different biochemical families of VOCs, it is very difficult to comprehensively remediate all VOC compounds. Three of the most common methods utilized by IVF clinics include potassium permanganate-impregnated activated carbon, PCO, and the LifeAire System. The combination of potassium permanganate and activated carbon allows certain VOCs to be adsorbed and others to be oxidized but this method is unable to comprehensively remediate all families of VOCs that exist within the IVF laboratory. PCO technology allows VOCs to be adsorbed onto a titanium dioxide catalyst where they are then oxidized by UV light. This technology can be effective in remediating VOCs but is known to produce embryotoxic byproducts and the catalysts used degrade over time, decreasing the effectiveness of the technology. The LifeAire System is a multi-stage air purification system that remediates all three components of airborne contamination through the use of specially formulated VOC filtration media, high dose UVC and HEPA filtration. This technology does not produce any byproducts and has been clinically verified by independent studies involving many independent IVF facilities. The presence of VOCs and airborne contamination within the IVF laboratory is a topic that must be thoroughly understood and controlled to provide the optimal environment for successful embryogenesis.

REFERENCES

1. Anand SS, Philip BK, Mehendale HM. Volatile organic compounds. In: Wexler P, editor. *Encyclopedia of Toxicology*. 3rd Edition. Amsterdam, The Netherlands: Academic Press; 2014. pp. 967–970.
2. Cui P, Schito G, Cui Q. VOC Emissions from Asphalt Pavement and Health Risks to Construction Workers. *J Clean Prod*. 2020 Jan 20;244:118757.
3. Kim BR. VOC emissions from automotive painting and their control: a review. *Environ Eng Res*. 2011 Mar;16(1):1–9.
4. Wang H, Xian Z, Wang L, et al. Emissions of volatile organic compounds (VOCs) from cooking and their speciations: a case study for Shanghai with implications for China. *Sci Total Environ*. 2018 Apr 15;621:1300–1309.
5. Conboy NJA, McDaniel T, George D, et al. Volatile organic compounds as insect repellents and plant elicitors: an integrated pest management (IPM) strategy for glasshouse whitefly (Tiraleurodes vaporariorum). *J Chem Ecol*. 2020 Oct 27;46:1090–1104.
6. Xao G, Xu W, Wu R, et al. Non-thermal plasmas for VOCs abatement. *Plasma Chem Plasma Process*. 2014 Jun 21;34:1033–1065.
7. Huang R, Lee S, Bennett JW. Fungal volatile organic compounds and their role in ecosystems. *Appl Microbiol Biotechnol*. 2015 Mar 14;99:3395–3405.
8. Fincheira P, Quiroz A. Microbial volatiles as plant growth inducers. *Microbiol Res*. 2018 Jan 31;208:63–75.
9. Di Carlo P, Brune WH, Martinez M, et al. Missing OH reactivity in a forest: evidence for unknown reactive biogenic VOCs. *Science*. 2004 Apr 30;304:722–725.

10. Fumian F, Chierici A, Mianchelli M, et al. Development and performance testing of a miniaturized multi-sensor system combining MOX and PID for potential UAV application in TIC, VOC and CWA dispersion scenarios. *Eur Phys J Plus*. 2021 Sep 6;136:913.
11. Daum KA, Watrous MG, Neptune MD, et al. *Data for First Responder Use of Photoionization Detectors for Vapor Chemical Constituents*. ID: Idaho National Laboratory; 2006. 78 p. Report No.: INL/EXT-05–00165.
12. McClenny WA, Pleil JD, Evans GF, et al. Canister-based method for monitoring toxic VOCs in ambient air. *J Air Waste Manag Assoc*. 1991:1308–1318.
13. Mortimer D, Cohen J, Mortimer ST, et al. Cairo consensus on the IVF laboratory environment and air quality: report of an expert meeting. *Reprod Biomed Online*. 2018;36:658–674.
14. Szulczynski B, Gebicki J. Currently commercially available chemical sensors employed for detection of volatile organic compounds in outdoor and indoor air. *Environments*. 2017;4(21).
15. Wang DKW, Austin CC. Determination of complex mixtures of volatile organic compounds in ambient air: an overview. *Anal Bioanal Chem*. 2006 Jun 8;386:1089–1098.
16. Whitaker D, Oliver K, Shelow D, et al. *Method TO-15A Determination of Volatile Organic Compounds (VOCs) in Air Collected in Specially Prepared Canisters and Analyzed by Gas Chromatography-Mass Spectrometry (GC-MS)*. Washington, DC: U.S. Environmental Protection Agency; 2019. 112 p. Report No.: Method To-15A.
17. Morbeck DE. Air quality in the assisted reproduction laboratory: a mini-review. *J Assist Reprod Genet*. 2015 Aug 4;32:1019–1024.
18. Agarwal N, Chattopadhyay R, Ghosh S, et al. Volatile organic compounds and good laboratory practices in the in vitro fertilization laboratory: the important parameters for successful outcome in extended culture. *J Assist Reprod Genet*. 2017 May 24;34:999–1006.
19. Cohen J, Gilligan A, Esposito W, et al. Ambient air and its potential effects on conception in vitro. *Hum Reprod*. 1997;12(8):1742–1749.
20. Missia DA, Demetriou E, Michael N, et al. Indoor exposure from building materials: a field study. *Atmos Environ*. 2010 Nov;44(35):4388–4395.
21. Brown SK. Chamber assessment of formaldehyde and VOC emissions from wood-based panels. *Indoor Air*. 1999;9:209–215.
22. Hang B, Sarker AH, Havel C, et al. Thirdhand smoke causes DNA damage in human cells. *Mutagenesis*. 2013 Mar 5;28(4):381–391.
23. McDermott C, Allshire A, van Pelt FNAM, Heffron JJA. Sub-chronic toxicity of low concentrations of industrial volatile organic pollutants in vitro. *Toxacol Appl Pharmacol*. 2007;219:85–94.
24. Pariselli F, Sacco MG, Rembges D. An optimized method for in vitro exposure of human derived lung cells to volatile chemicals. *Exp Toxicol Pathol*. 2009;61:33–39.
25. Dezest M, Le Bechec M, Chavatte L, et al. Oxidative damage and impairment of protein quality control systems in keratinocytes exposed to a volatile organic compounds cocktail. *Sci Rep*. 2017 Sep 6;7(1):1–4.
26. Khoudja RY, Xu Y, Li T, Zhou C. Better IVF outcomes following improvements in laboratory air quality. *J Assist Reprod Genet*. 2012 Dec 16;30:69–76.
27. Rubes J, Selevan SG, Evenson DP, et al. Episodic air pollution is associated with increased DNA fragmentation in human sperm without other changes in semen quality. *Hum Reprod*. 2005 Jun 24;20(10):2776–2783.
28. Boone WR, Johnson JE, Locke AJ, et al. Control of air quality in an assisted reproductive technology laboratory. *Fertil Steril*. 1999 Jan;7(1):150–154.
29. Worrilow KC, Huynh HT, Gwozdziewicz JB, et al. A retrospective analysis: the examination of a potential relationship between particulate (P) and volatile organic compound (VOC) levels in a class 100 IVF laboratory cleanroom (CR) and specific parameters of embryogenesis and rates of implantation (IR). *Fertil Steril*. 2001 Sep 1;76(3):S15–S16.
30. Worrilow KT, Huynh HT, Bower JB, et al. A retrospective analysis: seasonal decline in implantation rates (IR) and its correlation with increased levels of volatile organic compounds (VOC). *Fertil Steril*. 2002 Sep 1;78(1):S39.
31. Ritz B, Wilhelm M. Ambient air pollution and adverse birth outcomes: methodologic issues in an emerging field. Basic Clin Pharmacol Toxicol. 2008;102:182–190.
32. Cubillos VV, Capuano F, Beltran D, et al. *Evaluation of the Effects Produced by Styrene (Volatile Organic Compound-VOC) Over the Human Pre- Embryo Development*. In: 35th Annual Meeting of the European-Society-of-Human-Reproduction-and-Embryology (ESHRE) Conference, Vienna, Austria. Oxford: Oxford University Press; 2019 Jul 1. pp. 223–223.
33. Munch EM, Sparks AE, Duran HE, et al. Lack of carbon air filtration impacts early embryo development. *J Assist Reprod Genet*. 2015 May 24;32:1009–1017.
34. Forman M, Sparks AET, Degelos S, et al. Statistically significant improvements in clinical outcomes using engineered molecular media and genomically modeled ultraviolet light for comprehensive control of ambient air (AA) quality. *Fertil Steril*. 2014 Sep 1;102(3):e91.
35. Palter S, DiPaola K, Sparks AE, et al. Multi-center study: innovative control of ambient air quality in multiple IVF laboratories is associated with statistically significant improvements in clinical outcomes – analysis of 5319 cycles. *Fertil Steril*. 2016 Sep 1;106(3):e27–e28.
36. Fox JT, Ni P, Urrutia AR, et al. Modelling the equilibrium partitioning of low level airborne volatile organic compounds (VOCs) in human in vitro fertilization (IVF) laboratories. *Reprod Biomed Online*. 2023 Jan 1;46(1):54–68.
37. Price DL, Simmons RB, Crow SA, Ahearn DG. Mold colonization during use of preservative-treated and untreated air filters, including HEPA filters from hospitals and commercial locations over an 8-year period (1996–2003). *J Ind Microbiol Biotechnol*. 2005 Apr 26;32:319–321.
38. Brais N. Air Disinfection for ART clinics using ultraviolet germicidal irradiation. In: Esteves SC, Varghese AC, Worrilow KC, editors. *Clean Room Technology in ART Clinics a Practical Guide*. Boca Raton: CRC Press; 2017. pp. 119–132.
39. Sherertz RJ, Belani A, Kramer BS, et al. Impact of air filtration on nosocomial aspergillus infections unique risk of bone marrow transplant recipients. *Am J Med Open*. 1987 Oct;83:709–718.

40. Eckmanns T, Ruden H, Gastmier P. The influence of high-efficiency particulate air filtration on mortality and fungal infection among highly immunosuppressed patients: a systematic review. *J Infect Dis.* 2006;193:1408–1418.
41. United States Environmental Protection Agency. *What is a HEPA filter? [Internet].* Place Unknown: United States Government; 2022 [updated 2022 Apr 26; cited 2022 May 25]. Available from: www.epa.gov/indoor-air-quality-iaq/what-hepa-filter.
42. Kowalski W. *Ultraviolet Germicidal Irradiation Handbook.* New York: Springer-Verlag Berlin Heidelberg; 2009. Chapter 1, Introduction; pp. 1–16.
43. Kowalski W. *Ultraviolet Germicidal Irradiation Handbook.* New York: Springer-Verlag Berlin Heidelberg; 2009. Chapter 2, UV Inactivation; pp. 17–50.
44. Esteves SC, Bento FC. Air quality control in the ART laboratory is a major determinant of IVF success. *Asian J Androl.* 2016;18:596–599.
45. Chiang Y-C, Chiang P-C, Huang C-P. Effects of pore structure and temperature on VOC adsorption on activated carbon. *Carbon.* 2001;39(4):523–534.
46. Schnelle KB, Dunn RF, Ternes ME. *Air Pollution Control Technology Handbook.* Boca Raton: CRC Press; 2001. Chapter 10, Introduction to Control of Gaseous Pollutants.
47. Mahmoodlu MG, Hartog N, Hassanizadeh SM, Raoof A. Oxidation of volatile organic vapours in air by solid potassium permanganate. *Chemosphere.* 2013;91:1534–1538.
48. Hodgson AT, Destaillats H, Sullivan DP, Fisk WJ. Performance of ultraviolet photocatalytic oxidation for indoor air cleaning applications. *Indoor Air.* 2007;17:305–316.
49. Chen W, Zhang JS, Zhang Z. Performance of air cleaners for removing multiple volatile organic compounds in indoor air. *ASHRAE Trans.* 2005 Jan;111:1101–1114.
50. Disdier J, Pichat P, Mas D. Measuring the effect of photocatalytic purifiers on indoor air hydrocarbons and carbonyl pollutants. *J Air Waste Manage Assoc.* 2005;55:88–96.
51. Ginestet A, Pugnet D, Rowley J, Bull K, Yeomans H. Development of a new photocatalytic oxidation air filter for aircraft cabin. *Indoor Air.* 2005 Oct 1;15(5):326–334.
52. Qing Y, Krechmer JE, Shutter JD, et al. Real-time laboratory measurements of VOC emissions, removal rates, and byproduct formation from consumer-grade oxidation-based air cleaners. *Environ Sci Technol Lett.* 2021;8(12):1020–1025.

3

Laboratory Equipment and Consumables

Louise Best and Walid E. Maalouf

Setting up an ART laboratory requires consideration of many factors to ensure safe, efficient and optimal handling of biological material. IVF laboratories are under constant pressure to maintain and improve the quality of their services, as well as the percentage of successful clinical outcomes. There are a lot of careful considerations required when choosing the specialized equipment and consumables used in the laboratory to minimize the stress on gametes and embryos and maximize success of the standard operating procedures. When planning and designing a laboratory consideration of equipment in relation to each other should be well-thought-out in order for the work flow to operate effectively, whilst considering gas inlet and power supply accessibility. There should be minimal congestion around, microscopes, incubators and work areas. Lab design should include futureproofing with spare data ports, electric sockets and gas supply inlets where possible.

All equipment and consumables purchased should be certified and validated for use in an ART environment. The validation process should result in documented evidence that the process and piece of equipment or consumable will consistently meet its pre-determined specification. This process should be carried out at the specification stage, as well as the installation and performance stages. These documents should also be accompanied by a set of risk assessments to identify any significant risks related to the use of the item, and control measures that can be put in place to mitigate the risks.

3.1 Equipment

The number of staff, the space available and the number/complexity of the treatment cycles all feeds in to the amount of equipment required in the IVF laboratory. The selection of the equipment is based on factors relating to the minimum specifications and standards expected, but also based on the standard operating procedures that are planned to use as part of the treatment.

Space, and budget, are often limiting factors when deciding on which type of equipment to use, however, there are some essential pieces of equipment that are the minimum requirement: laminar flow hoods, heated stages, CO_2 incubator, centrifuge, microscopes and micromanipulators.

3.1.1 Laminar Flow Hoods

ART flow hoods are designed for both protection of the operator, but also to assist in the aseptic handling of spermatozoa, oocytes and culture media throughout from the dish preparation procedure to the embryo transfer or cryopreservation. Air quality of the laboratory is discussed in a different chapter (Chapter 2), but laminar flow hoods are expected to provide at least a grade C air, within a laboratory of air quality of at least grade D. Laminar flow hoods act to minimize the chance of microbial contamination. Workstations designed for oocyte and embryo handling have stages heated to 37°C +/- 0.2. Modern IVF workstations include built-in stereomicroscopes with integrated light source, although these can be purchased separately. Considerations when choosing a flow hood include minimal noise level, controlled and validated heated stage, air HEPA filtration and if necessary built-in gas and humidifying systems. There must be enough work areas to allow only a single patients samples to be handled at any one time. At least one andrology and one embryology workstation are essential in small IVF laboratories, adding one workstation for every 200–300 cases. Commonly, the stereomicroscope is integrated with a heated stage, and which may also incorporate an electronic witnessing system.

Open fronted class II flow hoods provide easier access and flexibility; however an enclosed style is an option to maintain environmental conditions during handling of eggs and embryos. These are known as modified isolette workstations. The closed nature of these workstations means there is less chance of pH and temperature drift during the handling process. An added advantage is that in some cases these are mobile and so can be used in areas adjacent to the laboratory. The disadvantage of these workstations is that they are more awkward to use, and often require the embryologist to stand during the procedure due to the location of the access ports.

3.1.2 Microscopes

The volume, and organization, of the workload will dictate the number of microscopes required. There should be a satisfactory number to avoid procedure delays. Stereo microscopes for required for the majority of the oocyte and embryo manipulations. As discussed, they are ideally located within flow hoods, and are used in conjunction with an adequately heated surface. Whilst upright microscopes are required for semen analysis and preparation. Polarization contrast is needed to view sperm.

Inverted microscopes with anti-vibration tables, equipped with micro-manipulators tool holders are required for ICSI, embryo biopsy, or to observe embryos at higher magnification. As well as a carefully controlled heated stage, these microscopes should include differential interference contrast (DIC)

DOI: 10.1201/9781003269502-3

or Hoffmann modulation contrast (HMC) to give relief contrast for unstained, low contrast specimens. HMC is suitable for use with plastic dishes. In addition, a laser module and objective on the inverted microscope is needed for assisted hatching and biopsy, or collapse prior to vitrification.

3.1.3 Incubators

Incubators are used to culture the embryos in an optimized environment, with carefully controlled temperature with or without humidification. Active humidification is needed by some incubator models to maintain consistent humidity levels and minimise media evaporation. The atmosphere within the incubators is controlled, in terms of carbon dioxide and oxygen levels. The carbon dioxide concentration acts to buffer the pH in the culture media by reacting with water (H_2O) to generate bicarbonate (HCO_3). The optimum concentration of CO_2 for pH maintenance is 5 to 6.5%. The oxygen concentration recreates the partial pressure normally found in human blood, normally at 5%, which is considered beneficial for blastocyst culture. Incubator atmosphere is controlled by the supply of pure CO_2 and pure N_2, or by the supply of premixed gas, depending on the requirements of the incubator.

A minimum of two incubators are advised for better workflow, even in small IVF labs – one for culturing embryos and one for oocyte retrieval and/or equilibrating dishes, which also acts as an emergency backup. There are several types of incubators available to choose from, from a wide range of suppliers. The main variations between incubators are the size, and methods used to control humidity, temperature, and gas flow – all of which are crucial for maintaining the steady state of culture media. Only a few studies have compared the effects of incubators with various features on embryo development and clinical outcomes, however, selection of incubator should consider: gas availability and supply, recovery rates, sensors for environment conditions, alarm compatibility, humidification options, easy calibration, cleaning and maintenance.

Large box incubators are affordable and convenient choice for equilibrating dishes, and tubes of media or oil. On the other hand, benchtop style incubators are preferred over large box style incubators as they provide a more stable environment for embryos culture in vitro. The small individual chambers enable rapid recovery of optimal culture conditions after door opening, lessening environmental stress. In addition, portable or transport incubators will be required if offering transport IVF with satellite facilities, or when the operation room is not adjacent to the IVF laboratory. Since around 2010, time-lapse incubation started being used increasingly in the IVF laboratory and is discussed in more detail in Chapter 36. They are increasingly used in IVF labs, as they provide the ability to constantly monitor the embryos via an internal integrated camera, and the annotation of division events can provide extra information that can be used for embryo selection.

3.1.4 Cryostorage

Dewars are vacuum-insulated, double-walled containers used for cryostorage of gametes and embryos. They are used for long- and short-term storage, as well as for temporary benchtop storage used for immediate immersion of cryo-carriers following the vitrification procedure. IVF laboratories will generally keep a number of dewars. Samples may be stored directly in the nitrogen liquid, or in vapour phase storage, where the samples are stored within a chamber that is kept at -196°C without direct contact with liquid. This has the advantage of removing the theoretical risk of cross contamination within a liquid phase. Large dewars are generally used for long-term storage as small tanks require frequent topping up with LN_2. Some backup capacity should be factored in to the planning of the dewar purchase, to accommodate cryopreserved samples in the case of a failure emergency.

Auto-fill dewars are becoming more commonly used. These dewars are connected to a liquid nitrogen supply which allows automated demand for nitrogen filling when the sensor detects requirement for a top up. Systems are being developed that digitally store, track and retrieve cryosamples using automated robotics within a proprietary platform. Irrespective of the level of automation, all operators, or handlers of liquid nitrogen, must have carried out a recognized training program and must wear appropriate personal protective equipment – goggles, or face visor, and gloves suitable for purpose. As the liquid nitrogen warms to room temperature it evaporates and expands to almost 700 times its liquid volume. This means that there must be adequate oxygen monitoring systems, fan extraction installed and a thorough, documented evacuation procedure. Daily physical checks of the dewars should be recorded – to detect any early signs of potential tank failure. Finally, considerations when purchasing dewar storage are the available floor space in a dedicated cryoroom; the installation of low oxygen monitoring and fan extraction; the amount of liquid nitrogen that can be delivered and stored or generated; and the number of samples to be stored, for how long, and in which storage devices.

3.1.5 Centrifuges

Centrifuges are mainly used in andrology to prepare the sperm prior to assisted reproductive treatments. There is a wide choice of suitable centrifuges. Considerations when selecting a centrifuge are: size of the level, stable surface, within usable distance of the andrology area; capacity and speed required for SOPs; and style of bucket to fit the tube consumables, and whether lids are required for the buckets.

3.1.6 Refrigerators and Freezers

The size and number of refrigerators and freezers needed are based on patient and treatment volume. Refrigerators are required to store media at their required storage temperature. A freezer choice should be based on the type of material to be stored. Both should be designed specifically for IVF laboratory use, should be lockable, and be monitored by an alarm system.

3.1.7 Other Supplementary Equipment

There is a number of additional equipment that is required to support the workflow within an ART laboratory. These include tube warmer blocks, un-gassed warming ovens, spermatozoa counting chambers and pipettors, as well as the fundamentals of lab furniture, like lab chairs and computers.

3.1.8 Monitoring and Alarm Systems

Critical equipment such as culture incubators, cryostorage dewars, fridges holding media stock and freezers should be fitted with monitoring equipment that is linked with an autodial system that will alert lab staff in the event that parameters fall outside of set limits. An on-call system ensures that these alarms are responded to even out of hours. Adequate spare capacity of equipment should be available to enable the transfer of samples if the event of a failure, or malfunction.

3.1.9 Quality Management Equipment

A gas analyzer is used to measure the actual CO2 and 02, if applicable, within the incubators. The recorded value can be compared to the digital display on the incubator, and adjustments or off-setting can take place as required to maintain the optimized atmosphere for culture. A pH meter or blood gas analyzer are optional pieces of equipment that can be used in conjunction with the gas analyzer to maintain the optimal pH of the culture media. Commercially available media normally recommend a working range of pH7.2–7.4. In addition to the gas levels, thermometers, thermocouples or thermobuttons are required for the careful independent monitoring of heated surfaces, incubators and hot blocks.

An uninterrupted power supply (UPS) system should be installed to provide backup power for essential or critical equipment in the event of a power failure. UPS systems should be maintained with record of the battery performance and replacement schedule. Surge control systems should also be considered to protect the delicate electronics of the specialized equipment.

Regulatory frameworks mandate that procedures involving the manipulation of gametes or embryos are performed in a controlled environment with appropriate air quality[1]. The manipulation environment should be maintained at a minimum of Grade D, but ideally Grade C (as defined in the current European Guide to Good Manufacturing Practice (GMP) Annex 1). The risk of bacterial or other contamination should be minimized. The air quality of the IVF lab can be achieved and preserved by use of air filtration system and creating positive pressure within the lab. Volatile organic compounds (VOCs) should be avoided. Regular particle counts (either with own equipment or using an external contractor) will provide information on the environmental grade of air, as will sample microbiological testing, using swabs or settle plates.

3.2 Consumables

Wherever possible, consumables, like equipment, should be CE marked (or equivalent) medical devices for compliance for local regulation and suitable for IVF work. There are many types of consumables used in the IVF laboratory, and theatre, but this chapter focuses on those relevant to IVF work directly, or known to affect the environment around the gametes and embryos in vitro. To this end a certificate of validation should be provided with each batch received. All consumables must be sterile and single use disposables. Where no CE marked (or equivalent) consumable is available, each batch received of that consumable should be tested prior to use by means of a 24hour sperm survival test.

3.2.1 Plasticware

Plastic is the most common material used in producing labware in the IVF laboratory as it is easily mouldable. In particular, medical grade polystyrene provides clarity similar to glass and it is the plastic of choice for manufacturers of labware, which is usually followed by coating and sterilization processes before the final product is produced. There are currently over 30 pieces of plastic items that are used in every IVF procedure from egg collection to fresh, or frozen, embryo transfer. In order to avoid toxicity risk from plastic or plastic production' contaminants on *in vitro* cultured embryos (**1**), the quality and certification of the product for IVF used have to be verifiable. In the European Union, IVF labware have to be certified as class IIa category of medical devices for their eligibility to use with human embryos.

In addition to the quality and certification, the labware design is also critical in the optimization of the culture system. They can be custom made for use with a specific piece of equipment, like with time-lapse equipment, however, those will be tested individually and together with the respective equipment for their suitability for embryo culture or equivalent part of the IVF procedure. IVF plastics for general use as well have specific designs that can facilitate different applications such micro-droplet culture for easier individual embryo identification and tracking, multi-wells for applications such as vitrification and warming, low rim or tapered edges for easy access to embryos or micropipettes during ICSI or biopsy, and or designs that can allow easier labelling and handling. Another important design is the ability to provide consistency in temperature control, and this is usually achieved with IVF specific labware that are designed flat for direct contact with the heated surfaces. This is in contrast to a number of labware that inherited the design of microbiological plates that usually have raised edges to allow stacking of dishes in the incubator, but are sometimes used in IVF due to their lower cost.

3.2.2 Culture Media

Media used to culture preimplantation oocytes and embryos is considered to be one of the most important factors for the success of IVF treatments (**2**). There are many culture media commercially available, each with a slightly different composition. The first culture media in IVF/ICSI were balanced salt solutions to which glucose and phosphate were added. Subsequently, more complex culture media formulations with the addition of non-essential amino acids, chelators (EDTA), vitamins and antibiotics were introduced (**3**). Subsequently sequential, and single step, culture media were designed to take into account the changing metabolic needs of the embryo from the cleavage to the blastocyst stage. The choice of media is to an extent based on personal preference but it should be validated in each lab setting by comparison of embryo quality, clinical pregnancy rates and ultimately live birth rates. The factors that should also be taken into account when deciding on a culture media range is the availability of supply, ease and reliability of deliveries, cost and expiry periods. Embryo culture media must be stored according to the manufacturers' recommendations. Daily recording of storage temperatures should be recorded to highlight any deviation, and potential compromise to the stock.

3.2.3 Oil for Embryo Culture

Overlying culture media with mineral or paraffin oil is an important component of the embryo culture system. It acts to hold the gas concentrations within media which stabilizes pH. It provides temperature stability, helps avoid evaporation and harmful osmolality increases. Many different oils are available on the market, with differences in their viscosity, density and overall quality. The density of the oil is an important factor to consider in terms of media evaporation, especially in non-humidified incubators, or laboratories with very low environmental humidity. The use of a heavy oil may therefore provide a more stable and protective culture environment. Manufacturers should provide a certificate showing they have used a sensitive mouse embryo assay (MEA) protocol to detect toxicity in oils sample, this gives an indication of the oil quality.

3.2.4 Flushing Media

Flushing media is commercially available for washing and holding oocytes during an oocyte retrieval. It is a buffered media used to maintain stability outside of a CO2 regulated incubator. It is commercially available with or without heparin (that reduces blood clotting) and may also contain phenol red (as a pH indicator) and an antibiotic, usually gentamycin, to eliminate any bacterial contamination.

3.2.5 Cryopreservation Media and Consumables

Cryopreservation media has been developed to maximize gamete and embryo survival, and to maintain DNA integrity and function after cryopreservation. Components of the media vary for specific use with sperm, oocytes or embryos, and each manufacturer has their own preparation.

Sperm is typically cryopreserved in cryostraws or ampules, whereas there are a wide variety of holding devices for oocytes and embryos. These are discussed in Chapter 31 but they are categorized into those that expose the samples directly to liquid nitrogen (referred to as open system), or do not have direct contact (referred to as closed system). Media and consumables used in cryopreservation are also described in later chapters, but as with other media requirements, the supplier, protocol and results are major factors when considering which media to use within the laboratory.

3.2.6 Liquid Nitrogen

Liquid nitrogen is required for the vitrification process and the storage of gametes and embryos, as discussed above. Deliveries are scheduled according to the laboratory contract. Large pressurized holding tanks come in a range of sizes, depending on the laboratory needs. Liquid nitrogen generators are available, if these are more suitable for the laboratory needs, however the volume of liquid generated may not be sufficient for larger facilities.

This large volume liquid nitrogen storage must be maintained and managed carefully. There are many regulations relating to the safe and suitable location of the tank (also see *Cryostorage* section). These regulate safety distances, ventilation, gas detection, appropriate signage, marking and labelling. In addition, emergency procedures should be established and documented.

3.2.7 Micromanipulation Pipettes

There are three commonly used types of micropipettes. Holding, ICSI injection and biopsy needles are typically made of borosilicate glass. As they are used for handling single cells or single embryos then they are produced with a stringent quality control and assurance to make sure that the dimensions and mechanical integrity are guaranteed for precise control when performing an ICSI or an embryo biopsy. All three types are typically provided with angles that range from 20 to 35 degrees (or 0 degrees if straight) so they are used with a micromanipulator. Holding micropipettes have a rounded tip and polished opening to hold an oocyte or embryo when performing ICSI or a biopsy. They typically have an inner diameter of 15 to 30μm and an outer diameter of 85 to 150μm depending on the application. ICSI micropipettes have a sharper tip with or without a spike, and inner diameter of 4 to 5.5 μm, and used for an aspiration and injection of a single sperm into the oocyte. Biopsy pipettes can have a blunt smooth tip or bevelled, with a diameter that varies between 20 and 35 μm depending on the application, and are typically used for the invasive biopsy of an embryo.

A fourth type of pipette is used for handling of embryos and can be made of borosilicate glass or medical grade plastic depending on user preference. Glass usually results in less stickiness of embryos to its surface, whilst plastic polymer will result in less scratching of the petri dishes. The diameters will vary depending on the application, size or stage of the embryo handled, and typically this will be between 120 and 300μm.

3.2.8 Gases

The three typical gases used with the incubators to provide the required percent CO2 and O2 are either 100% CO2 and 100% N2 gases connected to incubators that have their own gas mixers. Alternatively, pre-mixed gases with a specific concentration of CO2 and O2 (balanced with Nitrogen) is used for the other type of incubators. As those will be used to create the environment around the embryo whilst in culture then only high-quality gases with very low impurities (ideally <1ppm). The role of the nitrogen gas is passive. It is used to balance the oxygen-carbon concentration.

Unless you have an in-house nitrogen gas generator, all gases will be supplied in small compressed gas cylinders.

These cylinders should be manually handled carefully after completing a recognized training course. As the gases can be corrosive only regulators, tubing and manifolds that are appropriate for the gas must be used as this will prevent compromising the purity of the supply, equipment failure or injury to laboratory staff. For safety, cylinders must be stored upright, and suitability chained to prevent them falling, and should be in a suitable ventilated storage area with appropriate signage, and a contact number to contact in the case of an emergency.

3.2.9 Oocyte Aspiration Needles

Oocyte aspiration or retrieval needles are used to aspirate oocytes from the ovarian follicles. These are not generally considered a laboratory consumable, but as a product that comes into contact with the gametes they should form part of the lab traceability system. They can be supplied in a variety of different gauges, the higher the gauge, the smaller the hole created by the needle. Typical dimensions are 16–17 G for conventional needles and 19–20 for ultrathin needles. The type of needles chosen depends on the preference of the clinician, but ultrathin needles are used to minimize penetration resistance of follicles and trauma, and ultimately improving patient comfort and clinical efficiency (**4**). Aspiration needles can be with double lumen that also allow the ability to flush the follicles. Other design features usually include appropriate needle and tubing length, echo marking for easier identification with ultrasound, and double sterile packing that meets surgical standards.

3.2.10 Embryo Transfer Catheters

An embryo transfer catheter is used to deliver the embryo from the culture dish to the uterus with minimal trauma or discomfort to the patient. This is most regularly through the transcervical route, however, in very rare cases the route maybe transabdominally, which requires a specialist catheter. There are many suppliers of transcervical catheters, with a wide choice of features – straight or pre-curved, soft or rigid, with or without a guiding stylet, and with varying lengths and levels of echogenicity which facilitates use of ultrasound guidance. These individual variables may not contribute significantly to the success of an IVF programme, but is an important factor to be discussed between the embryologist and the clinician.

3.3 Stock Management

Every laboratory should have an inventory system that ensures an adequate supply of media and consumables for the types and volume of treatments being carried out, as well as a rotation system so that stock is used in a chronological order and used before an expiry dates. The stock should be held in a clean, temperature-controlled environment, in line with the manufacturer's instructions.

When receiving deliveries of media, it is important that the shipment has maintained it cold environment throughout its journey, known as cold chain custody. Any shipment that is received at a temperature outside of the manufacturers recommended storage temperature range (above or below) should be rejected and a replacement shipment requested.

3.4 Contingency Equipment

All critical equipment should be logged on a register, with a contingency plan for repair or replace, to avoid any compromise to gametes or embryos, which may affect patient chance of success. Replacement equipment should be available, or a contingency plan in place – this will often involve having a reciprocal arrangement with a neighbouring laboratory, if possible. All equipment that is essential for the safe preparation and culture should be regularly serviced by a specialist, in accordance with the supplier's recommendation.

3.5 SOPs, Instruction Manuals and Cleaning Regimes

All equipment after validation should have associated SOPs setting out the correct and safe way to use, deviations to use, ways of recording incidents associated with equipment, ways of disposal or decommissioning, what regular checks or servicing are required, and details of how and when to clean, if applicable. Please refer to Chapter 6 for more details on quality control and management in the IVF laboratory.

3.6 Electronic Witnessing

Identification of patients and their gametes and embryos is a fundamental requirement within an IVF laboratory. A system of identifying, labelling and witnessing should be established. Electronic witnessing systems are available as an optional equipment item, which can be used to reduce the burden of manual witnessing and can be used as evidence and reassurance for patients during their treatment or following a period of cryostorage.

Manual verification of patients' identity should be performed at critical steps: before oocyte retrieval, at semen recovery, at insemination or ICSI, at cryopreservation and at embryo transfer procedures. This may be supplemented with electronic witnessing. Electronic systems use either RFID tags and/or barcodes, with readers, linked to a database system to monitor sample movements. These systems can also have the added advantage of linking an open batch of consumables to a process, hence creating a traceability system.

Whether electronic or manual, double checks are recommended at the very least at those steps that are considered non-reversible: insemination of oocytes, replacement of embryos, zygote or embryo freezing and thawing. In the UK witnessing of all gamete and embryo movements, is mandatory. The record of these must identify the practitioner and be date and time stamped. It is vital that all information regarding the patient treatment progress within the laboratory should be recorded in real time.

3.7 Final Word

The HFEA Code of Practice (**5**) in the UK for instance dictates that all critical equipment and technical devices must be identified and validated, and regularly inspected and maintained in accordance with the manufacturer's instructions. Where equipment or materials affect critical processing or storage parameters (eg, temperature, pressure, particle counts, microbial contamination levels) they must be identified and be the subject of appropriate monitoring, alerts, alarms and corrective action, as required, to detect malfunctions and defects, and to ensure that the critical parameters are maintained within acceptable limits at all times. New, repaired and recommissioned equipment must be tested and re-validated before use. Test results must be documented. Maintenance, servicing, cleaning, disinfection and sanitation of all critical equipment and premises must be performed regularly and recorded accordingly.

In the future as automation and use of artificial intelligence increases within the embryology laboratory, novel pieces of equipment may become more commonplace. These may include computer-assisted semen analysis (CASA) equipment, robotic solutions for routine processes (oocyte retrieval, ICSI, dish preparation), electronic tagging of all laboratory plasticware, image capture equipment to allow AI assessments, and even 'laboratory in a box' concept using microfluidics (**6**).

REFERENCES

1. Nijs M, Franssen K, Cox A, et al. Reprotoxicity of intrauterine insemination and in vitro fertilization-embryo transfer disposables and products: a 4-year survey. *Fertil Steril.* 2009;92(2):527–535.
2. Mantikou E, Youssef MA, van Wely M, et al. Embryo culture media and IVF/ICSI success rates: a systematic review. *Hum Reprod Update.* 2013;19(3):210–220.
3. Gardner DK, Lane M. Alleviation of the '2-cell block' and development to the blastocyst of CF1 mouse embryos: role of amino acids, EDTA and physical parameters. *Hum Reprod.* 1996;11(12):2703–2712.
4. Wikland M, Blad S, Bungum L, et al. A randomized controlled study comparing pain experience between a newly designed needle with a thin tip and a standard needle for oocyte aspiration. *Hum Reprod.* 2011;26(6):1377–1383.
5. HFEA. *Code of Practice.* 9th Edition. London: HFEA; 2021. Available from: https://portal.hfea.gov.uk/media/ihkjnfqq/2022-07-01-code-of-practice-2021.pdf.
6. Campbell A, Gardner DK, Meseguer M, et al. In vitro fertilization and andrology laboratory in 2030: expert visions. *Fertil Steril.* 2021;116(1):4–12.

4

Staffing in the IVF Laboratory

Alison Campbell

4.1 Training to Work in an IVF Laboratory

Originally, IVF laboratory staff were pyramid trained by a small number of early pioneers in practical aspects of IVF laboratory work and they learned, what was understood about *in vitro* culture and the biology of IVF, on an apprenticeship basis, or else they were self-taught, using a limited number of texts, or by undertaking their own research. Since the mid-1990s, there has been a rapid increase in our understanding of what matters in the IVF laboratory and a drive for continuous improvement. Scientific knowledge and expertise are a cornerstone of this, and high-quality training of IVF laboratory staff is essential.

Internationally, there are few official training programmes for reproductive scientists and technicians, but an increasing number of practical training programmes and postgraduate degree courses which aim to provide the scientific and academic foundation for IVF scientists, respectively. Some training programmes aim to combine both practical and academic aspects. In 2011, the UK Department of Health introduced 'Modernising Scientific Careers' (MSC) which is a career structure for healthcare scientists. Prior to this, embryologists were trained following the Association of Clinical Embryologists (ACE) Certificate. In October 2013 ACE withdrew this training certificate.

The MSC introduced training programmes including an equivalent programme that replaced ACE and referred to as the Scientist Training Programme (STP), but the places of the STP are limited. Trainees are recruited nationally by panels of experienced embryologists and placed, as supernumeraries, in IVF clinics who have been accredited as training centres. Training involves both academic and practical elements and takes place over three years, resulting in a master's degree and access to accreditation as a clinical embryologist.

In the United States, like many parts of the world, there is no official certification for staff in IVF laboratories. There are a few specific programs but an apparent lack of standardized training and no standardized way for reproductive scientists to demonstrate their training of competency.

ASRM Guidance of 2021 details minimum standards for practices offering assisted reproduction technologies (ART), and advises that embryology laboratory technologists, who perform ART laboratory procedures, should either meet the qualification requirements for laboratory supervisor or have a bachelor's or master's degree in chemical, physical, biological, or medical technology, or clinical or reproductive laboratory science from an accredited institution. In addition, they require documented training, which includes performing minimum numbers of procedures. The American Board of Bioanalysts (AAB) provides certification as a Technical Supervisor in embryology, specifying the number and type of procedures undertaken, and the need for specific degrees from accredited institutions with minimum periods of experience. Rules vary by state regarding andrology labs.

The European Society for Human Reproduction (ESHRE) offers certification for clinical embryologists. Stating that 'Today's clinical embryologists require a foundation to prepare for and adapt to the new technologies, understand the relevance and application of advances in cell biology and genetics and apply good clinical practice.' ESHRE certification provides formal recognition of the role of a clinical embryologist and provides two levels of certification: one for senior level clinical embryologists and one for clinical embryologists.

Despite such programmes being available, most IVF laboratory staff are trained in house. Providing the training and competency assessment is robust, and there are suitably qualified senior personnel available to support and supervise, as required, whilst it may not be ideal, this general principle can be largely effective. See Figure 4.1 for a sample index of laboratory tasks and processes requiring training and competency assessment.

4.2 Staff Numbers and Skills

Many factors play into the number of scientific staff required within an effective embryology team. These include: size of the clinic (number of treatments undertaken), services offered, case complexity, level of staff expertise, degree and level of training underway, scheduling and distribution of the clinical caseload, scientists' degree of involvement with indirect services (e.g. donor recruitment, management and administration), research projects, additional responsibilities of team members, number of diagnostic semen analyses etc.

DOI: 10.1201/9781003269502-4

Section	Title	Page No.	Date Completed
Section 1	**General Lab Maintenance and Administration**		
1.1	Laboratory Gowning	5	
1.2	Daily AM/PM, Weekly Checks	5	
1.3	Equipment Cleaning and Maintenance	5	
1.4	Gas Management System	6	
Section 2	**Stock Management**		
2.1	Stock Check/Rotation and Ordering	7	
2.2	Incoming Inspection of Temp Critical and Non-Critical Consumables	7	
Section 3	**Information Technology**		
3.1	CIS CARE Data Management Software	8	
3.2	Electronic Witnessing	9-11	
3.3	Continuous Monitoring	12	
3.4	Document Management	13	
Section 4	**Semen**		
4.1	Semen Analysis	14	
4.2	Sperm Prep for IUI/IVFI/ICSI	15	
4.3	Sperm Cryopreservation and Thawing	16	
4.4	Surgical Sperm Retrieval	17	
4.5	Receipt of Donor Sperm	18	
Section 5	**Oocytes**		
5.1	Oocyte Collection	19	
5.2	Oocyte Vitrification	20	
5.3	Oocyte Thawing	21	
5.4	Oocyte Denudation for ICSI	22	
Section 6	**Embryology**		
6.1	Assessing Consents	23	
6.2	Clinical Scheduling Meetings	24	
6.3	Manual Witnessing	25	
6.4	Dish and Media Preparation	27	
6.5	IVF Insemination	28	
6.6	Fertilization Assessment (IVF)	29-30	
6.7	Fertilization Assessment (ICSI)	31-32	
6.8	Embryoscope Annotation/CARE Maps	33	
6.9	Embryo Vitrification	34	
6.10	Embryo Thawing	35	
6.11	Embryo Selection, Grading, Loading and Transfer	36	
6.12	Embryo/Egg/Sperm Disposal (Post Cycle)	37	
6.13	Embryo/Egg/Sperm Disposal (No longer required)	38	
6.14	Patient Communication	39	
Section 7	**ICSI**		
7.1	ICSI Rig Set-Up	40	
7.2	Sperm Immobilisation	40	
7.3	Egg Injections	40	
7.4	Split Cases	41	
7.5	Full ICSI Cases	41	
Section 8	**Embryo Biopsy**		
8.1	Assisted Hatching	43	
8.2	Aneuploid Embryo/3PN	44	
8.3	Split Cases	45-46	
8.4	Full Clinical Cases	46-47	
Section 9	**Quality Management**		
9.1	Final Release of Tissues and Cells	48	
9.2	Distribution/Import/Export of Tissues and Cells	49	
9.3	Reporting of Non-Conformances/Adverse Events	50	

FIGURE 4.1 Sample index of IVF laboratory tasks and processes requiring training and competency assessment.

Section	Title	Page No.	Date Completed
9.4	Change Control	51	
9.5	Process/Equipment Validation	52	
9.6	Document Review	53	
Section 10	Lab Management (Where applicable)		
10.1	Attendance at Management Meeting	54	
10.2	Attendance at Clinical Review Meetings	55	
10.3	Lab Staff Roster and Resource Coordination	56	
10.4	NEQAS Coordination	57	
10.5	Environmental Monitoring	58	
10.6	Equipment Servicing Coordination and Oversight	59	
10.7	Generation and Investigation of KPIS	60	
10.8	Generation of Broad Shoulder Report and Review	61	
10.9	Protocol Generation and Update	62	

FIGURE 4.1 *(Continued)*

TABLE 4.1

The IVF Laboratory Team Categorized into 4 Levels or Groups

Level	Example role/title	
A. Management	Lab Manager/Director	Deputy Lab Manager
B. Qualified/Competent Scientist	Senior Clinical Embryologist/Andrologist	Clinical Embryologist/Andrologist
C. Pre-Qualified Scientist	Junior Embryologist/ Andrologist	Trainee Embryologist/ Pre-Registrant Embryologist/ Practitioner
D. Support	Technician/ Assistant	Administrator

Many of these factors may not be controlled by the IVF laboratory team, such that they may need to up skill or adapt to changing circumstances or new technologies.

The estimated staff numbers and roles required, described in this chapter, are based on experience of the author and the few, somewhat outdated, published guidelines available.

4.3 IVF Laboratory Team Roles and Ratios

For ease and example, clinics may be categorised as small, medium or large, based on the number of primary cycles they undertake annually. Primary cycles can be defined as oocyte recoveries for IVF or ICSI (including egg freeze, egg recipient and surrogacy). This is a useful measure for a typical IVF laboratory as, in general, other treatments, such as the number of semen analyses or frozen embryo transfers, are proportionally related to the number of primary cycles. Certainly, this is the case within a network of clinics like Care Fertility.

The embryology department at Care Fertility generally has low staff turnover and offers an active program of staff development and training. These factors are also important when considering staffing. Utilising a tool, or blueprint, which indicates the ideal ratios of staff at different levels can be helpful when recruiting or altering team structure. It can also aid best practice, efficiency and workload management. These proportions are designed to allow sufficient flexibility and supervision within the teams and to ensure an appropriate number of suitably qualified clinical scientists to provide safe and effective practice, in line with the legal and ethical boundaries of our profession. Prior to registration, scientists do not act as autonomous professionals; exercising their own professional judgement, and so a sufficient proportion of registered embryologists (levels A and B, see Table 4.1) are required to ensure they are accessible to more junior staff at all times.

For simplicity, three clinic sizes have been specified with working examples in Table 4.2 to show the optimal proportions of staff at different levels. It is not always practical or

TABLE 4.2

Clinic Sizes

Large Clinic	>900 primary cycles
	A:B:C:D = 1:2:2:1.5 (e.g. 1LM, 1DLM, 4 State Reg, 4 Pre Reg/training, 3 support staff)
Medium Clinic	~550–750 A:B:C:D = 1:1.5:1:1 (e.g. 1LM, 1DLM, 3 State Reg, 2 Pre Reg, 2 support staff)
Small Clinic	~350–450 A:B:C:D = 1:2.5:2:1 (e.g. 1LM, 2.5 State Reg, 2 Pre Reg, 1 support staff)

possible to continuously maintain these ratios but they may be used as a guide to ensure the team is appropriately balanced and skilled.

4.4 Calculating the IVF Lab Staff Required Based on Workload and Other Factors

Several attempts have been made to publish guidelines or tools to discuss the number of staff required in an IVF laboratory. However, with varied roles and duties, clinic management, regulation and laws dictating the types of treatments offered and sometimes setting limits of the number of oocytes which can be inseminated, whether embryos can be biopsied or cryopreserved, there are large practice variances across the world. Scheduling of treatments, working patterns and contracted hours, can complicate calculations on the number of 'full time equivalent' staff required.

The most up to date report on this subject relates to a Spanish survey which looked at the embryologists' time required to perform processes within a classic IVF cycle with and without time lapse. The average time reported was 8.11 h for a standard cycle and 10.27 h with time lapse. The calculations included all documentation, preparation, database management and manual double witnessing. In their published tool, an average of 1.81 h is added for every vitrification episode. In addition, the time to undertake a semen analysis, with all associated tasks with partner sperm was 2.7 h and an additional hour was required for donor sperm. The tool can be adapted using an online calculation platform.

Different changes in IVF laboratory practices, over the past decade or so, may have increased or decreased the ideal staff number. For example, the implementation of electronic witnessing, and automated systems (such as live data entry) would likely lead to a reduction in the average amount of time required because the IVF scientist can work more autonomously and continuously, and not need to pause to call a witness; disturbing them from their current duties. Whereas, the introduction of preimplantation genetic testing of embryos, requiring embryo biopsy, tubing and detailed patient communications may have the opposite effect. Time lapse imaging, in the Spanish study was considered to add a time requirement to the embryologist, but this will depend on how it is utilised and whether full annotation is used, or whether automated assessment is performed. The latter bringing efficiencies and improved reproducibility.

Scheduling of treatment cycles makes preparing and managing the workload much easier for the IVF lab team and equipment, but many IVF clinics do not attempt to strictly manage the caseload, and the clinic teams have to adapt at short notice. As with any team, there can be unpredictable complexities in the work being undertaken (e.g. requiring a second semen sample or surgical sperm recovery), or staff sickness or leave which increase the workload demand on the remaining team. The IVF laboratory team benefits greatly from a flexible and adaptable approach, and this is in the best interest of the patients whose gametes and embryos are in our care.

In general, an IVF team member, will be most effective and efficient if their role is clearly defined, there are established and proven operating procedures and sufficient supervision and leadership. As a rough gauge, and based on experience and reports in the literature, approximately one full time qualified and competent IVF scientist is required for around 125 primary cycles per annum. Primary cycles are defined as oocyte recoveries for IVF or ICSI, including egg freeze, egg recipient and surrogacy. This number is in line with the limited information and consensus documentation published internationally on embryology staffing. However, for a very small clinic performing up to 150 cycles per annum, for example, it is not recommended that they rely on only one person. This is a gauge and if the laboratory undertakes a high proportion of complex cases, such as PGT-A, vitrification or egg banking, numbers and skills would need adjustment.

Support staff are essential within the IVF laboratory team. There are a high number of tasks and duties, such as quality control, quality assurance, equipment monitoring, ordering and results analyses, which can often be undertaken by technical staff or administrators. This model ensures that the competent embryologists or andrologists spend much of their time at the bench, with patients or training and supervising more junior staff, whilst being supported with the housekeeping and administration required for the IVF laboratory. Approximately one full time support person (technician/administrator) is required for around 300 primary cycles per annum. Technical or embryology administration support is necessary and can be cost effective. In addition, trainees are an important part of the IVF laboratory team and are involved in day-to-day activities within the lab as part of their training and development. Having trainees also puts demand on the experienced staff particularly early in the training, when they should be considered supernumerary and require protected study time.

As the number of primary cycles increases, there are often further efficiencies and flexibilities. Such that, in a large clinic (>900 primary cycles), approximately one full time qualified and competent IVF scientist is required for approximately 150 primary cycles, and 1.0 FTE support for approximately 350 primary cycles. The aforementioned guidelines can therefore be used to establish the full time equivalent required per embryology team before adjustments for the impact of training, supervision, and other duties, which can impact how the actual full time staff complement feels.

Introducing a 'feels like' figure for laboratory staffing may aid secondary benchmarking for team management, productivity and development. An example 'feels like' adjustment factor may be used to account for the impact of training. During the course of an IVF scientist training, their contribution to the workload, as they gain experience, increases. In order to compare the workload demands and enable workload management across a team, the Care Fertility-derived 'feels like' deduction (to the actual FTE) in the first year is -0.8, second year 0.5 and third year is 0.2. The experience and competencies gained during their training will vary depending on the setting and clinic/laboratory culture for training, but an adjustment like this helps manage the wider team's expectation.

Whilst the headcount of the team is actual, and the optimal full time equivalent required is formulaic, the impact of having a training program, which may bring in multiple staff with no experience; and take experienced staff away from their normal workload – for supervision, should be considered when benchmarking clinics against each other and in order to understand the capacity of the team to manage the workload and participate in supervision and training effectively and efficiently. Teams which feel stretched but do not appear to have a staff shortfall based on the simplistic 'staff calculator' could benefit from independent assessment by another embryology staff member to look for differences and efficiencies in practice which may have a positive impact.

4.5 Finally on Recruitment and Retention

Being a relatively young discipline, there have been recent reports of an aging embryology workforce and a forthcoming lack of talented staff being trained to take on responsibility for the IVF laboratory, as the experienced leaders are set to retire. In some regions, recruitment of competent staff is challenging and in others staff turnover is high; as they move between clinics for a better package, or work-life balance. The concerns appear to be greater where there is a lack of structure and IVF provision is under resourced.

Managing to obtain a healthy staff turnover; not too high and not too low, can be difficult – especially in a standalone clinic, as opposed to a network where opportunities for promotion and relocation may be more available. But building an effective team, which brings a range of skills and talent, and works well together can have positive effects on individuals within it, the team as a whole, the clinic and the patients. Creating a working environment within the IVF laboratory which is motivating, comfortable, organised and successful is important for the recruitment and retention of talent. And important for the remarkable work that IVF laboratory staff do.

REFERENCES

Alikani M, Go KJ, McCaffrey C, et al. Comprehensive evaluation of contemporary assisted reproduction technology laboratory operations to determine staffing levels that promote patient safety and quality care. *Fertility and Sterility*. 2014 Nov 1;102(5):1350–1356.

American Association of Bioanalysts (AAB). Certification options, available at: www.aab.org/aab/ALSELS_Certification_Option_to_TS(ABB).asp

Campbell A, Cohen J, Ivani K, et al. The in vitro fertilization laboratory: teamwork and teaming. *Fertility and Sterility*. 2022 Jan 1;117(1):27–32.

ESHRE, European Society for Human Reproduction & Embryology. Certification for clinical embryologists, available at: www.eshre.eu/Accreditation-and-Certification/Certification-for-embryologists

ESHRE Guideline Group on Good Practice in IVF Laboratories: De los Santos MJ, Apter S, Coticchio G, et al. Revised guidelines for good practice in IVF laboratories (2015). *Human Reproduction*. 2016 Apr 1;31(4):685–686.

Go KJ. 'By the work, one knows the workman': the practice and profession of the embryologist and its translation to quality in the embryology laboratory. *Reproductive Biomedicine Online*. 2015 Oct 1;31(4):449–458.

Practice Committee of the American Society for Reproductive Medicine, Practice Committee of the Society for Assisted Reproductive Technology. Minimum standards for practices offering assisted reproductive technologies: a committee opinion. *Fertility and Sterility*. 2021 Mar 1;115(3):578–582.

Veiga E, Olmedo C, Sánchez L, et al. Recalculating the staff required to run a modern assisted reproductive technology laboratory. *Human Reproduction*. 2022 Aug 1;37(8):1774–1785.

5

Evidence-Based Practice in Reproductive Medicine

Alison Richardson and Kanna Jayaprakasan

5.1 Introduction

Reproductive medicine is a rapidly evolving specialty and has now progressed well beyond mere fertility treatments. This is despite the fact that human reproduction research has always been fraught with both scientific and ethical challenges to the extent that the development of treatments for infertility was initially hindered. Since the birth of Louise Brown in 1978, the fertility sector has experienced massive growth and change. In this sentinel IVF birth, the mother had a natural menstrual cycle, physicians laparoscopically retrieved a single pre-ovulatory oocyte from her ovary, fertilised it *in vitro*, and then transferred the resulting eight-cell embryo into her uterus. Since then, advances in science and technology have continued to improve outcomes and there is much to celebrate about the sector and the progress that has been made.

Firstly, the number of IVF cycles undertaken, and the success rates associated with them, have increased significantly. IVF now accounts for millions of births worldwide and 1–3% of all births every year in the United States and Europe. In 1991, around 6700 IVF cycles were recorded at licensed fertility clinics in the UK and the average live birth rate per embryo transferred was only 7%. By 2019, the number of cycles had increased tenfold to over 69,000 and the average live birth rate was 24% (**1**).

One of the main drivers for the markedly improved success rates was the introduction of controlled ovarian stimulation regimens. At its inception, IVF was undertaken in a natural menstrual cycle, which yielded on average 0.7 oocytes per retrieval procedure and a 6% per cycle pregnancy rate (**2**). The advent of controlled ovarian stimulation using gonadotropins to stimulate multiple ovarian follicles to produce oocytes in the 1980s improved average oocyte yields to 2.1–2.6 and average pregnancy rates to 23.5% per cycle in 1982 and 30% in 1983 (**2, 3**). In early IVF procedures an important concern was premature ovulation, which would make retrieving oocytes impossible despite careful and labour intensive controlled ovarian stimulation. However, two innovations to IVF practice, including the use of GnRH agonists in the 1980s and GnRH antagonists in 2001 made it possible to prevent premature ovulation and reliably control oocyte retrieval.

Another reason for the improved success rates has been the evolution of embryo culture. Initially embryo culture media was fashioned from media intended for culture of somatic cells and supplemented with serum (**4, 5**). Since then, efforts have been directed toward improving culture systems to optimise embryo development and increase the number of high-quality embryos available for transfer by supplementing it with various different macromolecules, altering the energy substrate composition and amino acid balance and adding growth factors. For many years, laboratories made their own culture media, but it is now commercially produced, resulting in improved consistency and quality control between different laboratories and practices (**6**). These improvements in embryo culture have enabled the *in vitro* culture of embryos to be extended to the blastocyst stage, thereby facilitating detailed morphological assessment of embryos and better selection of embryos for transfer. This has enabled us to maximise pregnancy rates in IVF while minimising the number of embryos transferred and thus minimising the risk of multiple pregnancies.

In 1991 more than 80% of IVF cycles involved the transfer or two or more embryos and the multiple birth rate was around 28% as a consequence (**1**). Since then, numerous clinical advancements including those described above, combined with guidelines regarding the number of embryos to be transferred, have ensured that live birth rates can be maintained, and multiple birth rates significantly reduced, following the transfer of a single embryo. In 2019, for example, a single embryo was transferred in 75% of IVF cycles and the multiple birth rate was only 6% (**1**). This is an extremely important development because multiple pregnancy is the single biggest risk of fertility treatment and efforts to reduce it substantially improve the safety and acceptability of IVF as a treatment modality.

Thirdly, cryopreservation techniques have improved meaning that following a fresh IVF cycle, surplus embryos of suitable quality can be stored for use in subsequent cycles. As a result, 41% of all IVF cycles in the UK in 2019 involved the transfer of a frozen embryo compared to only 10% in 1991 (**1**). This increased utilisation of frozen embryos again means that IVF is becoming safer because it effectively maximises the number of live births possible from a single cycle of ovarian stimulation (which carries risks of ovarian hyperstimulation and those associated with the oocyte retrieval procedure every time it is undertaken). Improvements in cryopreservation have also made it more feasible for more patients to freeze their eggs or embryos for medical or social reasons. The use of egg freezing has increased tenfold in the past 10 years from just under 230 cycles in 2009 to almost 2400 cycles in 2019 (**1**).

The introduction of ICSI in the mid-1990s revolutionised the treatment of male factor infertility such that the number of cycles involving patient eggs and donor sperm decreased from around 2000 in 1993 to consistently just over 1000 cycles per year between 2001 and 2007 (**1**). This means that more couples are able to have children that are genetically related to both of them. The ability, availability and acceptability of using donor sperm and/or donor eggs has however increased significantly

DOI: 10.1201/9781003269502-5

in the last 10 years such that in 2019, in the UK alone, almost 10,000 cycles involved their use (**1**). This means that there is greater reproductive choice for all individuals, be they older or single women or couples in same sex relationships.

Finally, the introduction of pre-implantation genetic testing (PGT) means that people who have serious inherited diseases in their family and want to avoid passing the disease on to their children, now have options. In the past, such couples might be offered invasive prenatal testing in the form of chorionic villus sampling or amniocentesis (but these procedures carry a risk of miscarriage) or more recently, non-invasive prenatal testing using free fetal DNA (which eliminates the risk of miscarriage), but if an affected baby is identified, the couple would then face the difficult decision of whether or not to terminate the pregnancy. Another alternative might be that such couples consider using donated sperm, eggs or embryos in treatment or exploring adoption. PGT means that embryos can be tested during IVF so that only those that do not carry the gene for the specific condition being tested for are transferred. In this way, couples can have unaffected genetically related children. Initially this involved screening cleavage stage embryos using fluorescent in-situ hybridisation but that was subsequently found to reduce live birth rates and be generally detrimental (**7, 8**). Nowadays embryos are biopsied at the blastocyst stage and PCR is used for the analysis. Genetic testing can also be used to look for embryonic aneuploidy, which although not routinely recommended, may have a role in certain select patient populations e.g. older women or those with a history of recurrent miscarriage.

The increasing demand for fertility treatment drives research and development of technologies to optimise IVF regimens and success. Developments in science and technology have meant that in the UK alone, in the last 30 years, almost 595,000 people have had around 1.3 million IVF cycles and 260,000 donor insemination cycles, resulting in the birth of over 390,000 babies (**1**). None of this would have been possible without the sector embracing evidence-based practice, which is the focus of the remainder of this chapter.

5.2 What Is Evidence-Based Practice?

The term 'evidence-based medicine' was first introduced in the medical literature in the early 1990s. Although initially set within the context of medicine, many professions allied to health and social care subsequently embraced the advantages of an evidence-based approach to their work hence the term 'evidence-based practice' (EBP) is now considered to be a more accurate description of the phenomenon. It also better reflects the fact that in most clinical scenarios, including in the IVF context, many practitioners work together in multi-disciplinary teams and the provision of high-quality care is not solely the responsibility of the medics.

EBP refers to the application of the best available research to clinical care, which requires the integration of evidence with clinical expertise and patient values. Practitioners must use their clinical skills and prior experience to rapidly identify each patient's unique clinical situation, applying the evidence tailored to the individual's risks versus benefits of potential interventions. The ultimate goal of EBP is to support patients by contextualising the evidence with their preferences, concerns and expectations. This avoids a one-size-fits-all approach to clinical management and results in a process of shared decision-making, in which the patient's values, circumstances and setting, dictate the best care. The decisions should be made by those receiving care, informed by the tacit and explicit knowledge of those providing care, within the context of the available resources (**9**).

All health care specialists must therefore be able to gain, assess, apply, and integrate new knowledge and have the ability to adapt to changing circumstances throughout their professional life. Without the skills, professionals and organisations will find it difficult to provide 'best practice'.

In this chapter, we explore the components of EBP based on a consensus statement conceived by the delegates of the second international conference of Evidence-Based Health Care Teachers and Developers held in Sicily in 2003, with selected studies and examples relevant to specialists in the field of reproductive medicine. The statement proposed a five-step model of EBP, often referred to as 'the 5 As of EBP', which we will now go on to consider in turn.

5.3 Step 1: Translation of Uncertainty into an Answerable Question (Ask)

Asking a well-structured question is of paramount importance in EBP. Several tools exist to help develop structured questions to enable an effective literature search (**10**). Any data retrieved therefore should then be relevant to the specific clinical question. The PICOS tool, which focuses on the population, intervention, comparison, outcomes and study design of an article, is commonly used for asking clinical questions. An example based on the recent SCRaTCH trial (**11**) is illustrated in Table 5.1 below.

TABLE 5.1

The PICOS Summary Based on the SCRaTCH Trial (Using Data from [**11**])

Participants/ Population	**Women with one failed IVF/ICSI cycle**
Intervention	A single endometrial scratch in the mid-luteal phase of the menstrual cycle prior to the start of stimulation for IVF/ICSI
Comparator	No endometrial scratch or sham intervention
Outcome(s)	Primary: Live birth after a fresh transfer from the second IVF/ICSI treatment (i.e. the first cycle after randomisation) Secondary: Implantation rate after the second fresh IVF/ICSI treatment; biochemical pregnancy loss and miscarriage rate after the second fresh IVF/ICSI treatment; cumulative live birth after the full second IVF/ICSI treatment (i.e. including all fresh and frozen transfers); cumulative biochemical-, clinical-, ongoing pregnancy rate, ongoing pregnancy leading to live birth rate and multiple pregnancy rate within 12 months after randomisation; and the time to biochemical pregnancy leading to live birth.
Study design	Randomised controlled trial

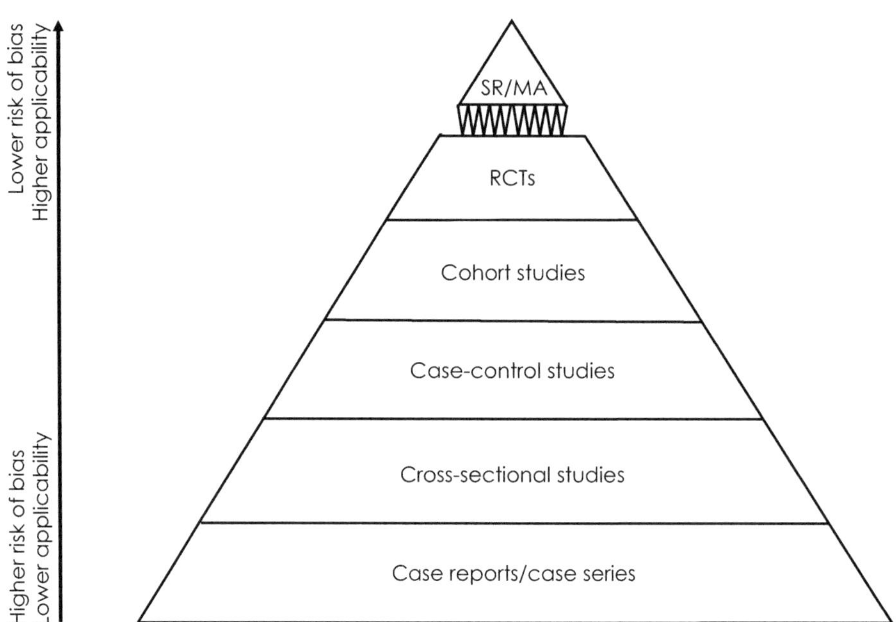

FIGURE 5.1 The pyramid of evidence (adapted from [**12**]).

5.4 Step 2: Systematic Retrieval of Best Evidence Available (Acquire)

Whilst studies of any design have the potential to change practice, not all evidence that is generated is equal. The early adopters of EBP indicated a hierarchy of evidence, giving rise to the 'pyramid of evidence' which depicts weaker study designs, for example, case series, at the bottom and systematic reviews and meta-analyses at the top, with case-control and cohort studies and randomised controlled trials (RCTs) in the middle (Figure 5.1).

A general description of the different study designs as well as some pertinent examples related to the field is given in Table 5.2.

Systematic reviews seek to collate evidence that fits prespecified eligibility criteria in order to answer a specific research question. They aim to minimise bias by using explicit, systematic methods documented in advance with a protocol. The results can then be used to inform decisions about health and social care. A systematic review can be performed with or without a meta-analysis, which uses statistical methods to combine and summarise numerical data from multiple separate studies collated in a systematic review. The Cochrane Database of Systematic Reviews is the leading journal and database for systematic reviews of RCTs in healthcare. They have published over 80 systematic reviews and meta-analyses pertaining to various stages of the ART cycle, of which 39 include interventions that were effective or promising and 22 were ineffective or possibly ineffective. For a further 22 interventions, the reviews were unable to draw conclusions owing to the lack of evidence. The main findings of these Cochrane reviews, as well as several other key systematic reviews and meta-analyses, have been summarised in Table 5.3.

Considerable effort has been put into improving the methodology and reporting of systematic reviews and meta-analysis (**12**). Established guidance exists to support the conduct of systematic reviews. The EQUATOR (Enhancing the QUAlity and Transparency Of health Research) Network is an international initiative that aims to improve the reliability of research by improving the reporting of published reports (www.equator-network.org/). The network has published reporting guidelines for all main study types, including systematic reviews. Additionally, the Preferred Reporting Items for Systematic Reviews and Meta-Analyses (PRISMA) guidelines suggest a minimum set of items for reporting in different types of systematic reviews and meta-analyses (www.prisma-statement.org/). Despite these efforts, the inclusion of systematic reviews and meta-analyses at the top of the 'pyramid of evidence' has been challenged and the suggestion to use these as a lens through which other types of studies should be seen has been proposed (**13**). Even when systematic reviews employ comprehensive literature searches and rigorous study selection processes, the certainty of the evidence provided within them can still be questionable. In other words, a meta-analysis of well-conducted RCTs at low risk of bias cannot be equated with a meta-analysis of observational studies at higher risk of bias. For example, a meta-analysis of 19 observational studies showed that ART increased the risk of major malformation with an OR of 1.29 (95% CI 1.01–1.67) (**14**). Clearly this meta-analysis should not be on the top of the pyramid similar to a meta-analysis of RCTs. After all, the evidence remains consistent of non-randomised studies and likely subject to numerous confounders.

TABLE 5.2

A General Description of Different Study Designs

Study Design	Description	Best Use	Advantages	Disadvantages	Example(s)
Cross-sectional	Assesses the prevalence of an outcome in a broad population at a specific point in time	To quantify the prevalence of a disease or risk factor or to quantify the accuracy of a diagnostic test	• Cheap and simple • Ethically safe	• Establishes association at most, not causality • Susceptible to recall and Neyman bias • Confounders may be unequally distributed • Group sizes may be unequal	The impact of IVF on birthweight from 1991 to 2015: *Singleton birthweight has increased markedly over the past 25 years. Such a change is not seen in the general population of live born singletons in the UK or other developed countries and seems to be specific to this IVF population* (**52**) Prevalence of uterine anomalies and their impact on early pregnancy in women conceiving after ART: *Women who are referred for ART have a high prevalence of congenital uterine anomalies, the most common anomaly being an arcuate uterus* (**53**)
Case-control	Patients with a certain outcome or disease and an appropriate group of controls without the outcome or disease are selected and then information is obtained on whether the subjects have been exposed to the factor under investigation	To investigate outbreaks or studying rare diseases or outcomes	• Quick and cheap • Only feasible method for very rare disorders or those with a long lag between exposure and outcome • Fewer subjects needed than for cross-sectional studies	• Reliance on recall or records to determine exposure status • Confounders • Selection of control groups is difficult • Potential bias: recall, selection	Obstetric outcome among women with unexplained infertility after IVF: *The overall obstetric outcome among couples with unexplained infertility treated with IVF was good, with similar outcome compared with spontaneous pregnancies and IVF pregnancies generally* (**54**)
Cohort	Data are obtained from groups who have been exposed, or not exposed, to the new technology or factor of interest. No allocation of exposure is made by the researcher.	To study the effect of predictive factors an outcome	• Ethically safe • Subjects can be matched • Can establish timing and directionality of events • Eligibility criteria and outcome assessments can be standardised • Administratively easier and cheaper than an RCT	• Controls may be difficult to identify • Exposure may be linked to a hidden confounder • Blinding is difficult • Randomisation is not present • Large sample sizes and/or long follow up required for rare diseases	Outcome of ART in women with congenital uterine anomalies: *Congenital uterine anomalies as a whole do not affect clinical pregnancy or live birth rates in women following IVF but do increase the incidence of preterm birth. The presence of uterine anomalies more severe than arcuate uterus significantly worsens all pregnancy outcomes* (**55**) The effect of deprivation on IVF outcome: *More socioeconomically deprived women are significantly less likely to achieve a live birth than less deprived women independent of the number of cycles of IVF undertaken* (**56**)
Randomised controlled trials	An experimental comparison study in which participants are allocated to treatment/intervention or control/placebo groups using a random mechanism. Participants are then followed up in the same way to compare the benefits and harms observed in each group.	To study the effect of an intervention	• Unbiased distribution of confounders • Blinding more likely • Randomisation facilitates statistical analysis	• Expensive: time and money • Volunteer bias • Ethically problematic at times	Comparing direct and afterload techniques of embryo transfer: *Difficult transfer rate was significantly higher in the direct ET group than in the afterload group. However, no differences in pregnancy and live birth rates between the two groups were observed* (**57**) Ultrasound guided embryo transfers: *No difference in clinical pregnancy or live birth rates were observed between those that did and did not have abdominal ultrasound to guide replacement at the time of embryo transfer* (**58**) Assessing the effectiveness and safety of the endometrial scratch procedure prior to first-time IVF±ICSI: *An endometrial scratch is safe but does not improve pregnancy outcomes when performed in the mid-luteal phase prior to first IVF± ICSI cycle* (**59**) Assessing the effectiveness of physiological, hyaluronan-selected ICSI for infertility treatment: *Compared with ICSI, use of hyaluronan-based sperm selection for ICSI (i.e. physiological ICSI or PICSI) does not significantly improve term live birth rates* (**60**) Single fresh and frozen-thawed blastocyst transfer using hyaluronan-rich transfer medium: *Pregnancy rates after fresh elective and frozen-thawed single blastocyst transfer were similar when comparing hyaluronan-rich and conventional transfer medium* (**61**)

TABLE 5.3

A Summary of Results from all Cochrane Reviews Related to Assisted Reproductive Technology

	Effective	Promising (more evidence needed)	Possibly ineffective (more evidence needed)	Ineffective	No conclusions possible due to lack of evidence
Indication for ART		• In women with unexplained subfertility, IVF may be associated with higher LB rates than both unstimulated and stimulated IUI[4] (**62**) • In women with unexplained subfertility, IVF was associated with higher LB rates than stimulated IUI overall, but in women <38yrs old, LB rates were similar between the two groups (findings from more recent, non-Cochrane SR) (**63**)			• In women with unexplained subfertility, there was no conclusive evidence of a difference in LB rates between IVF and expectant management[6] and in those who were treatment naïve, there was insufficient evidence to determine whether there was a difference in LB rates between IVF and stimulated IUI[3] (**62**) • IVF versus tubal reanastomosis for subfertility after tubal sterilisation: no RCTs found (**64**) • IVM in subfertile women with PCOS: no properly conducted RCTs found (**65**) • Thyroxine for subfertile women with auto-immune thyroid disease or subclinical hypothyroidism: insufficient evidence (**66**)
Pre-ART and adjuvant strategies	• Endometrial injury in the mid-luteal phase of the preceding cycle increases CP and LB rates following IVF[3] (**67**) • Use of GH increases the no. of oocytes retrieved and CP rates in poor responders but has an uncertain effect in normal responders[6] (**68**) • Laparoscopic tubal occlusion prior to IVF is an acceptable alternative to salpingectomy in women with hydrosalpinges[3] (**69**)	• Oral antioxidants given to men in couples with male factor or unexplained subfertility may improve LB rates[5] (**70**) • Limited evidence in support of supplemental oral antioxidants for subfertile women[6] (**71**) • Vasodilators may increase CP rates in women undergoing IVF[5]. Insufficient evidence regarding LB rates (**72**) • Pre-treatment with DHEA or testosterone may be associated with increased LB rates in poor responders who are undergoing IVF[3] (**73**) • GH appears to increase CP and LB rates in poor responders who are undergoing IVF[2] (**74**)	• Endometrial injury in the mid-luteal phase of the preceding cycle does not increase LB rates (findings from more recent, non-Cochrane SR) (**75**) • Insufficient evidence to show whether acupuncture improves CP or LB rates[5] (**76**) • Pre-conceptual lifestyle advice on a combination of topics may result in little to no difference in LB rate[5] (**77**) • Insufficient evidence to show whether there was any effect on reproductive outcomes following interventions for women with endometrioma prior to undergoing IVF[6] (**78**) • Insufficient evidence to show whether ovarian cyst aspiration before IVF affects CP or LB rates[6] (**79**) • In antagonist protocols, metformin may reduce LB rates in women with PCOS. It may however reduce the risk of OHSS[5] (**80**)		• Aspirin for IVF: insufficient evidence from adequately powered RCTs (**81**) • Insufficient evidence regarding the routine use of NSAIDs as co-treatments in infertile women undergoing IVF[6] (**82**)

Down-regulation with agonist or antagonist	• The CP rate is higher when GnRH agonists are used in long protocols compared to short protocols[3] (**83**) • Compared to long GnRH agonist protocols, GnRH antagonist protocols significantly reduce the risk of OHSS without compromising LB rates[3] (**84**)	• Uncertain as to whether long-term GnRH agonist therapy prior to IVF in women with endometriosis affects LB rate[6] (**85**)	• Insufficient evidence to show a difference in CP or LB rates using depot versus daily administration of GnRH agonists for pituitary desensitisation[4] (**86**)		
Ovarian stimulation	• Recombinant and urinary gonadotrophins are equally effective and safe for COS in IVF[2] (**87**) • Use of a medium dose (150–180µg) of long acting FSH is as safe and effective as daily FSH in women with unexplained subfertility[3] (**88**) • A decreased dose of FSH in predicted high responders reduces the risk of moderate or severe OHSS[5] (**89**)	• In GnRH agonist protocols, co-administration of rLH and rFSH may improve CP and ongoing pregnancy rates but not LB rates[3] (**90**) • Use of CC or letrozole for COS (with or without gonadotrophins) reduced the quantity of gonadotrophins required, and the incidence of OHSS. Evidence was insufficient to determine an effect on CP or LB rates. It may be associated with an increased risk of cycle cancellation and reduced number of oocytes retrieved[4] (**91**) • FSH replaced by low dose hCG in the late follicular phase does not appear to affect CP and ongoing pregnancy rates compared to FSH alone. Insufficient evidence to comment on LB, OHSS and miscarriage rates[6] (**92**) • No difference in natural cycle IVF and standard IVF in terms of CP, LB, OHSS and multiple pregnancy[6] (**93**)	• Cycle monitoring by US and serum E2 is no more efficacious than by using US alone[5] (**94**) • Pre-treatment with the COCP is associated with a lower LB rate than no pre-treatment[3]. Insufficient evidence to show whether pre-treatment with progestogens or oestrogens affect CP or LB rates[4] (**95**) • Glucocorticoids may increase CP but not LB rates[5] (**96**) • Current evidence does not provide clear justification for adjusting the standard dose of 150iu in the case of poor or normal responders[5] (**89**)		• Evidence was insufficient to support the routine use of any particular intervention for pituitary down-regulation, ovarian stimulation or adjuvant therapy in the treatment of poor responders to COS in IVF[6] (**97**)

(Continued)

TABLE 5.3 ***(Continued)***

A Summary of Results from all Cochrane Reviews Related to Assisted Reproductive Technology

	Effective	Promising (more evidence needed)	Possibly ineffective (more evidence needed)	Ineffective	No conclusions possible due to lack of evidence
Ovulation triggering	• Recombinant hCG and rLH are as effective as final oocyte maturation triggers as urinary hCG[3] **(98)** • Compared to hCG, use of a GnRH agonist as a trigger in GnRH antagonist cycles is associated with decreased CP[5] and LB[3] rates and increased miscarriage[3] rates. However, OHSS rates are reduced[3] **(99)**				
Oocyte retrieval	• Various approaches for pain relief for women undergoing TVOR are all associated with a high degree of satisfaction in women[6] **(100)**		• Insufficient evidence to show whether hCG priming has an effect on LB or miscarriage rates on oocyte maturation in vivo[5] **(101)**	• Follicular flushing during TVOR has little or no effect on CP or LB rates compared with aspiration alone[3] **(102)**	
Sperm retrieval			• Advanced sperm selection strategies in ART may not increase LB rates[6]. Sperm selection using hyaluronic acid binding may reduce miscarriage rates[5] **(103)**		• Insufficient evidence to support any specific SSR technique for azoospermic men undergoing ICSI[5] **(104)** • Insufficient evidence to show whether sperm selected by hyaluronic acid binding improves CP or LB rates[5] **(105)** • Insufficient evidence to support using IMSI over ICSI in clinical practice **(106)**
Lab phase	• Embryo culture with low oxygen concentrations increases LB rates[3] **(107)**	• Brief co-incubation of sperm ad oocytes may improve CP rates for women undergoing IVF compared to standard overnight insemination protocols[5] **(108)** • Vitrification probably increases CP rates compared to slow freezing[3] **(109)**	• Insufficient evidence to show that metabolomic assessment of embryos before implantation has any meaningful effect on CP, LB or miscarriage rates[5] **(110)** • Assisted hatching appears to increase CP[5] but not LB rates[3]. Multiple pregnancy rates may also be increased[5] **(111)**	• PGT-A using FISH decreases LB rates among women of AMA and those with RIF[3] **(112)**	• Insufficient evidence to support ICSI versus conventional techniques for oocyte insemination during IVF in non-male factor subfertility[5] **(113)** • Insufficient good quality evidence regarding benefit of time-lapse systems versus conventional embryo incubation on CP and LB rates[5] **(114)**

					• Insufficient evidence to support the use of any specific culture medium[6] (**115**) • Insufficient evidence as to whether growth factor supplemented culture media (GM-CSF) is more effective than culture media not supplemented with GM-CSF[6] (**116**) • Insufficient evidence to suggest incubating at a lower temperature improves pregnancy outcomes[6] (**117**) • Insufficient good quality evidence of a difference in cumulative LB rate, LB rate after first ET or miscarriage rate between IVF with and IVF without PGT-A[4] (**118**)
Embryo transfer	• US guidance improves CP and LB rates compared to clinical touch[4] (**119**) • ET media containing HA increases CP and LB[3] rates and may slightly decrease miscarriage rates[5] (**120**) • ET on day 2 and day 3 are equally effective[6] (**121**) • In a single IVF cycle, LB rates are lower following SET compared with DET but SET results in fewer multiple pregnancies[1] and the cumulative LB rate is comparable[4] (**122**) • ET at the blastocyst stage is associated with higher CP[3] and LB[5] rates than at the cleavage stage (**123**)	• Pregnancy outcomes for cleavage stage ET using an intrauterine hCG dose of 500iu or greater are promising[7] (**124**) • Insufficient evidence to show whether application of seminal plasma to the genital tract influenced rates of LB or miscarriage but it may increase CP rates[5]	• Insufficient evidence to show whether benefit was observed with any of the following interventions at the time of ET: full bladder, removal of cervical mucus, flushing the endocervical canal or endometrial cavity[4] (**125**) • Antibiotic administration before ET reduced upper genital tract microbial contamination but had no clear effect on CP rates[3] (**126**) • Insufficient evidence to show whether endometrial injection of embryo culture supernatant prior to ET improves CP and LB rates[6] (**127**) • Oxytocin antagonists at the time of ET do not appear to improve CP or LB rates[7] (**128**)	• ET media containing HA does not improve CP or LB rates in recipients of donor oocytes (findings from recent non-Cochrane review)(**129**)	• The margin of benefit between cleavage stage and blastocyst stage ET is unclear[6] (**130**) • Insufficient evidence to support a certain amount of time for women to remain recumbent following ET or to support the use of fibrin sealants[6] (**131**) • Insufficient evidence that giving granulocyte colony stimulating factor improves outcomes in women undergoing IVF[6] (**132**)

(Continued)

TABLE 5.3 ***(Continued)***

A Summary of Results from all Cochrane Reviews Related to Assisted Reproductive Technology

	Effective	Promising (more evidence needed)	Possibly ineffective (more evidence needed)	Ineffective	No conclusions possible due to lack of evidence
Luteal phase support	• Progesterone has higher CP rates than placebo[6] and lower OHSS rates than hCG[5]. Addition of one or more doses of GnRH agonists was associated with higher LB rates. Addition of hCG or oestrogen did not improve outcomes. The route of progesterone administration did not seem to matter[5] **(133)**	• Peri-implantation LMWH may improve LB rates in women undergoing IVF[6] **(134)**			• No clear evidence to suggest that administration of peri-implantation glucocorticoids significantly improves clinical outcomes in IVF[3] **(135)**
Prevention of OHSS	• Dopamine agonists are effective at preventing moderate or severe OHSS in women at high risk[5] **(136)** • Compared to GnRH agonist protocols, GnRH antagonist protocols are associated with a large reduction in OHSS risk and no difference in LB rates[3] **(84)** • Compared to hCG, GnRH agonist triggers in antagonist protocols are associated with a significant reduction in OHSS but this is accompanied by a lower CP and LB rate and increased miscarriage rate[3] **(99)**	• Human albumin, HES and mannitol reduce incidence of moderate and severe OHSS in women at high risk[6] **(137)**	• Insufficient evidence to support routine cryopreservation and the relative merits of intravenous albumin versus cryopreservation[5] **(138)** • Evidence suggests coasting may reduce rates of moderate to severe OHSS compared to no coasting[3] but this is not as effective as early unilateral follicular aspiration, using a GnRH antagonist trigger or cabergoline[6] **(139)**		

Frozen embryo transfer	• Elective freeze-all strategies are no superior in terms of cumulative LB rates than conventional strategies but they do lower the risk of OHSS in women at risk[5] (**140**)				• Insufficient evidence to support the use of any particular cycle regimen for women undergoing FET (**141**) • Insufficient evidence to support any particular protocol for women undergoing ET with embryos derived from donor oocytes (**142**)

Note: As the Cochrane review was published in 2018, we have incorporated recent reviews for some relevant topics, for which the evidence base has changed

[1]high quality evidence [2]moderate-high quality evidence [3]moderate quality evidence [4]low-moderate quality evidence [5]low quality evidence [6]very low quality evidence [7]variable quality evidence

AMA: advanced maternal age; COCP: combined oral contraceptive pill; COS: controlled ovarian stimulation; CP: clinical pregnancy; DET: double embryo transfer; DHEA: dehydroepiandrosterone; E2: oestradiol; ET: embryo transfer; FET: frozen embryo transfer; FISH: fluorescent in situ hybridisation; FSH: follicle stimulating hormone; GH: growth hormone; GnRH: gonadotropin releasing hormone; HA: hyaluronic acid; hCG: human chorionic gonadotropin; HES: hydroxyethyl starch; ICSI: intracytoplasmic sperm injection; IMSI: intracytoplasmic morphologically selected sperm injection; IUI: intrauterine insemination; IVF: in vitro fertilisation; IVM: in vitro maturation; LB: live birth; LMWH: low molecular weight heparin; OHSS: ovarian hyperstimulation syndrome; PCOS: polycystic ovary syndrome; PGT-A: pre-implantation genetic testing for aneuploidy; rFSH: recombinant follicle stimulating hormone; RIF: recurrent implantation failure; rLH: recombinant leutenising hormone; SET: single embryo transfer; SSR: surgical sperm retrieval; TVOR: transvaginal oocyte retrieval; US: ultrasound

Another version of a pyramid describing the sources of evidence that can be used for answering questions has been developed (Figure 5.2). This shows a hierarchy ranging from studies, synopses of single studies (abstracts), synthesis and synopses of synthesis (i.e. systematic reviews), summaries (i.e. guidelines) and systems (**15**). Whilst this may also imply some sort of increasing validity and applicability, its main purpose is to emphasise that the lower sources of evidence are the least preferred in practice because they require more expertise and time to identify, appraise and apply.

Guidelines are often the first resource clinicians will seek out when making decisions about the care of their patients. The recommendations they contain are not intended to dictate an exclusive course of care or treatment. They must be evaluated with reference to each individual's needs as well as resources and limitations unique to the institution, and variations in local populations. Multiple organisations including the Royal College of Obstetricians and Gynaecologists, the British Fertility Society, the National Institute for Health and Care Excellence and international fertility societies like the European Society of Human Reproduction and Embryology and American Society of Reproductive Medicine (ASRM) have produced various guidelines to aid practitioners in the field of reproductive medicine (**16–23**).

Unfortunately, guidelines can be somewhat out of date by the time or shortly after they are published depending on how rapidly the evidence in a particular area is evolving. In such situations, synthesised summaries may be useful. These are frequently updated summaries of evidence and systematically derived recommendations, but existing resources for providing synthesised summaries for clinical reference, for example BMJ Best Practice and UpToDate, vary in quality and comprehensiveness (**15**).

At the top of the pyramid, evidence and guidance are integrated within computerised decision support systems and electronic health records so that the features of individual patients are automatically linked with the information best suited to their care, rendering unnecessary 'the search' as a practitioner action. This is a challenge to implement in a reliable and extensive way but remains very much the ideal.

5.5 Step 3: Critical Appraisal of Evidence for Validity, Clinical Relevance, and Applicability (Appraise)

Once the evidence has been acquired, it needs to critically appraised. This is the process of assessing and interpreting the evidence by systematically considering (i) the validity of the study (ii) the results and (iii) the relevance to the specific clinical context. Full instruction on how to critically appraise a paper is beyond the remit of this book chapter but there are numerous publications on this topic (**24–28**) as well as multiple on-line and face-to-face training opportunities.

The risk of bias is not solely dependent on the design of the study, hence it is also important to take into consideration the quality of the study (**29**). This can be assessed using a variety of different tools, depending on the design of the study (**30–34**). In addition, various different checklists or toolkits exist to aid the process. The Critical Appraisal Skills Programme (CASP), Centre for Evidence-Based Medicine (CEBM) and Scottish Intercollegiate Guidelines Network (SIGN) for example all have checklists that can be downloaded from their websites free of charge that help to ensure a comprehensive assessment of the evidence has been undertaken.

GRADE (Grading of Recommendations, Assessment, Development and Evaluations) is a transparent framework for developing and presenting summaries of evidence and provides a systematic approach for making clinical practice recommendations (**35–38**). It is the most widely adopted tool for grading the quality of evidence and for making recommendations. The GRADE Working Group developed a framework to evaluate the quality or certainty of evidence (Table 5.2). The certainty of evidence can be rated down for the risk of bias, imprecision,

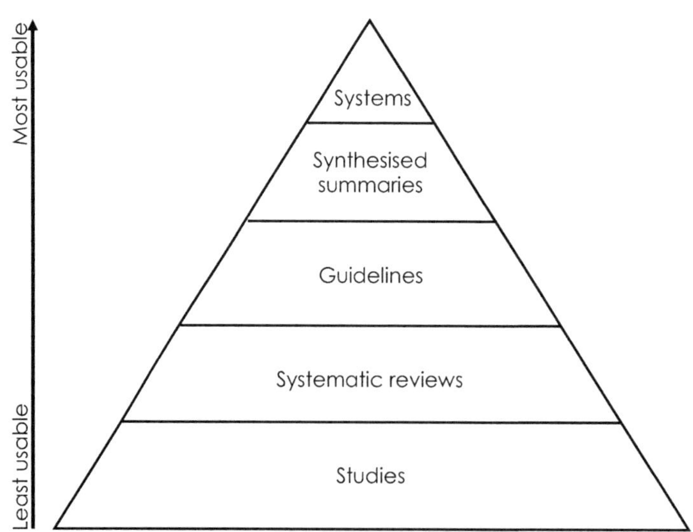

FIGURE 5.2 Evidence-based healthcare pyramid for finding pre-appraised evidence and guidance (adapted from [**15**]).

TABLE 5.4

GRADE Certainty Ratings

Certainty	Summary
High	True effect is similar to the estimated effect
Moderate	True effect is probably close to the estimated effect
Low	True effect might be markedly different from the estimated effect
Very low	True effect is probably markedly different from the estimated effect

inconsistency, indirectness, and publication bias but rated up for a large magnitude of effect, dose-response gradient and when all residual confounding would decrease the magnitude of the effect. Depending on the certainty of the evidence as well as the balance between desirable and undesirable consequences and the resources required for the intervention in question, strong or weak recommendations can then be made.

In a similar way, the Human Fertilisation and Embryology Authority (HFEA), in agreement with other professional and patient bodies, have devised traffic light ratings for various different IVF 'add-ons' (Figure 5.3). The intention is to provide patients with useful information regarding optional additional treatments that usually involve an additional cost on top of the cost of a routine cycle of proven fertility treatment. It is an attempt to make it easier for patients to understand the scientific evidence related to each intervention. It is important to note however that some interventions may have other benefits for specific patient groups, for example, an elective freeze all approach for a woman at high risk of developing OHSS or PGT-A for an older woman who has had several failed cycles previously. The evidence that supports the use of add-ons in a specific clinical context may not be as high quality as that used to decide the traffic light ratings and this should be discussed with patients so that they can make informed decisions about the treatment that they receive.

5.6 Step 4: Application of the Results in Practice (Apply)

Some evidence is easy to apply in clinical practice. For example, bed rest following embryo transfer, which for many years was fairly standard practice, has since been shown to significantly reduce clinical pregnancy rates in numerous individual randomised controlled trials (**39–43**) and subsequent meta-analysis (**44**). Encouraging immediate ambulation by asking women to walk out of the procedure room themselves rather than wheeling them out on a trolley can be implemented quickly without any major challenges in most units. Unfortunately, not all changes are so easy to introduce. Applying the evidence in practice often requires careful consideration and manipulation of numerous different factors including local clinical expertise, available resources, and patient expectations.

It is important that evidence-based practice is encouraged at both an individual and organisational level. This is aided by the publication of guidelines from national and international governing bodies, for example the British Fertility Society (BFS), the Association of Reproductive and Clinical Scientists (ARCS), European Society of Human Reproduction and Embryology (ESHRE) and American Society of Reproductive Medicine (ASRM). In addition to the generation of evidence-based guidelines and standard operating procedures, individuals and Units can benefit from evidence-based journal clubs to discuss relevant questions supported by presentation of clinical scenarios and critical appraisal toolkits. For those who do not have access to a local journal club, virtual journal clubs, which are becoming increasingly popular, are suitable alternatives. ESHRE for instance has a monthly virtual journal club which is advertised and available to join on social media #ESHREjc.

In this digital age, the high volume of information published makes it more difficult for individuals to always maintain an evidence-based approach. Whilst the publication of 'overview reviews' such as those by the Cochrane group (**45**) and more

Rating	Description	Examples
+	Findings from high quality evidence shows **this add-on is effective at improving the treatment outcome**	• ICSI for male factor infertility • Blastocyst culture
±	It **is not clear whether this add-on is effective at improving the treatment outcome**. This is because there is conflicting moderate/high quality evidence	• Elective freeze all cycles • Endometrial scratching • EmbryoGlue
?	**We cannot rate the effectiveness of this add-on at improving the treatment outcome** as there is insufficient moderate/high quality evidence.	• Assisted hatching • Intralipids • Intracytoplasmic morphologic sperm injection (IMSI) • Intrauterine culture
0	The evidence from moderate/high quality evidence shows that **this add-on has no effect on the treatment outcome**.	• Physiological intracytoplasmic sperm injection (PICSI) • Time-lapse imaging and incubation
!	**There are potential safety concerns and/or**, on balance, the findings from moderate/high quality evidence shows that this **add-on may reduce treatment effectiveness**.	• Preimplantation Genetic Testing for Aneuploidy (PGT-A) • Steroids • Endometrial receptivity testing • Intravenous immunoglobulin

FIGURE 5.3 HFEA traffic light ratings for IVF 'add-ons'.

- Viable intrauterine pregnancy confirmed by ultrasound
  - o Accounting for singleton, twin, and higher order multiple pregnancy
- Pregnancy loss
  - o Accounting for ectopic pregnancy, miscarriage, stillbirth, and termination
- Live birth
- Gestational age at delivery
- Birth weight
- Neonatal mortality
- Major congenital anomaly
- Time to pregnancy leading to live birth (when applicable)

FIGURE 5.4 A core outcome set for future infertility research.

recently Holt-Kentwell et al. (**46**) makes it easier for practitioners to synthesise the data and thus keep up to date, the evidence is constantly evolving and hence institutional support is crucial.

In addition to providing resources and organising expert panels to generate evidence-based guidance, institutions could do more to support evidence-based decision-making. Although computerised decision support systems are already being incorporated into day-to-day practice in many IVF units, for example, with EmbryoScope™ and Violet™, there is the potential for this to be explored further.

Finally, ensuring the collection of relevant outcomes is pivotal for supporting future decision-making with the results. The Core Outcome Measures in Effectiveness Trials (COMET) initiative aims to facilitate the development and application of core outcome sets, which are minimum standardised sets of outcomes that should be measured and reported in all clinical trials on specific healthcare topics (**47**). In the past, many studies evaluating interventions in the field of ART have reported many different outcomes (**48**) which makes it difficult to compare, contrast and combine individual trials, limiting the ability of the research to inform clinical practice (**49**). A core outcome set for future infertility research has now been developed (**50**) which will help to standardise outcome selection, collection, and reporting across future infertility research and institutions should ensure that these are utilised by individual researchers when designing or reporting on studies (Figure 5.4).

5.7 Step 5: Evaluation of Performance (Audit)

Acquiring and appraising the evidence and generating guidelines or standard operating procedures as a consequence is insufficient on its own. Practice needs to be constantly evaluated to make sure that it follows the local, national and, where relevant, international evidence-based recommendations. At a local level, audits of outcomes and adherence to guidelines should be an integral part of practice.

More importantly, systematic effort should be made at national and international levels to evaluate clinical practice across different units. In the UK, the HFEA Code of Practice states that all centres must put in place a quality management system and implement this system to continually improve the quality and effectiveness of the service provided. Centres must audit all activities and processes against compliance with the regulatory requirements and their own approved protocols and quality indicators. The audits must be performed at least every two years, by trained and competent staff and in an independent way. Findings and corrective actions must be documented and implemented. Unlike in other areas of healthcare in the UK, where this behaviour would be encouraged but not necessarily enforced and certainly no penalties would be incurred if not completed, it is a legal requirement borne out of the Human Fertilisation and Embryology Act 1990.

This is not to say that continuous evaluation and adherence to evidence-based practice are without challenges. The applicability of existing evidence is particularly difficult when the research is not directly aligned with the clinical scenarios for example in older women, women with recurrent implantation failure, in BAME women or those from more socioeconomically deprived areas or with certain conditions such as polycystic ovary syndrome or endometriosis. These challenges, and our desire to improve clinical care, should incentivise clinicians to put systems in place for evaluating clinical performance as an integral part of practice.

Other challenges that relate to implementing EBP in reproductive medicine perhaps more so than in other specialties is the fact that not only is the fertility sector an intensely competitive market (with up to 60% of treatments being funded privately by the patients themselves) but also information about various treatment options is becoming increasingly available online. Many patients are frequently being offered and charged for optional extras to their treatment which claim to improve their chances of having a baby. These additional therapies cover a range of interventions and are collectively known as treatment 'add-ons'. Offered responsibly, they can be a sign of healthy innovation in the fertility sector. However, there is currently little evidence that any of the add-ons offered increase the chance of a clinical pregnancy or live birth and these, often vulnerable, patients should not be exploited. Practitioners have a duty of care to patients which should separate pressure from patients and commercial interests from their best practice advice. A consensus statement on the responsible use of treatment add-ons in fertility services, endorsed by all the key UK societies, has set out principles of responsible innovation which should help guide professionals in the UK (and beyond). These give clinics the space to innovate but also ensure systems are in place to allow new treatment add-ons to be introduced through pre-clinical and clinical testing to confirm safety and efficacy (**51**).

5.8 Conclusion

In conclusion, reproductive medicine is a rapidly evolving specialty that has benefited enormously from EBP. Advances in science and technology continue to occur and by incorporating EBP into our day-to-day clinical care, we can ensure that our patients continue to benefit from these so that further improvements in the efficacy and safety of IVF will continue to occur. We hope that this chapter will inspire and encourage the readers to start or continue to use EBP in their clinical work.

REFERENCES

1. HFEA. *Fertility Treatment 2019: Trends and Figures.* Human Fertilisation and Embryology Authority; 2021.
2. Edwards RG, Steptoe PC, Purdy JM. Establishing full-term human pregnancies using cleaving embryos grown in vitro. *Br J Obstet Gynaecol.* 1980;87(9):737–756.
3. Beall SA, DeCherney A. History and challenges surrounding ovarian stimulation in the treatment of infertility. *Fertil Steril.* 2012;97(4):795–801.
4. Quinn P, Kerin JF, Warnes GM. Improved pregnancy rate in human in vitro fertilization with the use of a medium based on the composition of human tubal fluid. *Fertil Steril.* 1985;44(4):493–498.
5. Menezo Y, Testart J, Perrone D. Serum is not necessary in human in vitro fertilization, early embryo culture, and transfer. *Fertil Steril.* 1984;42(5):750–755.
6. Swain JE, Carrell D, Cobo A, et al. Optimizing the culture environment and embryo manipulation to help maintain embryo developmental potential. *Fertil Steril.* 2016;105(3):571–587.
7. Fritz MA. Perspectives on the efficacy and indications for preimplantation genetic screening: where are we now? *Hum Reprod.* 2008;23(12):2617–2621.
8. Mastenbroek S, Twisk M, van der Veen F, Repping S. Preimplantation genetic screening: a systematic review and meta-analysis of RCTs. *Hum Reprod Update.* 2011;17(4): 454–466.
9. Dawes M, Summerskill W, Glasziou P, et al. Sicily statement on evidence-based practice. *BMC Med Educ.* 2005;5(1):1.
10. Methley AM, Campbell S, Chew-Graham C, et al. PICO, PICOS and SPIDER: a comparison study of specificity and sensitivity in three search tools for qualitative systematic reviews. *BMC Health Serv Res.* 2014;14:579.
11. van Hoogenhuijze NE, Mol F, Laven JSE, et al. Endometrial scratching in women with one failed IVF/ICSI cycle-outcomes of a randomised controlled trial (SCRaTCH). *Hum Reprod.* 2021;36(1):87–98.
12. Page MJ, McKenzie JE, Bossuyt PM, et al. The PRISMA 2020 statement: an updated guideline for reporting systematic reviews. *BMJ.* 2021;372:n71.
13. Murad MH, Asi N, Alsawas M, et al. New evidence pyramid. *Evid Based Med.* 2016;21(4):125–127.
14. Rimm AA, Katayama AC, Diaz M, et al. A meta-analysis of controlled studies comparing major malformation rates in IVF and ICSI infants with naturally conceived children. *J Assist Reprod Genet.* 2004;21(12):437–443.
15. Alper BS, Haynes RB. EBHC pyramid 5.0 for accessing preappraised evidence and guidance. *Evid Based Med.* 2016;21(4):123–125.
16. NICE. *Fertility Problems: Assessment and Treatment [CG156].* London: National Institute for Health and Care Excellence; 2017.
17. Bosch E, Broer S, Griesinger G, et al. ESHRE guideline: ovarian stimulation for IVF/ICSI. *Hum Reprod Open.* 2020;2020(2):hoaa009.
18. Anderson RA, Amant F, Braat D, et al. ESHRE guideline: female fertility preservation. *Hum Reprod Open.* 2020;2020(4).
19. D'Angelo A, Panayotidis C, Amso N, et al. Recommendations for good practice in ultrasound: oocyte pick up(dagger). *Hum Reprod Open.* 2019;2019(4).
20. ESHRE Working Group on Time-Lapse Technology, Apter S, Ebner T, Freour T, Guns Y, Kovacic B, Le Clef N, Marques M, Meseguer M, Montjean D, Sfontouris I. Good practice recommendations for the use of time-lapse technology. *Hum Reprod Open.* 2020;2020(2):hoaa008.
21. De los Santos MJ, Apter S, Coticchio G, et al. Revised guidelines for good practice in IVF laboratories (2015). *Hum Reprod.* 2016;31(4):685–686.
22. RCOG. *The Management of Ovarian Hyperstimulation Syndrome.* London: Royal College of Obstetrics and Gynaecologists; 2016.
23. Mascarenhas M, Jeve Y, Polanski L, et al. Management of recurrent implantation failure: British Fertility Society policy and practice guideline. *Hum Fertil.* 2022;25(5):813–837.
24. Greenhalgh T. Assessing the methodological quality of published papers. *BMJ.* 1997;315(7103):305–308.
25. Greenhalgh T. How to read a paper. Getting your bearings (deciding what the paper is about). *BMJ.* 1997;315(7102): 243–246.
26. Greenhalgh T. How to read a paper. Statistics for the non-statistician. I: different types of data need different statistical tests. *BMJ.* 1997;315(7104):364–366.
27. Greenhalgh T. How to read a paper. Statistics for the non-statistician. II: "Significant" relations and their pitfalls. *BMJ.* 1997;315(7105):422–425.
28. BMJ. *Best Practice: EBM Toolkit.* Available from: https://bestpractice.bmj.com/info/toolkit/learn-ebm/.
29. Guyatt GH, Oxman AD, Sultan S, et al. GRADE guidelines: 9. Rating up the quality of evidence. *J Clin Epidemiol.* 2011;64(12):1311–1316.
30. Schunemann HJ, Oxman AD, Brozek J, et al. Grading quality of evidence and strength of recommendations for diagnostic tests and strategies. *BMJ.* 2008;336(7653):1106–1110.
31. Whiting PF, Rutjes AW, Westwood ME, et al. QUADAS-2: a revised tool for the quality assessment of diagnostic accuracy studies. *Ann Intern Med.* 2011;155(8):529–536.
32. Shea BJ, Reeves BC, Wells G, et al. AMSTAR 2: a critical appraisal tool for systematic reviews that include randomised or non-randomised studies of healthcare interventions, or both. *BMJ.* 2017;358:j4008.
33. Jadad AR, Moore RA, Carroll D, et al. Assessing the quality of reports of randomized clinical trials: is blinding necessary? *Control Clin Trials.* 1996;17(1):1–12.
34. Altman DG, Schulz KF, Moher D, et al. The revised CONSORT statement for reporting randomized trials: explanation and elaboration. *Ann Intern Med.* 2001;134(8):663–694.
35. Guyatt GH, Oxman AD, Kunz R, et al. What is "quality of evidence" and why is it important to clinicians? *BMJ.* 2008;336(7651):995–998.
36. Guyatt GH, Oxman AD, Vist GE, et al. GRADE: an emerging consensus on rating quality of evidence and strength of recommendations. *BMJ.* 2008;336(7650):924–926.
37. Guyatt G, Oxman AD, Akl EA, et al. GRADE guidelines: 1. Introduction-GRADE evidence profiles and summary of findings tables. *J Clin Epidemiol.* 2011;64(4):383–394.
38. Guyatt GH, Oxman AD, Kunz R, et al. GRADE guidelines: 2. Framing the question and deciding on important outcomes. *J Clin Epidemiol.* 2011;64(4):395–400.
39. Botta G, Grudzinskas G. Is a prolonged bed rest following embryo transfer useful? *Hum Reprod.* 1997;12(11): 2489–2492.

40. Rezabek K, Koryntova D, Zivny J. Does bedrest after embryo transfer cause a worse outcome in in vitro fertilization? *Ceska Gynekol.* 2001;66(3):175–178.
41. Amarin ZO, Obeidat BR. Bed rest versus free mobilisation following embryo transfer: a prospective randomised study. *BJOG.* 2004;111(11):1273–1276.
42. Purcell KJ, Schembri M, Telles TL, et al. Bed rest after embryo transfer: a randomized controlled trial. *Fertil Steril.* 2007;87(6):1322–1326.
43. Gaikwad S, Garrido N, Cobo A, et al. Bed rest after embryo transfer negatively affects in vitro fertilization: a randomized controlled clinical trial. *Fertil Steril.* 2013;100(3):729–735.
44. Tyler B, Walford H, Tamblyn J, et al. Interventions to optimize embryo transfer in women undergoing assisted conception: a comprehensive systematic review and meta-analyses. *Hum Reprod Update.* 2022;28(4):480–500.
45. Farquhar C, Marjoribanks J. Assisted reproductive technology: an overview of Cochrane reviews. *Cochrane Database Syst Rev.* 2018;8:CD010537.
46. Holt-Kentwell A, Ghosh J, Devall A, et al. Evaluating interventions and adjuncts to optimize pregnancy outcomes in subfertile women: an overview review. *Hum Reprod Update.* 2022;28(4):583–600.
47. Prinsen CA, Vohra S, Rose MR, et al. Core outcome measures in effectiveness trials (COMET) initiative: protocol for an international Delphi study to achieve consensus on how to select outcome measurement instruments for outcomes included in a 'core outcome set'. *Trials.* 2014; 15:247.
48. Wilkinson J, Bhattacharya S, Duffy J, et al. Reproductive medicine: still more ART than science? *BJOG.* 2019;126(2):138–141.
49. Duffy JMN, Ziebland S, von Dadelszen P, et al. Tackling poorly selected, collected, and reported outcomes in obstetrics and gynecology research. *Am J Obstet Gynecol.* 2019;220(1):71. e1–e4.
50. Duffy JMN, Bhattacharya S, Bhattacharya S, et al. Standardizing definitions and reporting guidelines for the infertility core outcome set: an international consensus development study. *Fertil Steril.* 2021;115(1):201–212.
51. HFEA. *The Responsible Use of Treatment Add-Ons in Fertility Services: A Consensus Statement.* 2019. Available from: www.eshre.eu/Guidelines-and-Legal/Position-statements/Treatment-addons.
52. Castillo CM, Horne G, Fitzgerald CT, et al. The impact of IVF on birthweight from 1991 to 2015: a cross-sectional study. *Hum Reprod.* 2019;34(5):920–931.
53. Jayaprakasan K, Chan YY, Sur S, et al. Prevalence of uterine anomalies and their impact on early pregnancy in women conceiving after assisted reproduction treatment. *Ultrasound Obstet Gynecol.* 2011;37(6):727–732.
54. Isaksson R, Gissler M, Tiitinen A. Obstetric outcome among women with unexplained infertility after IVF: a matched case-control study. *Hum Reprod.* 2002;17(7):1755–1761.
55. Prior M, Richardson A, Asif S, et al. Outcome of assisted reproduction in women with congenital uterine anomalies: a prospective observational study. *Ultrasound Obstet Gynecol.* 2018;51(1):110–117.
56. Richardson AL, Baskind NE, Karuppusami R, et al. Effect of deprivation on in vitro fertilisation outcome: a cohort study. *BJOG.* 2020;127(4):458–465.
57. Levi Setti PE, Cirillo F, Morenghi E, et al. One step further: randomised single-centre trial comparing the direct and afterload techniques of embryo transfer. *Hum Reprod.* 2021;36(9):2484–2492.
58. Drakeley AJ, Jorgensen A, Sklavounos J, et al. A randomized controlled clinical trial of 2295 ultrasound-guided embryo transfers. *Hum Reprod.* 2008;23(5):1101–1106.
59. Metwally M, Chatters R, Dimairo M, et al. A randomised controlled trial to assess the clinical effectiveness and safety of the endometrial scratch procedure prior to first-time IVF, with or without ICSI. *Hum Reprod.* 2021;36(7):1841–1853.
60. Miller D, Pavitt S, Sharma V, et al. Physiological, hyaluronan-selected intracytoplasmic sperm injection for infertility treatment (HABSelect): a parallel, two-group, randomised trial. Lancet. 2019;393(10170):416–422.
61. Korosec S, Virant-Klun I, Tomazevic T, et al. Single fresh and frozen-thawed blastocyst transfer using hyaluronan-rich transfer medium. *Reprod Biomed Online.* 2007;15(6):701–707.
62. Pandian Z, Gibreel A, Bhattacharya S. In vitro fertilisation for unexplained subfertility. *Cochrane Database Syst Rev.* 2015(11):CD003357.
63. Nandi A, Raja G, White D, et al. Intrauterine insemination + controlled ovarian hyperstimulation versus in vitro fertilisation in unexplained infertility: a systematic review and meta-analysis. *Arch Gynecol Obstet.* 2022;305(4): 805–824.
64. Yossry M, Aboulghar M, D'Angelo A, et al. In vitro fertilisation versus tubal reanastomosis (sterilisation reversal) for subfertility after tubal sterilisation. *Cochrane Database Syst Rev.* 2006(3):CD004144.
65. Siristatidis CS, Maheshwari A, Vaidakis D, et al. In vitro maturation in subfertile women with polycystic ovarian syndrome undergoing assisted reproduction. *Cochrane Database Syst Rev.* 2018;11:CD006606.
66. Akhtar MA, Agrawal R, Brown J, et al. Thyroxine replacement for subfertile women with euthyroid autoimmune thyroid disease or subclinical hypothyroidism. *Cochrane Database Syst Rev.* 2019;6:CD011009.
67. Nastri CO, Lensen SF, Gibreel A, et al. Endometrial injury in women undergoing assisted reproductive techniques. *Cochrane Database Syst Rev.* 2015(3):CD009517.
68. Sood A, Mohiyiddeen G, Ahmad G, et al. Growth hormone for in vitro fertilisation (IVF). *Cochrane Database Syst Rev.* 2021;11:CD000099.
69. Johnson N, van Voorst S, Sowter MC, et al. Surgical treatment for tubal disease in women due to undergo in vitro fertilisation. *Cochrane Database Syst Rev.* 2010(1):CD002125.
70. de Ligny W, Smits RM, Mackenzie-Proctor R, et al. Antioxidants for male subfertility. *Cochrane Database Syst Rev.* 2022;5:CD007411.
71. Showell MG, Mackenzie-Proctor R, Jordan V, et al. Antioxidants for female subfertility. *Cochrane Database Syst Rev.* 2020;8:CD007807.
72. Gutarra-Vilchez RB, Bonfill Cosp X, Glujovsky D, et al. Vasodilators for women undergoing fertility treatment. *Cochrane Database Syst Rev.* 2018;10:CD010001.
73. Nagels HE, Rishworth JR, Siristatidis CS, et al. Androgens (dehydroepiandrosterone or testosterone) for women undergoing assisted reproduction. *Cochrane Database Syst Rev.* 2015(11):CD009749.

74. Duffy JM, Ahmad G, Mohiyiddeen L, et al. Growth hormone for in vitro fertilization. *Cochrane Database Syst Rev*. 2010(1):CD000099.
75. Metwally M, Chatters R, White D, et al. Endometrial scratch in women undergoing first-time IVF treatment: a systematic review and meta-analysis of randomized controlled trials. *Reprod Biomed Online*. 2022;44(4):617–629.
76. Cheong YC, Dix S, Hung Yu Ng E, et al. Acupuncture and assisted reproductive technology. *Cochrane Database Syst Rev*. 2013(7):CD006920.
77. Boedt T, Vanhove AC, Vercoe MA, et al. Preconception lifestyle advice for people with infertility. *Cochrane Database Syst Rev*. 2021;4:CD008189.
78. Benschop L, Farquhar C, van der Poel N, et al. Interventions for women with endometrioma prior to assisted reproductive technology. *Cochrane Database Syst Rev*. 2010(11):CD008571.
79. McDonnell R, Marjoribanks J, Hart RJ. Ovarian cyst aspiration prior to in vitro fertilization treatment for subfertility. *Cochrane Database Syst Rev*. 2014(12):CD005999.
80. Tso LO, Costello MF, Albuquerque LET, et al. Metformin treatment before and during IVF or ICSI in women with polycystic ovary syndrome. *Cochrane Database Syst Rev*. 2020;12:CD006105.
81. Siristatidis CS, Basios G, Pergialiotis V, et al. Aspirin for in vitro fertilisation. *Cochrane Database Syst Rev*. 2016;11:CD004832.
82. Nyachieo A, Siristatidis CS, Vaidakis D. Nonsteroidal anti-inflammatory drugs for assisted reproductive technology. *Cochrane Database Syst Rev*. 2019;10:CD007618.
83. Siristatidis CS, Gibreel A, Basios G, et al. Gonadotrophin-releasing hormone agonist protocols for pituitary suppression in assisted reproduction. *Cochrane Database Syst Rev*. 2015(11):CD006919.
84. Al-Inany HG, Youssef MA, Ayeleke RO, et al. Gonadotrophin-releasing hormone antagonists for assisted reproductive technology. *Cochrane Database Syst Rev*. 2016;4:CD001750.
85. Georgiou EX, Melo P, Baker PE, et al. Long-term GnRH agonist therapy before in vitro fertilisation (IVF) for improving fertility outcomes in women with endometriosis. *Cochrane Database Syst Rev*. 2019;2019(11).
86. Albuquerque LE, Tso LO, Saconato H, et al. Depot versus daily administration of gonadotrophin-releasing hormone agonist protocols for pituitary down regulation in assisted reproduction cycles. *Cochrane Database Syst Rev*. 2013(1):CD002808.
87. van Wely M, Kwan I, Burt AL, et al. Recombinant versus urinary gonadotrophin for ovarian stimulation in assisted reproductive technology cycles. *Cochrane Database Syst Rev*. 2011(2):CD005354.
88. Pouwer AW, Farquhar C, Kremer JA. Long-acting FSH versus daily FSH for women undergoing assisted reproduction. *Cochrane Database Syst Rev*. 2015(7):CD009577.
89. Lensen SF, Wilkinson J, Leijdekkers JA, et al. Individualised gonadotropin dose selection using markers of ovarian reserve for women undergoing in vitro fertilisation plus intracytoplasmic sperm injection (IVF/ICSI). *Cochrane Database Syst Rev*. 2018;2:CD012693.
90. Mochtar MH, Danhof NA, Ayeleke RO, et al. Recombinant luteinizing hormone (rLH) and recombinant follicle stimulating hormone (rFSH) for ovarian stimulation in IVF/ICSI cycles. *Cochrane Database Syst Rev*. 2017;5:CD005070.
91. Kamath MS, Maheshwari A, Bhattacharya S, et al. Oral medications including clomiphene citrate or aromatase inhibitors with gonadotropins for controlled ovarian stimulation in women undergoing in vitro fertilisation. *Cochrane Database Syst Rev*. 2017;11:CD008528.
92. Martins WP, Vieira AD, Figueiredo JB, et al. FSH replaced by low-dose hCG in the late follicular phase versus continued FSH for assisted reproductive techniques. *Cochrane Database Syst Rev*. 2013(3):CD010042.
93. Allersma T, Farquhar C, Cantineau AE. Natural cycle in vitro fertilisation (IVF) for subfertile couples. *Cochrane Database Syst Rev*. 2013(8):CD010550.
94. Kwan I, Bhattacharya S, Woolner A. Monitoring of stimulated cycles in assisted reproduction (IVF and ICSI). *Cochrane Database Syst Rev*. 2021;4:CD005289.
95. Farquhar C, Rombauts L, Kremer JA, et al. Oral contraceptive pill, progestogen or oestrogen pretreatment for ovarian stimulation protocols for women undergoing assisted reproductive techniques. *Cochrane Database Syst Rev*. 2017;5:CD006109.
96. Kalampokas T, Pandian Z, Keay SD, et al. Glucocorticoid supplementation during ovarian stimulation for IVF or ICSI. *Cochrane Database Syst Rev*. 2017;3:CD004752.
97. Pandian Z, McTavish AR, Aucott L, et al. Interventions for 'poor responders' to controlled ovarian hyper stimulation (COH) in in-vitro fertilisation (IVF). *Cochrane Database Syst Rev*. 2010(1):CD004379.
98. Youssef MA, Abou-Setta AM, Lam WS. Recombinant versus urinary human chorionic gonadotrophin for final oocyte maturation triggering in IVF and ICSI cycles. *Cochrane Database Syst Rev*. 2016;4:CD003719.
99. Youssef MA, Van der Veen F, Al-Inany HG, et al. Gonadotropin-releasing hormone agonist versus HCG for oocyte triggering in antagonist-assisted reproductive technology. *Cochrane Database Syst Rev*. 2014(10): CD008046.
100. Kwan I, Wang R, Pearce E, et al. Pain relief for women undergoing oocyte retrieval for assisted reproduction. *Cochrane Database Syst Rev*. 2018;5:CD004829.
101. Reavey J, Vincent K, Child T, et al. Human chorionic gonadotrophin priming for fertility treatment with in vitro maturation. *Cochrane Database Syst Rev*. 2016;11:CD008720.
102. Georgiou EX, Melo P, Brown J, et al. Follicular flushing during oocyte retrieval in assisted reproductive techniques. *Cochrane Database Syst Rev*. 2018;4:CD004634.
103. Lepine S, McDowell S, Searle LM, et al. Advanced sperm selection techniques for assisted reproduction. *Cochrane Database Syst Rev*. 2019;7:CD010461.
104. Van Peperstraten A, Proctor ML, Johnson NP, et al. Techniques for surgical retrieval of sperm prior to intracytoplasmic sperm injection (ICSI) for azoospermia. *Cochrane Database Syst Rev*. 2008(2):CD002807.
105. McDowell S, Kroon B, Ford E, et al. Advanced sperm selection techniques for assisted reproduction. *Cochrane Database Syst Rev*. 2014(10):CD010461.
106. Teixeira DM, Hadyme Miyague A, Barbosa MA, et al. Regular (ICSI) versus ultra-high magnification (IMSI) sperm selection for assisted reproduction. *Cochrane Database Syst Rev*. 2020;2:CD010167.
107. Bontekoe S, Mantikou E, van Wely M, et al. Low oxygen concentrations for embryo culture in assisted reproductive technologies. *Cochrane Database Syst Rev*. 2012(7):CD008950.

108. Huang Z, Li J, Wang L, et al. Brief co-incubation of sperm and oocytes for in vitro fertilization techniques. *Cochrane Database Syst Rev*. 2013(4):CD009391.
109. Glujovsky D, Riestra B, Sueldo C, et al. Vitrification versus slow freezing for women undergoing oocyte cryopreservation. *Cochrane Database Syst Rev*. 2014(9):CD010047.
110. Siristatidis CS, Sertedaki E, Vaidakis D, et al. Metabolomics for improving pregnancy outcomes in women undergoing assisted reproductive technologies. *Cochrane Database Syst Rev*. 2018;3:CD011872.
111. Lacey L, Hassan S, Franik S, et al. Assisted hatching on assisted conception (in vitro fertilisation (IVF) and intracytoplasmic sperm injection (ICSI)). *Cochrane Database Syst Rev*. 2021;3:CD001894.
112. Twisk M, Mastenbroek S, van Wely M, et al. Preimplantation genetic screening for abnormal number of chromosomes (aneuploidies) in in vitro fertilisation or intracytoplasmic sperm injection. *Cochrane Database Syst Rev*. 2006(1):CD005291.
113. van Rumste MM, Evers JL, Farquhar CM. Intracytoplasmic sperm injection versus conventional techniques for oocyte insemination during in vitro fertilisation in patients with non-male subfertility. *Cochrane Database Syst Rev*. 2003(2):CD001301.
114. Armstrong S, Bhide P, Jordan V, et al. Time-lapse systems for embryo incubation and assessment in assisted reproduction. *Cochrane Database Syst Rev*. 2019;5:CD011320.
115. Youssef MM, Mantikou E, van Wely M, et al. Culture media for human pre-implantation embryos in assisted reproductive technology cycles. *Cochrane Database Syst Rev*. 2015(11):CD007876.
116. Armstrong S, MacKenzie J, Woodward B, et al. GM-CSF (granulocyte macrophage colony-stimulating factor) supplementation in culture media for women undergoing assisted reproduction. *Cochrane Database Syst Rev*. 2020;7:CD013497.
117. Baak NA, Cantineau AE, Farquhar C, et al. Temperature of embryo culture for assisted reproduction. *Cochrane Database Syst Rev*. 2019;9:CD012192.
118. Cornelisse S, Zagers M, Kostova E, et al Preimplantation genetic testing for aneuploidies (abnormal number of chromosomes) in in vitro fertilisation. *Cochrane Database Syst Rev*. 2020;9:CD005291.
119. Brown J, Buckingham K, Buckett W, et al. Ultrasound versus 'clinical touch' for catheter guidance during embryo transfer in women. *Cochrane Database Syst Rev*. 2016;3:CD006107.
120. Heymann D, Vidal L, Or Y, et al. Hyaluronic acid in embryo transfer media for assisted reproductive technologies. *Cochrane Database Syst Rev*. 2020;9:CD007421.
121. Brown J, Daya S, Matson P. Day three versus day two embryo transfer following in vitro fertilization or intracytoplasmic sperm injection. *Cochrane Database Syst Rev*. 2016;12:CD004378.
122. Kamath MS, Mascarenhas M, Kirubakaran R, et al. Number of embryos for transfer following in vitro fertilisation or intra-cytoplasmic sperm injection. *Cochrane Database Syst Rev*. 2020;8:CD003416.
123. Glujovsky D, Quinteiro Retamar AM, Alvarez Sedo CR, et al. Cleavage-stage versus blastocyst-stage embryo transfer in assisted reproductive technology. *Cochrane Database Syst Rev*. 2022;5:CD002118.
124. Craciunas L, Tsampras N, Coomarasamy A, et al. Intrauterine administration of human chorionic gonadotropin (hCG) for subfertile women undergoing assisted reproduction. *Cochrane Database Syst Rev*. 2016(5):CD011537.
125. Derks RS, Farquhar C, Mol BW, et al. Techniques for preparation prior to embryo transfer. *Cochrane Database Syst Rev*. 2009(4):CD007682.
126. Kroon B, Hart RJ, Wong BM, et al. Antibiotics prior to embryo transfer in ART. *Cochrane Database Syst Rev*. 2012(3):CD008995.
127. Siristatidis CS, Sertedaki E, Karageorgiou V, et al. Endometrial injection of embryo culture supernatant for subfertile women in assisted reproduction. *Cochrane Database Syst Rev*. 2020;8:CD013063.
128. Craciunas L, Tsampras N, Kollmann M, et al. Oxytocin antagonists for assisted reproduction. *Cochrane Database Syst Rev*. 2021;9:CD012375.
129. Heymann D, Vidal L, Shoham Z, et al. The effect of hyaluronic acid in embryo transfer media in donor oocyte cycles and autologous oocyte cycles: a systematic review and meta-analysis. *Hum Reprod*. 2022;37(7):1451–1469.
130. Glujovsky D, Farquhar C, Quinteiro Retamar AM, et al. Cleavage stage versus blastocyst stage embryo transfer in assisted reproductive technology. *Cochrane Database Syst Rev*. 2016(6):CD002118.
131. Abou-Setta AM, Peters LR, D'Angelo A, et al. Post-embryo transfer interventions for assisted reproduction technology cycles. *Cochrane Database Syst Rev*. 2014(8):CD006567.
132. Kamath MS, Kirubakaran R, Sunkara SK. Granulocyte-colony stimulating factor administration for subfertile women undergoing assisted reproduction. *Cochrane Database Syst Rev*. 2020;1:CD013226.
133. van der Linden M, Buckingham K, Farquhar C, et al. Luteal phase support for assisted reproduction cycles. *Cochrane Database Syst Rev*. 2015(7):CD009154.
134. Akhtar MA, Sur S, Raine-Fenning N, et al. Heparin for assisted reproduction. *Cochrane Database Syst Rev*. 2013(8):CD009452.
135. Boomsma CM, Kamath MS, Keay SD, et al. Peri-implantation glucocorticoid administration for assisted reproductive technology cycles. *Cochrane Database Syst Rev*. 2022;6:CD005996.
136. Tang H, Mourad SM, Wang A, et al. Dopamine agonists for preventing ovarian hyperstimulation syndrome. *Cochrane Database Syst Rev*. 2021;4:CD008605.
137. Youssef MA, Mourad S. Volume expanders for the prevention of ovarian hyperstimulation syndrome. *Cochrane Database Syst Rev*. 2016(8):CD001302.
138. D'Angelo A, Amso N. Embryo freezing for preventing ovarian hyperstimulation syndrome. *Cochrane Database Syst Rev*. 2007(3):CD002806.
139. D'Angelo A, Amso NN, Hassan R. Coasting (withholding gonadotrophins) for preventing ovarian hyperstimulation syndrome. *Cochrane Database Syst Rev*. 2017;5:CD002811.
140. Zaat T, Zagers M, Mol F, et al. Fresh versus frozen embryo transfers in assisted reproduction. *Cochrane Database Syst Rev*. 2021;2:CD011184.
141. Ghobara T, Gelbaya TA, Ayeleke RO. Cycle regimens for frozen-thawed embryo transfer. *Cochrane Database Syst Rev*. 2017;7:CD003414.
142. Glujovsky D, Pesce R, Sueldo C, et al. Endometrial preparation for women undergoing embryo transfer with frozen embryos or embryos derived from donor oocytes. *Cochrane Database Syst Rev*. 2020;10:CD006359.

6

Quality Control and Management

Amy Barrie

6.1 Introduction

Within an organisation, all processes and activities form part of the quality management system (QMS). The definition of the QMS, according to the International Organization for Standardization is, 'the organizational structure, defined responsibilities, procedures, processes and resources for implementing quality management (i.e., the co-ordinated activities to direct and control an organisation with regard to quality), including all activities which contribute to quality, directly or indirectly'. Quality management is all encompassing and is critical in an assisted reproduction laboratory to maintain the required standards of safety and effectiveness and to ensure continual improvement.

6.1.1 Quality Control and Quality Assurance

Both quality control and assurance are pivotal to maintenance of the QMS. Quality control follows a reactive methodology to identify defects and is largely focussed on the end result. An example of a quality control measure may be key performance indicators. This is in contrast to quality assurance which uses a proactive methodology seeking to prevent defects before they arise and is focussed on the process rather than the end point. An example of quality assurance is auditing. In this chapter, quality control is the focus and although some aspects of quality assurance will be discussed, this will be to inform discussions pertaining to quality control. In addition, even though the UK model is used as a main reference, the principles are universal.

6.1.2 Quality Management and Regulation

The UK regulator of fertility treatment, the Human Fertilisation and Embryology Authority (HFEA) indicates how clinics must maintain quality through a number of licence conditions, the compliance with which is a mandatory requirement for all clinics within the UK. In relation to quality, these are licence conditions T32, T33, T35 and T36 (**1**).

Licence condition T32 states, the centre must put in place a quality management system and implement this system to continually improve the quality and effectiveness of the service provided.

Licence condition T33 states, the following documentation must form part of the quality management system:

a. A quality manual
b. Standard operating procedures (SOPs) for all activities authorised by the licence and other activities carried out in the course of providing treatment services that do not require a licence
c. Guidelines
d. Training and reference manuals
e. Reporting forms

Licence condition T35 states, required standards of quality and safety, in the form of quality indicators for all activities authorised by the licence and other activities carried out in the course of providing treatment services that do not require a licence, must be established.

Licence condition T36 states, centres must audit the activities and processes authorised by this licence and other activities carried out in the course of providing treatment services that do not require a licence against compliance with the regulatory requirements and their own approved protocols and quality indicators. These audits must be performed at least every two years, by trained and competent staff and in an independent way. Findings and corrective actions must be documented and implemented.

Within the QMS, documentation must be developed, maintained and improved. This includes standard operating procedures (SOPs) and a quality manual, which should delineate the quality objectives and policy and guidelines for the service, among others.

6.2 The Quality Manual

The quality manual is the single document that contains the quality objectives and quality policy. In general, the quality manual should include all elements of the QMS which includes a description of the scope of the QMS, an organisational chart, a description of the roles and responsibilities of the laboratory management, a description of the structure and relationships of the documentation used in the QMS (**2**). The quality manual must be readily accessible by all staff and be reviewed

DOI: 10.1201/9781003269502-6

regularly. Any changes must be closely managed by the nominated staff (usually the laboratory manager and quality manager) to ensure integrity of the QMS.

As a guide, a standard quality manual would contain, but is not limited to, the following sections to comply with ISO 15189:

- Organisation and management responsibility
- Quality management system
- Quality policy
- Quality objectives
- Document control
- Third party agreements
- Examination by external laboratories
- External services and supplies
- Resolution of complaints
- Identification and control of non-conformances
- Corrective action
- Preventative action
- Continual improvement
- Control of reports
- Evaluation and audits
- Management review
- Personnel
- Accommodation and environmental conditions
- Laboratory equipment, reagents and consumables

6.3 The Quality Policy

For an effective QMS, a quality policy is vital. The quality policy provides the overall intentions and direction of a laboratory. It usually reflects the overall policy of the organisation and provides the basis on which quality objectives are devised (**2**).

Whilst the HFEA mandate licence conditions, within the Code of Practice there is also the provision of guidance for clinics in terms of the QMS. This guidance is an interpretation of the licence conditions and provides clarification where licence conditions may not be clear. The HFEA Code of Practice provides guidance in specific relation to the quality policy. It states that centre management should ensure the quality policy includes a commitment to:

a. providing a service that meets its users' needs and requirements. This should include ensuring that all staff who come into contact with patients, donors and their partners (where applicable) provide good quality supportive care before, during and after treatment, as outlined in the centre's patient support policy
b. meeting the provisions of this Code of Practice and statutory provisions and standard licence conditions
c. continually improving the effectiveness of the quality management system
d. upholding good professional practice, and
e. ensuring the health, safety and welfare of all staff and visitors to the centre.

It also states that the quality policy should be:

a. signed and issued by the person responsible
b. communicated, understood and available throughout the centre, and
c. reviewed for continuing suitability.

Generally, the quality policy need not be longer than one to two A4 pages of typed text.

6.4 Quality Objectives

Quality objectives define something sought, or aimed for, in relation to quality (**2**). They will usually be SMART objectives; specific, measurable, achievable, realistic and time-based. They form the basis for which an organisation maintains and improves quality standards.

The HFEA Code of Practice states that centre management should establish documented quality objectives which should:

a. include objectives needed to meet users' needs and requirements, including their need for supportive care and treatment from clinic staff, before, during and after treatment or donation (see guidance note 3.14)
b. be measurable and consistent with the quality policy, and
c. be reviewed regularly.

The HFEA Code of Practice also states that centre management should establish a plan to achieve and maintain the quality objectives and the plans should be reviewed regularly.

6.5 Establishing the QMS

One of the pillars of an effective QMS is documentation. All aspects of the QMS are kept in document form, whether it's the quality manual, the quality policy, the quality objectives or SOPs and audits. Once the basis for the service has been devised in the form of the manual, policy and objectives, the associated documentation can be developed.

6.5.1 Document Management

A document is defined as any written form used to instruct or inform service users or staff within an organisation which includes, SOPs, forms and posters, among others. It is vital that all documents kept within the QMS are subject to version control and a review schedule. This ensures that staff are performing optimal procedures for the service users. Documents should have basic identification information contained within them including, a document title, document identification number, date of issue, date of review, name of issuer, name or reviewer and version number. There must be a central repository where details of all documents are kept and maintained. All documents must be controlled to eliminate unauthorised changes which could introduce risk into the service provision to the service users. Hard copies of documents should be avoided. Where hard copies are available, photocopying is possible which can increase the risk of old documentation being used. All documents should have an indication that the document is not controlled when printed to avoid this possibility.

It's important to define the QMS surrounding documentation in terms tiers of documents. As a guide:

Tier 1: Quality Manual. This tier of documents should only be editable by a department manager.

Tier 2: Quality SOPs. This would include the quality policy itself and should only be editable by a department manager.

Tier 3: SOPs. These are separated into several functions; administration, clinical, laboratory and maintenance. Changes to these documents may be authorised by the most appropriate member of staff.

Tier 4: Forms. This would include laboratory paperwork. Changes to these documents may be authorised by any member of staff using them.

Tier 5: Posters. These are either staff or service user facing and changes to documents in this tier may be authorised by any member or staff using them.

Whilst documents in tiers 4 and 5 are able to be amended by any member of staff using them, they must be subject to the same control procedure for changes.

Where a document requires review, the following steps should be taken:

a. Perform full and complete review of the document.
b. Record the changes made either through the use of a change control document associated with the document under review, or by identification within the document itself. One method for this is to highlight the changes in the document using the highlighting function and releasing the document with these highlights visible to users.
c. Update the date of issue and the date of review along with the name of the reviewer.
d. Update the version number.
e. Save the editable version password protected.
f. Save a non-editable version for general use and disseminate.

Any changes that could have an impact on any element of information governance must be approved by the most appropriate department lead with consideration to security and confidentiality, data protection, validation, and privacy impact statements. Changes may be initiated as a result of corrective action notices from audits, management review, attendance at professional meetings or other evidence-based changes. Once the need for a change in a document is identified, depending on the tier, the change should be discussed at the appropriate meeting to fully explore the implications and benefits of the change. Authority for drawing a conclusion from a discussion lies with the author.

Where an immediate change needs to be made to a document, it should be communicated verbally and digitally, i.e., email, with a read receipt to ensure all staff are aware of the change.

Once a document has been changed or reviewed, where acknowledgement by staff is required, such as where the change involves an SOP, a system must be in place for ensuring all staff have read and acknowledged any change. Where this is not fulfilled, organisations are at risk of staff performing processes based on old, sub-optimal evidence thereby not providing a high-quality standard to the service users.

Documents should be reviewed at least every two years. This interval would be at the discretion of the department lead and it is expected that tiers 1, 2 and 3 documents are updated more regularly in line with industry developments.

6.5.2 Standard Operating Procedures

For a medical laboratory, the standard operating procedures are crucial. These must be clearly defined with a standard set of headings. They must be simple and contain only the crucial information required to complete the task described. Additional information, such as justification for selection of a certain process, should be described within an appendix or supporting policy.

SOPs should be written in the first person with actions to complete in the following form, for example, 'start the timer for 3 minutes', 'move the oocytes from dish 1 to dish 2'. The description of the protocol should be bulleted with each being no more than two sentences. The principle of a SOP is as an immediate reference for any member of staff completing the procedure, it must therefore be accessible and simple.

6.5.3 Audit Documentation

As a fundamental part of the QMS, the documentation used for performing audits must be subject to the same controls as those in tier 3. Audit documentation must cover the relevant standards of the regulatory framework to which the laboratory abides. As such, the regular review of the audit documentation is crucial and must be undertaken in accordance with those outlined above.

6.6 Implementing and Maintaining the QMS

In order for a QMS to be effectively implemented, maintained and improved, there must be an individual whose responsibility it is to do so. This person, and others through delegation, must communicate the QMS with all relevant staff, ensure staff are aware of the importance of maintaining the system and encourage responsibility for an effective QMS to all staff.

6.6.1 User Feedback

Staff should be encouraged to make suggestions on how the service could be improved for the service users as well as the environment. Staff should be able to submit these suggestions anonymously but should also be encouraged to bring suggestions to team meetings or directly to their line manager. Staff suggestions should be a standing item on team meetings to allow staff to make suggestions regularly. Staff suggestions should be recorded along with action taken, if any, and how any potential improvement will be measured, where possible.

Service users should be given the opportunity to provide suggestions and feedback regularly. It should be the aim of the organisation to record all contact and feedback from customers whether it's positive, negative or an observation. This feedback could be received verbally or in written form. This feedback should be recorded and reviewed regularly at team meetings. This feedback could result in a service improvement and, as such, corrective action which should also be recorded appropriately. The use of surveys for service user feedback is worthwhile in order to collate standardised information from a maximum number of service users.

Organisations must have procedures for dealing with official complaints. This should include the time frames for communication to the complainant. All complaints should be responded to promptly and courteously and recorded in the appropriate manner.

6.6.2 Audit

Audit, if performed correctly, is an invaluable tool for maintaining quality within a laboratory. A comprehensive audit schedule should be devised to determine whether the QMS conforms to the regulatory requirements associated with the service and is effectively implemented and maintained (**1**). Firstly, audits should not be performed by someone directly involved in the area to be audited. For example, where equipment and consumable traceability in the laboratory is to be audited, the member of staff who is responsible for the maintaining these systems must not be involved. In addition, only those who have been competency assessed for performing audits should do so. Auditors should be unobtrusive and the completion of audits should be viewed as a method to improve the service rather than find error or fault. Audits should be planned and scheduled to cover all aspects of the regulatory framework to which the laboratory adheres. The laboratory should aim to use a combination of horizontal, vertical and process audits with each area being audited no less than every two years.

For effective audit the HFEA state that the centre should establish a documented procedure to:

a. define the responsibilities for planning and conducting audits
b. define the audit criteria, scope, frequency and methods
c. ensure audits are carried out by trained staff
d. ensure action is taken promptly to start corrective action
e. check the effectiveness of the action taken, in a subsequent audit, and
f. keep records of audits, to include:
    i. the processes, areas or items audited
    ii. any areas that do not comply with the quality management system
    iii. recommendations and timescales for action
    iv. action taken and its effectiveness.

As well as an internal audit programme, organisations must engage with external audit by professional or regulatory bodies such as the HFEA or the UK Accreditation Service (UKAS). Inter-laboratory comparisons are also recommended. These are useful for sharing best practice and identifying areas of the service that could be improved. Inter-laboratory comparisons must be documented in the same way as any other audit with appropriate follow-up in corrective actions and re-audit where required.

An effective audit cycle will consist of Preparing for audit; leading to Selecting criteria for audit review; leading to Measuring level of performance; leading to Making improvements; leading to Sustaining improvements; leading to Preparing for the next audit. Compliance and continuous improvement are thereby ensured.

6.6.3 Key Quality and Performance Indicators

6.6.3.1 Key Quality Indicators

Key quality indicators (KQIs) are used to measure the quality of the task being performed. These are usually derived from data which is continuously collected and reviewed on a monthly basis. Examples of quality indicators may be:

- Turnaround times for patient services
- Appointment cancellation rates
- Workload
- Monthly referrals
- Documents overdue for review
- Outstanding audits to perform
- Incidents overdue for review
- Number of complaints
- Customer satisfaction
- Number of incidents reported
- Number of team meetings held
- Staff sickness rate
- Overdue mandatory training

To determine quality, it's usually necessary to use one or more of these KQIs together, and reviewing them in this way could reveal where the service could be improved. For example, if the workload increases, the number of incidents or the turnaround times may be expected to increase and as a result, the referrals or the customer satisfaction may reduce. Similarly, this could be the case if the staff sickness is high. However, if the number of incidents increases and the turnaround time increases but the workload and staff complement is unchanged there may be another systemic explanation such as staff competence or procedural inefficiencies. Performing trend analyses on these quality indicators can provide both proactive and reactive actions. It can also be used to determine the effectiveness of process changes such as new patient information.

6.6.3.2 Key Performance Indicators

Key performance indicators (KPIs) differ from KQIs where KQIs assess the quality, KPIs assess the performance. KPIs are more often a single, measurable variable and relate to pre-set goals such as blastocyst utilisation rate or ongoing pregnancy rate. Reviewing KPIs provides organisations with information about where processes may not be performing and, together with KQIs, could highlight where a system could be changed. Examples of KPIs may be:

- Mature oocyte rate
- Fertilisation rate
- Oocyte degeneration rate following ICSI
- Blastulation rate
- Biochemical pregnancy rate
- Clinical pregnancy rate
- Live birth rate
- Multiple birth rate

Similar to KQIs, regular review of KPIs using trend analysis can inform both reactive and proactive actions. They can be informative regarding recent procedural changes and their effectiveness, and if assessed on an individual basis, can provide intel on staff competence.

The review of both KQIs and KPIs are crucial for maintenance of the QMS and continual improvement of the service.

6.6.4 Change Control

Whenever a change to a process is made, the control of this change is crucial. The change, along with justification for the change should be recorded on a Change Control Record. This record should also include the method of internal communication of the change, staff training provided, external communication and notification to relevant stakeholders. Recording the date the change has taken effect is important. All changes should be validated prior to being brought into effect however, sometimes prospective validation may not be possible and in these cases, retrospective validation is acceptable. Once the change has taken effect, monitoring must take place in the form of review of KPIs and KQIs. An example may be a change to a critical process such as semen preparation where the associated KPIs should be reviewed to ensure there is no detrimental effect. These may include motility and concentration of the final sample used for treatment, as well as fertilisation rate, tripronculeate rate (IVF only), blastocyst formation rate and ongoing pregnancy rate, for example.

6.6.5 Continual Improvement

A key part, and consequence, of an effective QMS is continual improvement. This can be achieved through many means such as corrective actions and audits however, regular review of the QMS as a whole should be performed at least annually. A review of the QMS should take place more often than annually during initial establishment. During this review, all aspects of the QMS should be considered and the HFEA state that a review of the QMS should include the following:

a. the volume and scope of work
b. staff
c. premises
d. the performance of third parties that could affect the quality management system or the centre's services
e. the results of the following activities:
    i. quality indicators for monitoring the centre's performance in the provision of emotional support and patient care generally
    ii. assessment of user satisfaction, and the monitoring and resolution of complaints
    iii. staff suggestions
    iv. an internal audit of all elements of the quality management system, including assisted conception processes
    v. participation in external reviews, and inter-centre and inter-laboratory comparisons
    vi. identification, investigation, control, recording and notification of serious adverse events and reactions, and
    vii. continual improvement, including the status of corrective and preventive actions.

Following the review, the results should be recorded including any actions and who is responsible for completing them. All staff should then have the results of the review communicated with them.

As well as the annual review, regular meetings are critical for continual improvement. These regular meetings should usually include the department heads and any persons responsible for quality in the organisation. During these regular meetings, standing items such as incidents reported, audit results, document reviews, complaints received and staff suggestions should be discussed. Having regular meetings throughout the year prior to the annual review ensures proactivity in identification for opportunities for improvement.

6.7 Why Does Quality Management Matter?

An effective QMS is vital in order to provide a high-quality service, improve success rates and gain patient trust and loyalty. An important element of an effective QMS is continual improvement and proactive thinking. By adopting a risk-based thought process, issues can be identified before they become problems that will be reported via an incident, non-conformance at audit or by poor user feedback. Effective quality management also optimises the use of available resources, creates efficiencies, increases service provision proficiency and can reduce service costs.

Quality management encompasses all aspects of a service. For effective service provision, a quality manual containing quality objectives and a quality policy must be developed. The objectives of the service must be specific, measurable, achievable, realistic and time-bound. There must be responsibility and motivation for continual improvement via regular review, robust auditing, controlled documentation and the seeking of feedback from both staff and users. Through the methodologies provided by the UK Accreditation Service and the guidance from the HFEA, fertility clinics are able to provide a high-quality, patient-centric service focussed on improvement.

6.8 Appendix: Definitions

- Non-conformance; non-fulfilment of a requirement of standard
- Remedial action; action taken at the time of a non-conformance to mitigate its immediate effects
- Corrective action: action taken to remove the root cause of the problem that caused the non-conformance
- Preventative action; a proactive process for identifying opportunities for improvement rather than a reaction to the identification of problems or complaints. This could also include analysis of data and trend or risk analyses.
- Root cause; the initiating cause of a chain of event that resulted in an untoward outcome or an effect of interest
- Horizontal audit; the audit of one process across many departments in the organisation
- Vertical audit; the audit of all processes used by a department
- Process audit; the observation and audit of a process in a department in action

REFERENCES

1. HFEA Code of Practice, 9th Edition, 2018; available at www.hfea.gov.uk/media/2565/hfea-draft-code-of-practice-9th-edition-consultation-version.pdf
2. Medical Laboratory Accreditation Standards ISO 15189, UK Accreditation Service, 2007; available at www.ukas.com/accreditation/standards/medical-laboratory-accreditation/

7

Analysis, Reporting and Presentation of Findings

Amy Barrie

7.1 Analysis

7.1.1 The Null Hypothesis

The key to effective analysis is an effective research question. The research question should be concise and have a clear aim. It should be formed as a null hypothesis so that, upon the outcome of the analysis, the hypothesis can either be rejected or accepted. A null hypothesis would be formed as if the intervention had had no effect. For example, if the research sought to determine if there was an increase in success rates when using a new type of culture medium the following null hypothesis may be used, 'Culture Medium A has no effect on success rates in patients undergoing assisted reproduction.' However, there is ambiguity in this and the researcher must define what is meant by 'success rate' first and foremost. Success rate in the field of assisted reproduction can take many forms and is determined by the researcher's point of view. It may be that the success rate of interest is pregnancy rate. In this case, the type of pregnancy must be defined further; biochemical rate, clinical rate, implantation rate or, the gold standard, live birth rate. Once the primary outcome measure has been determined, along with the intervention, the null hypothesis can be formed appropriately.

7.1.2 Testing the Hypothesis

To test any hypothesis, a robust method of analysis is a prospective, randomised controlled trial (**1**). The quality of analyses can be illustrated using a pyramid, where the highest quality, most robust methodology is at the top of the pyramid and the poorest quality is at the bottom (see Figure 5.1). For a randomised controlled trial, the researcher would usually have a control group to whom the intervention is not applied, and an intervention group to whom the intervention is applied. Prior to the intervention, all participants will have been given information about the research trial and provided informed consent. Participants will have also been subject to inclusion criteria that they must fit to be allowed to take part in the trial. Once it has been determined that the participant fits the inclusion criteria, each would be randomised at a critical point in the pathway. For example, if the research question related to the use of a new culture medium in the laboratory, participants would usually require a certain number of oocytes or embryos to participate. It would be at this point, when the critical number of oocytes or embryos has been reached that they would be randomised to either the control arm or the intervention arm.

7.1.3 Sample Sizes

The use of a power calculation and the determination of the appropriate sample size to use for the analysis to ensure that any rejection of the null hypothesis is due to a true lack of significance rather than a methodology defect is important. Usually, a statistician would provide assistance on the formulation of a power calculation, and it is certainly beyond the scope of this chapter, however, for a randomised controlled trial to be deemed high quality, a power calculation is mandatory. The power calculation will indicate the sample size required to effectively determine significance for primary outcome measures (in the example null hypothesis above, live birth rate) but the researcher should also consider any secondary outcome measures. These may be additional measures such as embryo utilisation rate or miscarriage rate, that can offer insight into causal relationships, but if significance is found in any of these then these must be taken with caution by the reader and highlighted as such by the author. Secondary outcomes can be useful to help direct future research both for the author and reader.

7.1.4 Retrospective Analyses

In the field of assisted reproduction, randomised controlled trials are notoriously difficult to undertake. This is true for many areas of medicine however, in this field, not only are the patients involved but also their reproductive material. Patients undergoing assisted reproduction can be incredibly vulnerable and largely unwilling to be part of experimentation when undergoing treatment to create a family. There is also a strong drive from patients where novel techniques or technologies may be available to offer these without substantial evidence for their effectiveness. In these circumstances, clinics have a duty to ensure that the patients are completely and honestly appraised of the technique or technology and any associated evidence to substantiate potential claims that patients may have seen. This pressure from patients creates an environment where novel techniques and technologies are utilised in clinics far sooner than scientific evidence suggests is reasonable. Finally, there is a substantial lack of funding for undertaking randomised controlled trials in the assisted reproductive medicine field, and if there is funding, there is not widespread knowledge of its existence. These drivers mean that researchers in this area often resort to simpler analyses such as those of a retrospective nature.

Retrospective analyses can be an effective means to test a hypothesis if designed appropriately. These analyses describe

DOI: 10.1201/9781003269502-7

the methods used to determine if an intervention has had an effect after it has been used widely, usually clinically. They are often chosen where a clinic introduces a novel technique or technology that has all the necessary clinical data to be used appropriately, but the clinic wants to determine if the introduction of this new technology or technique has offered any benefit in their specific setting. As with randomised controlled trials the sample size must be adequate. This can be determined in the same way as for a prospective trial and will, depending on the measured difference the researcher wants to observe between the control and the intervention group, provide a sample size required in each arm to analyse. In essence, there are two methods for undertaking a retrospective analysis that will provide robust results. The first is to compare two datasets, a control and an intervention, using regression analyses to detect confounders. This type of analysis is easier for the researcher to complete because essentially, the statistical analysis does all the work and identifies how the data could be confounded and informs the conclusions drawn. The data set can be maximised, the researcher can use all data from all patients spanning a significant time frame. However, the confounders could be many making post-hoc analysis more difficult to complete. If the statistical analysis identifies half a dozen confounders, the researcher then needs to either control for these confounders or cite them as confounders in their report thus reducing the impact of any significant analyses.

The second method that can be employed in a retrospective analysis is a matched-pair analysis. In this method, the researcher selects the datasets using known confounders by matching a data point in the control group to a data point in the intervention group against common confounders. The researcher will start with a maximised set of data from the intervention group. For example, if the research question was to determine if the use of a new culture medium improved live birth rate, then the researcher will select a patient from the intervention group (i.e. new culture medium) noting their age, number of oocytes collected and treatment type, as examples common confounders. The same patient type must then be identified from the dataset of patients cultured in the original culture medium. Ideally, the treatments of each should be within one year of one another to control for any major laboratory process changes. Once all data points in the intervention group have been matched to a control group data point, the statistical analysis can be completed. In this way, the researcher has controlled for confounders prior to analysis and has created a dataset that could have some semblance to that which would be obtained after randomisation in a prospective trial. These data can then be subject to regression analyses to identify further confounders however, the researcher must bear in mind the eventual validity of the results if the data becomes too controlled.

7.1.5 Statistical Analyses

As scientists, there is an expectation that we know the basics of statistics. But we must remember that this is a branch of science in itself and there are experts to assist in decisions and analysis using statistics. To undertake effective statistical analysis, it is important to get the advice of a person in-the-know. Statisticians will make light work of the analysis that is to undertaken and also provide invaluable insight into the dataset that could be problematic for effective statistical analysis. As a starting point, a basic statistical test decision tree should be used to determine which statistical test would be most effective for the dataset. Simply put, firstly, work out if the data is normally distributed. If it isn't then a non-parametric test is required. If it is then a parametric test can be used. The next step in the decision-making is based on the type of data to be analysed; is it continuous numerical or categorical, for example. Finally, the number of groups to be compared needs to be considered. The majority of analyses are a basic control versus intervention methodology however, there may be multiple groups to compare to one another. Each of these characteristics of the data will determine which statistical test should be performed. At the very least, a second opinion should be sought from a statistician or a colleague who has a proven track record with effective statistical analysis.

When dealing with statistics, and study design, an understanding of the phrase 'statistical significance' is important. This, as well as the use of P-values alongside confidence intervals. A common mistake in many analyses is the notion of 'approaching significance'. This is a mathematical implausibility and must be avoided. Within the field of assisted reproductive research, a cut-off of 0.05 for a P-value to demonstrate 'significance' is often chosen. It is imperative that this cut-off be selected appropriately and not arbitrarily. Recently, a debate has erupted amongst researchers in the medical field as to the improper use of P-values and the phrase 'statistically significant'. Researchers have called for 'a stop to the use of P-values in the conventional dichotomous way – to decide whether a result refutes or supports a scientific hypothesis' (**2**). They prepared a comment which was signed by more than 800 scientists, including statisticians, clinical and medical researchers, biologists and psychologists from more than 50 countries calling for the removal of the label of statistical significance for $P<0.05$, or any other threshold (**3**). This debate is out with the bounds of this chapter, but nonetheless interesting and informative for our field. This supports that it is mandatory, at the very least sensible, to seek the assistance of a qualified statistician so as not to fall into the trap that many do when drawing conclusions from analyses.

7.1.6 Ethical Approval

There are very few occasions where ethical approval is not required where research is being undertaken. Local ethical approval can be sought from internal review boards or regional ethics committees however, where patients are to be randomised and subject to an intervention, formal ethical approval using the Integrated Research Application System is required. This applies to both research both within and without the NHS (a common misconception applies it only to the former). To determine if ethical approval of this type is required, the research decision tool can be used from the Health Research Authority (**4**). For retrospective analyses, where contact with the patient is not required and only their data will be used, the data must be anonymised by a member of the direct care team, not the researcher, and crucially, the patient must have consented to non-contact research on the relevant treatment consent form.

7.2 Reporting

Reporting findings is how the author presents the analyses carried out. Usually they would include an abstract, introduction, material and methods, discussion and conclusion. Depending on where the information is going to be presented, each section will adhere to pre-set word limits and guidelines. This will differ from journal to journal, if the aim is publication, or conference to conference, if the aim is for public presentation in poster or oral form. Similarly, work may be presented locally as a service improvement or audit. These pieces of work are usually presented differently but would still resemble the structure of a scientific analysis.

Within this work the abstract should summarise every section of the larger body of work including the introduction, materials and methods, results, discussion and conclusions. The abstract does not need to hold all of the results, only the pertinent ones. It should open with a sentence or two to introduce the work along with the aims, and finish with a sentence or two conclude. The introduction of any piece of scientific work should include a comprehensive literature review to set the scene and indicate why the work has been necessary; there is a paucity of evidence supporting the research question or the aim is to replicate another researchers' work in a specific setting. The introduction should be a substantial length and critically appraise existing research. The length should always be in line with the guidelines associated with the publishing body whether it is a conference or journal. The introduction should provide the reader with context for the research question and identify where research is lacking or where a particular question is yet to be answered.

The materials and methods section should contain enough information to allow the reader to replicate the research conducted. Often, this information does not fit within the bounds of the guidelines and so the use of appendices or supplementary material is advised. Any consumables should be cited appropriately within the text followed by the manufacturer and country of manufacture. The type of analysis must not be misquoted; the methodology reported is that which has been performed, such as retrospective cohort analysis, double-blinded prospective analysis or case series.

Results should be clear and easy to follow. The numbers cited must be accurate and, if multiple groups for analysis are used, the total sample size must reflect the collection of the size of the groups. The use of graphs and tables are helpful when the analyses are complex, but they can also overcomplicate if not utilised effectively. Any graphs and tables used must stand alone and be able to be understood by the reader without the need to read the main body of the results section.

The discussion must convey the results of the analyses in the context of the research question. The discussion can use the research also cited in the introduction if the analyses presented are adding to a pool of knowledge. The author should describe what results mean for the relevant field of application but it's important that the results not be extrapolated or over-interpreted. The discussion should elaborate on the limitations of the design of the study, if any. It is vital that the author provides the limitations of the investigation, to ensure the appropriate level of validity is realised by the reader and that future analyses can be informed by shortcomings of the current analyses.

In general, the language of the report must be scientific and pitched at the level appropriate for the audience. Basic English must be adhered to, such as the appropriate use of abbreviations and the correct use of numbers written form. Although the report is scientific in nature, it is also a piece of writing that should be in constant prose. The author must ensure consistency and use appropriate terminology, for example, the use of 'oocyte' rather than 'egg' and not changing between the terms throughout the text.

7.3 Presentation

Presentation of work comes in many forms, but for scientific works the primary place for presentation is either in a journal or at a conference. For conference presentation, an abstract is required to provide the reviewers with an overview of the work carried out to determine if it is of the appropriate scientific calibre and aligned with the conference theme, if there is one. Presentation in a journal requires adherence to presentation guidelines specific to the journal of choice which usually include order of sections and word count. Once submitted to the journal, the manuscript will be subject to peer review, usually by two reviewers, who will provide feedback and a decision to accept or reject the manuscript. There are associated time frames for each stage however, depending on the edits required, the process can take many months.

The presentation of work at a scientific conference usually forms the basis for analytical improvement and subsequent publication. When work is presented at a conference, the author is requesting critical, peer-review to provide feedback that will strengthen their work and validate it for further publication.

7.3.1 Writing an Abstract

The ability to present an entire research project in a modest word count (on average 300) is a valuable skill. Abstracts are often required for journal submissions and form the basis of conference submissions. Abstracts are usually formed of the basic investigation headers; introduction, materials and methods, results, conclusion. There are some conferences, such as the European Society for Human Reproduction and Embryology (ESHRE), where the abstract headings are different; study question (25 words), summary answer (25 words), what is known already (100 words), study design, size and duration (75 words), participants/materials, settings, method (75 words), main results and role of chance (200 words), limitations, reasons for caution (50 words), wider implications of the findings (50 words).

It is vital to check the guidelines for the conference to which the submission is to be made. It's likely that, if these guidelines are not adhered to, the submission will not be accepted. These guidelines can change with each conference therefore assumptions on previous years submissions should not be made.

For an abstract there are some basic rules that should apply. Firstly, the work must not have been presented or published elsewhere. This work will be published in the journal to which the conference is associated and therefore must not be published elsewhere. Next, abstracts that are audits, opinions or those that cite analyses that have not yet been carried out are not likely to be accepted. To increase the chance of the abstract being accepted, absolute clarity is key. The abstract must be easy to read, and the results informing any conclusions must be easy to follow. It is crucial that any conclusions made are supported by the results and they are not over-stated for effect. Reviewers have a large volume of abstracts to read so an uncomplicated abstract is likely to be viewed more favourably. Keep the abbreviations to a minimum and do not cut corners in English language just to keep the word count down. This can be frustrating to reviewers and makes the abstract a little harder to read. If abbreviations are used, they must be expanded on first use. Avoid publication bias and, if a piece of research is undertaken that is well-designed, all and any results should be published. Those without statistical significance are as important as those with. Finally, a golden rule is to double and triple check the spelling and grammar. Careless mistakes can undermine the perceived quality of the entire project and completely turn off the reviewer.

7.3.2 Presenting a Poster

Poster presentations form a large part of presenting scientific works at conferences. The quality and presentation of posters is crucial to ensure the reader is engaged and the message is adequately portrayed. As with all submissions, whether an abstract, manuscript or poster, the guidelines for presentation must be adhered to. These usually dictate the file type and layout. Most conference organisers request posters be made in PowerPoint to allow for easy editing and upload to the digital platforms now widely in use. Where printed versions of posters are requested, there is an allocated space for display at the conference therefore the layout must be as advised otherwise the poster will not fit on the display board.

Once the guidelines have been reviewed and the template for the poster devised, it can be populated with information. As with the abstract, abbreviations must be expanded on first use. There should not be an overuse of data in the text. Posters allow the author to use pictures to illustrate methodology, and importantly, results. It is important, as with any scientific writing, that graphs within the document are able to stand alone. At conferences, there is usually a huge volume of posters, and readers like to digest as many as possible. Having graphs or illustrations that tell the story to the reader in an instant are valuable. All of the content in the poster must be appropriate to the abstract submitted; unless stated otherwise, no further data can be included in the poster that was not cited in the abstract. It is important that the poster is not filled with text and that the text is not too small. It's always a good idea to view the poster in real size on PowerPoint (or whichever design software being used) so that the point of view of the reader can be assessed to determine if the text is too big or small. It is important to follow guidelines, not doing so can result in a poster not being displayed or, at the very least, not stand the author in good stead for future submissions. Once the poster has been devised, all co-authors should be allowed the opportunity to review and make amendments. Before submission, work should be reviewed with a critical eye once last time to identify careless errors in spelling and grammar.

7.3.3 Presenting Orally

Unlike poster presentations, there are not usually strict guidance for oral presentations. The author will ordinarily be provided a time limit within which they are required to present the entirety of their work within. Most conference organisers will request a slide dedicated to conflicts of interests and also request permission from the author to have their details and/or presentation shared on the conference website.

When formulating the presentation, a rough guide or length is to have one slide for one minute. Therefore, if the allotted time is ten minutes then the author should aim to have ten slides with substantial content. The presentation should follow a logical order and slides should not be filled with text. The listener should be predominantly listening to the speaker alongside a few key words, messages or images on the slides. The slides should be visually stimulating and easy to digest. The colour of the text against the colour of the background should be selected cautiously to ensure listeners do not have to strain thus causing them to disengage. Animations and transitions can help keep the audience interested but there is a balance where too many can overwhelm and the listeners spend more time wondering what the next animation will look like rather than the content of the presentation.

The key to an excellent presentation is clear, concise delivery in both verbal and written content. The delivery should not be rushed; the slides should not be packed with words that the listeners have to read whilst the speaker talks; it should be one or the other. It is advised that the author practice the presentation out loud to a group of peers, or to themselves; speaking the words aloud will help identify where sentences do not come easily and which could lead to confusion during the presentation.

7.3.4 Writing a Manuscript

Writing research for publication should follow the basic principles outlined above for presenting works in abstract, poster or oral form. Usually work for publication in a journal as a full manuscript have had preliminary analyses presented at a conference and have thus already been subject to peer review resulting in work that is high quality and ready for full publication.

The first step to writing for publication is to select the journal to which to submit the works to. These can be selected based on the association with a professional body, for example, Human Reproduction and associated journals are linked with ESHRE. Depending on the type of analysis undertaken (randomised controlled trial, cohort analysis, case report etc) a particular journal may be more suitable and this should be a consideration. It is usually worth aiming high for submission in terms of impact factor when selecting the journal for publication, however, there is a significant amount of work to do to prepare work for publication so this selection should also be realistic. Once the journal has been selected, prepare the manuscript according to the guidelines. Most dictate the layout, i.e. font size, line spacing, numbering and reference style. Not following the author guidance is ill-advised and could increase the chance of rejection. The author guidelines can usually be found on the journal website.

A strong introduction with a comprehensive literature review written concisely, scientifically and clearly will go a long way to set the scene for the reviewer. Outline why the analysis was performed, where the gaps in the knowledge are and what the analysis hopes to add to this knowledge base. For the results section, all the numbers must be accurate; it's an easy mistake to make especially when the sample sizes are large. Develop a discussion section that answers questions the reviewer might have; highlight limitations and why it was not possible to rectify these limitations for the current analyses. Justify the methodology selection, even if it has flaws. Being critical of the work carried out, seeking improvement and highlighting these, all favour acceptance for publication. It is best practice to make sure that references are as current as possible unless an original piece of work is being cited such as the first use of gamete cryopreservation in human subjects.

Formulate a strong conclusion that summarises the work; a sentence or two linking back to the introduction, the main results and concluding remarks regarding application, validity and reliability. Prior to submission, all co-authors must have visibility of the manuscript and approve its submission. As always, request a proof-read to identify careless spelling or grammatical errors which can easily change a reviewer's opinion of the quality of the work.

7.4 Conclusion

Preparation and attention to detail are key for all elements of these processes. It is crucial that a null hypothesis be formulated that reflects the work appropriately and thus informs the relevant statistical analyses, which should be supported by advice from a qualified statistician. Avoid publication bias and report findings either way; if the analysis has been well designed then the publication of 'non-significant' results is as valuable as those reported as 'significant'. Sample sizes must be appropriately calculated and relevant ethical approvals must be in place. The golden rule for reporting and presenting is to follow the guidelines set out by the journal or conference to which the work is to be submitted. It must be scientifically written using constant prose and observing basic English language rules. Terminology must be consistent and a thorough check of spelling and grammar should be completed prior to submission. All co-authors must have visibility of the work prior to submission, and importantly, agree to its submission.

Analysing, reporting and presenting research can be arduous, but incredibly rewarding. If the work is well designed, it should be the intention at the outset of a worthwhile investigation to share with the wider scientific community.

REFERENCES

1. Yetley E, MacFarlane A, Greene-Finestone L, et al. Options for basing dietary reference intakes (DRIs) on chronic disease endpoints. *Am J Clin Nutr.* 2016–2017;105(1):249S–285S.
2. Amrhein V, Greenland S, McShane B. Scientists rise up against statistical significance. *Nature.* 2019;567:305–307.
3. Indrayan A. Attack on statistical significance: a balanced approach for medical research. *Indian J Med Res.* 2020; 151(4):275–278.
4. Health Research Authority (HRA). 2017. Available from: www.hra-decisiontools.org.uk/research/docs/DefiningResearchTable_Oct2017-1.pdf accessed 10/2022.

8

The Human Fertilisation and Embryology Authority (HFEA)

Debra Bloor

To understand the regulatory framework and the role of the HFEA in fertility treatment in the UK it is useful to consider the wider ethics and societal concerns associated with ART and the treatment of infertility – particularly the arguments for and against IVF that were considered by the legislators at the time the law was first drafted (Table 8.1).

The Human Fertilisation and Embryology Act (the Act) was passed in the UK in 1990 with the law mandating the formation of the Human Fertilisation and Embryology Authority (HFEA) – the first statutory body to regulate and control assisted conception anywhere in the world (**1**). The rights and protections enshrined in the law can look outdated more than 30 years later but it can be argued that fertility treatment was able to grow and evolve *because* the public could be confident in the regulatory framework to prevent a slippery slope decline to designer babies, disregard for the special status of human embryos and the welfare of future children.

8.1 Licensing of ART Providers

By setting out the activities governed by the Act the law makes it a criminal offence for anyone to keep, process, procure, distribute or store eggs sperm or embryos intended for human application, or to place eggs, sperm or embryos in a woman without a licence from the HFEA

> In 2010 in the first case of its kind, two men who ran an online business to provide sperm were convicted of three counts of procuring gametes or reproductive cells without a licence or third-party agreement. They were sentenced to nine months each but their prison terms were suspended for two years at London's Southwark Crown Court and they were fined £15,000 each. The judge hearing the case noted they had been repeatedly told by health authorities that they required a licence. (See further in [**2**].)

(**3**). In this way the Act ensures fertility treatment is only ever provided in the UK by those who can clearly demonstrate they meet all the required standards of quality and safety and ethical practice,

The law makes it a requirement that every HFEA licence is issued to a Person Responsible (PR). As implied in the title,

TABLE 8.1

Arguments for and against IVF

For	Against
ART	**ART**
Childlessness is distressing and ART can alleviate the suffering	ART violates the unity of marriage by introducing third parties into an exclusive relationship.
ART provides people with the chance of having a child that is their genetic offspring	Although infertility may be distressing there are other options, such as adoption.
IVF and spare embryos	**IVF and spare embryos**
Embryos not used in treatment can be frozen and used later.	Immoral to produce embryos that will never be implanted and it is unacceptable to allow these unwanted embryos to die.
	Insufficient evidence of safety and efficacy of egg freezing and of long-term impact of freezing of sperm and embryos.
	Infertility treatment may be provided for couples without due regard for the interests of any child that may be born as a result
Gamete donation	**Gamete donation**
Egg or sperm donation or surrogacy is an altruistic act that can alleviate the suffering of infertility	A father may be more likely to not love a donor conceived child because it would not be his biologically. This child might therefore be stigmatised and the parents may feel obliged to keep the nature of their child's birth secret.
Embryo research	**Embryo research**
While respect might be owed to a developing human embryo, that respect can be balanced against the benefits of research.	Fertilised embryos have a right to life.
No animal model alternatives are suitable experimental subjects for disorders that occur only in humans.	Embryos cannot give consent,
	Eugenics and trans-species hybridization are the likely products of embryological experimentation.
	The moral worth of an embryo, and the moral law prohibiting their exploitation, outweighs any potential benefits of scientific research.

DOI: 10.1201/9781003269502-8

the PR is held personally accountable for ensuring that all of the conditions of the HFEA licence are complied with and if an HFEA inspection finds that standards have not been met and concludes that the PR has not 'discharged their duty' then HFEA has the power to revoke a licence and prevent a clinic from continuing to provide treatment.

Although revocations are rare, the law has been used effectively to prevent services like internet-based sperm donation being provided unlawfully,

8.2 The HFEA Code of Practice

The language of the Act makes it an impractical everyday source of guidance for clinics and their teams and the HFEA produces a Code of Practice (CoP) that translates the legislation into more practically applicable standard licence conditions (**4**) and directions (**5**) – both of which represent mandatory requirements for all those providing fertility treatment. Archived copies of the CoP can be accessed on the HFEA website (**6**).

Much of the CoP sets out standards – essentially a series of rules – that when followed ensure quality and safety for eggs, sperm, embryos and patients. These standards aren't reproduced or commented on here but the following sections aim to highlight how and where those standards link back to the ethical concerns that influence the provision of fertility services.

8.3 Consent: Enshrining the Rights of Egg and Sperm Providers

Fertility treatment is unlike any other healthcare treatment because the eggs and sperm of two people are used to create a third potential future life.

The law sets out strict consent requirements (set out at schedule 3 of the Act (**7**), to ensure that no-one can become the parent of a child without their explicit knowledge and consent.

8.4 Consent for Treatment

- must be in writing and signed by the person providing the eggs or sperm or a person acting at their request;
- specify the purposes for which gametes and or embryos can be used;
- specify the maximum period of storage;
- state should happen to the gametes or embryos if the person who gave the consent dies or becomes mentally incapacitated.

Gamete providers are further protected by the right to change or withdraw their consent at any time up until gametes or embryos are used in treatment.

Those giving consent must have capacity (**8**) and unlike organ or non-reproductive tissue donation; the law **does not** allow a person to give consent on another person's behalf to the use or storage of a person's eggs or sperm or stored embryos.

> In 1997 the Court of Appeal gave judgment in relation to the case of Diane Blood who was seeking to use sperm taken from her deceased husband when he was in a coma.
>
> The Court ruled that Mrs Blood could not lawfully be treated with the sperm of her late husband in the UK because he had not given his consent.
>
> Although next of kin can give consent for tissues and organs from a deceased person to be used in treatment, the law does **not** allow eggs or sperm retrieved from a deceased person to be stored or used unless the deceased gave their consent before their death.
>
> Any clinic approached to store gametes taken from a deceased person should alert the HFEA immediately – see guidance in (**9**).

8.5 Consent to Storage

Because treatment can include storage of cryopreserved eggs, sperm and or embryos there is the potential for a child to be born after the death of an egg or sperm provider. Again, to ensure that a person cannot be made the parent of a child without their explicit consent, even after death, consent forms issued by the HFEA and that all patients providing eggs or sperm for treatment or donation, give the opportunity to document what should happen of the gamete provider dies or becomes unable to make their own decisions (known as mental incapacity).

> It is the possibility of the birth of a future child after the death of the genetic parent of that child that is unique to fertility treatment and informs the strict consent and counselling requirements of the law.

To provide an opportunity for a future child born after the death of their genetic parent to have the name of their parent registered on their birth certificate, consent forms also allow a person to consent to be registered posthumously on their child's birth certificate if this is their wish,

8.6 Becoming the Legal Parent of a Child

In the UK the person giving birth to a child is always recognised in law as the legal mother of that child even where the woman giving birth did not provide the eggs; this means an egg donor is protected from being considered a child's legal mother. The law very specifically states that a sperm donor who gives their consent to donation as required by the Act is not to be treated as the father of a child. In this way, sperm donors are protected from being the legal parent of a child as a result of their donation.

The law is complex when it comes the legal parenthood of a child conceived as a result of treatment using donor sperm.

1. Firstly, the law recognises the spouse or civil partner of the birth mother as the legal father or second parent of their child.
2. If the birth mother is not married or in a civil partnership BUT her treatment partner provided the sperm for treatment then the sperm provider is recognised as their child's legal parent by registering the birth.
3. If the birth mother is **not** married or in a civil partnership and treatment used donated sperm treatment their treatment partner (regardless of gender) can become the legal second parent of their child but ONLY with the explicit consent of the birth mother and the treatment partner given on parenthood consent forms issued by the HFEA.

This legal hierarchy brings its own challenges. In the case of a person who is not married or in a civil partnership with their partner who is having treatment with donor sperm, any errors or anomalies in their respective consents to parenthood can only be resolved by a court. Clearly, clinic staff have a responsibility to ensure consent is documented accurately but where errors are identified the resulting lengthy legal process to seek a declaration of parenthood can cause significant distress. For this reason, it's crucially important that all clinic staff are fully trained, competent and confident in seeking consent to parenthood.

Finally, where a person wo is married or in a civil partnership seeks treatment using donor sperm **without** their spouse or civil partner the legal parenthood hierarchy puts the spouse or civil partner at risk of becoming a child's legal parent without their knowledge. In such cases clinics may sometimes decline to provide treatment until a divorce, dissolution or legal separation is in place to protect the rights of the spouse or civil partner.

8.7 Consent to Disclose of Identifying Information: Enshrining Privacy and Confidentiality

When the law was enacted in 1990, special provisions were included to protect the privacy and confidentiality of those having IVF treatment. While there is a general duty of confidentiality in healthcare settings which mean that a person can be disciplined or lose their job for breaching a patient's confidentiality, the Act makes it a criminal offence for someone working an HFEA licensed clinic to disclose information that would identify a person as having had treatment or storing their gametes. HFEA licensed clinics can't even communicate with a patient's GP without the explicit consent of the person themselves.

The HFEA issues a consent to disclosure (CD) form (**10**) to capture patients' consent wishes and all patients – even non gamete providing partners – complete the form. The CD form also provides an opportunity to specify whether identifying information about their treatment can be shared with researchers or whether they consent to being contacted by researchers. Consent to disclosure supports important research, such as examining the link between ovarian stimulation and miscarriage (**11**).

In a time when so much personal and private information is shared in the it is hard to reconcile the strict rules of confidentiality enshrined in the law. They do clearly afford all those accessing assisted conception services complete privacy – even from their own GP or treating doctor.

8.8 Counselling and Information: The Right to Be Fully Informed

In consideration of the unique nature of the decisions being made and consents being provided prior to fertility treatment, the law requires that before a person gives consent to use, storage or donation of eggs sperm or embryos or gives their consent to being a child's legal parent, they must be given the opportunity to receive counselling about the implications of taking the proposed steps and be provided with such relevant information as is proper.

The HFEA's CoP provides comprehensive guidance on what information should be provided to patients prior to their giving consent.

Counselling (as opposed to provision of information) is expected to be provided by a suitably qualified and experienced person and the HFEA's CoP provides guidance on the qualifications a person providing counselling is expected to have.

8.9 Welfare of the Child

To protect future children from risk of serious harm, the law includes a mandatory requirement that before treatment services are provided, there should be an assessment of the patient and their partner (if they have one) to determine whether there is a risk to the future child of significant harm or neglect. The assessment must also consider the need of a child for supportive parenting, and the risk of harm or neglect to any other child who may be affected by the birth. This is known as a welfare of the child or WOC assessment and the HFEA issues a self-assessment form that all those having licensed treatment and their partners should complete (**12**).

8.10 Treatment with Donated Eggs Sperm and Embryos

The gift of donated eggs, sperm and embryos changes lives and to enable donor conception within an ethical framework, the law and HFEA CoP standard licence condition enshrine protections for donors, recipients and donor conceived children and the section on legal parenthood above sets out some of those key protections.

HFEA standard licence conditions further protect the rights of donors by allowing them to add conditions to the use of their gametes. Notably though, these must be compatible with the Equality Act 2010. It would be in contravention of the Equality Act 2010 (**13**) for a clinic to recruit a donor who imposes conditions (restricting the use of their eggs or sperm for treatment of only married couples, for example) that would reduce the choice of donors for those with protected characteristics.

To preserve the spirit of altruistic donation and limit the risks of donors being financially incentivised to donate the HFEA also imposes mandatory requirements on what reimbursements can be made to gamete donors (**14**).

> **HFEA CoP INTERPRETATION OF MANDATORY REQUIREMENTS 20A**
>
> The centre must give patients seeking treatment with donor gametes and embryos information about the importance of telling any resultant children, at an early age, of their donor-conceived origins. The centre must also give patients information on suitable methods of informing children of their donor-conceived origins.

Licensed centres in the UK may not use the gametes or embryos of a donor to create more than 10 families (or any lower figure specified by the donor). In acknowledgment of any possible risk of donor conceived people meeting and establishing a co-sanguineous relationship the law allows a donor conceived person to contact the HFEA to find out if they are related to a person, they wish to marry or enter into an intimate relationship with.

Although between 1990 and 2005 gamete donors were assured of anonymity – their identity could not and cannot be revealed to a door conceived child unless they explicitly change their consent – in 2005 the law was changed and since children conceived using donated gametes can find out the identity and last known address of their donor once they reach age 18.

These provisions are only effective in supporting the rights of a donor conceived person but only if the person knows they are donor conceived. While the law can never force egg sperm or embryo recipients to reveal this information, the HFEA CoP does issue guidance to clinics that they should encourage and support donor gamete recipients to be open and transparent with their children. Arguably however, the strict laws of confidentiality offer protection for those who do choose not to reveal this information

8.11 Embryo Testing

Returning to the potential slippery slope of designer babies, in recognition of both the risks and benefits of embryo testing, the law permits pre-implantation genetic testing but only in very strict circumstances.

Pre-implantation genetic testing for aneuploidy (PGT-A) is only permitted to establish whether an embryo has a chromosomal abnormality that may affect its capacity to result in a live birth.

> The law requires that fertility clinics should not select embryos of a particular sex for social reasons. Information about the sex of an embryo obtained in the course of testing must not be used to select the sex of a future child for social reasons.

Pre-implantation genetic testing for conditions caused by single gene defects (known as PGT-M – conditions like cystic fibrosis, for example) can only be carried out when an embryo is at risk of being affected by a specific abnormality and where testing has been authorised by HFEA (**15**) because the HFEA is satisfied the condition is serious.

Chromosomal rearrangements like duplications, deletions and inversions, can significantly disrupt healthy embryo development resulting in pregnancy loss or the birth of a baby with significant developmental defects. The HFEA has authorised embryo testing for "chromosomal rearrangements (various)" – known as PGT-SR, if there is documented evidence that there is a risk of an embryo inheriting a chromosomal abnormality which can cause pregnancy failure or developmental defects.

The law also permits pre implantation tissue typing (PTT) but only where it is authorised by the HFEA on a case-by-case basis where parents are seeking treatment of a child with a life-limiting blood disorder that requires a transfusion of stem cells from a tissue-matched donor. Where a closely matched donor isn't available, parents can choose to have another child and use PTT to select embryos that are an exact tissue match to their affected sibling.

> The principal purposes for which human embryo research can be licensed:
>
> * increasing knowledge about serious disease or other serious medical conditions;
>   - developing treatments for serious disease or other serious medical conditions,
>   - increasing knowledge about the causes of any congenital disease or congenital medical condition that does not fall within paragraph (a);
>   - promoting advances in the treatment of infertility;
>   - increasing knowledge about the causes of miscarriage;
>   - developing more effective techniques of contraception;
>   - developing methods for detecting the presence of gene, chromosome or mitochondrion abnormalities in embryos before implantation, or;
>   - increasing knowledge about the development of embryos.

8.12 Training and Research

The special status of a human embryo is recognised in the requirement of the law that applies to the use of human embryos in research and training. As with all aspects or ART, embryos can only ever be used with the explicit and written consent of the egg and sperm provider and they have the right to change or withdraw that consent at any time before embryos are used,

Use of embryos in training is only permitted for those processes specifically authorised by the HFEA (**16**) and where eggs or sperm are used in training, the training must never result in the creation of an embryo. Human embryos cannot be used for the development or testing of new procedures.

All human embryo research is licensed on a case-by-case basis by the HFEA and is only permitted where the HFEA is satisfied that the research is "necessary or desirable" for any of the specific purposes for which embryo research is allowed.

8.13 Summary

Like other healthcare regulatory frameworks, the 1991 Human Fertilisation and Embryology Act and its interpretation as set out in the HFEA's Code of Practice sets standards designed to ensure that treatment practices, equipment and premises are suitable and protect the quality and safety of eggs sperm and embryos and the safety of patients and staff, and to ensure that services are provided by suitably qualified staff.

REFERENCES

1. The Human Fertilisation and Embryology Act 1990: www.legislation.gov.uk/ukpga/1990/37/contents accessed 24/1/2023.
2. Starza-Allen A. Directors of online sperm website on trial, *BioNews, PET*: www.progress.org.uk/directors-of-online-sperm-website-on-trial/ accessed 24/1/2023.
3. Activities governed by the Act: www.legislation.gov.uk/ukpga/1990/37/crossheading/activities-governed-by-the-act 24/1/2023.
4. Licence conditions: https://portal.hfea.gov.uk/knowledge-base/licence-conditions/ accessed 24/1/2023.
5. Directions: https://portal.hfea.gov.uk/knowledge-base/directions/ accessed 24/1/2023.
6. Code of practice: https://portal.hfea.gov.uk/knowledge-base/read-the-code-of-practice/ accessed 24/1/2023.
7. Schedule 3: www.legislation.gov.uk/ukpga/1990/37/schedule/3 accessed 24/1/2023.
8. Assessing capacity: www.nhs.uk/conditions/consent-to-treatment/capacity/ accessed 24/1/2023.
9. Other guidance and information: https://portal.hfea.gov.uk/knowledge-base/other-guidance/retrieval-and-storage-of-gametes-where-patients-are-unable-to-consent accessed 24/1/2023.
10. Consent form: https://portal.hfea.gov.uk/media/1500/cd-form-v10-16-october-2019.pdf accessed 24/1/2023.
11. Sunkara SM, Khalaf Y, Maheshwari A, et al., Association between response to ovarian stimulation and miscarriage following IVF: an analysis of 124 351 IVF pregnancies, *Hum Reprod*. 29(6); 2014: 1218–1224.
12. Welfare of the child: patient history form: https://portal.hfea.gov.uk/media/1405/welfare-of-the-child-form-v3.pdf accessed 24/1/2023.
13. Equality Act: www.legislation.gov.uk/ukpga/2010/15/contents accessed 24/1/2023.
14. HFEA, Directions given under the Human Fertilisation and Embryo Act 1990 (as amended): https://portal.hfea.gov.uk/media/1461/2017-04-03-general-direction-0001-version-4-final.pdf accessed 24/1/2023.
15. PGT-M conditions: https://portal.hfea.gov.uk/media/1461/2017-04-03-general-direction-0001-version-4-final.pdf accessed 24/1/2023.
16. Authorised purposes: https://portal.hfea.gov.uk/knowledge-base/other-guidance/authorised-processes/ accessed 24/1/2023.

9

Anatomy and Physiology of Mammalian Reproductive System

Dr. Ishita Mishra

9.1 Anatomy of Female Reproductive System

9.1.1 External Genitalia (Vulva)

The external genitalia or the vulva is bound by mons pubis anteriorly, perineum posteriorly, labia majora laterally and the vestibule in the centre (**1**). The labia majora are broad elevation of skin and subcutaneous tissue and form the lateral margin of the vulva (**2**). They unite anteriorly to form a pad of subcutaneous tissue called the mons pubis in front of the pubis (**1**). The labia majora are lined by squamous epithelium and contain sebaceous glands, sweat glands and hair follicles (**2**). Clitoris is a small cylindrical erectile body, measuring about 2.5cm situated in the anterior part of vulva (**2**). The glans (head) of the clitoris is richly supplied with nerves (**2**). Labia minora are two thin skin folds positioned medial to labia majora on either side (**2**). Anteriorly, they unite with each other in front and behind the clitoris to form the prepuce and frenulum of the clitoris respectively (**2**). Posteriorly, the labia minora join to form a transverse fold of skin called the fourchette (**2**).

The vestibule is a triangular space bound by the clitoris anteriorly, fourchette posteriorly and by labia minora on the either side (**2**). The vestibule consists of the urethral opening, Skene's glands, vaginal introitus and the Bartholin's gland. Urethral opening lies in the midline, just anterior to the vaginal introitus (**2**). The ducts of the Skene's (paraurethral) glands, one on each side, open into the skin crease between the urethra and the labia minora (**1**). Vaginal introitus lies posterior to the urethra and is ringed by remnants of the hymen that is usually ruptured during the first sexual intercourse (**2**). Vestibular bulbs are elongated masses of erectile tissues situated beneath the mucus membrane of vestibule on the either side of the vaginal introitus (**2**). Bartholin's (greater vestibular) glands are pea sized glands situated close to the posterior end of vestibular bulb (**2**). The Bartholin's gland ducts, one on each side, open at the junction of anterior two-third and posterior one-third into the crease between the hymen and labia minora (**2**). See Figures 9.1a and b.

9.1.2 Uterus and Cervix

The Uterus is a pyriform shaped muscular organ and lies in the pelvis between the bladder anteriorly and the rectum posteriorly (**2**). It is divided into three parts: Body or corpus, isthmus and the cervix (**2**). The body of the uterus consists of the fundus and the uterine cavity. The fundus is the rounded superior end of the uterus above the origin of the fallopian tubes (**2**). The shape of the uterine cavity is inverted triangular and measures approximately 3.5cm in length (**2**). The cornua of the uterus lies at the junction of the fundus and the uterine cavity body at superolateral angle of the body of the uterus (**2**). Isthmus is the constricted part approx. 0.5cm long and lies between the body and the cervix (**2**). The body of the uterus consist of 3 layers: Serosa which is the outermost coat, myometrium which is middle layer consisting of smooth muscle fibres and the endometrium, inner mucosal lining of the cavity. The endometrium consists of the surface epithelium (ciliated columnar) and the lamina propria consisting of stromal cells, simple tubular endometrial glands, vessels, and nerves (**2**). Endometrium is divided into two zones: stratum basalis, the basal layer which lies in contact with the myometrium and the superficial functional zone which undergoes cyclical changes under the influence of hormones during the menstrual cycle (**3**).

The broad ligament is a sheet- like fold of peritoneum extending from the lateral pelvic wall to the uterus (**1**). Three structures extend from the cornua of the uterus: fibromuscular band of tissue called the round ligament anteriorly followed by fallopian tube superolaterally and the ovarian ligament inferiorly (**1**). The round ligament courses through the inguinal canal to end in the connective tissue of labia majora (**1**).

The cervix is cylindrical shaped lowermost part of the uterus with a narrow central canal called the endocervical canal (**2**). The canal opens as internal os above into the uterine cavity and as the external os below into the vagina (**1**). It measures approximately 2.5cm in length (**2**). The dome shaped part of the cervix bulges into the vagina and forms a gutter at the top of the vagina (vault) (**1**). This is called the anterior, posterior and two lateral fornices at the junction of cervix and the vaginal wall anteriorly and posteriorly and laterally, respectively (**1**). The cervix is composed of fibrous connective tissue and the endocervical canal is lined by single layer of tall columnar epithelium (**2**). The part of the cervix in the vagina is covered by stratified squamous epithelium and extends up to the external os (**2**). The cervical glands secrete an alkaline mucus rich in fructose, glycoprotein and mucopolysaccharides contributing significantly to the normal vaginal discharge (**2**).

The position of the uterus normally is that of anteversion, where the body of the uterus arches forward over the superior surface of the emptied bladder and anteflexion where the cervix is angled forward on the vagina (**2**). In about 15–20% females, the uterus remains in retroverted position where the body of the uterus arches backward away from the superior surface of the bladder (**1, 2**). Uterine artery arising from the anterior division of the internal iliac artery is the major source

DOI: 10.1201/9781003269502-9

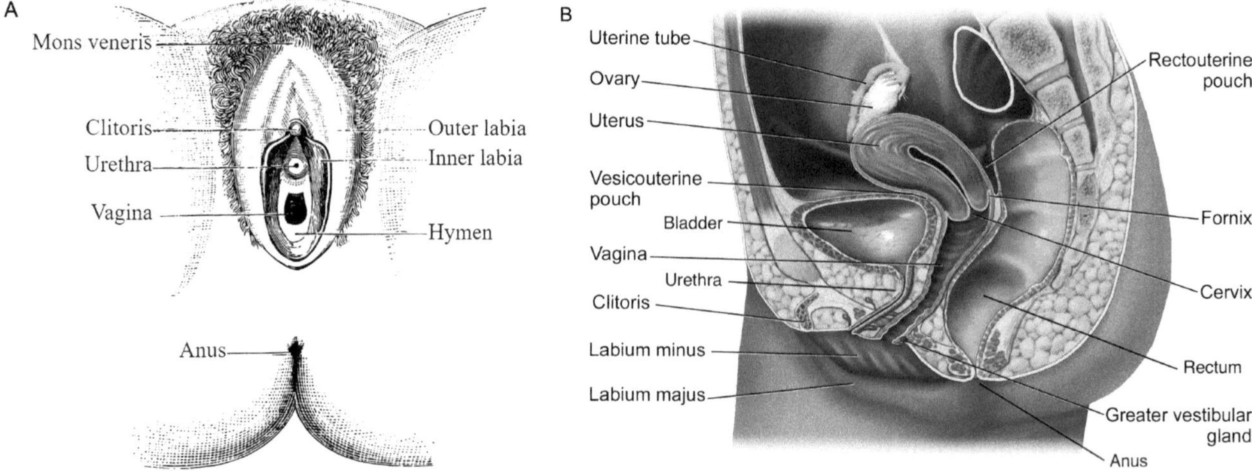

FIGURE 9.1 (a) External genitalia (from Haultain FWB, Ferguson JH, and book of Obstetric Nursing, 1902, via https://commons.wikimedia.org/w/index.php?curid=67138440 in the Public Domain); **(B)** Female reproductive system (from Blausen.com staff, Medical gallery of Blausen Medical 2014, WikiJournal of Medicine 1(2). DOI:10.15347/wjm/2014.010. ISSN 2002–4436, via https://commons.wikimedia.org/w/index.php?curid=56281677 in the Public Domain).

of arterial supply to the uterus (**2**). The ovarian and the vaginal artery are other sources and anastomose with the uterine artery (**2**). The veins drain into the internal iliac veins (**2**).

APPLIED ANATOMY

- There is rich venous plexus in the adipose tissue layer of the labia majora, which if damaged can cause haematoma formation (**2**).
- During sexual excitement, Bartholin's gland secretes alkaline mucus which helps in lubrication (**2**).
- Implantation of the blastocyst normally occurs in the body of the uterus.
- After shedding of the superficial part of endometrium during menstruation, the regeneration of endometrium occurs from the basal layer (**3**).
- The normal length of the uterine cavity including the cervical canal is usually 6–7cm (**2**).
- The cervical secretion undergoes cyclical changes with the menstrual cycle, under oestrogenic stimulation, the glycoprotein network is arranged parallel to each other thus facilitating sperm ascent. Progesterone produces interlacing bridges thereby preventing sperm penetration (**2**).

9.1.3 Fallopian Tubes (Uterine Tubes)

Fallopian tubes are paired structures projecting laterally form each side of cornua of the uterus (**1**). They open into the peritoneal cavity immediately adjacent and superior to the ovaries (**1**). The fallopian tubes measure approximately 10cm in length and is divided into four parts from medial to lateral end – 1. Intramural or interstitial part in the uterine wall, 1.25cm long and the narrowest part; 2. isthmus, 2.5 cm long 3. ampulla, tortuous and 5cm long 4. Infundibulum expanded trumpet-shaped end 1.25cm long curving around the superolateral pole of the ovary (**2**). The margin of the infundibulum is rimmed by small finger like projections called fimbriae. The fallopian tube consists of 3 layers from outer to inner: serosa, muscular and inner mucosal folds lined by columnar epithelium (**2**). The main arterial supply is from the uterine and ovarian arteries and the venous drainage is through the pampiniform plexus into the ovarian veins (**2**).

9.1.4 Ovaries

Ovaries are oval shaped paired gonads approximately 3cm long and are situated adjacent to the lateral pelvic wall (**1, 2**). The two essential functions of ovary are 1. Germ cell maturation, storage and release (oogenesis) and 2. Steroidogenesis (**1**). Ovaries are intraperitoneal structures attached to the posterior aspect of the broad ligament by the mesovarium containing ovarian vessels and nerves, to the lateral pelvic wall by infundibulopelvic ligament and to the uterus by the ovarian ligament (**1**). The ovary is lined by a single layer of cuboidal cells called the germinal epithelium (**2**). The substance of the ovary consists of the outer cortex and inner medulla (**2**). The cortex consists of stromal cells which are thickened beneath the germinal epithelium to form tunica albuginea and the functional units called the follicles in various phases of development during the menstrual cycle (**2**). Medulla consists of loose connective tissue, hilus cells, blood vessels and nerves (**2**). The arterial supply is from a branch of abdominal aorta, the ovarian artery and the venous drainage is through pampiniform plexus into the inferior vena cava on the right side and left renal vein on the left side (**2**).

9.1.5 Vagina

The vagina is a fibromuscular tube-like structure extending from the inferior part of the uterus to the vaginal introitus at the vulva (**2**). The vaginal canal is directed upward and backward and has 4 walls: an anterior, a posterior and two lateral walls (**2**). The anterior wall is approximately 7cm long and the posterior wall is 9cm long (**2**). The layers of vaginal wall from within outwards consists of the mucosa lined by stratified squamous epithelium, submucous layer of loose areolar vascular tissue, muscular layer and fibrous coat (**2**). The pH of the vagina is acidic (4 to 5.5) and varies with menstrual cycle (**2**). Under the influence of oestrogen, glycogen in the exfoliated squamous cells is converted into lactic acid by Doderlein's bacilli (**2**). This acidic pH prevents the growth of pathogenic organisms (**2**). The arterial supply is from cervicovaginal, vaginal, middle rectal and internal pudendal arteries and venous drainage into internal iliac and internal pudendal veins (**2**).

APPLIED ANATOMY

- The fallopian tube has important reproductive functions: transport and survival of the gametes including collection of mature ovulated egg from the ovary and facilitation of fertilisation in the ampulla (**1**).
- The abnormal implantation of fertilised in the fallopian tube is called as tubal ectopic pregnancy.
- During intercourse, semen is deposited in the vaginal vault. Spermatozoa swim up into the cervical canal and through the uterine cavity into the uterine tubes where fertilization takes place in the ampulla.

9.2 Anatomy of Male Reproductive System

See Figures 9.2a and b.

9.2.1 Testes

Testis are ellipsoid shaped structures measuring 4cm in length and 2.5cm in diameter and is enclosed within the end of an elongated musculofascial pouch which is continuous with the anterior abdominal wall and projects into the scrotum (**1, 4**). The testis develops high on the posterior abdominal wall and descends through the inguinal canal into the scrotum by the end of fetal life (**1**). The sides and the anterior aspect of testis are covered by a closed sac of peritoneum called the tunica vaginalis (**1**). The thick connective tissue capsule surrounding the testis is called the tunica albuginea (**1**). The testis consists of seminiferous tubules and interstitial tissue. Spermatozoa are produced in the seminiferous tubules. The 400–600 highly coiled seminiferous tubules are modified at each end to become straight tubules, which connect to a collecting chamber called the rete testis in a thick, vertically oriented linear wedge of connective tissue (mediastinum testis) (**1**). 12–20 efferent ductules originate from the upper end of the rete testis, penetrate the capsule and connect with the epididymis (**1**).

9.2.2 Epididymis

Epididymis is a single, long coiled duct along the posterolateral margin of the testis. It is divided into three parts: head (caput), body (corpus) and tail (cauda) (**1**). The head of the

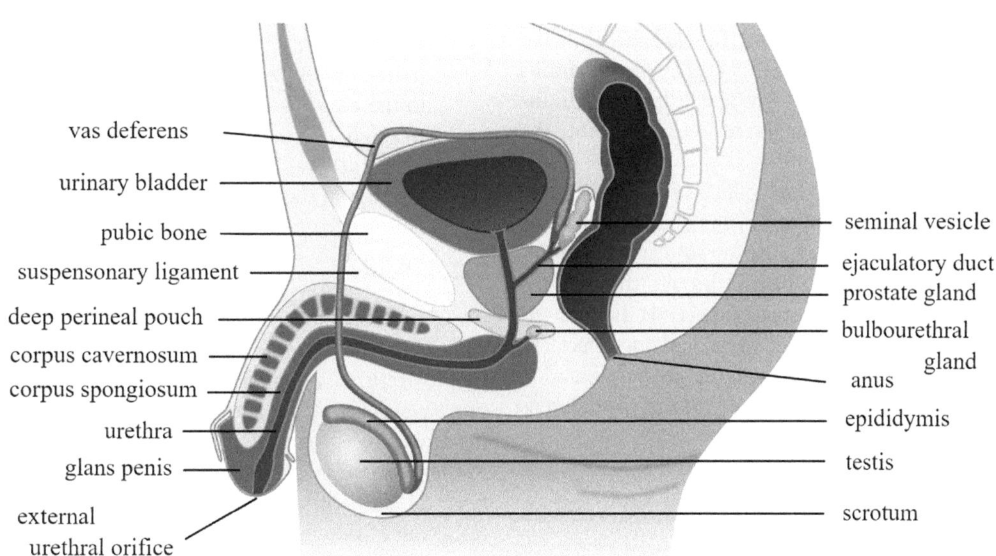

FIGURE 9.2a Male reproductive system (from Wumingbai, https://commons.wikimedia.org/w/index.php?curid=102958455 under Creative Commons licence).

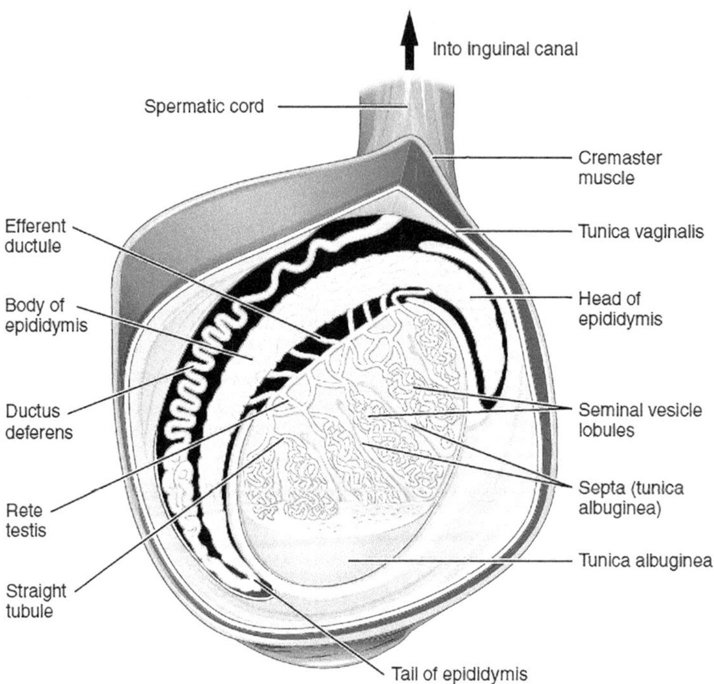

FIGURE 9.2b Section of testis (from OpenStax College – Anatomy & Physiology, Connexions Website., http://cnx.org/content/col11496/1.6/ via https://commons.wikimedia.org/w/index.php?curid=30132978 under Creative Commons licence).

epididymis lies on the posterosuperior pole of the testis and consists of enlarged coiled mass of efferent ductules (**1**). The efferent ductules drain into a single, long coiled duct called the true epididymis and this continues as the body of the epididymis along the posterolateral aspect of the testis and enlarges to form the tail of the epididymis at the inferior pole of the testis (**1**). The end of the epididymis is continuous with ductus deferens. The testicular arteries arising from the aorta supply blood to the testes and epididymis (**4**). The dense vascular plexus, the pampiniform plexus, lies just beneath the tunica vaginalis surrounding the testes (**4**). The plexus drains into the testicular veins and the right testicular vein drains into the inferior vena cava, and the left testicular vein into the left renal vein (**4**)

The ductus deferens is a 45 cm long muscular duct that transports spermatozoa from the tail of the epididymis to the ejaculatory duct (**1, 4**). It ascends in the scrotum at the posterosuperior margin of the testis and passes through the inguinal canal to enter the anterior abdominal wall (**1, 4**). It joins the duct of the seminal vesical to form the ejaculatory duct (**1**). The ejaculatory duct penetrates through the prostate gland to connect with the urethra (**1**). Blood supply to the vas deferens is from the inferior vesicular artery (**4**).

9.2.3 Accessory Glands

1. *Seminal vesicle*: Seminal vesicles are 5cm long paired sac-like structures situated lateral to the ductus deferens at the base of the bladder (**4**).
2. *Prostrate*: Prostrate is an unpaired accessory structure and is situated immediately inferior to the bladder (**1**). It is inverted rounded cone shaped that surrounds the urethra in the pelvic cavity and separates it from the ejaculatory duct (**1**). The peripheral zone of the glandular tissue of the prostate is composed of 50 lobules and each lobule contains minute ducts that empty directly into the urethra just above the ejaculatory ducts (**4**).
3. *Bulbourethral gland*: Bulbourethral glands are paired pea-shaped mucous glands situated lateral to the membranous part of the urethra which passes through the deep perineal pouch (**1**). Their ducts open into the bulb of the spongy part of urethra at the root of the penis (**1**).

9.2.4 Penis

The penis is composed of erectile tissue in form of two corpus cavernosa and single corpus spongiosum which is traversed by the urethra (spongy urethra) (**1**). The proximal part of corpus cavernosa attached to the pubic arch form the root of the penis and the proximal part of corpus spongiosum anchored to the perineal membrane form the bulb of the penis (**1**). The body of the penis is covered by the skin and is formed by tethering of two proximal free parts of corpus cavernosa and related free part of corpus spongiosum (**1**). The corpus spongiosum expands to form the head of the penis (glans penis) (**1**). The glans is covered with a retractable folded layer of thin skin, called the prepuce or foreskin (**4**). The external urethral orifice is the sagittal slit at the end of the penis (**1**). The arterial blood supply to the penis is from the internal pudendal arteries (**4**). The venous drainage is through the prostatic plexus either directly or through the dorsal vein of the penis (**4**). Penile nerve supply is derived from the pudendal nerve (2nd, 3rd, 4th sacral nerves) and from the pelvic autonomic plexuses (**4**).

APPLIED ANATOMY

- The testis is the site of spermatogenesis and steroidogenesis
- The pampiniform venous plexus around the testis dissipates heat out of the scrotum by vasodilatation and thereby has a key role in maintaining a lower intratesticular temperature than the core body temperature (**4**)
- Vas deferens can be easily palpated in the spermatic cord between the testis and the superficial inguinal ring (**1**)
- Secretions from the seminal vesicle contribute to 50–60% of volume of seminal fluid whereas prostrate secretions contribute to 15% of the volume (**4**).
- Important seminal vesicle-derived semen components include fructose and prostaglandins (**4**).
- Prostate-derived components, acid phosphatases, zinc, citrate and proteases aid in semen liquefaction. Liquefaction enables sperm to escape the very viscous initial ejaculate (**4**).
- The bulbourethral glands contribute to the pre-ejaculatory emission from the penis (**1**)
- The function of the penis is penetration of the vagina which allows deposition of the semen near the cervix (**4**)

9.3 Physiology of the Female Reproductive System

Menstruation is the visible manifestation of cyclical physiological uterine bleeding due to shedding of the endometrium following hormonal changes through the hypothalamic-pituitary-ovarian axis (**3**). This depends on three key factors: Active coordination of the hypothalamic-pituitary-ovarian axis, a hormone responsive endometrium and a patent outflow tract (**3**). Menstruation occurs cyclically at intervals of 24–35 days with median duration of 28 days (**5**). The onset of menstruation is called as menarche which occurs between 11–15 years of age (**3**). Menstruation ceases 45–50 years of age and this is called as menopause (**3**). Menstrual cycle is divided into four phases: follicular, ovulation and luteal and menstrual phase.

9.3.1 Regulation of Menstrual Cycle

9.3.1.1 Formation of Primordial Follicles from the Primordial Germ Cells

See Figure 9.3.

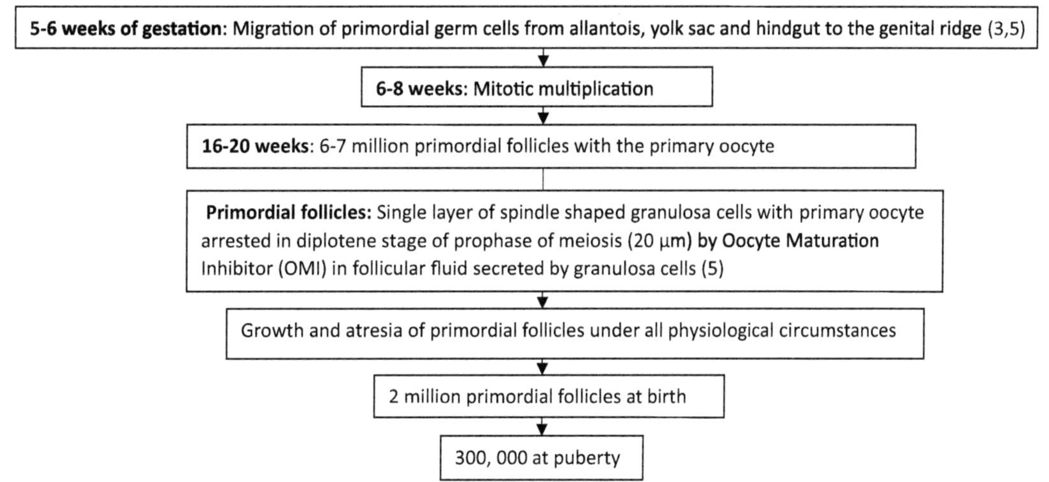

FIGURE 9.3 Formation of primordial follicle.

9.3.1.2 *Follicular Phase: Making the Follicle Ready to Ovulate (Day 5–14)*

9.3.1.2.1 Follicle Variation

Period of initial growth of the follicle destined to ovulate from primordial follicle to pre-ovulatory follicle with series of hormones and autocrine and paracrine peptides acting on the follicle. This occurs over a period of 10–14 days (**3, 5**). Out of the reservoir of 300,00 follicles at puberty, 400 will ovulate in one's reproductive years (**3, 5**). Which follicle would be singled out to grow and play a leading role depends on: Follicle readiness, which depends on the paracrine and autocrine microenvironment (Transforming growth factor (TGF-B), Neurotrophins and Connexin protein) and the hormone stimulation (**3, 5**; see Figure 9.4).

A. **Recruitment (rescue from atresia)**: It involves maturation and growth of the ovulatory cohort of primordial follicles that have been rescued from apoptosis under the influence of FSH:
   1. Increase in size of oocyte from 20μm to 80μm and formation of acellular glycoprotein coat produced by follicular cells. This is called as Zona pellucida (**3, 5**)
   2. Transformation of granulosa cells shape from spindle to cuboidal (**3, 5**)
   3. Formation of antrum by coalescing of follicular fluid. Follicular fluid is ultra-filtrate of blood from vessels in theca interna (**3, 5**).
B. **Development of primordial follicles into pre-antral follicle:**
   1. Multiplication of granulosa cells (**3, 5**)
   2. Basement membrane formation between granulosa and stromal cells (**3, 5**)
   3. Formation of theca cells into theca interna and externa after the formation of 3–6 layered granulosa cells (**3, 5**)

   The pre-antral follicle consists of enlarged oocyte with presence of zona pellucida, multi-layered granulosa cells with FSH receptors and theca cells.
C. **Development of antra follicle from pre-antral follicle**: This is dependent on gonadotrophin (FSH) and oestrogen (**3, 5**). At low concentrations, androgen enhance their own aromatization into oestrogen (**3, 5**). If the androgen concentration is high, aromatisation is inhibited and androgen micro-environment causes atresia of the follicles (see Figure 9.5)
D. **Selection of Dominant follicle:** At day 5–7 of the menstrual cycle, the follicle with highest antral concentration of oestrogen and lowest androgen oestrogen ratio with maximum FSH receptors in the granulosa cells becomes the dominant follicle (**3, 5**). In the dominant follicle, there is an increase in FSH receptors in the proliferated granulosa cells and hence oestrogen allows the follicle to respond at lower concentration of FSH (**3, 5**). The increased vascularity of theca cells allows for preferential delivery of gonadotrophins (**3, 5**). The fully mature Graafian/ Dominant follicle just prior to ovulation measures about 20mm and consists of:
   1. Vacuolated and vascular theca interna and externa (**3**).
   2. Membrana granulosa separating theca cells from granulosa cells (**3**).
   3. Enlarged granulosa cells with FSH and LH receptors (**3**).
   4. Cumulus oophorous: Granulosa cells surrounding the oocyte and anchoring it to the follicle wall. The radially arranged cells around the oocyte are called corona radiata (**3**).
   5. Antrum containing follicular fluid (**3**).

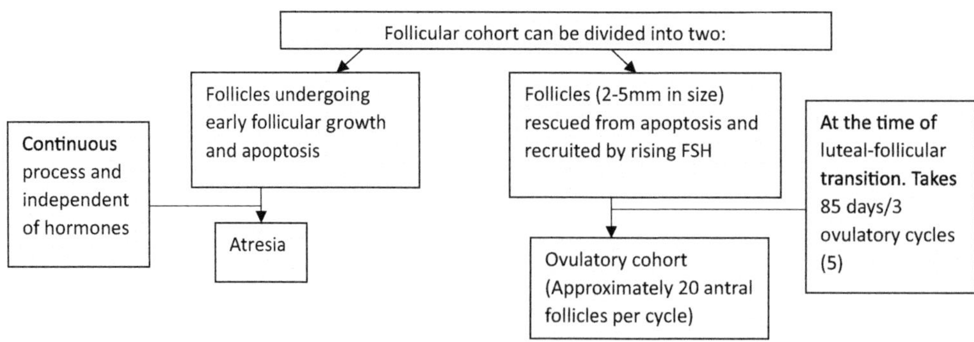

FIGURE 9.4 Types of primordial follicle cohort.

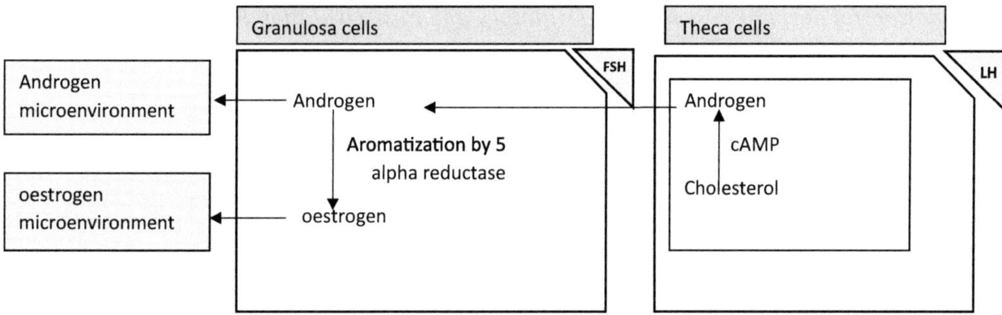

FIGURE 9.5 Hormonal control during antral follicle development.

9.3.1.3 *Ovulation*

9.3.1.3.1 Follicle Variation during Ovulation (3, 5; See Figure 9.6)

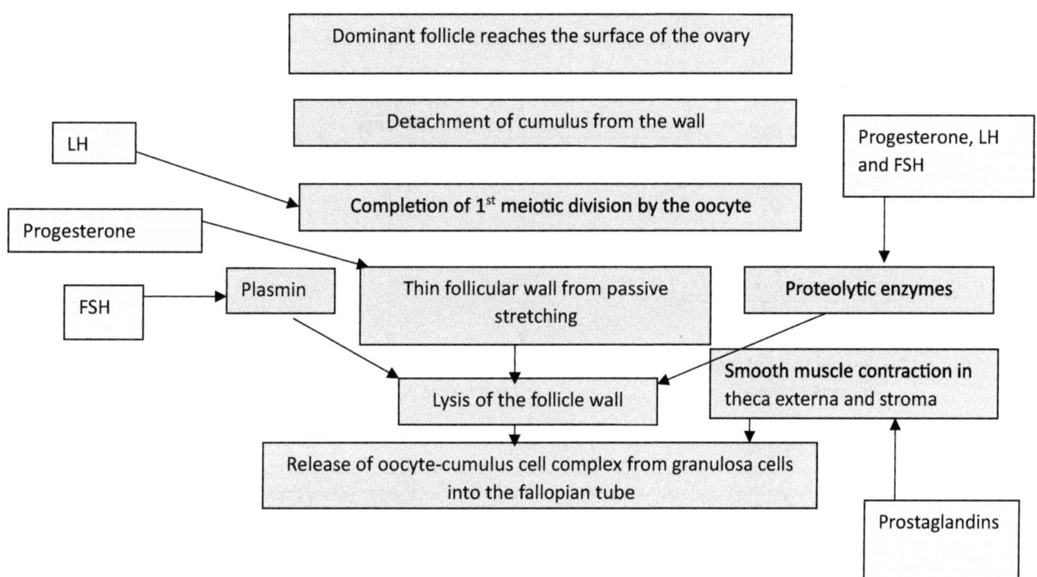

FIGURE 9.6 Follicle variation during ovulation.

9.3.1.3.2 Hormonal Control during Periovulatory, Ovulatory and Post-Ovulation Phase (3, 5; see Figure 9.7)

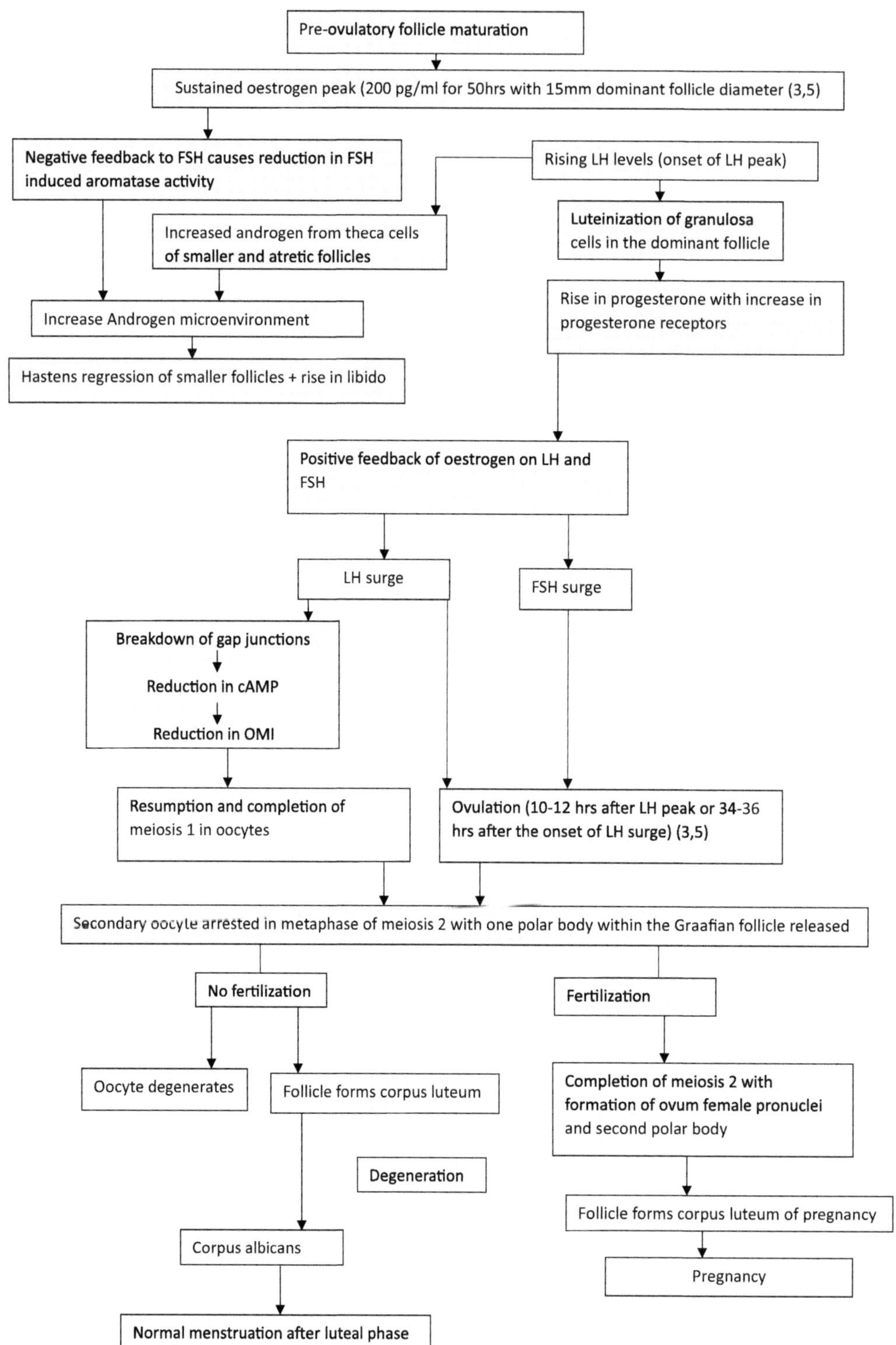

FIGURE 9.7 Hormonal control during periovulatory, ovulatory and post-ovulation phase.

9.3.1.3.3 Endometrial Lining Variation (Proliferative Stage)

Epithelium: Transformation of epithelium to columnar type with basal nuclei (**3**)

Glands: Tubular glands perpendicular to the surface (**3**)

Stroma: Compact spindle shaped cells with evidence of mitosis. Spiral vessels form loose capillary network just below the epithelium (**3**)

9.3.1.4 Luteal Phase

Following ovulation, the ruptured Graafian follicle develops into corpus luteum which has a life span of 12–14 days in absence of fertilisation (**3, 5**). The oocyte is picked up into the fallopian tube and it undergoes degeneration if not fertilized or maturation if fertilization occurs (**3, 5**).

9.3.1.4.1 Hormonal Variation

After midcycle LH surge, the LH secretion causes luteinization of the granulosa cells causing formation of corpus luteum (**3**). Progesterone is the predominant hormone secreted by corpus luteum along with oestrogen (**3, 5**). Oestrogen induces the progesterone receptors in the endometrium. Hence, the progesterone can act only on oestrogen primed endometrium (**3**). Progesterone reaches its peak level about 8 days after LH peak whereas oestrogen maintains a plateau at low levels (**3**). Subsequently, oestrogen and progesterone exert negative feedback on LH and FSH leading to low levels of LH and FSH (**5**). This causes lysis of corpus luteum and fall in oestrogen and progesterone levels (**3**). This removes the negative feedback on the Gonadotrophin releasing hormone (GnRH) and FSH and increased FSH starts the recruitment of follicles for the next cycle (**3**).

9.3.1.4.2 Follicle Variation

1. Proliferation: Collapsed wall of empty follicle forms convolutions (**3**). The granulosa cells undergo hypertrophy without multiplication and are polyhedral in shape, attaining the maximum size on day 4 after ovulation (**3**).
2. Vascularization: Growth of capillaries into the granulosa layer towards the lumen which can sometimes bleed in the cavity (**3**).
3. Maturation: 7–8 days after ovulation at the peak of secretory phase, the corpus luteum measures 1–2cm, theca interna cells undergo hypertrophy, invasion of granulosa cells by theca lutein cells (K cells), lipid inclusion in the lutein cells (**3**).
4. Regression: On day 22–23 of menstrual cycle, degeneration starts due to withdrawal of tonic support of LH (**3**). There is presence of vacuolation in the cells, atrophy of lutein cells and presence of hyaline tissue between them (**3**). Corpus luteal cyst transforms into corpus albicans (**3**). Through negative feedback on the Hypothalmo-pituatary axis, progesterone suppresses new follicular growth (**3, 5**).

9.3.1.4.3 Endometrial Lining Variation (Secretory Phase)

Epithelium: Further transformation of epithelium to columnar and ciliated type (**3**).

Glands: Increase in size with taller lining epithelium and appearance of subnuclear vacuolation from glycogen secretion between the nuclei and the basement membrane (**3**). Shape of the glands changes to corkscrew shaped (**3**).

Stroma: Superficially placed swollen, large and polyhedral stromal cells (**3**). Marked spiralling of blood vessels 93)

Five to six days prior to menstruation, the endometrial growth ceases (**3**). The regressive changes in form of dehydration of the glands and engorgement of vessels are marked (**3**). The withdrawal of oestrogen and progesterone causes spasm of the spiral arteries leading to stasis and tissue anoxemia (**3**).

9.3.1.5 Menstrual Phase

See Figure 9.8.

9.3.1.5.1 Follicle Variation

Regression of corpus luteum (**3**). Rescue of follicle from atresia and recruitment of ovulatory cohort (**3**). This starts 2 days before the onset of menses (**3**).

9.3.1.5.2 Hormone Variation

Low level of oestrogen and inhibin-A release from degenerating corpus luteum with a high level of FSH from lack of negative feedback of oestrogen (**3, 5**).

9.3.1.5.3 Epithelial Lining Variation

Prostaglandins cause spasm of the basal spiral arterioles leading to stasis and damage of the arteriolar walls (**3**). Proteolytic enzymes cause destruction of the functional layer (**3**). As a result, the menstrual blood consists of blood from the damaged arteriolar walls and the shed superficial functional endometrial layer (**3**). This ends with prolonged vasoconstriction, myometrial contraction and local aggregation of platelets with fibrin (**3**).

9.4 Physiology of the Male Reproductive System

9.4.1 Spermatogenesis

Spermatogenesis is the complete process of formation of a spermatozoon from a spermatogonium (**6**). It includes the first and second meiotic divisions and spermiogenesis (**6**). The spermatogenesis starts at puberty and is initiated by pulsatile GnRH release from the hypothalamus (**6**). The entire cycle takes 74 days and is a continuous process (**6**).

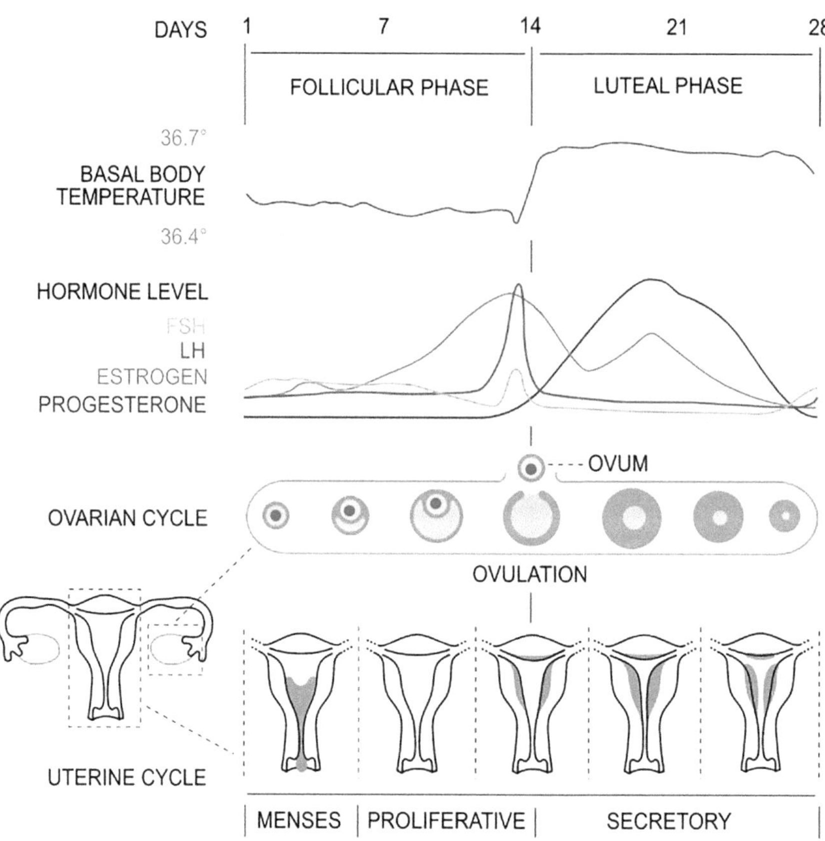

FIGURE 9.8 Menstrual Cycle (from Isometrik via https://commons.wikimedia.org/w/index.php?curid=8703107 under Creative Commons licence).

9.4.2 Spermiogenesis

The process of transformation of round spermatid into spermatozoa is called as spermiogenesis (**6**). The spermatid consists of nucleus, golgi apparatus, centriole and mitochondria (**6**). During the process of spermatogenesis, the nucleus forms the head and the Golgi apparatus is transformed into acrosomic cap (**6**). The centriole divides into two parts and the axial filament grows out of them (**6**). One centriole lies in the neck and the other forms the terminal disc in the distal part of the middle piece (**6**). The part of the axial filament between the head and the terminal disc is surrounded by the mitochondria and together they form the middle piece (**6**). The remaining part of axial filament elongates to form the tail (**6**). Most of the cytoplasm is shed during this process and this is facilitated by the sertoli cells (**6, 7**). Sperm are released into the lumen of seminiferous tubule in testis (**7**).

Acrosome helps in binding to the zona pellucida of the egg through release of hydrolytic enzymes and aid penetration (**6**). Flagellum aids with sperm movement through the female tract and penetration of the oocyte (**6**). Mitochondria arranged around the middle-piece provides energy for motility of the sperm (**6**).

See Figures 9.9 and 9.10.

9.4.3 Maturation

The spermatozoa are propelled into the epididymis by fluid secretions from sertoli cells and peristalsis from testicular tunica and connective tissue (**6**). Sperm undergoes maturation in the epididymis. It acquires motility and fertilising ability in the head and body of the epididymis, respectively (**6**). Sperm acquires its ovum penetrating and fertilizing ability in the female genital tract and this is called as capacitation (**6**).

9.4.4 Hormonal Regulation of Spermatogenesis and Steroidogenesis

See Figure 9.11.

The seminiferous tubule in the testis consists of 2 cell types: Sertoli cells which nurture the germ cells in the testis and the developing germ cells which undergo the process of spermatogenesis and spermiogenesis to produce spermatozoa (**7**). The compartment in between the seminiferous tubules consists of interstitial or Leydig cells which produce androgen, mainly testosterone (**7**).

Two cell, two gonadotrophin theory of female regulation of hypothalamic-pituitary gonadal axis applies to the male reproductive system as well. GnRH is secreted from the hypothalamus in a pulsatile fashion and stimulates the release of the

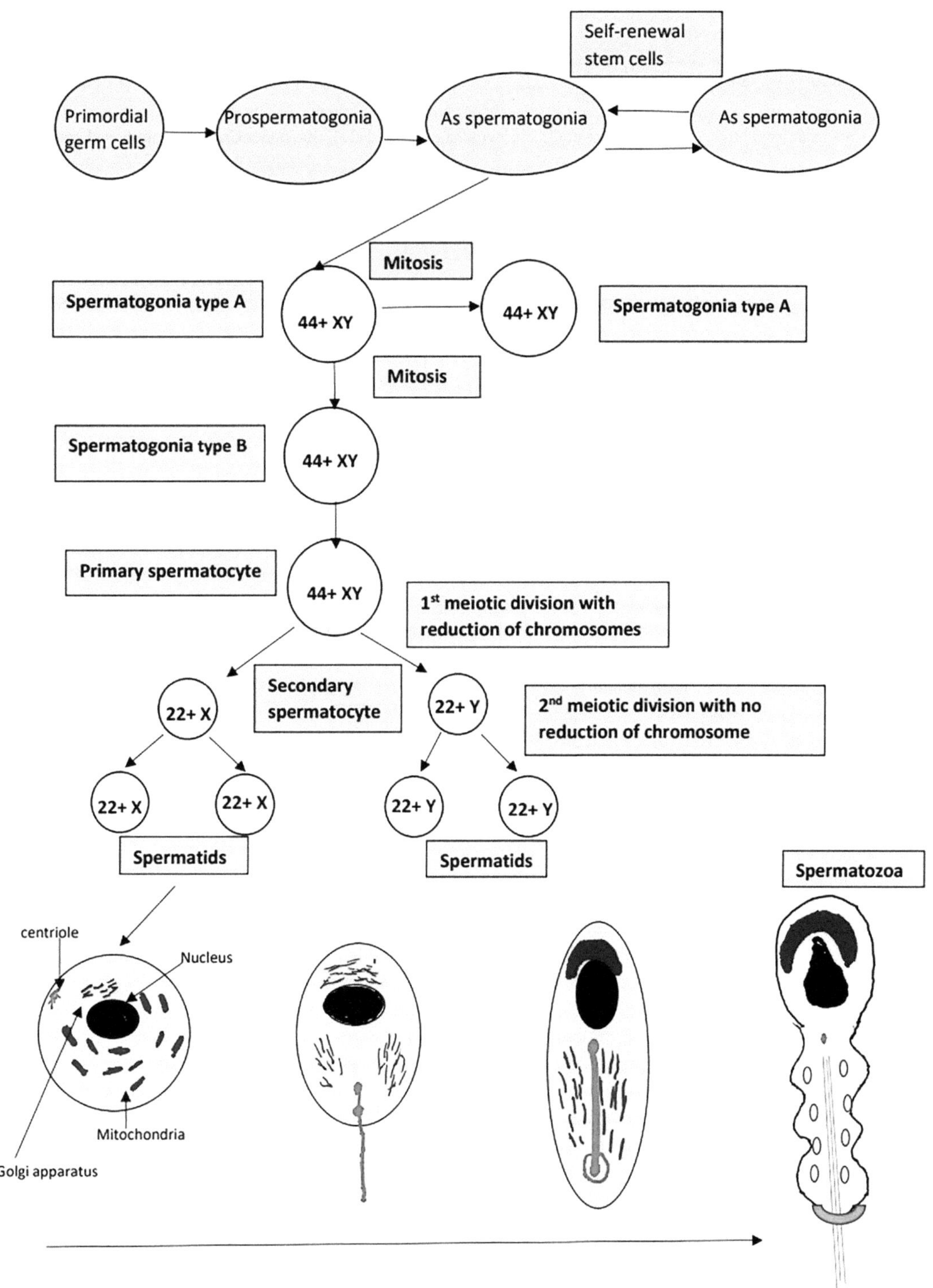

FIGURE 9.9 Process of spermatogenesis.

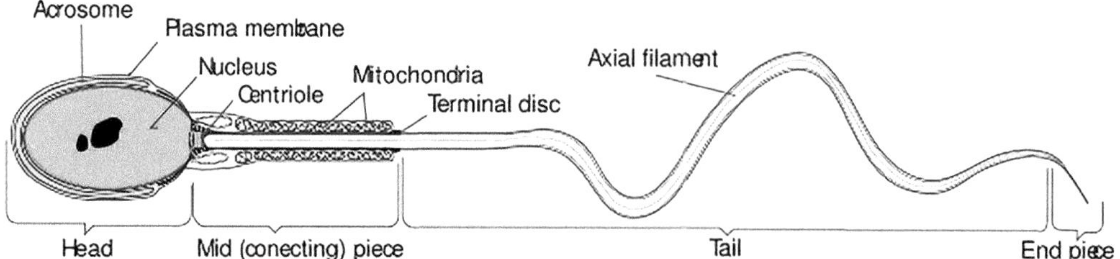

FIGURE 9.10 Spermatozoa (from https://commons.wikimedia.org/w/index.php?curid=1713008 under Creative Commons licence).

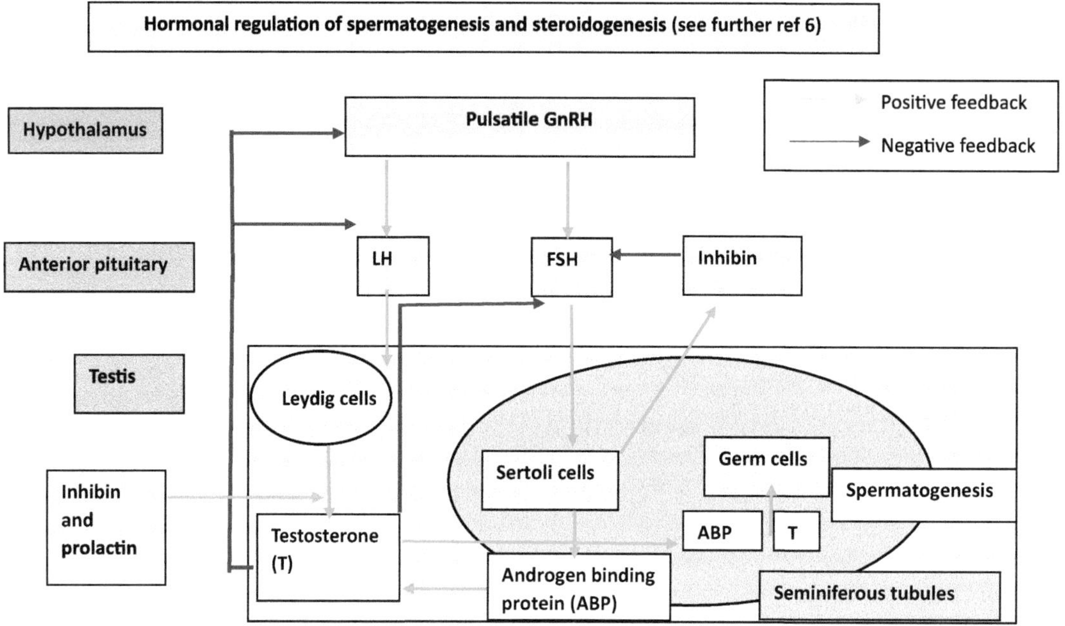

FIGURE 9.11 Hormonal regulation of spermatogenesis and steroidogenesis.

gonadotropins, FSH and LH (**7**). FSH binds to and activates the FSH receptors on Sertoli cells in the seminiferous tubules (**7**). This leads to production of androgen receptors and androgen binding protein (ABP) (**7**). LH on the other hand binds to and activates the LH receptors on the interstitial Leydig cells in the testis and along with prolactin and inhibin stimulation lead to androgen primarily testosterone production in a dose dependent manner (**7**). Testosterone binds to ABP secreted by Sertoli cells and diffuse into the seminiferous tubules from the interstitial site (**7**). Testosterone activates the androgen receptors on the germ cells and spermatogenesis is maintained (**7**). Inhibin secreted by Sertoli cells and testosterone inhibit FSH and testosterone inhibits LH by reducing the frequency of GnRH pulses (**7**).

9.4.5 Erection and Ejaculation

9.4.5.1 Erection

Erection of the penis occurs when the extensive cavernous spaces of the corpora cavernosa and corpus spongiosum fill with blood (**4**). Engorgement of the penis inhibits venous return and allows maintenance of erection (**4**). Innervation of the penis is critical for its erection in form of parasympathetic activation and sympathetic inhibition (**7**).

9.4.5.2 Ejaculation

Ejaculation consists of the synchronized succession of physiological events that form two distinct phases: emission and expulsion (**8**). Emission describes the secretion of the seminal plasma and spermatozoa into the urethra (**8**). This is mediated by adrenergic sympathetic fibres through hypogastric nerve causing phasic smooth muscle contraction of prostate, vas deferens and seminal vesicles (**7**). Ejaculation describes the ejection of semen from the posterior urethra (**7**). This is mediated by the pudendal nerve and spinal nerves 2, 3 and 4 causing the contraction of the smooth muscles of the urethra and bulbocavernosus and ischiocavernosus muscles (**7**).

APPLIED ANATOMY

- The post pubertal male has continuous gametogenesis and testosterone production whereas the post pubertal female has cyclic functions (**6**).
- In anovulatory cycle, there is no selection of dominant follicle. This results in unopposed secretion of oestrogen from growing follicles with suppression of GnRH and absence of ovulation (**3**).
- Symptoms experienced at the time of ovulation: Unilateral iliac fossa pain (Mittelschmerz pain), mild vaginal bleeding and mucoid vaginal discharge (**3**).
- Within a few years after menarche, the luteal phase becomes extremely consistent (13–15 days) and cycle length reflects difference in length of follicular phase (**5**).
- Once the spermatogenesis is initiated by FSH, ongoing spermatogenesis in the testes can be maintained qualitatively by testosterone alone (**7**).

REFERENCES

1. Drake RL, Vogl W, Mitchell AW. Pelvis and perineum. In: Drake RL, Vogl W, Mitchell AW, editors. *Gray's Anatomy for Students*. 1st Edition. Philadelphia, USA: Elsevier; 2005. pp. 364–457.
2. Dutta DC. Anatomy of female pelvic organs. In: Konar H, editor. *D.C. Dutta's Textbook of Gynaecology*. 6th Edition. Kolkata, India: New Central Book Agency (P) Ltd; 2013. pp. 1–14.
3. Chakravorty BN. Menstruation. In: Konar H, editor. *D.C. Dutta's Textbook of Gynaecology*. 6th Edition. Kolkata, India: New Central Book Agency (P) Ltd; 2013. pp. 80–94.
4. Heffner LJ, Schust DJ. Gross anatomy of the male reproductive tract. In: Heffner LJ, Schust DJ, editors. *The Reproductive System at a Glance*. 4th Edition. Chichester, UK: John Wiley & Sons Ltd; 2014. pp. 22–23.
5. Fritz MA, Speroff L. Regulation of the menstrual cycle. In: Fritz MA, Speroff L, editors. *Clinical Gynecologic Endocrinology and Infertility*. 8th Edition. Philadelphia: Wolters Kluwer; 2010. pp. 199–242.
6. Singh IB. Reproductive system, gametogenesis, ovarian and menstrual cycles. In: Subhadra Devi V, editor. *Inderbir Singh's Human Embryology*. 11th edition. New Delhi, India: Jaypee Brothers Medical Publishers (P) Ltd; 2018. pp. 22–32.
7. Heffner LJ, Schust DJ. Male reproductive physiology. In: Heffner LJ, Schust DJ, editors. *The Reproductive System at a Glance*. 4th Edition. Chichester, UK: John Wiley & Sons Ltd; 2014. pp. 34–35.
8. Clément P, Giuliano F. Physiology of ejaculation. In: Mulhall J, Incrocci L, Goldstein I, et al., editors. *Cancer and Sexual Health: Current Clinical Urology*. 1st Edition. New York, NY: Humana Press, Springer Science+Business Media LLC; 2011. pp. 77–89.

10

Epigenetics and ARTs

Lessly Pilar Sepulveda-Rincon, Giles Watts and Walid E. Maalouf

10.1 Introduction

Over the years, both the clinical need to provide new assisted reproductive technologies (ARTs) to alleviate infertility and the agricultural need to produce better livestock to meet the needs of the booming world population have led to the development of several *in vitro* production techniques. In farm animals, collecting pre-ovulatory oocytes from ovaries and further *in vitro* fertilization (IVF) has become a common method of breeding for cattle (**1**), sheep (**2**), pigs (**3**) and goats (**4**). ART *in vitro* procedures expose the gametes (sperm and oocyte) and the developing embryo to a variety of stressors such as temperature, pH, light and sub-optimal culture conditions, during manipulation and culture, and whilst early crucial developmental processes are ongoing. Diverse mammalian species have been a crucial tool to develop and optimise procedures and reagents used in human ART. Livestock animals and ruminants have also been used as models to study possible effects of ART on future offspring. In cattle, it has been reported that increased supplementation of serum in the *in vitro* embryo culture medium can contribute towards a higher average birth weight in cattle offspring compared to the *in vivo* controls – a disorder called "large offspring syndrome" (LOS) (**5, 6**). From these studies, interest regarding the possible mechanisms of how ART could affect the offspring health has increased. Molecular mechanisms affecting gene expression have been investigated.

The three-dimensional structure of deoxyribonucleic acid (DNA) was first described by James Watson and Francis Crick in 1953. It has the form of a double helix with two complementary polynucleotide chains running opposite strand polarity (anti-parallel). They are held to each other through hydrogen bonding between the bases on the inside, while the phosphate backbone is on the outside of the helix. Adenine (A) always pairs with thymine (T), and cytosine (C) always pairs with guanine (G) (**7**). Most of the DNA is packaged in the cell nucleus, while the rest is mitochondrial. The DNA in the nucleus is arranged as a set of different chromosomes. The basic structural unit of DNA is a nucleosome, which is composed of a core of histone proteins, wrapped with two rounds of DNA of about 146 nucleotide pairs long. Core histone proteins are small, abundant in a cell, basic (rich in lysine and arginine), and highly conserved among most eukaryotic proteins. The core structure consists of a complex of pairs of histone proteins – two histone H2A-H2B dimers and histone $(H3\text{-}H4)_2$ tetramer. Nucleosomes are united together through DNA linking stretches of about 40 nucleotide pairs. The structure is further stabilised via the linker histone protein H1 (**8**). A long N-terminal amino acid 'tail' extends from every core histone, which can be subject to further modifications such as acetylation, methylation, phosphorylation and ubiquitination. The different epigenetic modifications of the nucleosome make the chromatin a highly dynamic entity, important for the complex control of differential gene expression (**9**). Genes are defined segments of DNA that contains a specific sequence of nucleotides; a regulatory sequence which regulates the time and amount of expression, followed by a coding sequence. Genes contain exons and introns that are part of the coding sequence, the first being the coding fragments of the sequence, while the others are non-coding intervening sequences. The first product of genes is ribonucleic acid (RNA), and the ultimate product is usually a protein. In the nucleus of a eukaryotic cell, the packaging of DNA is facilitated by its association with other histone and non-histone proteins to form chromatin, or the more condensed form, chromosome. Chromatin can be classified into two main forms, a highly condensed form, called heterochromatin, and a less condensed form, called euchromatin. Heterochromatin usually lacks active genes, while euchromatin is rich in active genes.

Epigenetics, a term coined in 1957 by Conrad Warrington, is defined as the inheritance of a gene function through mitosis and meiosis, without changes occurring in the DNA sequence itself. Different cell types in different organs and tissues in the human body will have different functions, while they all still have the same genes. This is because cells in the same organism have the same genotypic DNA inheritance, but due to epigenetic differences, they acquire different phenotypic inheritance or cellular identity. The variability of epigenetic information between such cells is dictated mainly by the enzymatically catalysed post-translational modifications of core histone tails, changing the charge and conformation of core histones. The resulting epigenetic network reflects which genes are expressed or silenced, and if paternal or maternal alleles are expressed, also known as genomic imprinting (the imprinted gene is usually the silent parental allele) (**10**). Those histone modifications are achieved by enzymes such as acetylases, phosphorylases, methyl-transferases, and ADP-ribosylates (**11**), in addition to the enzymes that can reverse those processes. Some of the modifications occur on the DNA itself such as by the methylation of the CpG dinucleotides or to other non-histone proteins.

DOI: 10.1201/9781003269502-10

10.2 Epigenetics and Development

An important mechanism for gene silencing, and for maintaining this silent state in animal and plant cells, is DNA methylation, which constitutes a long-term epigenetic mark. In some other organisms, such as yeast, fruit-flies and fungi, little or no DNA methylation occurs, and therefore not a crucial adaptation for their survival. Another important role for DNA methylation and chromatin compaction in multicellular organisms is the evolutionary advantage of this mechanism in its roles in protection against retroviruses and transposable elements (**12**). The methylation status changes depend on whether genes are active or silent. The upstream promoter is methylated in inactive genes, and un-methylated in active ones (**13**). Methylated CpG binding protein MeCP1 and MeCP2 are protein complexes that include a DNA binding subunit (MBD). These proteins preferentially bind to methylated DNA so they can suppress transcription. Both MeCP1 and MeCP2 are linked with other protein silencing complexes such as the histone de-acetylases (HDAC) 1 and HDAC2 (**12**). Histone acetylation is also another integral modification that plays an important role in gene regulation. The ε-amino terminals of specific lysine residues of the core histone tails are acetylated through the transfer of an acetyl-group from acetyl-CoA by means of histone acetyl transferases, and the process is balanced by HDACs (**14**). The modulation of histone acetylation has also been reported to have major roles in cell function including gene expression or silencing (**15–17**), control of cell cycle progression (**18, 19**), epigenetic memory (**20, 21**), DNA repair mechanisms and apoptosis (**22, 23**), and it is also found important in the remodelling of the embryonic genome during normal development (**24**).

Initial hypothesis on the developmental origins of health and disease (DOHaD) theory was initially proposed by David Barker based on his epidemiological studies linking certain adult diseases such as hypertension to early events in utero (**25, 26**). Medical ART procedures are carried out during developmental periods when genomic imprints have been shown to be vulnerable in mammalian studies. Epigenetic markings on the parental gametes are necessary for parental specific genomic imprinting, re-establishment of totipotency, and for development to proceed (**27**). It is believed that genomic imprinting affects more than 1% of the proteins produced in the humans (**28**). Loss of DNA methylation in a specific allele leads to loss of imprinting. Research on DNA methylation of imprinted genes has been a topic that gained a lot of attention in the last three decades. Imprinting gene disorders associated with ARTs are Angelman, Silver-Russel and Beckwith-Wiedeman syndromes. In less than 10% of Angelman syndrome and around 50% of the sporadic cases of Beckwith-Wiedeman, the syndromes are due to an epigenetic defect related to loss of methylation on the maternal allele (**29**).

Both methylation and de-methylation take place during gametogenesis and in early embryo development and play a major role in the final imprinting of genes. Oogenesis and spermatogenesis represent a critical stage because genomic imprints are erased and re-established in developing gametes. One example of imprinting genes would be the insulin growth factor 2 (*IGF2*) gene which is methylated in oocytes but not in the spermatozoon. In the offspring, the paternal allele is expressed whereas the maternal one is silenced. This however, is not a general rule as *IGF2* receptor (*IGF2R*) has an opposite parental allelic methylation pattern, and the maternal copy is expressed (reviewed in (**30**)). Most imprinted genes and repetitive DNA elements are only partially de-methylated during spermatogenesis, but are completely re-methylated in the mature sperm (**31, 32**). Nevertheless, little has been reported or considering the effects of the lifestyle habits and age of the paternal side in further embryo development. Different paternal lifestyle habits like alcohol consumption, tobacco smoking, drug use, overweight or obesity, type 2 diabetes mellitus and others have been related to different DNA methylation patterns in sperm or offspring (reviewed on (**33, 34**)). It is worth noting that most of these aberrant DNA methylation patterns have been observed in imprinting genes such as *IGF2* and *PEG3* among others and have also been related to poor sperm quality and recurrent pregnancy loss (**35–37**). In regards with the effects of sperm cryopreservation on DNA methylation, just a couple of studies with small sample sizes have reported no effects on DNA methylation in imprinting genes after freezing (**38, 39**).

10.3 Epigenetics and ART

As mentioned before, the paternal allele imprints are established earlier during gametogenesis than the maternal allele imprints, hence it is likely that ARTs would affect maternal allele imprints, especially during ovulation induction. The epigenetic mark of oocytes is also remodelled during oogenesis. Most imprinted genes are de-methylated during the development of female germ cells, and remain so in oocytes at metaphase of the second meiotic division (**32**). Therefore, the importance of studying the effects of superovulation protocols and their effect on oocyte epigenetic modification and further embryo development is paramount. It has been reported that methylation patterns of maternal imprinting genes as *MEST*, *KCNQ1OT1* and *ZAC* and paternal imprinting gene *H19* in oocytes obtained from superovulation protocols in mouse and humans differed from those obtained on natural cycles (**40**). Additionally, different DNA methylation levels were observed between children from superovulation protocols using clomifene and those without (**41**). It is worth noting that while male offspring presented differences in methylation levels of *PEG3* and *MEG3* imprinting control regions (ICRs), *IGF2* ICR was affected in female offspring. Furthermore, with the increased use of cryopreserved oocytes, the effects of oocyte vitrification on epigenetics should be studied as even in bovine and murine species the literature is limited but suggests that epigenetic changes are induced by oocyte vitrification protocols (reviewed on (**42**).

Furthermore, studies on epigenetic reprogramming in the early embryo has further extended the origins to the early pre-implantation embryo (**43**). There are scarce reports on epigenetic differences caused by different oocyte fertilisation methods, but it has been suggested that children born after intracytoplasmic sperm injection (ICSI) treatment present hypomethylation levels in comparison with IVF children ((**44**),

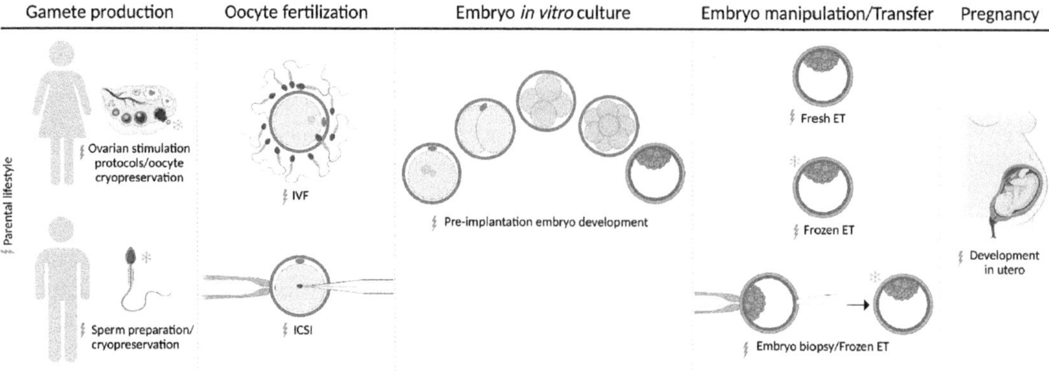

FIGURE 10.1 Assisted reproductive technologies affecting offspring epigenetics (created with BioRender.com).

reviewed on (**45**)). Regardless the fertilisation method, higher methylation rates of *IGF2* were observed in foetuses after IVF or ICSI when compared with those produced after controlled ovarian hyperstimulation (**46**).

After fertilisation, there is a second critical phase during which there is global de-methylation of non-imprinted sequences, and with maintenance of imprinted sequences. Both genomes undergo a de-methylation process, followed by de novo methylation of genes in the early stages of mammalian embryo development (**47, 48**). DNA methyltransferase Dnmt1 is also essential for X chromosome inactivation and genomic imprinting in the mammalian embryo (**49**). *In vitro* manipulation or sub-optimal embryo culture conditions can lead to incorrect fetal programming. For instance, non-physiological ovine embryo culture conditions result in reduced methylation of the *IGF2R* gene, and that was associated with fetal overgrowth (**50**). Even though differences in global DNA methylation levels have been found between conceived ART children versus naturally conceived children (**51–53**), no differences have been observed in DNA methylation levels in children born after ART using different embryo culture media (**51, 52, 54, 55**). On the other hand, differences in global DNA methylation profiles have been observed in placentas from embryos cultured in normoxic versus hypoxic conditions and after fresh or frozen embryo transfers (**56, 57**).

Moreover, different DNA methylation profiles detected in umbilical cords of newborns have suggested that lifestyle habits and maternal exposure to certain substances during pregnancy might be the cause of these patterns in the newborns (reviewed on (**33**)). Similarly, significant differences in differently methylated regions (DMR) of *KCNQ1, SNRPN, H19 and PEG1/MEST* imprinting genes based on natural conception or IVF treatment (**58, 59**). Additionally, DNA methylation differences in *H19*, *IGF2* and *MEST* imprinting genes have been found in placentas from ART and naturally conceived newborns ((**45, 57**), further reviewed on (**60**)).

10.4 Conclusion

In summary, ARTs are a combination of very complex variables and processes prone to epigenetic changes in the future offspring (Figure 10.1) ranging from maternal and paternal health status to the different *in vitro* protocols for gamete and embryo production/cryopreservation and pregnancy. This makes it difficult to isolate single factors contributing to the reported epigenetic changes caused after ARTs. With new developing and more affordable genetic testing, further studies will be needed to determine if ARTs might be linked to further epigenetic modifications during embryo development and further offspring health. It is paramount to identify crucial timepoints that are perhaps more prone to cause epigenetic imbalances in the offspring (Figure 10.1). In the future, epigenetic marks might not only be used as diagnostic biomarkers for ART successful rates but as possible targets to improve successful rates as previously reported in farm animals (**61**).

REFERENCES

1. Brackett BG, Bousquet D, Boice ML, et al. Normal development following in vitro fertilization in the cow. *Biol Reprod.* 1982;27(1):147–58.
2. Crozet N, Huneau D, Desmedt V, et al. In vitro fertilization with normal development in the sheep. *Gamete Res.* 1987;16(2):159–70.
3. Yoshida M. In vitro fertilization of pig oocytes matured in vivo. *Jpn J Vet Sci.* 1987;49(4):711–8.
4. Keskintepe L, Darwish G, Kenimer A, Brackett B. Term development of caprine embryos derived from immature oocytes in vitro. *Theriogenology.* 1994;42(3):527–535.
5. Kruip TA, Den Daas J. In vitro produced and cloned embryos: effects on pregnancy, parturition and offspring. *Theriogenology.* 1997;47(1):43–52.
6. Walker S, Hartwich K, Seamark R. The production of unusually large offspring following embryo manipulation: concepts and challenges. *Theriogenology.* 1996;45(1):111–120.
7. Van De Sande JH, Ramsing NB, Germann MW, et al. Parallel stranded DNA. *Science.* 1988;241(4865):551–557.
8. Hayes JJ, Tullius TD, Wolffe AP. The structure of DNA in a nucleosome. *Proc Natl Acad Sci.* 1990;87(19):7405–7409.
9. Tsunaka Y, Furukawa A, Nishimura Y. Histone tail network and modulation in a nucleosome. *Curr Opin Struct Biol.* 2022;75:102436.
10. Turner BM. Cellular memory and the histone code. *Cell.* 2002;111(3):285–291.

11. Mazzio EA, Soliman KF. Basic concepts of epigenetics: impact of environmental signals on gene expression. *Epigenetics*. 2012;7(2):119–130.
12. Turner BM. *Chromatin and Gene Regulation: Molecular Mechanisms in Epigenetics*. 1st Edition. Cornwall, UK: Blackwell Science; 2008.
13. Bird A. DNA methylation patterns and epigenetic memory. *Genes Dev*. 2002;16(1):6–21.
14. Wolffe AP, Pruss D. Targeting chromatin disruption: transcription regulators that acetylate histones. *Cell*. 1996;84(6): 817–819.
15. Wolffe AP, Hayes JJ. Chromatin disruption and modification. *Nucleic Acids Res*. 1999;27(3):711–720.
16. Tse C, Sera T, Wolffe AP, et al. Disruption of higher-order folding by core histone acetylation dramatically enhances transcription of nucleosomal arrays by RNA polymerase III. *Mol Cell Biol*. 1998;18(8):4629–4638.
17. Allfrey VG, Faulkner R, Mirsky A. Acetylation and methylation of histones and their possible role in the regulation of RNA synthesis. *Proc Natl Acad Sci*. 1964;51(5):786–794.
18. Vogelauer M, Rubbi L, Lucas I, et al. Histone acetylation regulates the time of replication origin firing. *Mol Cell*. 2002;10(5):1223–1233.
19. Aoki F, Schultz RM. DNA replication in the 1-cell mouse embryo: stimulatory effect of histone acetylation. *Zygote*. 1999;7(2):165–172.
20. Turner BM. Histone acetylation and an epigenetic code. *Bioessays*. 2000;22(9):836–845.
21. Jenuwein T, Allis CD. Translating the histone code. *Science*. 2001;293(5532):1074–1080.
22. Georgieva E, Lopez-Rodas G, Sendra R, et al. Histone acetylation in Zea mays. II. Biological significance of post-translational histone acetylation during embryo germination. *J Biol Chem*. 1991;266(28):18751–18760.
23. Carrozza MJ, Utley RT, Workman JL, et al. The diverse functions of histone acetyltransferase complexes. *Trends Genet*. 2003;19(6):321–329.
24. Xu W, Edmondson DG, Evrard YA, et al. Loss of Gcn512 leads to increased apoptosis and mesodermal defects during mouse development. *Nat Genet*. 2000;26(2):229–232.
25. Barker DJ, Osmond C, Golding J, et al. Growth in utero, blood pressure in childhood and adult life, and mortality from cardiovascular disease. *BMJ*. 1989;298(6673):564–567.
26. Barker D, Osmond C. Low birth weight and hypertension. *BMJ*. 1988;297(6641):134.
27. McGrath J, Solter D. Completion of mouse embryogenesis requires both the maternal and paternal genomes. *Cell*. 1984;37(1):179–183.
28. Argyraki M, Damdimopoulou P, Chatzimeletiou K, et al. In-utero stress and mode of conception: impact on regulation of imprinted genes, fetal development and future health. *Hum Reprod Update*. 2019;25(6):777–801.
29. Gicquel C, Gaston V, Mandelbaum J, et al. In vitro fertilization may increase the risk of Beckwith-Wiedemann syndrome related to the abnormal imprinting of the KCN1OT gene. *Am J Hum Genet*. 2003;72(5):1338–1341.
30. Lewin B, Krebs J, Kilpatrick ST, Goldstein ES. *Lewin's Genes X*. Burlington, NJ: Jones & Bartlett Learning; 2011.
31. Lees-Murdock D, De Felici M, Walsh C. Methylation dynamics of repetitive DNA elements in the mouse germ cell lineage. *Genomics*. 2003;82(2):230–237.
32. Li J-Y, Lees-Murdock DJ, Xu G-L, et al. Timing of establishment of paternal methylation imprints in the mouse. *Genomics*. 2004;84(6):952–960.
33. Greeson KW, Crow KMS, Edenfield RC, et al. Inheritance of paternal lifestyles and exposures through sperm DNA methylation. *Nat Rev Urol*. 2023 Jun;20(6):356–370.
34. Jazayeri M, Alizadeh A, Sadighi M, et al. Underestimated aspects in male infertility: epigenetics is a new approach in men with obesity or diabetes: a review. *Int J Fertil Steril*. 2022;16(3):132–139.
35. Song B, Chen Y, Wang C, et al. Poor semen parameters are associated with abnormal methylation of imprinted genes in sperm DNA. *Reprod Biol Endocrinol*. 2022;20(1):155.
36. Khambata K, Raut S, Deshpande S, et al. DNA methylation defects in spermatozoa of male partners from couples experiencing recurrent pregnancy loss. *Hum Reprod (Oxford, England)*. 2021;36(1):48–60.
37. Sciorio R, Tramontano L, Rapalini E, et al. Risk of genetic and epigenetic alteration in children conceived following ART: is it time to return to nature whenever possible? *Clin Genet*. 2023;103(2):133–145.
38. Kläver R, Bleiziffer A, Redmann K, et al. Routine cryopreservation of spermatozoa is safe – evidence from the DNA methylation pattern of nine spermatozoa genes. *J Assist Reprod Genet*. 2012;29(9):943–950.
39. Khosravizadeh Z, Hassanzadeh G, Tavakkoly Bazzaz J, et al. The effect of cryopreservation on DNA methylation patterns of the chromosome 15q11-q13 region in human spermatozoa. *Cell Tissue Bank*. 2020;21(3):433–445.
40. Sato A, Otsu E, Negishi H, et al. Aberrant DNA methylation of imprinted loci in superovulated oocytes. *Hum Reprod*. 2007;22(1):26–35.
41. Lloyd DT, Skinner HG, Maguire R, et al. Clomifene and assisted reproductive technology in humans are associated with sex-specific offspring epigenetic alterations in imprinted control regions. *Int J Mol Sci*. 2022;23(18).
42. Barberet J, Barry F, Choux C, et al. What impact does oocyte vitrification have on epigenetics and gene expression? *Clin Epigenetics*. 2020;12(1):121.
43. Sinclair KD, Singh R. Modelling the developmental origins of health and disease in the early embryo. *Theriogenology*. 2007;67(1):43–53.
44. Penova-Veselinovic B, Melton PE, Huang RC, et al. DNA methylation patterns within whole blood of adolescents born from assisted reproductive technology are not different from adolescents born from natural conception. *Hum Reprod*. 2021;36(7):2035–2049.
45. Penova-Veselinovic B, Wijs LA, Yovich JL, et al. Cohort profile: the growing up healthy study (GUHS)-a prospective and observational cohort study investigating the long-term health outcomes of offspring conceived after assisted reproductive technologies. *PLoS One*. 2022;17(7):e0272064.
46. Lou H, Le F, Hu M, et al. Aberrant DNA methylation of IGF2-H19 locus in human fetus and in Spermatozoa from assisted reproductive technologies. *Reprod Sci*. 2019;26(7):997–1004.
47. Reik W, Santos F, Dean W. Mammalian epigenomics: reprogramming the genome for development and therapy. *Theriogenology*. 2003;59(1):21–32.
48. Maalouf WE, Alberio R, Campbell KH. Differential acetylation of histone H4 lysine during development of in vitro

fertilized, cloned and parthenogenetically activated bovine embryos. *Epigenetics*. 2008;3(4):199–209.
49. Li E, Bestor TH, Jaenisch R. Targeted mutation of the DNA methyltransferase gene results in embryonic lethality. *Cell*. 1992;69(6):915–926.
50. Young LE, Fernandes K, McEvoy TG, et al. Epigenetic change in IGF2R is associated with fetal overgrowth after sheep embryo culture. *Nat Genet*. 2001;27(2):153–154.
51. Barberet J, Binquet C, Guilleman M, et al. Do assisted reproductive technologies and in vitro embryo culture influence the epigenetic control of imprinted genes and transposable elements in children? *Hum Reprod*. 2020;36(2):479–492.
52. Ducreux B, Frappier J, Bruno C, et al. Genome-wide analysis of DNA methylation in Buccal cells of children conceived through IVF and ICSI. *Genes (Basel)*. 2021;12(12).
53. Cannarella R, Crafa A, Mongioì LM, et al. DNA methylation in offspring conceived after assisted reproductive techniques: a systematic review and meta-analysis. *J Clin Med*. 2022;11(17).
54. Koeck RM, Busato F, Tost J, et al. At age 9, the methylome of assisted reproductive technology children that underwent embryo culture in different media is not significantly different on a genome-wide scale. *Hum Reprod (Oxford, England)*. 2022;37(11):2709–2721.
55. Mulder CL, Wattimury TM, Jongejan A, et al. Comparison of DNA methylation patterns of parentally imprinted genes in placenta derived from IVF conceptions in two different culture media. *Hum Reprod*. 2020;35(3):516–528.
56. Ghosh J, Coutifaris C, Sapienza C, et al. Global DNA methylation levels are altered by modifiable clinical manipulations in assisted reproductive technologies. *Clin Epigenetics*. 2017;9:14.
57. Barberet J, Romain G, Binquet C, et al. Do frozen embryo transfers modify the epigenetic control of imprinted genes and transposable elements in newborns compared with fresh embryo transfers and natural conceptions? *Fertil Steril*. 2021;116(6):1468–1480.
58. Rancourt RC, Harris HR, Michels KB. Methylation levels at imprinting control regions are not altered with ovulation induction or in vitro fertilization in a birth cohort. *Hum Reprod*. 2012;27(7):2208–2216.
59. Barberet J, Ducreux B, Guilleman M, et al. DNA methylation profiles after ART during human lifespan: a systematic review and meta-analysis. *Hum Reprod Update*. 2022;28(5):629–655.
60. Schroeder M, Badini G, Sferruzzi-Perri AN, et al. The consequences of assisted reproduction technologies on the offspring health throughout life: a placental contribution. *Front Cell Dev Biol*. 2022;10:906240.
61. Saraiva NZ, Oliveira CS, Almeida NNC, et al. Epigenetic modifiers during in vitro maturation as a strategy to increase oocyte competence in bovine. *Theriogenology*. 2022;187:95–101.

11

Folliculogenesis and Oogenesis

Juan Hernandez-Medrano and Marianna Belmpa

11.1 Introduction

After sex determination, further proliferation of stroma cells is observed, which leads to the formation of ovigerous cords, consisting of pre-granulosa cells and oogonia that will give rise to the primordial follicles (PF) (**1**). Shortly after ovigerous cord formation, oogonia recruit somatic cells from the surface epithelium, ancestors of granulosa cells (GCs). In these structures, oogonia are mitotically active and reach their highest number of around 7,000,000 in human and 850,000 in sheep (**1**). During mitosis, oogonia remained linked together by cytoplasmatic bridges (**2**). When these bridges break and oogonia separate, pre-granulosa cells surround them and the oogonia enter meiosis induced by an increase in retinoic acid (**2**). Once this meiosis phase starts, there is a rapid decline in the numbers of oogonia by apoptosis (i.e., 85–90%) resulting in the formation of PF (**1, 2**). Although recently challenged (**3**), the total number of PF (500,000 to 1 million in humans), also known as the ovarian reserve, is established at birth, with the number depleting thereof until menopause (**2**).

The PF is the female reproductive unit comprised of an oocyte surrounded by a single layer of flattened GCs and a basal lamina, separating it from surrounding tissues (**4**). PF remain in a dormant condition with the oocyte and GCs arrested at prophase I of meiosis I (i.e., primary oocyte) and in phase G0/G1 of mitosis, respectively (**5**). In this phase of meiosis, the oocyte has completed recombination between maternal and paternal homologous chromosomes and remains in the diplotene stage of prophase I until meiosis is resumed after puberty (**6**). The PF has a limited blood supply until its activation to enter folliculogenesis (**5**). It is evident at this stage of development that oogenesis and folliculogenesis are intrinsically linked, but once the primary oocyte is arrested, oogenesis is paused until the signal to reactivate meiosis arrives after puberty: preovulatory LH surge (Fig 1).

Endocrinologically speaking, there are two levels of control for folliculogenesis and oogenesis: local and systemic (**7, 8**). At the local level, the oocyte-somatic cell communication (GC and theca cells (TC)) is central because even meiotically arrested the oocyte is able to grow in size and impinge on surrounding somatic cell function as the follicle moves through the different developmental stages (**9, 10**). At the systemic level, the gonadotrophins (i.e., Luteinising (LH) and Follicle-stimulating hormones (FSH)) and the feedback mechanisms established with ovarian steroids and other factors (e.g., inhibin) drive follicular development. In this chapter, we will briefly review folliculogenesis and oogenesis as separate processes based on the information generated in model species (i.e., sheep and mice) and humans.

11.2 Folliculogenesis

Folliculogenesis can be described as the process of development and growth of ovarian follicles. It begins early in fetal life and comprises the development of follicles from the PF to the preovulatory stages (Figure 11.1). According to the stage of growth, follicles are categorized as PF (i.e., not activated), preantral (i.e., primary and secondary) and antral (tertiary and preovulatory or Graafian (**10**). These stages can be grouped depending on their dependency on gonadotrophins into dependent, responsive and independent (**7, 11**). Preantral phase includes the growth of an activated PF to a secondary stage mostly independent of gonadotrophin input but controlled by local factors (**2, 8, 10**). While the antral phase starts when a fluid-filled cavity appears within the follicle: the antrum (i.e., tertiary follicle), and at this point follicles are dependent on gonadotrophins for their growth (**4**). During the transition from preantral (secondary) to early antral (tertiary), follicles acquire specific receptors to gonadotrophins (mainly FSH) which makes them responsive to these hormones to promote their development (**12**).

11.2.1 Primordial Follicle Activation

Activation refers to the series of events that culminate with the commitment of a PF to enter folliculogenesis (**2**). Once the PF is activated or committed, it cannot return to the dormant state, and only two fates are possible, ovulation or atresia (**2, 7, 11**).

Only a small number of PF will be able to ovulate (~400 during a woman's life), with most undergoing atresia (99.9%; 2, 12). Although the process it still under research in humans, it has been reported that in mice GCs drive activation (**13**) through the mammalian Target of Rapamycin Complex 1 (mTOR1). mTOR1 is activated in the flattened GCs of the PF, causing them to transform into cuboidal cells and express KIT ligand, which, through its receptor c-kit, stimulates the phosphatidylinositol-3-kinase (PI3K)/AKT serine/threonine kinase pathway activating the oocyte (**13**). Oocyte activation is a subtle event shown by an increase in volume (3–10 fold), an increase in intracellular organelles volume (e.g., smooth

DOI: 10.1201/9781003269502-11

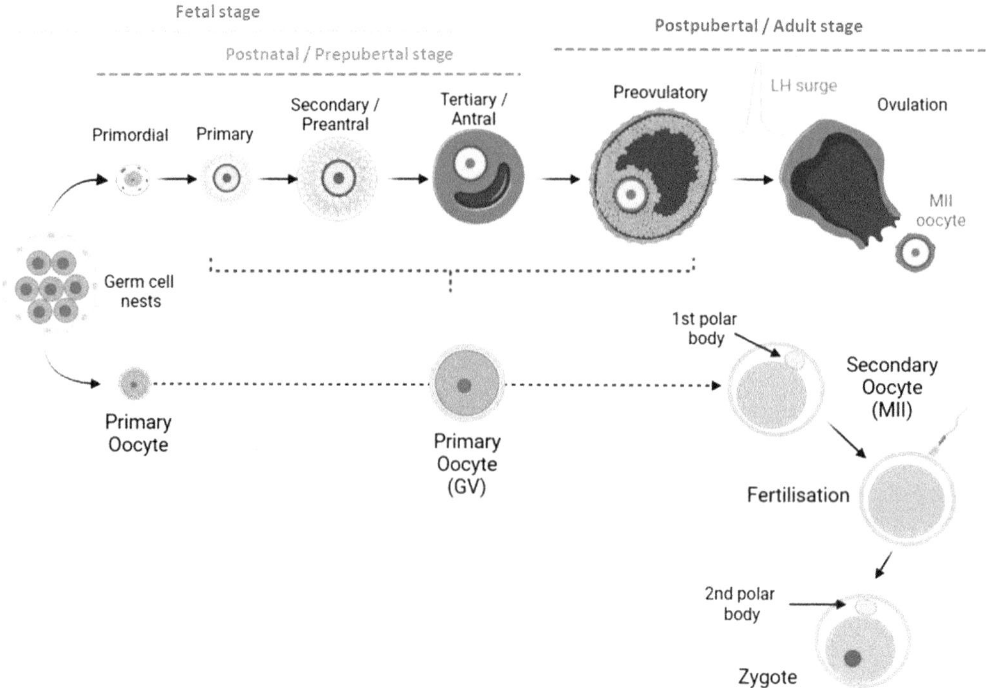

FIGURE 11.1 Schematic representation of the simultaneous events that encompass folliculogenesis and oogenesis. Early follicle formation takes place during fetal development with folliculogenesis progressing throughout female life, but final follicle growth and ovulation only occur after puberty, with the preovulatory LH surge. Diagram created using BioRender.com.

endoplasmic reticulum, ribosomes and mitochondria) and activation of genes associated with mitochondrial activity and cell signalling and communication (**12, 14**).

From studies in rodents, several growth factors from the transforming growth factor-β (TGF-β) superfamily, such as gonadal differentiating factor-9 (GDF-9), bone morphogenetic proteins (BMP)-4, and -15, anti-Mullerian hormone (AMH) and their putative receptors, are directly or indirectly implicated in the PF to primary follicle transition (**8, 12, 15, 16**). It has been reported that several of these factors can act, through intermediaries (e.g., FOXL2, LHX8, NOBOX; (**2**)), on the PI3K/AKT/mTOR pathway. Activation of this pathway ultimately results in the differentiation of cuboidal granulosa cells and formation of the primary follicle.

11.2.2 Preantral Follicular Development: Primary to Secondary Follicle

During this stage, the GC layer grows from a single layer of cuboidal cells in the primary follicle to a multilayer GC structure in the secondary follicle. In humans, the diameter of the follicle increases from 55–75 um (primary) to 185–200 um (large preantral), with the oocyte also increasing in diameter from 40 um to 90 um on average (**14**). The transition from primary to preantral follicle takes around 150 days in humans (**14**) and 130 days in sheep (**12**), making this the longest stage of folliculogenesis. It is during this stage that the zona pellucida and the TC layers develop in the follicles. Furthermore, cytoplasmic bridges appear between the oocyte and surrounding GC, which are essential to oocyte-GC communication (**8, 14**). It is through this direct interaction that the oocyte can regulate GC metabolic and endocrine activities (**12**), controlling directly or indirectly preantral and early antral follicular development (**12**).

The primary to secondary follicle transition includes two key events: replication of GC layers and the appearance of TC. When a follicle develops a second layer to 7–8 layers of cuboidal GCs, it is considered at the secondary stage (**7, 12, 17**). In sheep, a large preantral follicle (late secondary stage) has between 1,000 and 3,500 GCs, representing a 7 to 8-fold increase in number (**12**). Furthermore, TCs separate into two layers: theca externa and theca interna (TIC) (**7, 14, 17**). TIC development occurs around the basal lamina and is accompanied by angiogenesis which means that secondary follicles can be affected by hormones in circulation (**4**). Theca externa mainly consists of fibroblasts, and its role is still not clear while TIC is highly vascularized, and its main characteristic is its steroidogenic capacity which includes the production of specific androgens that are necessary for oestrogen production by GCs (**1**). Although TIC first appears in small preantral follicles with 2 to 4 layers of GCs, the responsible enzymes for steroid synthesis are expressed in large preantral follicles, which contain 4 to 8 layers of GCs (**18**). Therefore, due to the appearance of luteinizing hormone (LH) receptors in theca interna cells, circulating LH can reach the ovary, bind to its receptors and stimulate androgen synthesis (**19**).

Similar to ruminants, in humans, at the early pre-antral stage (2–3 GC layers), follicles express mRNA for FSH receptor (**7, 10**) followed by LH receptor mRNA when the TIC layer is developed (**20, 21**). At this latter stage, levels of mRNA for steroidogenic enzymes such as cytochrome P450 side chain cleavage (P450scc), 17α-hydroxylase/lyase (P450c17) and 3β-hydroxysteroid dehydrogenase (3β-HSD) are expressed in TIC (**11, 20, 21**). Human TICs are the main site for androstenedione production, the aromatisable substrate for oestradiol synthesis by the aromatase enzyme (**14**). Expression of mRNA for the steroid acute regulatory protein (StAR) and aromatase enzymes in GCs are evident at the late preantral stage (**16, 20, 21**). Even though during the preantral stage of development, follicles do not rely on gonadotrophin support, these may help follicle growth in close interaction with growth factors produced locally (**7, 21**).

11.2.3 Antral Follicular Development

Although still disputed and similar to other species studied (i.e., ruminants), human follicular growth occurs in a wave-like pattern, defined as a periodic and synchronous growth of a group of antral follicles (**22**). The follicle starts to accumulate liquid and form an antrum when they reach a diameter of about 0.2–0.4mm in ruminants (**7**). During a wave, a group of follicles of >4mm in diameter emerges (recruitment phase) in a period of 1 or more days, driven by increases in FSH release (**12, 22**). They enter a phase of continuous growth for 3–6 days until they reach ~8–10mm in diameter when one of the follicles is selected (selection phase) to grow further and develop ovulatory capacity (dominance phase), while the rest undergo atresia (**7, 23, 24**). Usually, 2 or 3 waves of follicular growth occur during the menstrual cycle (**22, 25**), with an average duration of the cycle of 28 days (2-wave cycles= 27 days and 3-wave cycles= 29 days) (**22, 25**). In women with 2-waves, emergence of the first follicular wave takes place at the time of ovulation (i.e., mid-luteal stage) which is an anovulatory, followed by a second ovulatory wave during the follicular phase (**25**). In the case of 3-waves, a second anovulatory wave occur during the late-luteal phase, with the ovulatory wave also taking place during the follicular phase (**25**).

11.2.4 Antral Follicular Recruitment

This stage refers to the recruitment of 2–3mm antral follicles to continue growing under the influence of gonadotrophins with a duration of around 50 days (**4**). Before the emergence of a new wave, a transient surge increase in FSH concentrations is required (**14, 22**). The FSH threshold needed to initiate the gonadotrophin-dependent growth is highly variable between individuals and even between follicles (**22, 26**). Follicles recruited during the surge grow while FSH concentrations decrease steadily (**7, 9, 14, 22**). Recent studies (**7**) have shown that the expression of FSH receptors during follicular development is constitutive and that this hormone is required to induce its own receptors in GCs. In addition, the surge in FSH induces the expression of P450scc and aromatase in GCs and P450c17 in TIC, which increases the production of oestradiol and inhibin within the follicle (**20, 21**).

As the follicle grows and GCs numbers increase, production of oestradiol and inhibin (B in humans and A in ruminants) rises, activating the negative feedback to the hypothalamus and pituitary, decreasing the release and circulatory concentrations of FSH (**7, 9, 11, 22, 27**). Studies in humans (**14**) and ruminants (**12, 28**) using GnRH agonists to suppress peripheral gonadotrophin concentrations have shown that early antral follicles do not grow further than 2–4mm in the absence of FSH. But when FSH is supplemented, follicles are able to reach 8–10mm in diameter, but further growth is arrested in the absence of LH (**28**). This indicates that follicles are recruited to grow under FSH influence, which is a self-limiting event, because as the follicle grows and produces higher concentrations of oestradiol and inhibin, FSH decreases, removing the support. Only those follicles (usually 1 or 2) developmentally more advanced continue to grow under LH influence (**7, 9**). This is consistent with the information regarding the switch of gonadotrophin dependence, from FSH to LH, during the selection phase.

11.2.5 Selection of the Dominant Follicle

Selection of the dominant follicle takes place during the early or mid-follicular phase of the cycle (**22**). When follicles reach ~8–10mm diameter, one or two of this group are selected to continue growing and become the dominant and subordinate follicle (**14, 21–24, 29**). It is at this stage of development that FSH reaches its lowest concentrations. This decrease in FSH suppresses the recruitment of a new antral follicular wave (**11, 30–33**). When FSH decreases, the growth of subordinate follicles gradually stops, and all undergo atresia (**29**). If the FSH concentrations decrease below basal levels, the development of the dominant follicle can also be impaired (**33**). It has been proposed that the future dominant follicle acquires several properties that enable its growth under low FSH conditions (**29, 33**). Therefore, the follicle that is functionally more developed continues growing due to a gradual change in its gonadotrophin-dependency from FSH to LH (**7, 21, 29, 34**).

The events described above correspond to follicular recruitment during the follicular phase in humans and other animals. Similar events occur during the mid-luteal or late-luteal waves of recruitment, but due to the negative gonadotrophin feedback of progesterone, follicular growth slows down as FSH concentrations decrease. In addition to progesterone, the human CL produces oestradiol and inhibin (A mainly), which further decreases FSH concentrations causing a low number of healthy follicles >4mm to be present (**22**). This may be the reason why follicular waves in humans are not as evident as in other animals, but it confirms that the physiological mechanisms driving early antral follicular development are conserved among different species.

11.2.6 Follicular Dominance

After selection, the dominant follicle continues growing for about 14 days to reach a preovulatory diameter of 16–29mm at a rate of 1–4mm/day (**25**). At the dominant stage, expression of mRNA encoding for gonadotrophin receptors, steroidogenic enzymes and StAR protein are enhanced, causing oestradiol concentrations to increase further (**21, 35**). The start of dominance is linked to the expression of mRNA for LH receptor and 3βHSD in GCs of the dominant follicle (**7, 33, 35, 36**). In fact, in ruminants, it was demonstrated that GCs of selected follicles expressed LH receptors while subordinate follicles did not (**37**). There is consensus on the need for LH for development to the preovulatory stage with an increase in the frequency of LH release as ovulation approaches. In sheep it was reported that threshold concentrations of LH were needed for pre-ovulatory follicle development (**7**), but overall concentration may be more important because continuous infusion of LH supported follicular growth. These data support the importance of LH for the growth of the dominant follicle and the change of dependency as part of the selection process (**7, 33**). The effects of both gonadotrophins on the selection of the dominant follicle are directly and indirectly linked to the changes in intra-ovarian factors (see below).

11.2.7 Intra-Ovarian Factors

Several local or paracrine factors have been implicated during antral-follicle development such as oestradiol, members of the TGF-β superfamily and insulin-like growth factor (IGF) system (**7, 33**). IGF system is comprised by IGFs (I and II), IGF receptor-1, IGF binding proteins (IGFBP) and the enzymes that control IGFBP concentration (**7, 21, 33, 38**). IGFs (IGFI and II) acting on the IGF receptor-1 in GCs estimulates proliferation, FSH sensitivity, steroidogenesis, inhibin/activin production and androgen production in TIC (**33, 39, 40**). The actions of IGFs are controlled by IGFBPs that bind them and control their bioavailability (**41**). Low concentrations of IGFBP-2, -4 (**42**) and -5 (**43**), coupled to an increased proteolytic activity (i.e., pregnancy associated plasma protein A) (**44**) and subsequent increase in free IGFs, have been implicated in the selection of the dominant follicle (**7, 29**). Furthermore, concentrations of these factors in the subordinate and non-selected follicles are higher (**33, 45, 46**). FSH and IGF act synergistically to stimulate proliferation, steroidogenesis and activin and inhibin production in granulosa cells (**29, 33**).

Several members of the TGF-β superfamily have been implicated during the selection of the dominant follicle and are considered partly responsible for the processes that lead to selection and ovulation (**8**). Local autocrine/paracrine effects of oocyte-derived factors, such as GDF-9, BMP-15 and BMP-6, and GC factors, such as BMP-6 and activin, have been reported to increase GC proliferation and modulate growth during FSH-dependent stage (**8**). In fact, activin appears to be the main factor involved in follicular recruitment because its absence (thorough increased follistatin or absence of its receptor (**47, 48**) arrested follicular development. In small follicles, the synthesis of activin is higher than inhibin, while in larger follicles, the opposite is observed (**8**). Because both factors (and follistatin) have opposite effects on cellular proliferation, gonadotrophin-receptor expression and steroidogenesis, it is evident that a balance between them must exist within the follicle to allow growth and development (**8**).

Anti-Mullerian hormone, a member of the TGF-β superfamily, is also involved in antral follicular development. As mentioned before, AMH is produced during preantral stages with a decrease as the antral follicle increases in size, inversely associated with steroidogenic activity in GCs and theca cells (**49**). Furthermore, it has been reported that AMH decreases GC meiotic activity (**27**). Other members of this superfamily, such as several BMPs and BMP binding proteins, have different roles during the selection and dominance phases of folliculogenesis (**8**). Apart from the numerous local factors and their interaction within the follicle, the local extra-follicular environment and blood supply are fundamental to sustaining and allowing follicular development.

Vascularisation of the follicle is observed during the late pre-antral follicular stage when two capillary networks interconnect at the level of the theca layer surrounding the follicle (**50**). This event has been implicated in the selection of the dominant follicle since an increase in the blood supply would increase the access of this follicle to gonadotrophins, growth factors, steroid precursors and other nutrients (**51, 52**). The most important factors involved in this process are the vascular endothelial growth factor (VEGF) and the basic fibroblast growth factor (bFGF) produced in the granulosa and theca cells, respectively (**51, 53**). During follicular development, concentrations of VEGF and bFGF increase in the follicular fluid as the diameter of the follicle increases (**53**). This could lead to an increment in the blood vessels and blood supply for the dominant follicle giving it an advantage over the subordinates (**36, 52**). However, more research needs to be done regarding vascular support during the selection of the dominant follicle in cattle.

11.3 Oogenesis

The process of oogenesis encompasses the differentiation of primordial germ cells into oogonia; these into primary oocytes arrested in meiosis I during the formation of primordial follicles; the reactivation of meiosis to originate the mature oocyte (oocyte arrested in metaphase II or secondary oocyte); and, after fertilisation, the formation of the zygote (Fig 1). As described in a previous chapter, primordial germ cells arrive at the genital ridges (precursor of the ovaries in females) around day 25–30 of pregnancy. At this time, primordial germ cells enter an intense period of replication by mitosis and become oogonia (Fig 1). Around days 60–90 of pregnancy, these cells enter meiosis, a process driven by retinoic acid, and the formation of primordial follicles initiates (Fig 1). When oogonia enter meiosis I, they complete chromatid exchange and crossover and are arrested at the diplotene stage of prophase I. At this stage, oogonia become primary oocytes. The primary oocytes contained within the primordial follicle can remain arrested in prophase I for several years, up to 40 years in humans, until the onset of ovulatory cycles during adolescence (i.e., LH preovulatory surge; Fig 1).

It is well established that although oocytes are in meiotic arrest during preantral follicle development (i.e., primary oocytes or germinal vesicle stage, GV), they are still highly active and able to control surrounding GC metabolic and endocrine function through the production of specific oocyte-derived growth factors, among which GDF9 and BMP15 seem to be central (**10**). In this way, the oocyte obtains energy metabolites and growth factors from GCs necessary for its growth during folliculogenesis (**54**). As the latter process progresses, the oocyte grows and undergoes a series of cytoplasmic and nuclear changes and reorganisation necessary to allow reactivation of meiosis (i.e., meiotic competence) and support early embryo development (i.e., developmental competence) (**55**). In fact, oocytes in mid-sized to pre-ovulatory follicles are still meiotically arrested but developmentally competent (**56**).

As mentioned in the previous section, a direct connection between the oocyte and the surrounding cumulus cells (CC) is paramount for adequate oocyte development (**54**). These connections are known as transzonal projections (**54**) and are important to preserve the oocyte in the arrested state in prophase I (GV). It has been reported that these connections are dependent on cyclic nucleotides, such as cyclic adenosine monophosphate (cAMP), which in turn are modulated by FSH concentrations (**57**). Moreover, cAMP in the oocyte can control factors involved in transcription and chromatin remodelling processes observed in full-size oocytes about to undergo reactivation of meiosis (**56**). Therefore, moderate to high concentrations of cAMP in the oocyte are necessary to keep the meiotic arrest (**56**).

Although the oocyte can synthesise cAMP, most cAMP is produced in the surrounding CCs and transported into the oocyte (**54, 56**). Intra-oocyte high levels of cAMP activate the protein-kinase A enzyme which is necessary to prevent the activation of a maturation-promoting factor preventing meiotic reactivation (**56**). Additionally, cyclic guanosine monophosphate (cGMP) has been implicated in maintaining high levels of cAMP in the oocyte. cGMP produced in the surrounding CCs in response to natriuretic peptide C (NPC) from GCs, inhibits the actions of phosphodiesterase enzyme (PDE) 3A (oocyte-specific PDE), a potent cAMP hydrolysing enzyme, therefore maintaining a high cAMP environment (**56**). Therefore, it is clear that the follicular somatic cells provide the signals and factors necessary to prevent premature meiotic activation, this is preventing GV breakdown via the transzonal communication established early during folliculogenesis (**54, 56**).

Once the follicle reaches a preovulatory size and oestradiol concentrations are maximal, the LH preovulatory surge occurs, which is the signal to remove the brake on oocyte meiosis. The LH surge signalling through its receptors in GCs induces an increase in the cAMP in follicular fluid and a decrease in NPC production which reduces cGMP synthesis, releasing the blockage on PDE3A enzyme (**54, 56**). Moreover, the LH surge also causes a degradation of the gap junctions between the CCs and the oocyte, decreasing the communication between these cells (**54**). This loss of communication and activation of the PDE3A cause a rapid decrease in intra-oocyte cAMP, resulting in activation of the meiotic-promoting factor (**56**). This decrease in cAMP also causes a breakdown of the nuclear envelope and chromosome condensation completing meiotic activation (i.e., known as GV breakdown, GVBD). Once activation occurs, the oocyte completes meiosis I resulting in the expulsion of the first polar body (**58**). Simultaneously, the LH surge causes changes in the follicular wall, which result in the formation of the stigma that will become the ovulatory side.

The oocyte enters meiosis II and proceeds until metaphase II (i.e., secondary oocyte), at which point the oocyte is arrested again. At this stage, the follicle is known as a mature oocyte or MII oocyte (**58**). Most mammalian species ovulate an MII oocyte which is still surrounded by the CCs that undergo expansion at this stage. During this stage, the oocyte undergoes cytoplasmic maturation involving translational, post-translational and organellar reorganisation events important for the completion of meiosis, prevention of polyspermy and required to support early embryo development (**54**). At this point, the oocyte is developmentally competent and is awaiting the final signal that will allow the completion of meiosis II, which is fertilisation (**54**). When fertilisation occurs (sperm-oocyte fusion), a spike in intracellular calcium triggers the reactivation of meiosis, resulting in the release of the second polar body and the formation of the zygote (**58**). These latter stages are not within the scope of this chapter and will be discussed in other sections.

11.4 Conclusions

It is evident that folliculogenesis and oogenesis are parallel and interlinked processes that start during fetal development, with some follicles and oocytes able to reach full maturity and development at ovulation, an event that can only take place after puberty. Because of this close link, oocytes and follicular somatic cells are in constant communication, and it is reported that the oocyte can control somatic cell proliferation, metabolism and differentiation. This control confers the oocyte nutrients and factors necessary for its growth and development to reach meiotic and developmental competence. Therefore, both processes' final aim is to develop a competent oocyte that can be fertilised and support early embryo development. Although advances in the understanding of both processes have been seen in recent years, there are still aspects of oocyte maturation that require more research to improve assisted reproduction protocols.

REFERENCES

1. Hummitzsch K, Hatzirodos N, Irving-Rodgers HF, et al. Morphometric analyses and gene expression related to germ cells, gonadal ridge epithelial-like cells and granulosa cells during development of the bovine fetal ovary. *PLoS One*. 2019;14(3):e0214130.
2. Ford EA, Beckett EL, Roman SD, et al. Advances in human primordial follicle activation and premature ovarian insufficiency. *Reproduction*. 2020 Jan;159(1):R15–R29.
3. Horan CJ, Williams SA. Oocyte stem cells: fact or fantasy? *Reproduction*. 2017 Jul;154(1):R23–R35.
4. Conti M, Chang RJ. Folliculogenesis, ovulation, and luteogenesis. In: Jameson JL, editor. *Endocrinology: Adult and Pediatric*. 7th Edition. Philadelphia, PA: Elsevier Saunders; 2016. 2 p.
5. Cordeiro MH, Kim SY, Woodruff TK. Chapter 1 – ovarian follicle biology and the basis for gonadotoxicity. In: Anderson RA, Spears N, editors. *Cancer Treatment and the Ovary [Internet]*. Boston: Academic Press; 2015. pp. 3–20.
6. Andersen CY, Childs AJ, Anderson RA. 150 – differentiation of the ovary. In: Polin RA, Abman SH, Rowitch DH, Benitz WE, Fox WW, editors. *Fetal and Neonatal Physiology*. 5th Edition. Amsterdam, The Netherlands: Elsevier; 2017. pp. 1520–1528. e2.

7. Webb R, Campbell BK. Development of the dominant follicle: mechanisms of selection and maintenance of oocyte quality. *Soc Reprod Fertil Suppl.* 2007;64:141–163.
8. Knight PG, Glister C. TGF-beta superfamily members and ovarian follicle development. *Reproduction.* 2006;132(2):191–206.
9. Hernandez-Medrano JH, Campbell BK, Webb R. Nutritional influences on folliculogenesis. *Reprod Domest Anim.* 2012 Aug;47(Suppl. 4):274–282.
10. Webb R, Buratini J, Hernandez-Medrano JHH, et al. Follicle development and selection: past, present and future. *Anim Reprod.* 2016;13(3):234–249.
11. Campbell BK, Souza C, Gong J, et al. Domestic ruminants as models for the elucidation of the mechanisms controlling ovarian follicle development in humans. *Reprod Suppl.* 2003;61:429–443.
12. Scaramuzzi RJ, Baird DT, Campbell BK, et al. Regulation of folliculogenesis and the determination of ovulation rate in ruminants. *Reprod Fertil Dev.* 2011;23(3):444.
13. Zhang H, Risal S, Gorre N, et al. Somatic cells initiate primordial follicle activation and govern the development of dormant oocytes in mice. *Curr Biol.* 2014 Nov 3;24(21):2501–2508.
14. Gougeon A. Human ovarian follicular development: from activation of resting follicles to preovulatory maturation. *Ann Endocrinol Paris.* 2010 May;71(3):132–143.
15. Skinner MK. Regulation of primordial follicle assembly and development. *Hum Reprod Update.* 2005;11(5):461–471.
16. McNatty KP, Reader K, Smith P, et al. Control of ovarian follicular development to the gonadotrophin-dependent phase: a 2006 perspective. *Soc Reprod Fertil Suppl.* 2007;64:55–68.
17. Fortune JE. The early stages of follicular development: activation of primordial follicles and growth of preantral follicles. *Anim Reprod Sci.* 2003 Oct 15;78(3–4):135–163.
18. Logan KA, Juengel JL, McNatty KP. Onset of steroidogenic enzyme gene expression during ovarian follicular development in sheep. *Biol Reprod.* 2002 Apr;66(4):906–916.
19. Erickson GF, Shimasaki S. The physiology of folliculogenesis: the role of novel growth factors. *Fertil Steril.* 2001 Nov;76(5):943–949.
20. Bao B, Garverick HA. Expression of steroidogenic enzyme and gonadotropin receptor genes in bovine follicles during ovarian follicular waves: a review. *J Anim Sci.* 1998 Jul;76(7):1903–1921.
21. Webb R, Campbell BK, Garverick HA, et al. Molecular mechanisms regulating follicular recruitment and selection. *J Reprod Fertil Suppl.* 1999;54:33–48.
22. Baerwald AR, Adams GP, Pierson RA. Ovarian antral folliculogenesis during the human menstrual cycle: a review. *Hum Reprod Update.* 2012 Jan;18(1):73–91.
23. Ginther OJ, Beg MA, Donadeu FX, et al. Mechanism of follicle deviation in monovular farm species. *Anim Reprod Sci.* 2003;78(3–4):239–257.
24. Adams GP, Jaiswal R, Singh J, et al. Progress in understanding ovarian follicular dynamics in cattle. *Theriogenology.* 2008 Jan;69(1):72–80.
25. Baerwald AR, Adams GP, Pierson RA. A new model for ovarian follicular development during the human menstrual cycle. *Fertil Steril.* 2003 Jul;80(1):116–122.
26. Fauser BC, Van Heusden AM. Manipulation of human ovarian function: physiological concepts and clinical consequences. *Endocr Rev.* 1997 Feb;18(1):71–106.
27. Hsueh AJW, Kawamura K, Cheng Y, et al. Intraovarian control of early folliculogenesis. *Endocr Rev.* 2015 Feb;36(1):1–24.
28. Garverick HA, Baxter G, Gong J, et al. Regulation of expression of ovarian mRNA encoding steroidogenic enzymes and gonadotrophin receptors by FSH and GH in hypogonadotrophic cattle. *Reproduction.* 2002;123(5):651–661.
29. Mihm M, Evans AC. Mechanisms for dominant follicle selection in monovulatory species: a comparison of morphological, endocrine and intraovarian events in cows, mares and women. *Reprod Domest Anim.* 2008;43(Suppl. 2):48–56.
30. Campbell BK, Scaramuzzi RJ, Webb R. Control of antral follicle development and selection in sheep and cattle. *J Reprod Fertil Suppl.* 1995;49:335–350.
31. Gibbons JR, Wiltbank MC, Ginther OJ. Functional interrelationships between follicles greater than 4 mm and the follicle-stimulating hormone surge in heifers. *Biol Reprod.* 1997;57(5):1066–1073.
32. Bleach EC, Glencross RG, Feist SA, et al. Plasma inhibin A in heifers: relationship with follicle dynamics, gonadotropins, and steroids during the estrous cycle and after treatment with bovine follicular fluid. *Biol Reprod.* 2001;64(3):743–752.
33. Webb R, Nicholas B, Gong JG, et al. Mechanisms regulating follicular development and selection of the dominant follicle. *Reprod Suppl.* 2003;61:71–90.
34. Campbell BK, Engelhardt H, McNeilly AS, et al. Direct effects of ovine follicular fluid on ovarian steroid secretion and expression of markers of cellular differentiation in sheep. *J Reprod Fertil.* 1999;117(2):259–269.
35. Bao B, Garverick HA. Expression of steroidogenic enzyme and gonadotropin receptor genes in bovine follicles during ovarian follicular waves: a review. *J Anim Sci.* 1998;76(7):1903–1921.
36. Beg MA, Ginther OJ. Follicle selection in cattle and horses: role of intrafollicular factors. *Reproduction.* 2006;132(3):365–377.
37. Beg MA, Bergfelt DR, Kot K, et al. Follicular-fluid factors and granulosa-cell gene expression associated with follicle deviation in cattle. *Biol Reprod.* 2001;64(2):432–441.
38. Spicer LJ. Proteolytic degradation of insulin-like growth factor binding proteins by ovarian follicles: a control mechanism for selection of dominant follicles. *Biol Reprod.* 2004;70(5):1223–1230.
39. Spicer LJ, Echternkamp SE. The ovarian insulin and insulin-like growth factor system with an emphasis on domestic animals. *Domest Anim Endocrinol.* 1995;12(3):223–245.
40. Glister C, Tannetta DS, Groome NP, et al. Interactions between follicle-stimulating hormone and growth factors in modulating secretion of steroids and inhibin-related peptides by nonluteinized bovine granulosa cells. *Biol Reprod.* 2001;65(4):1020–1028.
41. Armstrong DG, Webb R. Ovarian follicular dominance: the role of intraovarian growth factors and novel proteins. *Rev Reprod.* 1997;2(3):139–146.
42. Nicholas B, Scougall RK, Armstrong DG, et al. Changes in insulin-like growth factor binding protein (IGFBP) isoforms during bovine follicular development. *Reproduction.* 2002;124(3):439–446.

43. Fortune JE. Selection and maintenance of the dominant follicle: an introduction. *Biol Reprod.* 2001;65(3):637.
44. Monget P, Fabre S, Mulsant P, et al. Regulation of ovarian folliculogenesis by IGF and BMP system in domestic animals. *Domest Anim Endocrinol.* 2002 Jul;23(1–2):139–154.
45. Armstrong DG, Baxter G, Hogg CO, et al. Insulin-like growth factor binding protein -2 and -4 messenger ribonucleic acid expression in bovine ovarian follicles: effect of gonadotropins and developmental status. *Endocrinology.* 1998;139(4):2146–2154.
46. Austin EJ, Mihm M, Evans AC, et al. Alterations in intrafollicular regulatory factors and apoptosis during selection of follicles in the first follicular wave of the bovine estrous cycle. *Biol Reprod.* 2001;64(3):839–848.
47. Guo Q, Kumar TR, Woodruff T, et al. Overexpression of mouse follistatin causes reproductive defects in transgenic mice. *Mol Endocrinol.* 1998;12(1):96–106.
48. Nishimori K, Matzuk MM. Transgenic mice in the analysis of reproductive development and function. *Rev Reprod.* 1996;1(3):203–212.
49. Campbell BK, Clinton M, Webb R. The role of anti-Müllerian hormone (AMH) during follicle development in a monovulatory species (sheep). *Endocrinology.* 2012 Sep;153(9):4533–4543.
50. Findlay JK. Angiogenesis in reproductive tissues. *J Endocrinol.* 1986;111(3):357–366.
51. Robinson RS, Woad KJ, Hammond AJ, et al. Angiogenesis and vascular function in the ovary. *Reproduction.* 2009 Dec;138(6):869–881.
52. Hunter MG, Robinson RS, Mann GE, et al. Endocrine and paracrine control of follicular development and ovulation rate in farm species. *Anim Reprod Sci.* 2004;82–83:461–477.
53. Berisha B, Schams D, Kosmann M, et al. Expression and localisation of vascular endothelial growth factor and basic fibroblast growth factor during the final growth of bovine ovarian follicles. *J Endocrinol.* 2000;167(3):371–382.
54. Li R, Albertini DF. The road to maturation: somatic cell interaction and self-organization of the mammalian oocyte. *Nat Rev Mol Cell Biol.* 2013 Mar;14(3):141–152.
55. Gilchrist RB, Thompson JG. Oocyte maturation: emerging concepts and technologies to improve developmental potential in vitro. *Theriogenology.* 2007 Jan;67(1):6–15.
56. Gilchrist RB, Luciano AM, Richani D, et al. Oocyte maturation and quality: role of cyclic nucleotides. *Reproduction.* 2016 Nov;152(5):R143–R157.
57. El-Hayek S, Clarke HJ. Follicle-stimulating hormone increases gap junctional communication between somatic and germ-line follicular compartments during murine oogenesis. *Biol Reprod.* 2015 Aug;93(2):47.
58. Pangas SA, Rajkovic A. Chapter 21 – follicular development: mouse, sheep, and human models. In: Plant TM, Zeleznik A, Knobil E, editors. *Knobil and Neill's Physiology of Reproduction.* 4th Edition. London: Academic Press; 2015.

12

Spermatogenesis, Spermiation and the Human Sperm

Vipul Batra, Nader Eid, Hannah L. Morgan and Adam J. Watkins

12.1 Introduction

The role of the spermatozoon is to deliver the male genome into the oocyte at the point of fertilisation. The mammalian spermatozoon has evolved into a specialised structure which, in humans, takes approximately 72 days to make. Spermatogenesis is a highly coordinated process that occurs within the testes and results in the differentiation of diploid spermatogonial stem cells into haploid spermatozoa which are capable of traversing the female reproductive tract. In a healthy man, millions of sperm are produced every single day. In this chapter, we will provide an overview of spermatogenesis and the structure and function of the mature sperm.

12.2 Physiology of the Testis and Seminiferous Tubule

In men, the testes are approximately 4–5 cm in length and 2.5–4 cm in width (**1**). Unlike the ovaries in women, the testes reside in the scrotum, outside of the main abdominopelvic cavity, covered with a strong connective tissue capsule, the tunica albuginca (**1**). This exterior location, in addition to several physiological adaptations such as highly folded scrotal skin, a venous counter current exchange system in the spermatogenic cord and a high number of scrotal sweat glands, results in a testicular temperature of approximately 35°C. Each testicle is divided into approximately 350 lobules and within each lobule are the highly folded seminiferous tubules. In men, the seminiferous tubules make up approximately 60–70% of the testis volume. Each tubule is approximately 200 µm in diameter and is surrounded by a layer of peritubular myoid cells and connective extracellular matrix (see Figure 12.1). The peritubular myoid cells maintain the structural integrity of the tubules and are capable of tubular contractility and sperm transport (**2**). The intratubular compartment comprises the seminiferous epithelium and is the site of spermatogenesis. Outside of the tubules lies the peritubular compartment comprising vascular, connective and immune cells as well as the endocrine Leydig cells. Each tubule connects to the rete testis, which facilitates the transport of sperm from the testis and into the head (caput) of the epididymis. From here, the sperm are transported into the body (corpus) and tail (cauda) of the epididymis where the sperm are stored and mature further.

12.3 Spermatogenesis and Spermiogenesis

Within each tubule lies the seminiferous epithelium which is comprised of two cell types; (i) sperm cells at different stages of spermatogenesis and; (ii) Sertoli cells which are the nurse cells of the tubule and are central in regulating spermatogenesis (see Figure 12.1). Spermatogonial stem cells lie at the basal levels of the seminiferous tubule. Like other stem cells, spermatogonial stem cells divide mitotically enabling them to both maintain the stem cell population (Type A spermatogonia) and produce a large number of daughter (Type B spermatogonia) cells, thus amplify the population. Type B spermatogonia are ultimately committed to meiosis and so will give rise to primary spermatocytes, secondary spermatocytes and spermatids. During their meiotic division, Type B spermatogonia remain connected by intracellular, cytoplasmic bridges. These connections are essential in allowing each germ cell to exchange material and to remain synchronised, resulting in a clonal population of sperm cells (**3**).

As they start to undergo meiosis, the spermatogonia migrate away from the basal compartment and move towards the luminal region. During the first meiotic prophase, a hallmark event in the production of genetically distinct sperm occurs through the processes of synapsis, crossing-over, chiasmata formation and cellular disjunction (**4**). During anaphase of meiosis, each chromosome is comprised of two chromatids which migrate to opposite poles. In telophase, cell division occurs forming two secondary spermatocytes, each containing half the number of chromosomes of the parent cell. Prophase of the second meiotic division is very rapid (approximately just 20 minutes), reducing the cellular DNA content by half. The two chromatids of each chromosome migrate to opposite poles but the two spermatids do not separate completely, retaining some fine intercellular connections. Following the second meiotic division, the round spermatids undergo a dramatic cellular re-organisation under a process known as spermiogenesis. Under this phase, many of the organelles within the spermatid are degraded or remodelled (**5**) to enable the sperm to have the correct structure and morphology. The DNA of the sperm is remodelled through the substitution of histones with protamines (**6**) enabling the sperm head to become highly compact. Other changes include the remodelling of the Golgi apparatus into the sperm acrosomal cap (**7**) and the creation of the perinuclear theca from the cytosol (**8**). Additionally, microtubules of one of the spermatid's centrioles elongates to become the tail. At this point, the spermatids are orientated in such a manner that their tails are directed towards the lumen of the tubule.

DOI: 10.1201/9781003269502-12

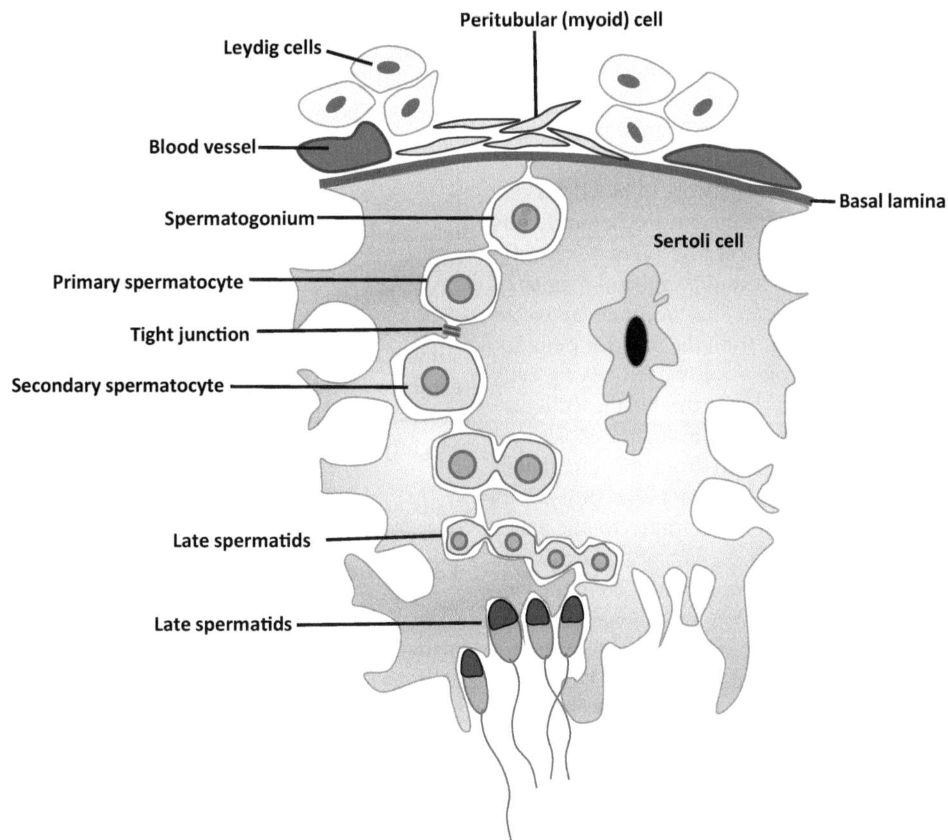

FIGURE 12.1 Seminiferous epithelium. Spermatogonial stem cells undergo mitosis enabling the stem cell pool to be maintained as well as a pool of daughter cells which differentiate into primary spermatocytes. These primary spermatocytes undergo a first round of meiosis to become secondary spermatocytes followed by a rapid second meiotic division to become haploid spermatids. Through the process of spermiogenesis, spermatids mature into mature spermatozoa. A series of inter-Sertoli cell tight junctions form the blood-testis barrier which regulates the movement of molecules from outside of the seminiferous tubule and separates the spermatogonia from the primary spermatocytes. Outside of the seminiferous tubules lie a dense network of blood vessels, peritubular cells and the Leydig cells, whose main role is in the production of testosterone.

The final phase of spermiogenesis involves the phagocytosing of the remaining cytoplasm by the Sertoli cells. In order to protect the paternal genome as the sperm transits through the male and female reproductive tracts, the mammalian sperm head and DNA undergo dramatic cellular and nuclear changes. Under this process, the round spermatids become polarised, with an elongated head at one end and the flagellum at the other. Additionally, the mitochondria become accumulated within the midpiece of the developing spermatozoa while the centriole pair begin to elongate to form the flagellum of the tail.

Post meiotically, the sperm genome becomes transcriptionally quiescent due to increased condensation of the chromatin. The nucleosome-bound DNA becomes destabilised through hyperacetylation of the histones. The histones are then replaced largely, but not completely by two protamines, protamine 1 (P1) and protamine 2 (P2), which are expressed in a roughly equal ratio (**9**). Changes in the P1/2 ratio have been associated with reduced sperm DNA compaction, increased DNA fragmentation and reduction in male fertility (**10**). Finally, the tight associations between the spermatozoa and the Sertoli cell are lost and the sperm are released into the lumen of the tubule. From here, the sperm are transported to the rete testis where they continue their journey and maturation through the male reproductive system.

In men, the process of spermatogenesis takes approximately 72 days, with cohorts of spermatogonial stem cells entering into the cycle every 16 days. This results in a staggered process of spermatogenesis that takes place along the whole length of the seminiferous tubule. This prevents the whole testis starting, and completing, the spermatogenic cycle at the same time while ensuring there is a constant production of sperm from multiple sites within the testis. Histological analysis of the testis in men, and other mammalian species, have revealed distinct stages and morphological characterises of the spermatogenic cycle. The stages of the cycle can be differentiated by the stages of meiosis under way, the location of the spermatids within the seminiferous epithelium and the nature and extent of the cellular nuclear and modifications of the spermatids. In men, there are 6 stages with each stage lasting approximately 16 days. The process of spermatogenesis is regulated by an intricate endocrine loop (**11**). The hypothalamus secretes gonadotrophin releasing hormones (GnRH) which act on the pituitary gland. GnRH stimulates the production of follicle stimulating hormone (FSH) which, in men, primarily acts on the Sertoli cells. The pituitary also secretes luteinising hormone (LH) which acts on the Leydig cells to promote the production and secretion of testosterone.

12.4 The Leydig Cell

The Leydig cells reside within the peritubular compartment of the testis and so are also known as the interstitial cells (see Figure 12.1). This region of the testis is composed of loose connective tissue and a highly dense network of blood vessels. These vessels not only provide nutrients to the seminiferous tubules, and so to the Sertoli cells, but also allow for Leydig cell-derived testosterone to be carried to peripheral regions of the body. It is this part of the testes that becomes activated in response to luteinising hormone from the anterior pituitary at puberty. Once activated, the main role of the Leydig cells is the production of testosterone. Here, the Leydig cells use cholesterol, either synthesised *de novo* through a cholesterol hormone-sensitive lipase, or taken up from the circulation through the low-, and high-density-lipoprotein receptors. This cholesterol is then transported from the outer to the inner mitochondrial membrane in a steroidogenic acute regulatory protein (StAR) controlled manner. Once within the mitochondria, free cholesterol is converted to pregnenolone (P5) and then progesterone (P4). Following this, 3β-hydroxysteroid dehydrogenase type 2 (3β-HSD2) and cytochrome P450 family 17 subfamily A member 1 (CYP17A1) convert progesterone to 17α-hydroxyprogesterone and androstenedione respectively. Finally, a Leydig cell-specific isoform of 17β-hydroxysteroid dehydrogenase (17β-HSD13) converts androstenedione to testosterone. As the Leydig cells are in such close proximity to the seminiferous tubules, much of the testosterone they produce is transported into the adluminal compartment of the tubules and maintained there at levels much higher than in the general circulation (**12**).

12.5 The Sertoli Cell

Within the seminiferous tubule, the Sertoli cell extends from the basal lamina to the lumen and represents the epithelial component of the tubule. During perinatal and neonatal life, the Sertoli cells undergo periods of proliferation, prior to undergoing a second round prior to puberty (**13**). Regulation of Sertoli cell proliferation and function is enacted through a range of factors including FSH and androgens, TGF-beta, BMPs, activins, oestrogens and TNF- alpha (**14**). The primary roles of the Sertoli cells are to support the developing sperm, regulate the hormonal environment within the seminiferous tubule and contribute to the formation of the blood-testis barrier (BTB). At any one time, each Sertoli cells is in contact with approximately 30–50 spermatogonial stem cells which can be at distinctly different stages of progression through the spermatogenic cycle (**15**). The Sertoli cells surround the developing sperm cells, giving structural support and guiding the sperm towards the tubule lumen as they progress through spermatogenesis. In the basal compartment of the seminiferous tubule, the Sertoli cell are critical in regulating the self-renewal of the spermatogonial stem cells (**16**). As the sperm develop, the Sertoli cells regulate the process of meiotic cell division while in the adluminal regions, the Sertoli cells are responsible for remodelling the spermatids, resorbing any residual cytoplasm and regulating the process of spermiation (**17**).

The Sertoli cells have multiple additional roles such as converting Leydig derived testosterone to the potent estrogen, estradiol 17-β which may have a role in enhancing spermatogenesis. The Sertoli cells are also important for the production of androgen-binding protein (ABP). ABP is critical in the maintenance of higher levels of testosterone within the tubule than outside. Sertoli cells also secrete a large volume of fluid into the lumen of the tubule. This is necessary for transporting the sperm towards the rete testes and epididymis as the spermatozoa at this time are immotile. Finally, the Sertoli cell secretes a range of endocrine factors such as inhibin. FSH stimulates the production of inhibin, which then has a negative feedback on the secretion of the pituitary to reduce the production of inhibin, so keeping inhibin and spermatogenesis within a tightly regulated range (**18**).

12.6 The Blood-Testis Barrier (BTB)

Critical to ensuring the tight spatiotemporal regulation of spermatogenesis is the association between the spermatogonial cells and the Sertoli cells (**19**). As indicated already, the Sertoli cells are in close contact with the spermatogonial stem cells, the maturing spermatids and the final spermatozoa. While the Sertoli cells interact with the developing sperm cells, they are also in direct contact with other Sertoli cells within the tubule to form the blood-testis barrier (BTB). The BTB is formed almost exclusively from inter-Sertoli cell interactions and connections. The BTB exists at the apposing membranes of two Sertoli cells, which forms the barrier between the basal and adluminal compartments of the tubule (**20**). Spermatogonia and pre- leptotene primary spermatocytes reside on the basal compartment while later-stage primary spermatocytes, spermatids and spermatozoa reside on the adluminal side. The BTB is formed from an array of different cell junctions along with a diversity of structural and polarity conferring, scaffolding, signalling and adaptor proteins, creating a tubular environment favourable to germ cell development (**21**). The presence of a range of tight junctions, desmosomes, gap junctions and testis-specific adherens junctions results in one of the tightest tissue barriers in the mammalian body and which creates an immunologically safe microenvironment for the developing sperm. However, as early primary spermatocytes develop and move towards the adluminal compartment, the inter-Sertoli cell tight junctions are disassembled and re-assembled (**22**). Recently, it has been shown that a structurally and functionally intact BTB is essential for germ cell development-associated differentiation events during mammalian spermatogenesis (**23, 24**). In rats, this axis is responsible for the coordinated release of last stage spermatids aligned at the luminal edge while the basal elongating spermatids and BTB undergo remodelling. Furthermore, a range of active biomolecules such as cytokines including TGF β-2 and β-3, TNFα, IL-1α, under hormonal regulation, contribute to conferring and maintaining the dynamic nature of the BTB.

The BTB also regulates the paracellular flow of vital and toxic molecules such as amino acids, sugars, androgens, drugs, and chemicals into the adluminal compartment thus creating a milieu conducive to post-meiotic germ cell development.

Additionally, the mediation of transcellular flow results in the compartmentalization of the seminiferous epithelium (**23, 25**). This morphological segregation allows the required access to vital bioactive molecules for renewal, proliferation and differentiation of the early-stage germ cells in the basal compartment. Both of these functions are indispensable for shielding the transiently expressed auto – antigens residing on the germ cells undergoing meiosis and developing spermatids in the adluminal compartment (**26, 27**). As such, the BTB creates an immunological barrier that in concert with local (testicular) immunoregulatory mechanisms (e.g. immunosuppression by Sertoli cell-secreted cytokines) operates not only to confer immune privilege to the testis but also to prevent testis-specific auto-immune diseases (**28, 29**).

It is noteworthy that the regulation of the transcellular flow of molecules by the BTB leads to the asymmetric distribution of biomolecules and cytoskeletal components and/or arrangement at the basal and adluminal compartments. Within the seminiferous epithelium there are distinct adherent junctions between adjacent Sertoli cells including heterotypic-basolateral junctions, homotypic and heterotypic-apical junctions (**25**), resulting in one of the tightest barriers in the body. The main constituents of the BTB are tight junctions and divide the seminiferous epithelium into the basal (containing the spermatogonial stem cells and spermatocytes) and the adluminal (containing elongating spermatocytes and spermatids) regions. Additionally, gap junctions, desmosomes, and other proteins such as occludins and cadherins, form the remaining components of the BTB.

12.7 The Structure of the Mature Sperm

As indicated previously, the mature spermatozoa are highly differentiated cells that consists of a head, midpiece and tail regions that are all contained within a single plasma membrane (see Figure 12.2a). The 'typical' human sperm has an oval head which is covered by a clearly defined acrosome. The tail connects to the midpiece and is symmetrical in shape and devoid of any cytoplasmic droplets or residue. The sperm head is approximately 4–5 µm in length and 2–3 µm in width (**30**). The midpiece is typically longer than the sperm head and approximately 1 µm wide while the tail is approximately 45–50 µm in length.

The head contains the highly condensed DNA which is largely inactive in its levels of transcription and DNA repair. This makes the DNA within the sperm more prone to damage in response to adverse environmental conditions. The sperm head is also covered with the acrosome, derived from the spermatid's Golgi apparatus. The acrosome lies underneath the plasma membrane and covers 40–70% of the anterior region of the sperm head. The acrosome contains a mix of hydrolytic enzymes and receptors that are required for the sperm's penetration and interaction with the oocyte's zona pellucida (**31**). When the sperm comes into contact with the zona pellucida proteins (ZP3 and ZP4 in humans and ZP3 mice) it undergoes the acrosome reaction. The plasma membrane of the sperm fuses with the membrane surrounding the acrosome allowing the contents of the acrosome to be exposed. Within the acrosome are numerous sperm antigens which are essential for

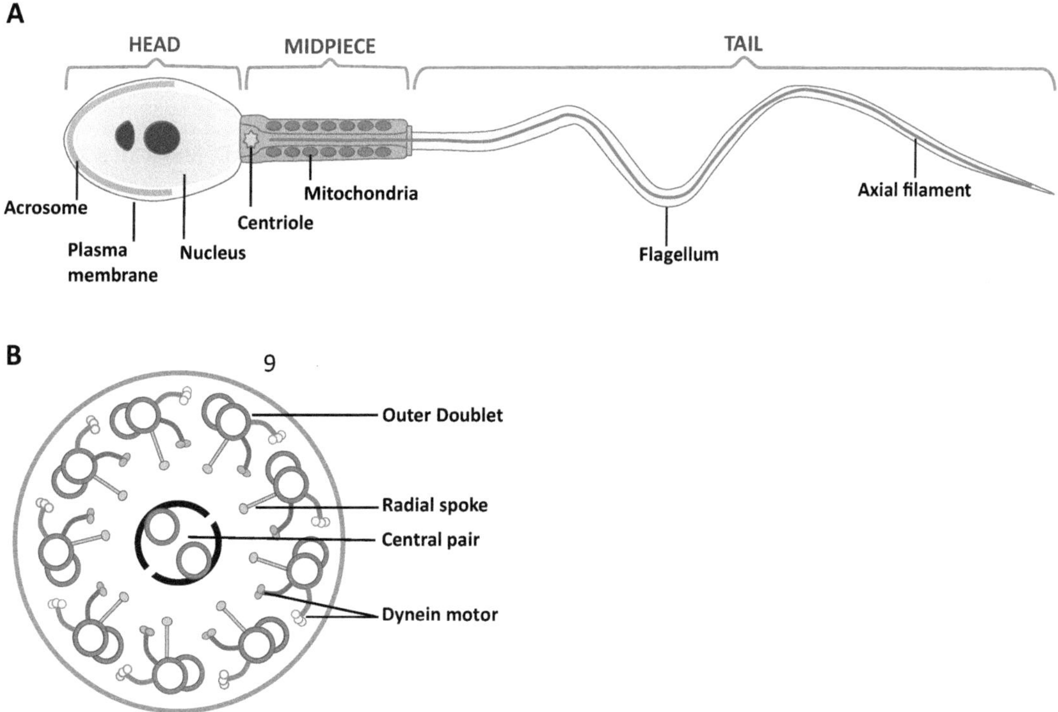

FIGURE 12.2 Structure of the mature spermatozoa. (a) The mature spermatozoon is comprised of three main sections termed the head, midpiece and the tail. The head contains the densely packaged DNA as well as the acrosome. Within the midpiece are the mitochondria and the centriole while the tail comprises the central microtubule axoneme. (b) Cross section through the sperm tail showing typical 9 + 2 microtubule structure common to flagella and which is responsible for sperm motility.

binding to the zona as well as enzymes such as hyaluronidase and acrosin, which are essential for the sperm to penetrate their way through the zona and into the oocyte. Sperm which do not initiate the acrosome reaction are not able to penetrate the zona. While the majority of the acrosome undergoes the acrosome reaction, an equatorial region remains intact, as it is this region of the sperm that initiates fusion with the oocyte at fertilisation. Some studies also suggest that region of the sperm head which lies below the acrosome, the post-acrosomal sheath, contains a sperm-derived activating factor which triggers calcium oscillations within the oocyte and pronuclear formation (**32**). Other studies, in both humans and mice, have also indicated a role for phospholipase C zeta (PLCζ) in activating the oocyte and triggering calcium oscillations (**33**). In human sperm, PLCζ has been identified in the equatorial and post-acrosomal sheath regions, while in mice, PLCζ is required to prevent fertilisation by multiple sperm (**34**).

Connecting the head and the tail of the sperm is the midpiece, containing mitochondria and axial filaments of the flagellum. In a typical human sperm, there are approximately 50–70 mitochondria which are arranged helically around the central axoneme. These mitochondria provide ATP to the axoneme which is used to drive the mechanical movement of the flagellum. Changes in the amounts of mitochondria, or copies of their DNA (mtDNA) have been associated with impairments in male fertility (**35**). The sperm tail comprises the typical 9 + 2 microtubule structure of flagella and cilia (see Figure 12.2b). Here, there are nine symmetrically arranged doublets around the outer section and which are connected to the two central doublets. This structure is regulated by a series of additional dynein motor proteins and microtubule-associated proteins which are believed to help control the motion of the flagella and so regulate the direction of the swimming sperm. The coordinated asynchronous movement of the dynein arms allows for the flagella movement and the beating of the tail. Outside of the outer doublets are a series of nine dense fibres which give the flagella additional flexibility and support during movement.

12.8 Post-Ejaculation Changes

At ejaculation, sperm are transported from the epididymis, through the vas deferens and to the urethra. While being transported through the male reproductive tract, secretions from the seminal vesicles and the prostate are added to the sperm and this constitutes the semen (sperm and seminal plasma). The role of the seminal plasma is to support and nourish the sperm while in the female reproductive tract (**36**). For example, the seminal fluid is alkaline in nature which helps to neutralise the acidic pH of the vagina. However, additional roles for the seminal plasma in mediating and directing maternal post-copulation reproductive tract responses which may influence subsequent embryonic development have recently been identified (**37**).

As the sperm progress through the female reproductive tract, they also undergo the additional processes of capacitation and hyperactivation. Both of these processes are essential to enable the sperm to fertilise the oocyte. During capacitation, the sperm undergo several changes including cholesterol efflux, lipid remodelling in the sperm head and an increase permeability to calcium ions (**38**). The increase in calcium results in an elevation in cAMP which aids the increased movement seen during hyperactivation. Under hyperactivation, sperm become more motile with more rapid beating of the flagella. Sperm become hyperactivated as they approach the oocyte. Within the sperm, the selective calcium ion channel located within the tail allow for a rapid rise in intracellular calcium which induces deeper bends within the sperm tail (**39**).

12.9 Conclusions

Spermatogenesis is a highly coordinated process resulting in a highly specialised cell, the mature spermatozoa. The intricate process of spermatogenesis can become disrupted by a range of environmental and lifestyle factors such as smoking, excessive alcohol intake or obesity. All of these can impact on the quality of the sperm produced and therefore male fertility. Studies are now also identifying long-term associations between paternal well-being at the time of conception and the development and long-term health of his offspring (**40**). Therefore, understanding the fundamental process of spermatogenesis and what constitutes a 'good quality' sperm is of utmost importance for ensuring male fertility and the health of his offspring.

12.9.1 Funding

This work was supported by Biotechnology and Biological Sciences Research Council (BBSRC) grant (BB/V006711/1) awarded to AJW.

REFERENCES

1. Middendorff R, Muller D, Mewe M, et al. The tunica albuginea of the human testis is characterized by complex contraction and relaxation activities regulated by cyclic GMP. *J Clin Endocrinol Metab.* 2002;87(7):3486–3499.
2. Potter SJ, DeFalco T. Role of the testis interstitial compartment in spermatogonial stem cell function. *Reproduction.* 2017;153(4):R151–R162.
3. Dym M, Fawcett DW. Further observations on the numbers of spermatogonia, spermatocytes, and spermatids connected by intercellular bridges in the mammalian testis. *Biol Reprod.* 1971;4(2):195–215.
4. Breuss MW, Yang X, Gleeson JG. Sperm mosaicism: implications for genomic diversity and disease. *Trends Genet.* 2021;37(10):890–902.
5. Bedard N, Yang Y, Gregory M, et al. Mice lacking the USP2 deubiquitinating enzyme have severe male subfertility associated with defects in fertilization and sperm motility. *Biol Reprod.* 2011;85(3):594–604.
6. Moritz L, Hammoud SS. The art of packaging the sperm genome: molecular and structural basis of the histone-to-protamine exchange. *Front Endocrinol (Lausanne).* 2022;13:895502.

7. Moreno RD, Ramalho-Santos J, Sutovsky P, et al. Vesicular traffic and golgi apparatus dynamics during mammalian spermatogenesis: implications for acrosome architecture. *Biol Reprod.* 2000;63(1):89–98.
8. Oko RJ. Developmental expression and possible role of perinuclear theca proteins in mammalian spermatozoa. *Reprod Fertil Dev.* 1995;7(4):777–797.
9. Oliva R. Protamines and male infertility. *Hum Reprod Update.* 2006;12(4):417–435.
10. Garcia-Peiro A, Martinez-Heredia J, Oliver-Bonet M, et al. Protamine 1 to protamine 2 ratio correlates with dynamic aspects of DNA fragmentation in human sperm. *Fertil Steril.* 2011;95(1):105–109.
11. Sofikitis N, Giotitsas N, Tsounapi P, et al. Hormonal regulation of spermatogenesis and spermiogenesis. *J Steroid Biochem Mol Biol.* 2008;109(3–5):323–330.
12. Smith LB, Walker WH. The regulation of spermatogenesis by androgens. *Semin Cell Dev Biol.* 2014;30:2–13.
13. Sharpe RM, McKinnell C, Kivlin C, et al. Proliferation and functional maturation of Sertoli cells, and their relevance to disorders of testis function in adulthood. *Reproduction.* 2003;125(6):769–784.
14. Lucas TF, Nascimento AR, Pisolato R, et al. Receptors and signaling pathways involved in proliferation and differentiation of Sertoli cells. *Spermatogenesis.* 2014;4:e28138.
15. Risley MS, Tan IP, Farrell J. Gap junctions with varied permeability properties establish cell-type specific communication pathways in the rat seminiferous epithelium. *Biol Reprod.* 2002;67(3):945–952.
16. de Rooij DG. Proliferation and differentiation of spermatogonial stem cells. *Reproduction.* 2001;121(3):347–354.
17. Wakayama T, Yokota S, Noguchi K, et al. Quantitative evaluation of spermatogenesis by fluorescent histochemistry. *Histochem Cell Biol.* 2022;157(3):287–295.
18. Meachem SJ, Nieschlag E, Simoni M. Inhibin B in male reproduction: pathophysiology and clinical relevance. *Eur J Endocrinol.* 2001;145(5):561–571.
19. Griswold MD. 50 years of spermatogenesis: sertoli cells and their interactions with germ cells. *Biol Reprod.* 2018;99(1):87–100.
20. Franca LR, Hess RA, Dufour JM, et al. The Sertoli cell: one hundred fifty years of beauty and plasticity. *Andrology.* 2016;4(2):189–212.
21. Mruk DD, Cheng CY. The mammalian blood-testis barrier: its biology and regulation. *Endocr Rev.* 2015;36(5):564–591.
22. Stanton PG. Regulation of the blood-testis barrier. *Semin Cell Dev Biol.* 2016;59:166–173.
23. Cheng CY, Mruk DD. A local autocrine axis in the testes that regulates spermatogenesis. *Nat Rev Endocrinol.* 2010;6(7):380–395.
24. Hess RA, Renato de Franca L. Spermatogenesis and cycle of the seminiferous epithelium. *Adv Exp Med Biol.* 2008;636:1–15.
25. Cheng CY, Mruk DD. The blood-testis barrier and its implications for male contraception. *Pharmacol Rev.* 2012;64(1):16–64.
26. Fijak M, Bhushan S, Meinhardt A. Immunoprivileged sites: the testis. *Methods Mol Biol.* 2011;677:459–470.
27. Meinhardt A, Hedger MP. Immunological, paracrine and endocrine aspects of testicular immune privilege. *Mol Cell Endocrinol.* 2011;335(1):60–68.
28. Mital P, Kaur G, Dufour JM. Immunoprotective sertoli cells: making allogeneic and xenogeneic transplantation feasible. *Reproduction.* 2010;139(3):495–504.
29. Washburn RL, Hibler T, Kaur G, et al. Sertoli cell immune regulation: a double-edged sword. *Front Immunol.* 2022;13:913502.
30. Maree L, du Plessis SS, Menkveld R, et al. Morphometric dimensions of the human sperm head depend on the staining method used. *Hum Reprod.* 2010;25(6):1369–1382.
31. Aldana A, Carneiro J, Martinez-Mekler G, et al. Discrete dynamic model of the mammalian sperm acrosome reaction: the influence of acrosomal pH and physiological heterogeneity. *Front Physiol.* 2021;12:682790.
32. Aarabi M, Balakier H, Bashar S, et al. Sperm-derived WW domain-binding protein, PAWP, elicits calcium oscillations and oocyte activation in humans and mice. *FASEB J.* 2014;28(10):4434–4440.
33. Escoffier J, Yassine S, Lee HC, et al. Subcellular localization of phospholipase Czeta in human sperm and its absence in DPY19L2-deficient sperm are consistent with its role in oocyte activation. *Mol Hum Reprod.* 2015;21(2):157–168.
34. Gat I, Orvieto R. "This is where it all started" – the pivotal role of PLCzeta within the sophisticated process of mammalian reproduction: a systemic review. *Basic Clin Androl.* 2017;27:9.
35. Piomboni P, Focarelli R, Stendardi A, et al. The role of mitochondria in energy production for human sperm motility. *Int J Androl.* 2012;35(2):109–124.
36. Schjenken JE, Robertson SA. The female response to seminal fluid. *Physiol Rev.* 2020;100(3):1077–1117.
37. Morgan HL, Watkins AJ. The influence of seminal plasma on offspring development and health. *Semin Cell Dev Biol.* 2020;97:131–137.
38. Puga Molina LC, Luque GM, Balestrini PA, et al. Molecular basis of human sperm capacitation. *Front Cell Dev Biol.* 2018;6:72.
39. Lin M, Lee YH, Xu W, et al. Ontogeny of tyrosine phosphorylation-signaling pathways during spermatogenesis and epididymal maturation in the mouse. *Biol Reprod.* 2006;75(4):588–597.
40. Batra V, Norman E, Morgan HL, et al. Parental programming of offspring health: the intricate interplay between diet, environment, reproduction and development. *Biomolecules.* 2022;12(9).

13

Fertilisation and Pre-Implantation Embryo Development

Andrew Thomson, Lyndon Miles and Kimberly Higgins

13.1 Scientific Theory Underpinning Practice

Oocytes must be inseminated with sperm (conventional IVF) or undergo Intracytoplasmic sperm injection (ICSI) for fertilisation to occur (**1**). Fully mature oocytes are arrested in metaphase II (MII) of meiosis and must be activated by the fertilising spermatozoon containing a haploid complement of chromosomes to allow cell cycle progression, cell division, and embryogenesis to proceed (**2**). For conventional IVF cases, as sperm reaches the oocyte, it must bind to the zona pellucida. Changes occur in the sperm cell membrane so receptors are exposed through the removal of a glycoprotein layer. The oocyte's cumulus cells will emit progesterone which binds to an ion channel on the sperm cell called CatSper. This causes an influx of extracellular calcium, increase in cyclic AMP and decrease in intracellular pH. This influx of calcium ions to propel the sperm forward giving it an extra boost to aid fertilisation and chemotaxis. This is known as capacitation; spermatozoa hyperactivation allows sperm to move through the mass of cumulus cells and reach the zona pellucida to which it can bind (**3**).

The zona pelludica is composed of four glycoproteins known as ZP1, ZP2, ZP3 and ZP4. ZP2 binds to the inner acrosomal membrane of the sperm. ZP3 binds to plasma membrane of the acrosomal cap of the sperm and ZP4 binds the anterior head of the capacitated acrosome. This is known as the acrosome reaction (**4**). The acrosomal cap contains a number of enzymes that are required for fertilisation. Alterations occur on the cap which release hyaluronidase to breakdown of the cumulus matrix surrounding the oocyte. As the cumulus breaks down, it exposes an area of the oocyte for the sperm acrosome to come into contact with and bind to the zona pellucida. As the plasma membranes fuse, the acrosome contents are released. The enzymes dissolve the zona pellucida at the contact point allowing fusion of the sperm into the oocyte (**4**).

Following fusion of the spermatozoa with the oocyte, the sperm head is incorporated into the oocyte cytoplasm and the sperm nuclear envelope disperses. The fertilising spermatozoon enters the oocyte containing a haploid complement of chromosomes. MII arrest is alleviated, thereby allowing cell cycle progression, cell division, and embryogenesis to proceed. Concurrently, fertilisation triggers the cortical reaction which includes cortical granule (CG) exocytosis (to prevent polyspermy), extrusion of the second polar body, maternal RNA recruitment, male and female pro-nuclear (PN) formation, and the initiation of embryonic gene expression. The cortical reaction involves exocytosis of the oocytes' cortical granules which are secretory vesicles that reside just below the oocytes plasma membrane which block the further entry of spermatozoa (polyspermy) by digesting sperm receptor proteins ZP2 and ZP3. It is well documented that oocytes are activated by Ca^{2+} oscillations induced as a result of Inositol Trisphosphate (IP_3)-mediated Ca^{2+} release from intracellular Ca^{2+} stores (**2, 5**) such as the endoplasmic reticulum. It is accepted that the fertilising sperm releases a soluble sperm factor (SPF) into the oocyte triggering these oscillations. However, there is wide debate over the actual identity of this sperm factor but increasing research (**2, 6**) has indicated that it is a sperm specific protein called phospholipase C zeta (PLCζ).

Oocyte activation results in the meiotic spindle being activated. The spindles pull apart as the sister chromatids separate. This is the completion of meiosis II leading to the extrusion of the 2nd polar body. This occurs via the paternal chromosomes inducing cortical actomyosin assembly and spindle formation independently. The chromosome-induced cortical cap undergoes protrusion, the anaphase spindle midzone first induces a unilateral furrow, which works with the cap protrusion causing spindle rotation. After successful spindle rotation, the spindle midzone induces bilateral furrowing which leads to an abscission of the polar body (**1**).

13.1.1 Signs of Fertilisation

Pronuclei (PN) are the first observable signs of fertilisation (**7, 8**). For fertilisation to be considered normal, two pronuclei must be observed (one maternal and one paternal) and ideally two polar bodies (PB's). Male and female pronuclei are usually formed simultaneously where the paternal pronucleus generates at the site of sperm entry and the maternal pronucleus at the pole of the meiotic spindle. However, as they form, the two pronuclei migrate towards each other separated only by a small strip of ooplasm containing mitochondria and smooth ER. These pronuclei are formed from sperm and oocyte chromatin. As the pronuclei become closely associated, micronucleoli appear within each pronuclei and line up along the strip of ooplasm. The female pronucleus often dismantles and undergoes membrane breakdown slightly ahead of the male pronucleus. As they both breakdown and disappear, they enter syngamy (**9**).

DOI: 10.1201/9781003269502-13

13.1.2 Pronuclei Appearance

The timing of pronuclei appearance varies considerably and can appear anytime between 3–20 hours post insemination and 3–18 hours post IVF and ICSI (**10**). With ICSI patients, as the acrosome reaction is bypassed this process is accelerated. During conventional in vitro (cIVF) and natural fertilisation, the spermatozoa take time to reach the oocyte, the cumulus cells gets digested by hyaluronic acid secreted by those that make it, until the spermatozoon fuses to the zona pellucida and activates the oocyte. With ICSI the spermatozoa is directly injected into the oocyte, bypassing the fusion of the sperm head to the oocyte. The disappearance of pronuclei occurs around 20 hours after injection and cleavage of the zygote occurring approximately 4 hours after this (**11**). For the disappearance of PN in both cIVF and ICSI, the female pronucleus often dismantles and undergoes membrane breakdown slightly ahead of the male pronucleus (**9, 12**). Time lapse studies have enabled a better understanding of the timing of pronuclear appearance and fading and proposed more precise timing for the assessment of fertilisation, at around 16 hours post insemination for ICSI (**13**).

Within the pronuclei are 2–7 micronucleoli (Figure 13.1). Historically, PN were graded as part of embryo selection. Z1 or Z2 give rise to the highest implantation and pregnancy rates while Z4 were thought to have the lowest potential (**14**). With the introduction of blastocyst culture and time lapse imaging, this grading is no longer used in routine practice.

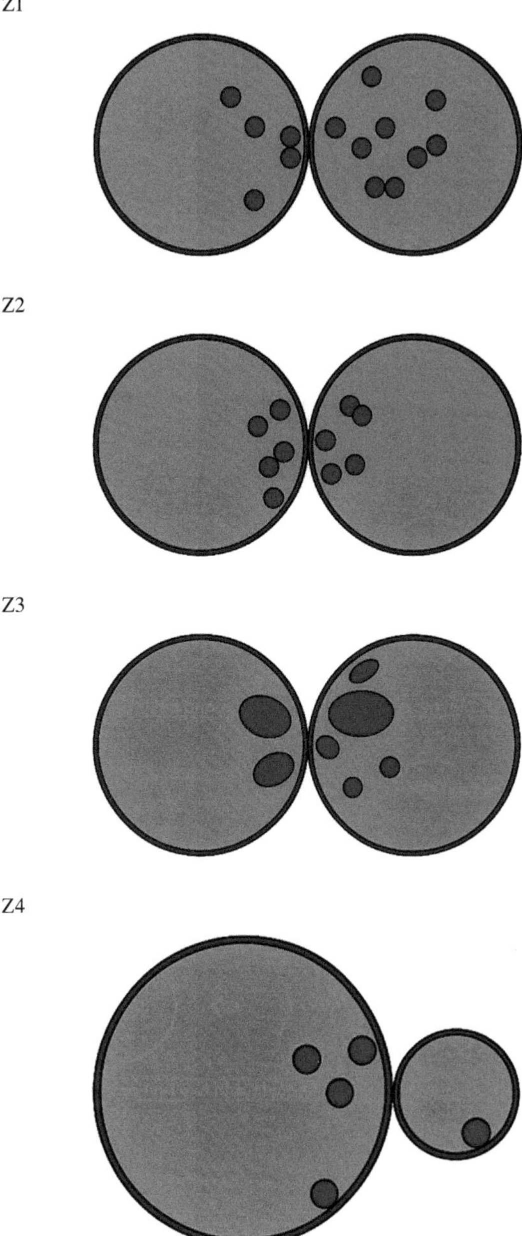

FIGURE 13.1 Pronuclei Z scores.

13.1.3 Laboratory Considerations

Failure to check the zygotes at an appropriate time can result in oocytes being included or excluded in error. Original studies suggested that the optimum time to perform fertilisation checks was 15–18 hours post insemination (**7**), but this has now been refined, as described above. In laboratories with no timelapse incubators, oocytes subjected to ICSI should be checked first followed by the cIVF inseminated oocytes. For those laboratories utilising time lapse, then the ICSI cases can be checked at any time point.

If pronuclear assessment is not carried out in the correct time frame, pronuclear development could be missed as they:

- If checked too early, 2PN may not have appeared yet and the oocyte may be incorrectly scored as not fertilised.
- If checked too late, single pronuclei may have appeared and disappeared (3PN or 1 PN).
- If checked too late, the zygote may have already entered syngamy (disappearance of PN prior to first cell division) and be incorrectly recorded as failed to fertilise and crucially 2PN may have been missed therefore excluding the embryo for consideration of embryo transfer.

13.1.4 Triploid Embryos

2PN embryos are selected for embryo transfer in preference over other embryos not displaying these features. However, in some IVF and ICSI cycles, valuable oocytes are lost due to the presence of ≥3PN (polypronuclei) forming a triploid embryo (Figure 13.2) in which the extra PN can be either maternal or paternal in origin (**8**). Triploid embryos are the most frequent (15–18%) cause of spontaneous abortion. If triploid embryos implant severe malformations to the foetus and patient may occur. This includes syndactyly of the fingers, syndactyly of the toes, and malformations of the genitals, urinary tract. Malformations to the heart and brain may be observed resulting in early postnatal death (**15**).

3PN's form more commonly in cIVF than with ICSI. Triploid embryos can be separated into two categories – diandric and

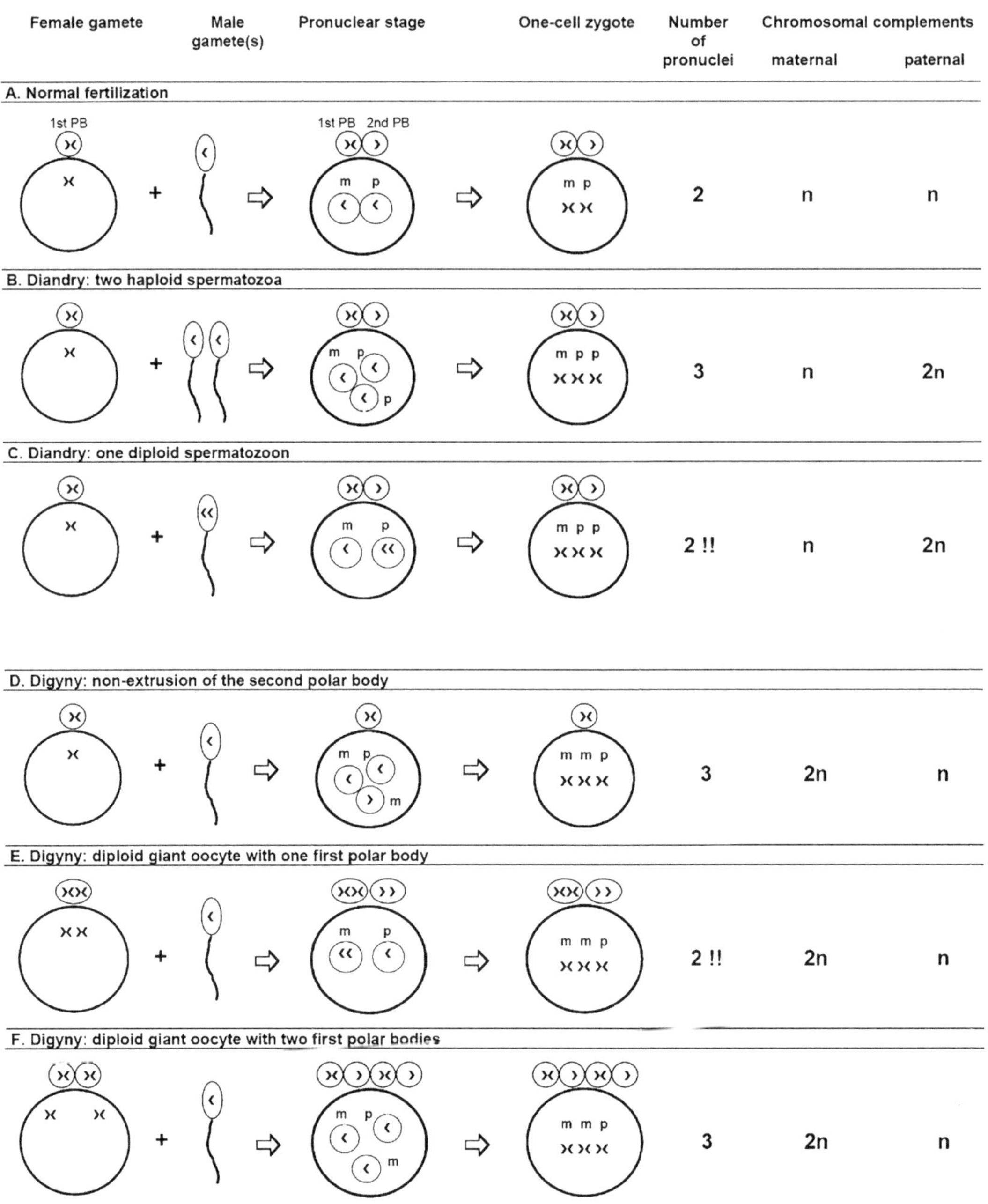

FIGURE 13.2 Mechanisms of triploidy in embryos (from [**14**] with permission).

digynic. Diandric embryos contain one maternal and two paternal PN whereas digynic embryos contain two maternal and one paternal PN (**16, 17**).

13.2 Diandric Embryos (1 Maternal, 2 Paternal PN)

In cIVF, embryos with 3PN and 2 polar bodies are nearly always due to entry of two spermatozoa into the oocyte (Figure 13.2b) resulting in diandric triploidy (**15**). This may be due to over insemination of sperm, delayed cortical reaction, thin zona pellucida, increased maternal age, insemination of immature or post-mature oocytes. A paternal haploid nucleus from each sperm will form along with a haploid maternal nucleus. A second PB will be extruded resulting in 3PN with 2PB visible (3n) (**18**).

Fertilisation of an oocyte with a diploid sperm (Figure 13.2c) is very rare *In-vivo* but occurs more commonly with ICSI (**19, 20**). Oocytes injected with sperm obtained from men suffering severe oligozoospermia have a much higher incidence (1.9%: 0.2%) of triploidy due to diploid sperm being injected

(**20**). A diploid paternal nucleus will form (2n) along with a haploid maternal nucleus (1n) and the second polar body will be extruded (**15**). However, 2PN will still be observed despite being triploid (3n). Diploid sperm cannot be identified via morphology such as abnormal head size, multiple tails etc (**20**). These rarer cases of triploidy were revealed by cytogenetic analysis of triploid embryos arising from ICSI demonstrating two Y chromosomes and a single X chromosome (**21**). They are further confirmed by cytoplasmic analysis of what were thought to be digynic triploid embryos. After failure to extrude the second body, 3PN was observed. Further analysis revealed four sets of chromosomes (4n), thereby, diandric and digynic fertilisation had occurred.

13.3 Digynic Embryos (2 Maternal and 1 Paternal PN)

Digynic embryos can also arise by the injection of a haploid sperm (1n) but demonstrate only 1PB (Figure 13.2d). This is due to the second PB being retained within the ooplasm and forming another maternal PN (2n) resulting in 3n. This is caused by disruption of the meiotic spindle during ICSI (**22**).

Digynic embryos can also arise with the use of giant oocytes as they are bi-nucleate at the germinal vesicle (GV) stage. This results in them always being diploid (2n) due to failure of cytoplasmic cleavage in an oogonium or fusion of two oogonia (**15**). Using giant oocytes, there are two ways of maturation to metaphase II that will alter the number of PN observed at fertilisation. Fertilisation of giant oocytes after fusion of a haploid spermatozoan, a paternal PN (1n) and a diploid female PN (2n) will be formed despite demonstrating 2PN (Figure 13.2e). It would be expected for a second PB containing two sets of chromatids to be extruded resulting in a digynic embryo. Alternatively, the bi-nucleate state can be maintained and the mature oocyte will contain two separate chromosome complements and carry two haploid first PBs. After fusion of a haploid spermatozoa, formation of three (two maternal and one paternal) PN, accompanied by extrusion of two second PBs, each one with a haploid chromatid set will occur (Figure 13.2f). Giant oocytes should be excluded from selection for embryo transfer due to their bi-nucleate status even if they appear with 2PN (Figure 13.2e) as they will still always be triploid (**15**).

13.4 Implications

Despite being triploid, embryo development may still continue and could lead to pregnancy. Cytogenetic analysis has shown that 61.8% of 3PN embryos have an abnormal chromosomal complement or complex mosaicisms and 12.6% of triploid embryos have been found to actually be diploid (**8, 23**). The rationale for this higher than expected value is that the third PN may have been misinterpreted and in reality could just be a vacuole or other cytoplasmic variation resulting in a diploid embryo being disregarded by user error. Due to the severe risks associated with triploid embryos, they should not be transferred, even if there are no alternatives for embryo transfer. Naturally occurring triploid pregnancies demonstrate the increased risk of fetal abnormalities, spontaneous abortions and neonatal deaths (**15**).

Other risks of transferring triploid embryos are not only that they pose a threat to the potential foetus but also to the mother. Androgenic triploid embryos are able to develop into non-malignant growths of trophoblast tissues (molar pregnancy) and chorionic villi which proliferate into a polycystic placental mass. This can be treated but it may become malignant and invade the uterine wall resulting in haemorrhage (**23**). However, molar pregnancies are rare and are estimated to occur in every 1 to 2 per 1000 pregnancies (**24**).

13.4.1 Artificial Oocyte Activation (AOA)

In an estimated 1–5% of ICSI cycles, severely reduced or failed fertilisation of oocytes will still occur (**6**). These cases can be potentially treated using AOA in a subsequent ICSI cycle. Recent studies (**2, 25, 26**) have shown that as oocyte activation requires Ca^{2+} oscillations. Calcium ionophores can be used to activate oocytes by utilising a single transient large dose of calcium (thereby, bypassing the need for PLCζ. This can yield high rates of activation in human oocytes and has resulted in a successful pregnancy and birth (**27**).

A prospective multi-centre trial investigating the use of a ready to use calcium ionophore investigated 101 patients who previously had <50% fertilisation in an ICSI cycle, 99% of patients had an improved outcome with 28% live birth rate (**25**). AOA increases fertilisation rates but concerns exist about one peak of Ca^{2+} influx rather than the oscillations seen in normal fertilisation which may affect gene regulation, hinder normal cellular development and gene expression as calcium channels are unable to regulate themselves. This can result in premature activation, reduced cleavage rates and an increase in triploid embryos (**6**).

Follow up studies on children born as a result of the use of AOA have been performed but the numbers are too limited to extrapolate definitive conclusions. One study investigated the neonatal and neurodevelopmental outcome of children between 3–10 years (**25**). They concluded that neonatal, developmental and behavioural outcome was reassuring but the results were considered preliminary and that AOA should still not be considered routine practice. Ebner and Montag (2015) looked at the neonatal outcomes of the children born from the use of CultActive and reported 1/35 livebirths had a malformation (anal atresia) but they concluded that this malformation has been observed in conventional IVF and ICSI without the use of AOA (**26**).

In 2012, the Scientific and Clinical Advances Advisory Committee discussed the use of gamete activation (both sperm and oocytes), as a result the artificial activation of oocytes was added to the list of licensed activities. However, its use is restricted to OAD patients as long as they are counselled in the theoretical risks relating to embryo viability. Centres are expected to document their rationale for using Calcium Ionophore for individual cases. Please refer to Chapter 32 in this book for more details on AOA.

13.4.2 Embryo Development

Historically, morphological evaluation of embryos has been the main method of choice to assess and select embryos (**28, 29**). As embryo quality is still the most predictive factor of IVF treatment outcome scoring embryos remains fundamental to IVF laboratories, but still remains open to intra- and interpersonal variability, despite efforts made to find more objective means (**30**).

Classical embryo morphological evaluation, has historically been performed by removing the embryos for a few minutes from the incubator on a daily basis daily to allow a static and single observation under a heated microscope. Continuous monitoring of embryo development from fertilization to blastocyst stage by automated time-lapse imaging has offered the possibility to appraise the timing of embryonic cell division (**31**). Payne et al. (1997) developed the first time-lapse system for studying morphokinetics in human embryos (**10**). This system overcame the limitations of such previous static observations. Images can now be taken several times per hour without being removal from the incubator. In addition, time-lapse allows observing exact time points of cell divisions, compaction and blastocyst formation, generation and absorption of fragments, and multinucleation. Blastocyst evaluation in conventional incubation systems is based on morphologic criteria only, for example, blastocoel formation and expansion, inner cell mass quality, and trophectoderm quality, whereas in time-lapse instruments, kinetic parameters can be evaluated besides pretransfer final morphology (**32**).

13.4.3 Pronuclei Disappearance and Mitotic Cleavage Divisions

Pronuclei disappear at syngamy and according to consensus, assessment of presence of pronucleus should be performed 17 ± 1 hours post insemination however recent time-lapse studies show that the highest proportion of oocytes exhibit pronuclei at 16–16.5 hours post insemination (**13**) so this may be preferable although may be subject to differing culture conditions between labs and therefore may be more accurately assessed on a lab specific basis, ideally following validation of similarly large in house data.

22–25 hours after IVF insemination or ICSI the pronuclei of the fertilised eggs break down and disappear ahead of the first division where the embryo splits to the 2-cell stage. We refer to these embryos in the first few days of development as "cleavage" stage embryos, because we can count the number of cleavage divisions under a microscope or via a computer screen when using time-lapse monitoring. Blastomeres often divide evenly, although asynchronously (**33**), so it is not uncommon for embryos to have an odd number of cells and uneven blastomeres. We can also see various indicators of poorer quality in the embryo at this stage such as fragments or multinucleation of blastomeres. Mitotic divisions continue as the two cells divide into four cells, then into eight cells and so on. Each division takes from 12 to 24 hours. Cleavage divisions in the first 4 days continue without any overall increase in size. This means that with each successive subdivision, the ratio of nuclear to cytoplasmic material increases (**34**). Initially, the dividing blastomeres are undifferentiated and aggregated into a sphere enclosed within the zona pellucida. At the 4–8 cell stage, a wave of embryonic genome activation occurs. When eight blastomeres have formed on day-3, the cells start to compact against one another. They begin to develop gap junctions, enabling them to develop in an integrated way and co-ordinate their response to physiological signals and environmental cues (**35**).

13.4.4 Morula and Blastocyst

When the cells number around 16–32, the solid group of cells within the zona pellucida is referred to as a morula. Cells then begin differentiate into an outer layer of cells called the trophectoderm, and an inner group called the inner cell mass. With further compaction the individual outer blastomeres, become indistinguishable. They are still enclosed within the zona pellucida. This compaction serves to make the structure watertight, containing the fluid that the cells will later secrete. The inner cells mass cells differentiate and polarise at one end of the embryo. They close together and form gap junctions, which facilitate cellular communication. This polarisation leaves a cavity, the blastocoel, creating a structure that is now termed the blastocyst. The trophectoderm cells secrete fluid into the blastocoel. The resulting increase in size of the blastocyst causes it to hatch through the zona pellucida, process is called zona hatching and it takes place on the sixth day of embryo development, immediately before the implantation process. The hatching of the human embryo is supported by proteases secreted by the cells of the blastocyst, which digest proteins of the zona pellucida, giving rise to a hole. Then, due to the expansion and contractions of the blastocyst, an increase of the pressure inside the blastocyst itself occurs, the hole expands and finally the blastocyst can emerge from the zona pellucida. The inner cell mass will give rise to the pre-embryo, the amnion, yolk sac and allantois, while the fetal part of the placenta will form from the outer trophoblast layer zona pellucida ultimately disappears completely, and the now exposed cells of the trophoblast allow the blastocyst to attach itself to the endometrium, where it will hopefully implant.

Yanhe Liu et al., 2015, using time-lapse videography showed that human early cleavage embryos were quicker following ICSI to reach developmental milestones compared to IVF when using insemination as the timing start point (t0), due to differences in the time taken for embryos to reach pronuclear fading (PNF) (**36**). These differences disappeared when PNF was used as t0. Using a biological rather than procedural t0 will allow a unified assessment strategy to be applied to all cycles irrespective of the insemination method, although some studies have not observed this phenomenon beyond the early developmental stages.

13.4.5 Aneuploidy and Morphokinetic Abnormalities

Aneuploidy (an abnormal number of chromosomes) in human embryos is surprisingly prevalent and increases drastically with maternal age, resulting in miscarriages, infertility and

ICM grade	Inner cell mass description
A	ICM prominent with many cells, tightly packed
B	Several cells, loosely grouped, larger in size
C	Very few cells
D	Cells of ICM appear degenerate or necrotic
E	No ICM discernible in any focal plane

TE grade	Trophectoderm description
A	Many cells, forming a cohesive layer
B	Few cells, forming a loose epithelium
C	Very few large cells

FIGURE 13.3 ICM and TE grading (adapted from [**46**]).

birth defects. Frequent errors during the meiotic divisions cause this aneuploidy, while age-independent errors during the first cleavage divisions of the embryo also contribute. Errors in mitotic cleavage divisions can lead to mosaic embryos where some cells are genetically normal whereas others are not. Such "mosaicism" in early embryos is attributed to errors during the mitotic divisions, because errors in meiosis would affect all blastomeres. This mitotic-origin mosaicism is not necessarily lethal, and birth of mosaic babies following transfer of mosaic embryos is rare because affected cells can be selected against during development. However, some individuals can be born with placental, somatic or germ line mosaicism. Chavez et al. (2012) were the first to observe that chromosomally normal embryos have strict and tightly clustered cell cycle parameters compared to aneuploid embryos (**37**).

Bamford et al. (2022) performed a systematic review and meta-analysis on embryo morphokinetic characteristics and euploidy (**38**). The main morphokinetic abnormalities exhibited by human embryos include:

Multinucleation: Presence of more than one nucleus in a single blastomere, including micronuclei. It is supposed that multinucleation arises from karyokinesis without subsequent cytokinesis or alternatively from errors during mitosis in chromosome segregation and packaging (**39**) quite often resulting in chromosomally abnormal cells. Detection of multinucleation is most reliable by time-lapse imaging (**40**).

Direct cleavage: Irregular cleavage where one blastomere divides directly into three or more daughter cells (**41**). It can be distinguished more precisely in direct and rapid cleavage (**40**) on the basis of the timing employed by the mother cell to divide into three: when t3-t2 = 0, it can be defined as direct and presumably originating from a trichotomous mitosis (**42**) caused by an irregular high number of centrioles that lead to aberrant chromosomes distribution; it can be defined as rapid when t3-t2 is less than 5.

Prolonged S2 phase: S2 phase (t4-t3) is the time for an embryo to cleave from three to four cells and it is called also the synchrony of the second cell cycle. Regarding the anomaly of prolonged S2 phase, researchers found this parameter reflective of euploidy at the cleavage stage (**35**) and reflective of gene expression. it was also considered a possible cause of mosaic embryos (**43**).

Reverse cleavage: is the phenomenon through which two or more blastomeres merge producing a hybrid cell. It could be because of defects in cell membrane (**44**).

This phenomenon is also called 'blastomere fusion' or 'failed cleavage' and considered as possible cause, which brings to mosaic embryos.

Absent cleavage: the presence of karyokinesis: it is the process by which a blastomere undergoes a pseudodivision without forming two discernible blastomeres with a single or multiple extra nuclei within the same blastomere (**44**).

Chaotic cleavage: this irregularity lies whenever blastomeres are arranged in various combinations with membrane ruffling, multiple cleavage furrows, divisions into unevenly sized blastomeres and several fragments (**44**).

13.4.6 Embryo Grading

The grading of cleavage stage embryos is based on their rate of growth, degree of fragmentation (the left-over pieces when a cell splits unevenly) and finally cell symmetry. An example of such grading may be the number of cells of the embryo followed by fragmentation and symmetry expressed in a scale from 1 to 4, with 4 being the highest grade and 1 the lowest. For example, an '844' (8-cell with grades 4 for fragmentation and symmetry) would be a top-quality day 3 8 cell with even cells and no fragmentation. A '422' (4-cell with grades 2 for symmetry and fragmentation) is an average quality 4-cell embryo with uneven cells and moderate fragmentation (**45**).

13.4.7 Blastocyst Grading

Blastocysts on the other hand can be graded on expansion, the quality of the inner cell mass and the quality of the trophectoderm. Blastocysts expansion is typically graded on a scale of 1 to 6. Early blastocysts, with fewer cells, are graded as 1 or 2 and are less 'inflated'. Because these have fewer cells and a poorly defined inner cell mass and trophectoderm they are not given any letter grades like more advanced blastocysts are. Once the blastocoel completely fills the embryo, it is considered a full blastocyst. The zona pellucida may still be thick (grade 3) but as the blastocoel continues to fill the embryo, the internal pressure will continue to build. This causes the zona pellucida to become very thin (grade 4). The zona pellucida will eventually fracture and the embryo will begin to hatch out (grade 5) and once fully hatched will be known as grade 6.

Blastocysts on day 5 and 6 of development can be graded using the same system, based on a number (based on expansion) followed by two letters, the first for ICM grade and the 2nd for TE grade. ICM is graded A-E dependent on size and TE is graded on the amount of cells present (Figure 13.3.)

With more applications of artificial intelligence and other novel technologies with time-lapse imaging and pre-implantation genetic testing of embryos, more knowledge and understanding of the different observations will be gained regarding fertilisation and the pre-implantation human embryo.

REFERENCES

1. Wang Q, Racowsky C, Deng M. Mechanism of the chromosome-induced polar body extrusion in mouse eggs. *Cell Div.* 2011;6(17):9.
2. Ramadan WM, Kashir J, Jones C, et al. Oocyte activation and phospholipase C zeta (PLCζ): diagnostic and therapeutic implications for assisted reproductive technology. *Cell Commun Signal.* 2012;10(1):12.
3. Lishko PV, Botchkina IL, Kirichok Y. Progesterone activates the principal Ca2+ channel of human sperm. *Nature.* 2011;471(10):387–391.
4. Ganguly A, Bansal P, Gupta T, et al. ZP domain of human zona pellucida glycoprotein-1 binds to human spermatozoa and induces acrosomal exocytosis. *Reprod Biol Endocrinol.* 2010;(8):110.
5. Berridge MJ. Inositol trisphosphate and calcium signalling mechanisms. *Biochim Biophys Acta.* 2009;1793(6):933–940.
6. Kashir J, Jones C, Chang Lee H, et al. Loss of activity mutations in phospholipase C zeta (PLCz) abolishes calcium oscillatory ability of human recombinant protein in mouse oocytes. *Hum Reprod.* 2011;26(12):3372–3387.
7. Gardner DK, Weissman A, Howles CM, et al. *Textbook of Assisted Reproductive Techniques: Laboratory and Clinical Perspectives.* 2nd Edition. London: Taylor and Francis, 2004.
8. Feenan K, Herbert M. Can "abnormally" fertilized zygotes give rise to viable embryos? *Hum Fertil (Camb).* 2006;9:157–169.
9. Veeck LL. *An Atlas of Human Gametes and Conceptuses.* Parthenon, Casterton Hall, Carnforth, Lancashire, UK: CRC Press, Boca Raton; 1999.
10. Payne D, Flaherty SP, Barry MF, et al. Preliminary observations on polar body extrusion and pronuclear formation in human oocytes using time-lapse video cinematography. *Hum Reprod.* 1997;12(3):532–541.
11. Zsolt PN. 'Timing of oocyte activation, pronucleus formation and cleavage in humans after intracytoplasmic sperm injection (ICSI) with testicular spermatozoa and after ICSI or in-vitro fertilization on sibling oocytes with ejaculated spermatozoa'. *Hum Reprod*, 1998;13, 6, 1606–1612.
12. Lawler C, Gordon-Baker HW, Edgar DH. Relationships between timing of syngamy, female age and implantation potential in human in vitro-fertilised oocytes. *Reprod Fertil Dev.* 2007;19(3):482–487.
13. Barrie A, Smith R, Campbell A, et al. Optimisation of the timing of fertilisation assessment for oocytes cultured in standard incubation: lessons learnt from time-lapse imaging of 78 348 embryos. *Biology Hum Reprod.* 2021;36(11):2840–2847.
14. Baczkowski T, Kurzawa R, Glabowski W. Methods of embryo scoring in in-vitro fertilisation. *Reprod Biol.* 2004;4(1):5–22.
15. Rosenbusch BE. Mechanisms giving rise to triploid zygotes during. *Fertil Steril.* 2008;50(1):49–55.
16. Dyban AP, Baranov VS. *Cytogenetics of Mammalian Embryonic Development.* Oxford, UK: Clarendon Press; 1987.
17. Baumer A, Balmer D, Binkert F, et al. Parental origin and mechanisms of formation of triploidy: a study of 25 cases. *Eur J Hum Genet.* 2000;8:911–917.
18. Zaragoza MV, Surti U, Redline RW, et al. Parental origin and phenotype of triploidy in spontaneous abortions: predominance of diandry and association with the partial hydatidiform mole. *Am J Hum Genet.* 2000;66: 1807–1820.
19. McFadden D, Jiang R, Langlois S, et al. Dispermy – origin of diandric triploidy: brief communication. *Hum Reprod.* 2002;17:3037–3038.
20. Egozcue S, Blanco J, Vidal F, et al. Diploid sperm and the origin of triploidy. *Hum Reprod.* 2002;17:5–7.
21. Guthauser B, Vialard F, Dakouane M, et al. Chromosomal analysis of spermatozoa with normal-sized heads in two infertile patients with macrocephalic sperm head syndrome. *Fertil Steril.* 2006;85:750. e5–e7.
22. Macas E, Imthurn B, Roselli M, et al. Chromosome analysis of single- and multipronucleated human zygotes proceeded after the intracytoplasmic sperm injection procedure. *J Assist Reprod Genet.* 1996;13:345–350.
23. Rosenbusch B, Schneider M, Kreienberg R, et al. Cytogenetic analysis of human zygotes displaying three pronuclei and one polar body after intracytoplasmic sperm injection. *Hum Reprod.* 2001;16:2362 2367.
24. Cunningham FG, Leveno KL, Bloom SL. Gestational trophoblastid disease. In: *Williams Obstetrics.* 23rd Edition. New York: McGraw Hill Co; 2010. pp. 257–265.
25. Vanden Meerschaut F, Nikiforaki D, et al. Assisted oocyte activation following ICSI fertilisation failure. *Reprod Biomed Online.* 2014;28:560–571.
26. Ebner T, Montag M. Live Birth after artificial oocyte activation using a ready to use ionophore: a prospective multicenter study. *Reprod Biomed Online.* 2015;30: 359–365.
27. Taylor SL, Yoon SY, Morshedi MS. et al. Complete globozoospermia associated with PLCzeta deficiency treated with calcium ionophore and ICSI results in pregnancy. *Reprod Biomed Online.* 2010;(20):559–564.
28. Pirkevi Çetinkaya C, Kahraman S. Morphokinetics of embryos – where are we now? *J Reprod Biotechnol Fertil.* 2016;5. doi: 10.1177/2058915816663858
29. Pinborg A. IVF/ICSI twin pregnancies: risks and prevention. *Hum Reprod Update.* 2005;11:575–593.
30. Shaulov T, Belisle S, Dahan MH. Public health implications of a North American publicly funded in vitro fertilization program; lessons to learn. *J Assist Reprod Genet.* 2015;32(9): 1385–1393.

31. Kirkegaard K, Agerholm IE, Ingerslev HJ. Time-lapse monitoring as a tool for clinical embryo assessment. *Hum Reprod*. 2012;27:1277–1285.
32. Gardner DK, Vella P, Lane M, et al. Culture and transfer of human blastocysts increases implantation rates and reduces the need for multiple embryo transfers. *Fertil Steril*. 1998;69:84–88.
33. Berrisford K, Cater E. Irregular cleavages. In: Campbell A, Fishel S, editors. *Atlas of Time Lapse Embryology*. Boca Raton, London: CRC Press; 2015. pp. 65–68.
34. Forgács G, Newman SA. *Cleavage and Blastula Formation: Biological Physics of the Developing Embryo*. Cambridge: Cambridge University Press, 2005. p. 27.
35. Brison DR, Sturmey RG, Leese HJ. Metabolic heterogeneity during preimplantation development: the missing link? *Hum Reprod Update*. 2014;20(5):632–640.
36. Liu Y, Chapple V, Feenan K, et al. Time-lapse videography of human embryos: using pronuclear fading rather than insemination in IVF and ICSI cycles removes inconsistencies in time to reach early cleavage milestones. *Reprod Biol*. 2015;15(2):122–125.
37. Chavez SL, Loewke KE, Han J, et al. Dynamic blastomere behaviour reflects human embryo ploidy by the four-cell stage. *Nat Commun*. 2012;3:1251.
38. Bamford T, Barrie A, Montgomery S, et al. Morphological and morphokinetic associations with aneuploidy: a systematic review and meta-analysis. *Hum Reprod Update*. 2022;28(5):656–686.
39. Desai N, Ploskonka S, Goodman LR, et al. Analysis of embryo morphokinetics, multinucleation and cleavage anomalies using continuous time-lapse monitoring in blastocyst transfer cycles. *Reprod Biol Endocrinol*. 2014;12:54.
40. Campbell A, Fishel S, Bowman N, et al. Modelling a risk classification of aneuploidy in human embryos using noninvasive morphokinetics. *Reprod Biomed Online*. 2013;26:477–485.
41. Hlinka D, Kalatova B, Uhrinova I, et al. Time-lapse cleavage rating predicts human embryo viability. *Physiol Res*. 2012;61:513–525.
42. Kola I, Trounson A, Dawson G, et al. Tripronuclear human oocytes: altered cleavage patterns and subsequent karyotypic analysis of embryos. *Biol Reprod*. 1987;37:395–401.
43. Lagalla C, Tarozzi N, Sciajno R, et al. Embryos with morphokinetic abnormalities may develop into euploid blastocysts. *Reprod Biomed Online*. 2017;34:137–146.
44. Barrie A, Homburg R, McDowell G, et al. Preliminary investigation of the prevalence and implantation potential of abnormal embryonic phenotypes assessed using time-lapse imaging. *Reprod Biomed Online*. 2017;34:455–462.
45. The Istanbul consensus workshop on embryo assessment: proceedings of an expert meeting. *Hum Reprod*. 2011 Jun;26(6):1270–1283. doi: 10.1093/humrep/der037. Epub 2011 Apr 18.
46. Schoolcraft WB, Gardner DK, Lane M, et al. Blastocyst culture and transfer: analysis of results and parameters affecting outcome in two in vitro fertilization programs. *Fertil Steril*. 1999;72(4):604–609.

14

The Endometrium, Implantation and Placental Development

Tom Bamford and Claudia Passaro

14.1 The Endometrium

14.1.1 Physiology of the Endometrium through the Menstrual Cycle

The endometrium is the mucosal lining of the uterus. It is a complex tissue, which during the woman's reproductive life undergoes cyclical changes coordinated by the hypothalamic-pituitary-ovarian axis. The function of the endometrium is to provide a nourishing immune privileged environment to support successful embryo implantation and pregnancy or to shed its superficial layer when implantation does not occur.

The endometrium comprises two layers, the outer functional layer and the underlying basal layer. The functional layer is a thick superficial layer, consisting of luminal epithelium, abundant vertical glands that penetrate into a stromal compartment and vasculature. This layer is shed and regenerated during each menstrual cycle. The basal layer consists of permanent stromal tissue, deep ends of uterine glands and vasculature. This layer remains through each cycle and provides most of the progenitor cells essential for regeneration of the functional layer (**1**). The health and function of the endometrium is vital to the success of natural conception and assisted reproduction.

In order to understand the cyclical changes the endometrium undergoes, it is important to have a clear understanding of the negative and positive feedback mechanisms the hypothalamic-pituitary-ovarian axis exerts on it during the menstrual cycle (Figure 14.1).

The menstrual cycle is composed of two systems: the ovarian cycle, that describes changes occurring in the ovaries; and the uterine cycle that describes changes occurring in the endometrium. These two systems operate in parallel, dividing the menstrual cycle into two phases: the follicular or proliferative phase and the luteal or secretory phase. During the proliferative phase the dominant ovarian hormone is oestradiol; in the secretory phase the dominant ovarian hormone switches to progesterone, secondary to the formation of the corpus luteum (CL).

The onset of menstruation signals the start of the cycle (day 1). Following menstruation, two hormones secreted by the anterior pituitary, the follicle stimulating hormone (FSH) and the luteinizing hormone (LH), stimulate follicular growth. This is coordinated by the release of gonadotrophic-releasing hormone (GnRH) in rhythmic pulses from the hypothalamus. Growing follicles secrete increasing quantities of oestrogens, which promote endometrial thickness. Indeed, under the influence of oestrogens, the endometrial basal layer undergoes development at the level of both glands and stroma (proliferative phase). Meanwhile, one large dominant follicle is recruited, secreting additional oestradiol which eventually will breach the threshold with a positive feedback on the anterior pituitary. This results in a LH surge (on day 14 of a 28-day cycle) lasting 48–72 hours, activating oocyte maturation, ovulation and stimulating progesterone production (**2**).

After ovulation, the luteal or secretory phase begins. The ovulated follicle forms a CL that secretes progesterone and some oestrogens that stimulate the secretory activity of the endometrial glandular epithelium. High concentration of progesterone inhibits FSH and LH by blocking GnRH secretion from the hypothalamus. Near the end of the cycle, around day 24–28, if pregnancy does not occur, the CL undergoes luteolysis with a decrease in progesterone secretion. The rapid drop in progesterone causes the functional layer to shed and the onset of the next menstrual cycle.

14.1.2 Endometrial Receptivity

A successful implantation requires a well-orchestrated cross-talk between a receptive endometrium and a functional blastocyst. Endometrial receptivity is the physiological state in which the endometrium allows blastocyst attachment and subsequent invasion into the stroma to access blood supply, inducing local changes that result in decidualization.

Decidualization is the process in which endometrial stromal cells begin to proliferate and differentiate into large, round, cytoplasmic-rich, multi-nucleated decidual cells (**3**). The function of decidualization is to maintain pregnancy by nutritionally supporting the embryo, allowing trophoblast invasion and recruitment and differentiation of immune cells and promotion of angiogenesis (**4–9**). Decidualization is triggered by an increased level of cyclic adenosine monophosphate (cAMP) in the endometrium, as a consequence of prolonged exposure to progesterone and oestrogen. In humans, unlike most other mammals, the onset of this reaction is cyclical and embryo-independent (**10**). This process occurs during each menstrual cycle; however, in the absence of an implanting embryo, progesterone and oestradiol levels will drop, halting decidualization. The time in which the endometrium is receptive to the embryo is around day 19–24 of the menstrual cycle, 6–10 days post ovulation, often termed the "window of implantation" (**11, 12**). Receptivity is driven by the sequential actions of the steroid hormones, oestradiol and progesterone. Critical shifts in expression of the receptors for these hormones are crucial events on which receptivity depends, particularly

DOI: 10.1201/9781003269502-14

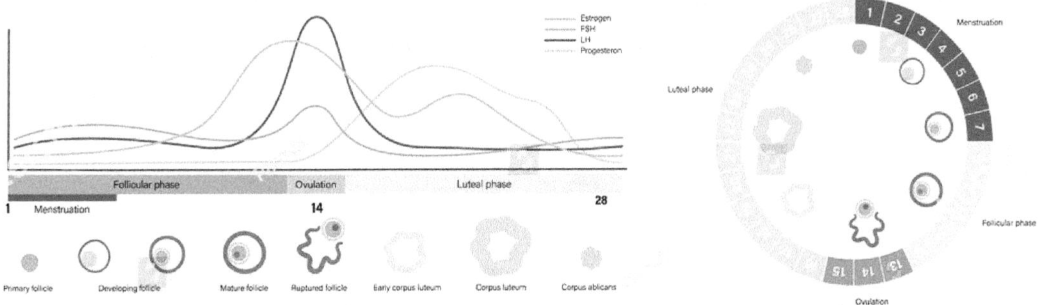

FIGURE 14.1 Ovulation and the menstrual cycle (from Shutterstock under license).

down-regulation of endometrial oestrogen receptor-alpha (ER-α) (**13–16**). Furthermore, morphological changes occur within the endometrium that are characteristic of endometrial receptivity. This includes the development of pinopodes, small microvilli on the apical surface of epithelial cells that project into the uterine lumen in response to progesterone (**17**). The adhesion of the blastocyst to the endometrium occurs at the top of the pinopodes (**18**). Since the presence of pinopodes are limited to the "implantation window", they are regarded as morphological markers for endometrial receptivity (**19**).

14.2 Embryo Implantation

Implantation is the period leading to the establishment of pregnancy, during which the embryo acquires a fixed position within the endometrium (Fig. 2). This process is characterised by three sequential phases: apposition, when the hatched blastocyst establishes its first contact with the endometrium; adhesion, when the association between the trophectoderm and the epithelium strengthens through the interaction of adhesion molecules; and invasion, when the trophoblast invades the stromal decidual tissue to reach the mother's capillaries and secure the blood supply.

The embryo enters the uterine cavity three to five days after fertilization. Once in the uterus, it starts to roll along the uterine lumen to find an appropriate site to appose (**20**). At apposition, the embryo stops moving freely inside the uterine cavity and it starts to show signs of polarity (**21**). The blastocyst adopts a specific orientation, with the inner cell mass directed towards the endometrium. At this point, the trophoblast cells adhere to the luminal epithelium, anchoring at the basal layer and starting the process of adhesion. This process is characterized by a stable interaction mediated by adhesion molecules (CAMs), which are a family of proteins consisting of integrins, cadherins, selectins and immunoglobulins (**22, 23**). Once the embryo is firmly attached to the endometrium, it starts to invade the stroma to access the maternal vascular system for nutrition (**24**).

During invasion the trophoblast cells differentiate into an inner layer of cytotrophoblasts and outer layer. Syncytiotrophoblast cells secrete human chorionic gonadotrophin (HCG) that maintains the CL. The CL in turn ensures the continued production of progesterone that sustains the decidua. The syncytiotrophoblasts form projections into the stroma, this polarized epithelium has specialised exchange processes to transport nutrients between maternal blood and the basal membrane (**25**).

Angiogenesis plays a significant role in embryo implantation. Decidualization of the endometrium triggers release of angiogenic factors which stimulate the development of fetal vessels and vascular remodelling of the maternal uterine spiral arterioles forming the feto-maternal circulatory interface (**26**). Haemorrhage is counteracted by the production of haemostatic mediators such as tissue factor and plasminogen activator inhibitor-I (**27**).

Interestingly, some evidence from literature suggest that the endometrium could have the ability to select competent and normal blastocysts by chemically mediated signals (**28, 29**). If abnormal, stromal cells could prevent implantation, leading to the expulsion of the blastocyst. Moreover, poor quality embryo could induce the release of inhibitors of pro-implantation modulators (**28**).

Genvacev et al. investigated the expression of a selectin adhesion system at the maternal-fetal interface, suggesting its importance in establishing human pregnancy. The author characterised the expression of L-selectin on trophectoderm cells of hatched human blastocysts and its ligand on the endometrium, hypothesising that this binding could initiate apposition (**30**). The three steps of apposition, adhesion and invasion arise due to a combination of coordinated molecular factors, receptiveness of the endometrium and signalling pathways between embryo and endometrium. Future research will aim to elucidate these mechanisms further and importantly how they translate into the clinical context of recurrent implantation failure (RIF) or miscarriage.

14.3 Placental Development

The placenta is the exchange organ between the mother and the fetus. The importance of this organ, not just for fetal development but also for long-term well-being of the child, cannot be overstated (**31**). Throughout pregnancy it covers a series of functions such as immunomodulation, it allows nutrient and waste exchange and has endocrine properties. Surprisingly, placental development is poorly understood, partly because basic science investigations in humans are limited by ethical

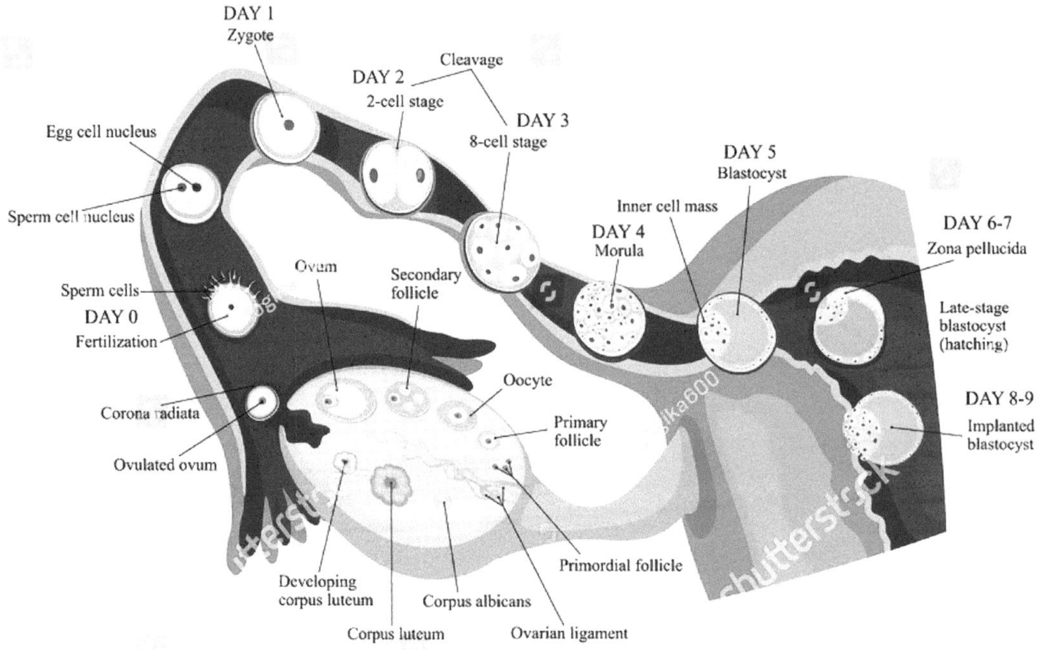

FIGURE 14.2 From ovulation to implantation (from Shutterstock under license).

and logistical challenges. A lack of analogous models compounds this problem, highlighted by the fact that placental conditions such as pre-eclampsia are only found in humans and possibly but not definitely, great apes (**32**).

The human placenta develops from the trophectoderm, the outer layer of the pre-implantation embryo. Implantation starts with the interaction of the polar trophectoderm, (the part continuous with the inner cell mass) and the uterine luminal epithelium. The placenta is derived from two cell lineages, the trophoblast and mesoderm. The cytotrophoblast cells eventually penetrate through the primary syncytium and grow to envelope the embryo in a shell. The cytotrophoblast cells are in contact with the decidua, i.e., the maternal-fetal interface. It is at this point that individual cytotrophoblast cells invade the decidua as extra-villous trophoblasts. They migrate deeply into the decidua where they transform the uterine vasculature in order to supply the placenta with maternal blood. The syncytiotrophoblasts are in direct contact with maternal glandular secretions and blood in the intervillous space, the site of nutrient extraction and gas exchange.

The membrane layer of trophectoderm and inner layer of mesoderm, derived from the epiblast, together form the chorion. This lines the chorionic cavity in which the embryo, amnion and yolk sac are enclosed. Importantly, it produces chorionic fluid which is essential for protecting the embryo. The chorionic villi form the placenta, the outer layer forms the chorion, and the amnion forms the inner layer. Chorionicity is important when assessing twin pregnancies, monochorionic twins for example, are twins that share the same placenta. This is a high-risk pregnancy and occurs when a split occurs on or after the third day of fertilization.

The placenta expresses imprinted genes, which are genes preferentially expressed from one parental allele. Epigenetics have an important role in regulating such gene expression in placental development through DNA methylation, histone modifications and non-coding RNAs (**33**). DNA methylation is the addition of a methyl group to a cytosine. Several studies have reported this mechanism of altering gene expression within the placenta (**34**). Non-coding RNAs are RNA molecules that are not translated into a protein, they have an important physiological role in proliferation and invasion of the trophoblasts (**35**). Finally, histone modification is the process whereby histone proteins are modified by enzymes, this can alter gene expression by modulating the degree of chromatin compaction (**33**). It has been demonstrated how environmental effects can disturb placental epigenetics and thus function (**36**).

Immune tolerance is vital to the process of placental invasion. Autoimmune reaction of the allogenic foetus is avoided is by syncytiotrophoblasts not expressing any human leukocyte antigens. There are also changes in the uterine environment, the most notable of which is the influx of uterine natural killer cells during invasion. It is thought that uterine NK cells may alter the structure of the uterine spinal arteries that supply the foetus and placenta (**37**). Possibly by affecting the structure of the microvasculature themselves or through trophoblast cell infiltration. Furthermore, trophoblast cells express a range of receptor of major histocompatibility complex (MHC) molecules which mediate the migration of leucocytes. It has been suggested that the interaction of the MHC molecules and NK cells induce immune tolerance to maternal T cells. Furthermore, a special type of cell, Hoffbauer cells are placental villous macrophages which are present throughout pregnancy and considered fetal in origin. They are thought to play a crucial role in placental development, although their functions are not completely understood (**38**). Further research into the interaction between the innate and adaptive immune response in the context of placental development is ongoing.

Abnormal placental development can give rise to a wide range of obstetric conditions such as pre-eclampsia, unexplained still birth, growth restriction, placental abruption, and preterm labour. This is ultimately due to defective trophoblast invasion into the decidua. If spiral arterioles are not converted and there is inadequate branching of the villi, reduced nutrients and oxygen are supplied to the foetus. Additionally, errors in chorion development can result in premature separation, resulting in placental abruption. Finally, pre-eclampsia is the result a poorly perfused placenta which triggers a systemic disorder which left untreated can lead to eclamptic seizures and adverse neonatal outcomes.

14.4 The Endometrium in Assisted Reproduction

During *in vitro* fertilization (IVF) cycles, superovulation is induced through the administration of hormones resulting in supraphysiological concentrations of oestrogen and progesterone. In fresh cycles luteal support is provided, usually in the form of vaginal progesterone. In frozen cycles, patients are administered oral oestrogen to build up the endometrial lining before starting progesterone pessaries. Manipulation of the menstrual cycle in such a way can displace the 'window of implantation', primarily through progesterone exposure (**39**). Therefore, controlled ovarian stimulation disrupts the natural physiological processes and is likely to alter key factors such as the rate of embryonic development and endometrial receptivity. Interestingly, Robert Edwards believed that the endometrium was the biggest barrier to progressing the success rates in assisted reproductive technology (ART) (**40**).

The endometrium can be assessed in ART in a variety of ways. Firstly, endometrial thickness assessed by ultrasound is correlated to serum oestradiol levels and has been directly related to treatment success in assisted reproduction (**41, 42**). The significance of a thin endometrium remains controversial, the majority of studies use <7mm or <8mm as cut off values, below which live birth rates are significantly reduced (**41**). Interventions for a thin endometrium include switching the route of administration or increasing the dose or altering the type of hormone replacement used.

Serum progesterone measurement has also been investigated as a potential biomarker of the competence of the endometrium. Since progesterone administration is integral in preparation for frozen embryo transfer (FET) cycles, and the number of such cycles are increasing, more attention has been given to the role of progesterone in treatment success. Progesterone allows the endometrium to become secretory and receptive. A recent systematic review suggests that there is a minimum threshold for serum luteal progesterone of 10ng/mL, above which there is significantly higher chances of pregnancy, live birth and a reduced miscarriage risk in FET cycles (**43**). Research is ongoing in this area; yet such findings have led to clinicians supplementing cycles with additional progesterone using subcutaneous or intramuscular routes.

The endometrium can also be assessed using more advanced methods, such as transcriptomic analysis of an endometrial biopsy taken in a mock frozen embryo cycle. This test is often referred to as endometrial receptivity analysis (ERA), utilising a transcriptomic panel of over 248 genes (**44**). This detects whether the window of implantation is displaced and if altering timing of progesterone exposure is required. The result is a more personalised protocol in the subsequent cycle, as the window of implantation is considered to stay constant between cycles. This approach has been predominantly indicated in patients who have had recurrent implantation failures (RIF) (**45, 46**).

The evidence supporting the ERA is largely derived from retrospective studies, with only one prospective controlled trial published at the time of writing (**47**). An original work identified that patients with a displaced window of implantation have significantly reduced chances of ongoing pregnancy (**48**). Furthermore, those with RIF were more likely to have a non-receptive endometrium (**49**). Interestingly, the aforementioned controlled trial reported a higher cumulative pregnancy rate in the personalised FET group versus standard FET (93% vs. 79%) and a higher pregnancy rate at first embryo transfer (57% vs. 43%) (**47**). These findings have been supported by several cohort studies (**50–53**), although limited by sample heterogeneity and size. The trial intention-to-treat analysis, however, reported a 14% and 11 % percentage points increase compared in the personalized embryo transfer to the frozen and fresh embryo transfer, but that was reported as non-significant as the study was powered to detect 15% point increase or more (**47**). A recent retrospective study with 488 patients demonstrated no clinical improvements with the use of the ERA in RIF (**45**), however, the study has been performed in patients with just one previous failed embryo transfer attempt, an unbalanced size groups and heterogeneity in the embryo quality and luteal support. At least one meta-analysis has been published since this latter study which included 11 studies in total that reported personalised embryo transfer for patients with RIF, with a 15.5% points increase compared to good prognosis patients (**54**). The complexity of endometrial receptivity cannot be overstated and therefore it seems that RIF is not attributed solely to gene expression (**55, 56**). Critics documented intra-patient variability in gene expression, although, such variability may also indicate non-adherence to test protocol such as incorrect timing of the biopsy (**57, 58**).

Other interventions to improve receptivity and implantation have previously been popular and are sometimes still offered to patients, including the endometrial scratch. This is endometrial injury performed using a pipelle biopsy. The hypothesis supporting this technique was that local inflammatory and repair mechanisms within the endometrium may improve implantation. There is now evidence from three RCTs in women with recurrent implantation failure indicating endometrial scratch does not significantly improve the pregnancy and live birth rates (**59–61**). Although the SCRatCH trial demonstrated 4.6% more live births in the intervention compared to the control group; however, the data is inconsistent and there are concerns this procedure could result in negative clinical outcomes (**62**).

The fourth aspect of the endometrium to consider in ART is the microbiome. There has now been a move from culturing the endometrium to sequencing bacterial DNA in order to understand the prevalence of different bacterial species. The lower reproductive tract is mainly dominated by lactobacillus species which are thought to keep the pH below 4.5, making it an inhospitable environment for pathogens (**63**). Several studies have positively associated a vaginal microbiota rich in Lactobacillus (without bacterial vaginosis) with success in ART (**64–67**). Similarly, altered endometrial and vaginal microbiota has been associated with poorer implantation rates in prospective studies (**68–71**). In addition to changes to microbiota, an inflammatory state of the endometrium called chronic endometritis has been associated with poorer outcomes. This is thought to result from an imbalance of the endometrial microbiome and an associated immune reaction. Treatment with antibiotics resulted in higher implantation rates and lower miscarriage rates in one study (**72**).

In the 1990s uterine natural killer cells were studied using immunohistochemistry; since then there has been a focus on the immune component of the endometrium (**73**). Natural killer cells are part of the innate immune system, in contrast to T and B lymphocytes which form part of the adaptive immune response. Uterine natural killer cells (uNK) appear to become more abundant in the secretory endometrium and there is evidence that they mediate implantation and tissue remodelling (**74, 75**). That said, both ‘too high’ and ‘too low’ uNK cells have been demonstrated to be harmful and a mechanism of action is yet to be precisely determined (**76**). The concept of ‘high’ uterine NK cell levels being associated with implantation failure led to the clinical introduction of measuring peripheral natural killer cells. Since, the measurement of peripheral natural killer cells in the serum has been demonstrated to not correlate with endometrial NK cells (**77, 78**). Of note, a meta-analysis of studies that evaluated peripheral and uterine natural killer cells in infertile versus fertile women showed no significant difference in predicting success (**79**). However, they did report higher levels in women with recurrent miscarriage (**79**). Patients are occasionally treated with therapies such as intravenous intralipid, steroids or other immunomodulatory drugs. The cellular mechanisms by which intralipids act are not fully understood, they are hypothesised to reduce the number of uNK cells. Their use remains controversial as there is a paucity of good quality evidence. It has been suggested that corticosteroids improve the uterine environment either by modulating uNK cells or altering cytokine activity. In a recent meta-analysis steroids use failed to improve live birth outcomes in 5 trials with 636 participants in the general infertility populations and no RCTs have been undertaken in the RIF population (**80**). A Cochrane review of twenty trials looked specifically at immunotherapy in those with recurrent miscarriage (not solely raised NK cells) and found there was no beneficial effect on the live birth rate over placebo (**81**). To summarise, there is a lack of consensus over the importance of raised natural killer cells, a reference range is yet to be defined and further studies are needed.

There may be an immune aetiology to recurrent implantation failures in some patients due to errors with the adaptive response, in particular the tolerance of the invasion of semi-allogenic material. The balance between type 1 helper T cells (Th1) and type 2 (Th2) has been studied for many years. These cells secrete distinct sets of cytokines, for example Th1 cells produce inflammatory cytokines such as interferon (IFN-y and IFN-a), promoting a cell mediated immunity compared to the humoral immunity induced by Th2 cells (**82, 83**). Several studies have demonstrated that successful pregnancy is associated with a predominant Th2 type immunity, while Th1 is associated with recurrent miscarriage (**7, 84**). Certain ratios such as IFN-y/IL4 ratio of ≥ 11.8 have been identified as being an indication for immunomodulatory therapies (**7, 84**). Such studies are small and reveal heterogenous results, therefore such an approach should strictly be experimental.

Low molecular weight heparins (LMWH) have become a commonly used adjuvant to aid implantation. The mechanisms by which heparin has been proposed to improve implantation are diverse, including the manipulation of certain growth factors (such as IGF-1, IGF-2 and HB-EGF) and improving blood flow. Meta-analysis of two RCTs failed to show a beneficial effect for all clinical outcomes (**85**). In an RCT of 83 women with a history of 3 or more implantation failures and a diagnosis of inherited or acquired thrombophilia, prophylactic LMWH from day of ET to delivery improved all clinical outcomes (**86**). A meta-analysis published in 2013 included three trials and found that in women with 3 or more implantation failures, LMWH significantly improved the clinical pregnancy rate (**87**). Similarly, a Cochrane review by Akhtar et al. (2018) assessed LMWH use in the general IVF population and reported an increase in live birth rate in the intervention group (OR 1.77 (95%CI 1.07–2.9, 3 RCTs, 386) (**88**). Whilst the evidence is mostly rated as low or very low-grade evidence, many clinicians see it as a valuable therapy in those patients with RIF. Aspirin was thought to work in a similar fashion, however no RCT’s (13 RCTs, 2653 participants) have demonstrated a benefit on live birth rate or ongoing pregnancy rate in the general IVF population or in the context of RIF (**89, 90**). In fact, there is a trend to it having a negative effect on live birth outcomes when 3 studies including 1053 participants were meta-analysed (OR 0.89 95% CI 0.66–1.19, moderate quality evidence) (**80, 90**)

A final barrier to implantation to be considered are fibroids and polyps, diagnosed on pelvic ultrasound. Fibroids are the most common benign tumour in women of reproductive age, prevalent in 20–50% of the population (**91**). Endometrial polyps have a similar prevalence and often present with intermenstrual bleeding; their effect on fertility is even more unclear. Proposed mechanisms by which polyps contribute to subfertility are: increase in plasma glycodelin concentrations, gland or stromal resistance, local inflammatory changes due to foreign body effects, abnormal vascularity cavity distortion and contractility (**92–94**). Large fibroids can obstruct tubes, result in endometrial atrophy, cause hyperplasia, inflammation, vascular alterations and release growth factors and adhesion molecules (**92, 93**). The evidence to guide management of infertile patients with fibroids is poor (**95**). The published data primarily consist of observational and largely retrospective studies with conflicting results. Subserosal fibroids do not appear to have a detrimental impact on fertility outcomes, whereas intramural fibroids are associated with reduced implantation and live birth rates (**95, 96**). There is insufficient evidence that removal by laparoscopic or abdominal myomectomy is beneficial however, such trials are scare due to difficulties in recruitment and sample size (**95, 96**). As a general approach, fibroids that are large (>5cm), symptomatic and the patient has otherwise unexplained infertility may warrant removal. Polyps can be removed more easily at hysteroscopy prior to IVF.

14.5 Conclusion

This chapter has illustrated the basic physiology involved in preparing the endometrium for implantation, the molecular mechanisms involved in receptivity and the way in which these can be manipulated in ART. It is clear there is great deal that we still do not understand; particular areas for further research include the role of the embryo-endometrium crosstalk, endometrial receptivity and microbiome investigations and the management options for those patients with recurrent implantation failure.

REFERENCES

1. Salamonsen LA, Hutchison JC, Gargett CE. Cyclical endometrial repair and regeneration. *Development*. 2021;148(17).
2. Duffy DM, Ko C, Jo M, et al. Ovulation: parallels with inflammatory processes. *Endocrine Reviews*. 2018;40(2):369–416.
3. Sang Y, Li Y, Xu L, et al. Regulatory mechanisms of endometrial decidualization and pregnancy-related diseases. *Acta Biochim Biophys Sin (Shanghai)*. 2020;52(2):105–115.
4. Oreshkova T, Dimitrov R, Mourdjeva M. A cross-talk of decidual stromal cells, trophoblast, and immune cells: a prerequisite for the success of pregnancy. *Am J Reprod Immunol*. 2012;68(5):366–373.
5. Bourdiec A, Ahmad SF, Lachhab A, et al. Regulation of inflammatory and angiogenesis mediators in a functional model of decidualized endometrial stromal cells. *Reprod Biomed Online*. 2016;32(1):85–95.
6. Yang H-L, Zhou W-J, Lu H, et al. Decidual stromal cells promote the differentiation of CD56brightCD16–NK cells by secreting IL-24 in early pregnancy. *Am J Reprod Immunol*. 2019;81(6):e13110.
7. Winger EE, Reed JL, Ashoush S, et al. Elevated preconception CD56+ 16+ and/or Th1:Th2 levels predict benefit from IVIG therapy in subfertile women undergoing IVF. *Am J Reprod Immunol*. 2011;66(5):394–403.
8. Ujvari D, Jakson I, Oldmark C, et al. Prokineticin 1 is upregulated by insulin in decidualizing human endometrial stromal cells. *J Cell Mol Med*. 2018;22(1):163–172.
9. Matsui N, Kawano Y, Nakamura S, et al. Changes in vascular endothelial growth factor production associated with decidualization by human endometrial stromal cells in vitro. *Acta Obstet Gynecol Scand*. 2004;83(2):138–143.
10. Ramsey EM, Houston ML, Harris JW. Interactions of the trophoblast and maternal tissues in three closely related primate species. *Am J Obstet Gynecol*. 1976;124(6):647–652.
11. Navot D, Scott RT, Droesch K, et al. The window of embryo transfer and the efficiency of human conception in vitro. *Fertil Steril*. 1991;55(1):114–118.
12. Domínguez F, Remohí J, Pellicer A, et al. Human endometrial receptivity: a genomic approach. *Reprod Biomed Online*. 2003;6(3):332–338.
13. Lessey BA, Killam AP, Metzger DA, et al. Immunohistochemical analysis of human uterine estrogen and progesterone receptors throughout the menstrual cycle*. *J Clin Endocrinol Metabol*. 1988;67(2):334–340.
14. Dorostghoal M, Ghaffari HO, Marmazi F, et al. Overexpression of endometrial estrogen receptor-alpha in the window of implantation in women with unexplained infertility. *Int J Fertil Steril*. 2018;12(1):37–42.
15. Lessey BA, Palomino WA, Apparao KBC, et al. Estrogen receptor-alpha (ER-alpha) and defects in uterine receptivity in women. *Reprod Biol Endocrinol*. 2006;4(1):S9.
16. Lee DK, Kurihara I, Jeong JW, et al. Suppression of ERalpha activity by COUP-TFII is essential for successful implantation and decidualization. *Mol Endocrinol*. 2010;24(5):930–940.
17. Stavreus-Evers A, Nikas G, Sahlin L, et al. Formation of pinopodes in human endometrium is associated with the concentrations of progesterone and progesterone receptors. *Fertil Steril*. 2001;76(4):782–791.
18. Usadi RS, Murray MJ, Bagnell RC, et al. Temporal and morphologic characteristics of pinopod expression across the secretory phase of the endometrial cycle in normally cycling women with proven fertility. *Fertil Steril*. 2003;79(4):970–974.
19. Adams SM, Gayer N, Hosie MJ, et al. Human uterodomes (pinopods) do not display pinocytotic function. *Hum Reprod*. 2002;17(8):1980–1986.
20. Ashary N, Tiwari A, Modi D. Embryo implantation: war in times of love. *Endocrinology*. 2018;159(2):1188–1198.
21. Ebner T, Maurer M, Shebl O, et al. Planar embryos have poor prognosis in terms of blastocyst formation and implantation. *Reprod Biomed Online*. 2012;25(3):267–272.
22. Lessey BA, Castelbaum AJ, Sawin SW, et al. Integrins as markers of uterine receptivity in women with primary unexplained infertility. *Fertil Steril*. 1995;63(3):535–542.
23. Lipari CW, Zhao Y, King JA, et al. Variations in L-selectin ligand expression in the luteal-phase endometrium after final oocyte maturation with human chorionic gonadotropin compared with a gonadotropin-releasing hormone agonist. *Fertil Steril*. 2008;90(3):876–878.
24. Yamakage S, Oe Y, Sekimoto A, et al. Protease-activated receptor 2 contributes to placental development and fetal growth in mice. *Thrombosis Research*. 2020;193:173–179.
25. Fuchs R, Ellinger I. Endocytic and transcytotic processes in villous syncytiotrophoblast: role in nutrient transport to the human fetus. *Traffic*. 2004;5(10):725–738.
26. Sherer DM, Abulafia O. Angiogenesis during implantation, and placental and early embryonic development. *Placenta*. 2001;22(1):1–13.
27. Lanir N, Aharon A, Brenner B. Haemostatic mechanisms in human placenta. *Best Practice Res Clin Haematol*. 2003;16(2):183–195.
28. Teklenburg G, Salker M, Molokhia M, et al. Natural selection of human embryos: decidualizing endometrial stromal cells serve as sensors of embryo quality upon implantation. *PLoS One*. 2010;5(4):e10258.
29. Teklenburg G, Salker M, Heijnen C, et al. The molecular basis of recurrent pregnancy loss: impaired natural embryo selection. *Mol Hum Reprod*. 2010;16(12):886–895.
30. Genbacev OD, Prakobphol A, Foulk RA, et al. Trophoblast L-selectin-mediated adhesion at the maternal-fetal interface. Science. 2003;299(5605):405–408.

31. Barker DJ. The fetal and infant origins of disease. *Eur J Clin Invest.* 1995;25(7):457–463.
32. Carter AM. Animal models of human pregnancy and placentation: alternatives to the mouse. *Reproduction.* 2020;160(6):R129–R143.
33. Nelissen ECM, van Montfoort APA, Dumoulin JCM, et al. Epigenetics and the placenta. *Hum Reprod Update.* 2010;17(3):397–417.
34. Koukoura O, Sifakis S, Spandidos DA. DNA methylation in the human placenta and fetal growth (review). *Mol Med Rep.* 2012;5(4):883–889.
35. Martinez VD, Cohn DE, Telkar N, et al. Profiling the small non-coding RNA transcriptome of the human placenta. *Sci Data.* 2021;8(1):166.
36. Januar V, Desoye G, Novakovic B, et al. Epigenetic regulation of human placental function and pregnancy outcome: considerations for causal inference. *Am J Obstet Gynecol.* 2015;213(4):S182–S196.
37. Moffett-King A. Natural killer cells and pregnancy. *Nat Rev Immunol.* 2002;2(9):656–663.
38. Zulu MZ, Martinez FO, Gordon S, et al. The elusive role of placental macrophages: the Hofbauer cell. *J Innate Immun.* 2019;11(6):447–456.
39. Venetis C, Kolibianakis E, Bosdou J, et al. Progesterone elevation and probability of pregnancy after IVF: a systematic review and meta-analysis of over 60 000 cycles. *Hum Reprod Update.* 2013;19(5):433–457.
40. Edwards RG. Human implantation: the last barrier in assisted reproduction technologies? *Reprod Biomed Online.* 2006;13(6):887–904.
41. Liu K, Hartman M, Hartman A, et al. The impact of a thin endometrial lining on fresh and frozen – thaw IVF outcomes: an analysis of over 40 000 embryo transfers. *Hum Reprod.* 2018;33(10):1883–1888.
42. Hershko-Klement A, Tepper R. Ultrasound in assisted reproduction: a call to fill the endometrial gap. *Fertil Steril.* 2016;105(6):1394–1402. e4.
43. Melo P, Chung Y, Pickering O, et al. Serum luteal phase progesterone in women undergoing frozen embryo transfer in assisted conception: a systematic review and meta-analysis. *Fertil Steril.* 2021;116(6):1534–1556.
44. Díaz-Gimeno P, Ruiz-Alonso M, Blesa D, et al. The accuracy and reproducibility of the endometrial receptivity array is superior to histology as a diagnostic method for endometrial receptivity. *Fertil Steril.* 2013;99(2):508–517.
45. Cozzolino M, Diaz-Gimeno P, Pellicer A, et al. Evaluation of the endometrial receptivity assay and the preimplantation genetic test for aneuploidy in overcoming recurrent implantation failure. *J Assist Reprod Genet.* 2020;37(12):2989–2997.
46. Díaz-Gimeno P, Ruiz-Alonso M, Blesa D, et al. The accuracy and reproducibility of the endometrial receptivity array is superior to histology as a diagnostic method for endometrial receptivity. *Fertil Steril.* 2013;99(2):508–517.
47. Simón C, Gómez C, Cabanillas S, et al. A 5-year multicentre randomized controlled trial comparing personalized, frozen and fresh blastocyst transfer in IVF. *Reprod Biomed Online.* 2020;41(3):402–415.
48. Díaz-Gimeno P, Ruiz-Alonso M, Sebastian-Leon P, et al. Window of implantation transcriptomic stratification reveals different endometrial subsignatures associated with live birth and biochemical pregnancy. *Fertil Steril.* 2017;108(4): 703–710. e3.
49. Ruiz-Alonso M, Blesa D, Díaz-Gimeno P, et al. The endometrial receptivity array for diagnosis and personalized embryo transfer as a treatment for patients with repeated implantation failure. *Fertil Steril.* 2013;100(3):818–824.
50. Hashimoto T, Koizumi M, Doshida M, et al. Efficacy of the endometrial receptivity array for repeated implantation failure in Japan: a retrospective, two-centers study. *Reprod Med Biol.* 2017;16(3):290–296.
51. Mahajan N. Endometrial receptivity array: clinical application. *J Hum Reprod Sci.* 2015;8(3):121–129.
52. Tan J, Kan A, Hitkari J, et al. The role of the endometrial receptivity array (ERA) in patients who have failed euploid embryo transfers. *J Assist Reprod Genet.* 2018;35(4):683–692.
53. Jia Y, Sha Y, Qiu Z, et al. Comparison of the effectiveness of endometrial receptivity analysis (ERA) to guide personalized embryo transfer with conventional frozen embryo transfer in 281 Chinese women with recurrent implantation failure. *Med Sci Monit.* 2022;28:e935634-1.
54. Liu Z, Liu X, Wang M, et al. The clinical efficacy of personalized embryo transfer guided by the endometrial receptivity array/analysis on IVF/ICSI outcomes: a systematic review and meta-analysis. *Front Physiol.* 2022;13:841437.
55. Macklon N. Recurrent implantation failure is a pathology with a specific transcriptomic signature. *Fertil Steril.* 2017;108(1):9–14.
56. Garcia-Velasco JA, Fassbender A, Ruiz-Alonso M, et al. Is endometrial receptivity transcriptomics affected in women with endometriosis? A pilot study. *Reprod Biomed Online.* 2015;31(5):647–654.
57. Stankewicz T, Valbuena D, Ruiz-Alonso M. Inter-cycle consistency versus test compliance in endometrial receptivity analysis test. *J Assist Reprod Genet.* 2018;35(7):1307–1308.
58. Cho K, Tan S, Buckett W, et al. Intra-patient variability in the endometrial receptivity assay (ERA) test. *J Assist Reprod Genet.* 2018;35(5):929–930.
59. Baum M, Yerushalmi GM, Maman E, et al. Does local injury to the endometrium before IVF cycle really affect treatment outcome? Results of a randomized placebo controlled trial. *Gynecol Endocrinol.* 2012;28(12):933–936.
60. Gürgan T, Kalem Z, Kalem MN, et al. Systematic and standardized hysteroscopic endometrial injury for treatment of recurrent implantation failure. *Reprod Biomed Online.* 2019;39(3):477–483.
61. Olesen MS, Hauge B, Ohrt L, et al. Therapeutic endometrial scratching and implantation after in vitro fertilization: a multicenter randomized controlled trial. *Fertil Steril.* 2019;112(6):1015–1021.
62. van Hoogenhuijze NE, Mol F, Laven JSE, et al. Endometrial scratching in women with one failed IVF/ICSI cycle-outcomes of a randomised controlled trial (SCRaTCH). *Hum Reprod.* 2021;36(1):87–98.
63. Ravel J, Gajer P, Abdo Z, et al. Vaginal microbiome of reproductive-age women. *Proc Natl Acad Sci USA.* 2011;108(Suppl. 1):4680–4687.
64. Babu G, Singaravelu BG, Srikumar R, et al. Comparative study on the vaginal flora and incidence of asymptomatic vaginosis among healthy women and in women with infertility problems of reproductive age. *J Clin Diagn Res.* 2017;11(8):DC18–DC22.

65. Eckert LO, Moore DE, Patton DL, et al. Relationship of vaginal bacteria and inflammation with conception and early pregnancy loss following in-vitro fertilization. *Infect Dis Obstetr Gynecol.* 2003;11(1):11–17.
66. Mangot-Bertrand J, Fenollar F, Bretelle F, et al. Molecular diagnosis of bacterial vaginosis: impact on IVF outcome. *Eur J Clin Microbiol Infect Dis.* 2013;32(4):535–541.
67. Moreno I, Codoñer FM, Vilella F, et al. Evidence that the endometrial microbiota has an effect on implantation success or failure. *Am J Obstet Gynecol.* 2016;215(6):684–703.
68. Koedooder R, Singer M, Schoenmakers S, et al. The vaginal microbiome as a predictor for outcome of in vitro fertilization with or without intracytoplasmic sperm injection: a prospective study. *Hum Reprod.* 2019;34(6):1042–1054.
69. Haahr T, Jensen JS, Thomsen L, et al. Abnormal vaginal microbiota may be associated with poor reproductive outcomes: a prospective study in IVF patients. *Hum Reprod.* 2016;31(4):795–803.
70. Moreno-Gallego JL, Chou S-P, Di Rienzi SC, et al. Virome diversity correlates with intestinal microbiome diversity in adult monozygotic twins. *Cell Host Microb.* 2019;25(2):261–272. e5.
71. Moreno I, Garcia-Grau I, Perez-Villaroya D, et al. Endometrial microbiota composition is associated with reproductive outcome in infertile patients. *Microbiome.* 2022;10:1–17.
72. Cicinelli E, Matteo M, Tinelli R, et al. Prevalence of chronic endometritis in repeated unexplained implantation failure and the IVF success rate after antibiotic therapy. *Hum Reprod.* 2014;30(2):323–330.
73. King A, Loke YW. On the nature and function of human uterine granular lymphocytes. *Immunol Today.* 1991;12(12):432–435.
74. Hanna J, Goldman-Wohl D, Hamani Y, et al. Decidual NK cells regulate key developmental processes at the human fetal-maternal interface. *Nature Med.* 2006;12(9):1065–1074.
75. Lash GE, Schiessl B, Kirkley M, et al. Expression of angiogenic growth factors by uterine natural killer cells during early pregnancy. *J Leukocyte Biol.* 2006;80(3):572–580.
76. Woon EV, Day A, Bracewell-Milnes T, et al. Immunotherapy to improve pregnancy outcome in women with abnormal natural killer cell levels/activity and recurrent miscarriage or implantation failure: a systematic review and meta-analysis. *J Reprod Immunol.* 2020;142:103189.
77. Laird SM, Mariee N, Wei L, et al. Measurements of CD56+ cells in peripheral blood and endometrium by flow cytometry and immunohistochemical staining in situ. *Hum Reprod.* 2011;26(6):1331–1337.
78. Huhn O, Zhao X, Esposito L, et al. How do uterine natural killer and innate lymphoid cells contribute to successful pregnancy? *Front Immunol.* 2021;12.
79. Seshadri S, Sunkara SK. Natural killer cells in female infertility and recurrent miscarriage: a systematic review and meta-analysis. *Hum Reprod Update.* 2014;20(3):429–438.
80. Holt-Kentwell A, Ghosh J, Devall A, et al. Evaluating interventions and adjuncts to optimize pregnancy outcomes in subfertile women: an overview review. *Hum Reprod Update.* 2022 Jun;28(4):583–600.
81. Wong LF, Porter TF, Scott JR. Immunotherapy for recurrent miscarriage. *Cochrane Database Syst Rev.* 2014(10).
82. Chaouat G. The Th1/Th2 paradigm: still important in pregnancy? *Semin Immunopathol.* 2007;29(2):95–113.
83. Lee S, Kim J, Hur S, et al. An imbalance in interleukin-17-producing T and Foxp3+ regulatory T cells in women with idiopathic recurrent pregnancy loss. *Hum Reprod.* 2011;26(11):2964–2971.
84. Kuroda K, Nakagawa K, Horikawa T, et al. Increasing number of implantation failures and pregnancy losses associated with elevated Th1/Th2 cell ratio. *Am J Reprod Immunol.* 2021;86(3):e13429.
85. Busnelli A, Somigliana E, Cirillo F, et al. Efficacy of therapies and interventions for repeated embryo implantation failure: a systematic review and meta-analysis. *Sci Rep.* 2021;11(1):1747.
86. Qublan H, Amarin Z, Dabbas M, et al. Low-molecular-weight heparin in the treatment of recurrent IVF – ET failure and thrombophilia: a prospective randomized placebo-controlled trial. *Hum Fertil.* 2008;11(4):246–253.
87. Potdar N, Gelbaya TA, Konje JC, et al. Adjunct low-molecular-weight heparin to improve live birth rate after recurrent implantation failure: a systematic review and meta-analysis. *Hum Reprod Update.* 2013;19(6):674–684.
88. Akhtar F, Wan X, Wu G, et al. Low-molecular-weight heparins: reduced size particulate systems for improved therapeutic outcomes. *Molecules.* 2018;23(7):1757.
89. Achilli C, Duran-Retamal M, Saab W, et al. The role of immunotherapy in in vitro fertilization: a guideline. *Fertil Steril.* 2018;110(3):387–400.
90. Siristatidis CS, Basios G, Pergialiotis V, et al. Aspirin for in vitro fertilisation. *Cochrane Database Syst Rev.* 2016 Nov;11(11):CD004832.
91. Downes E, Sikirica V, Gilabert-Estelles J, et al. The burden of uterine fibroids in five European countries. *Eur J Obstet Gynecol Reprod Biol.* 2010;152(1):96–102.
92. Ciarmela P, Islam MS, Reis FM, et al. Growth factors and myometrium: biological effects in uterine fibroid and possible clinical implications. *Hum Reprod Update.* 2011;17(6):772–790.
93. Purohit P, Vigneswaran K. Fibroids and infertility. *Curr Obstet Gynecol Rep.* 2016;5(2):81–88.
94. Munro MG. Uterine polyps, adenomyosis, leiomyomas, and endometrial receptivity. *Fertil Steril.* 2019;111(4):629–640.
95. Metwally M, Raybould G, Cheong YC, et al. Surgical treatment of fibroids for subfertility. *Cochrane Database Syst Rev.* 2020 Jan;1(1):CD003857.
96. Somigliana E, Vercellini P, Daguati R, et al. Fibroids and female reproduction: a critical analysis of the evidence. *Hum Reprod Update.* 2007;13(5):465–476.

15

Fetal Development and Sex Differentiation

Juan Hernandez-Medrano

15.1 Introduction

Sexual reproduction is based on the production of two different gametes with a complementary number of chromosomes that allows a species to proliferate and survive. During early embryo or fetal development, tissues associated with the reproductive function in the adult are sexually undifferentiated. Following a series of linked but independent events, differentiation of male and female gonads drive differentiation of the associated reproductive tissues and organs, culminating in the recognised male and female reproductive phenotypes and behaviours. Sexual differentiation can be separated into 1) sex determination that occurs at the time of fertilization when a zygote XX or XY is generated; 2) gonadal differentiation; 3) associated reproductive organ and tissue differentiation; and 4) hypothalamic differentiation. Most of the knowledge about sexual differentiation in humans has been generated and extrapolated from research carried out in animal models, i.e., rodents and sheep. Although the process is very similar, there are still some between species differences that are important to point out. Here we will attempt to present the general process of sexual differentiation and point out these species differences where information is available.

15.2 Sexual Determination

The precursor of the gonads, gonadal ridges, are present in the fetus during early pregnancy i.e., around day 32–40 in humans (**1, 2**). These structures contain precursor cells that will give rise to the somatic gonadal support (i.e., Sertoli and Granulosa) and steroidogenic cells (i.e., Leydig and Theca), and the primordial germ cells (PGCs). Recent studies using a single-cell approach, have determined that coelomic epithelial cells expressing GATA4, SF1 and WT1 seem to be the precursors of the supporting and steroidogenic gonadal cells (**1**). The PGCs originate in the yolk sac near the base of the allantois and migrate through the dorsal mesentery towards the gonadal ridges (**1**). The influence of the PGC on gonadal differentiation is sex-dependent because their absence in the bipotential gonads does not inhibit testes but is required for ovarian differentiation (**3**). This indicates that differentiation is mainly driven by the somatic supporting cells that are present in the undifferentiated gonad.

As in all eutherian species, in humans, sexual differentiation is determined by the establishment of genetic sex at fertilization, through X and Y chromosomes, process known as sext determination (**4, 5**). The presence of the male-specific gene SRY (Sex-Determining Region of the Y chromosome) is necessary to start the cascade of events that drives the differentiation of the gonadal ridges into the male gonad and phenotype, while the absence of SRY results in the formation of an ovary and a female phenotype (**4–6**).

15.3 Gonadal Differentiation: Testis

In mice and humans, it has been reported that SRY is expressed in somatic cells of the developing undifferentiated gonad around days 10.5 and 40–45, respectively (**2, 7**). SRY protein expression upregulates the synthesis of the transcription factor SOX-9 protein (**5, 8**) necessary to differentiate the supporting cells into Sertoli cells rather than granulosa cells (**6, 8**). Furthermore, an autocrine feed-forward loop is established within these pre-Sertoli cells via fibroblast growth factor-9 (FGF-9) and its receptor (FGFR2), which up-regulates synthesis of SOX-9, further supporting male differentiation of other pre-Sertoli cells and other cell types (**9**). A threshold number of pre-Sertoli cells are required to express SRY to ensure testis differentiation. Furthermore, a timely and dose manner expression of the downstream factors, i.e, SOX-9 and FGF-9, is needed to maintain testis differentiation (**9**). In mice, a 6-hour window following initial activation of SRY expression is necessary to maintain SOX9/FGF9 levels, if this window passes testicular development is compromised (**10**). This indicates that gonadal differentiation can be halted or regressed if the signals involved in the process are not produced adequately.

Differentiating Sertoli cells produce Anti-Mullerian Hormone (AMH) which drives the differentiation of the Leydig cells in the interstitial portion of the developing testis (**4, 5, 8**). In humans and mice, several factors have been implicated in Leydig cell differentiation such as the Dessert Hedgehog molecule produced by the pre-Sertoli cells (**11**) and the steroidogenic factor 1 (SF1), present during Leydig cell differentiation (**12**). In addition to Leydig cells, germ cells also follow a different pathway depending on the sex (**5**). In the mouse ovary, germ cells enter meiosis at day 13.5 of gestation after a period of mitosis, but in the male these cells are arrested as soon as mitosis concludes, associated to testosterone production (**4, 5**). This difference is not related to chromosomal sex but due to the gonadal environment present at the time of gonadal differentiation and development (**4, 5**). Therefore, factors and hormones produced during fetal gonadal development

DOI: 10.1201/9781003269502-15

may drive sexual differentiation of the gonads and other associated reproductive tissues.

Testicular differentiation is also influenced by vascular development. Around fetal day 50 in humans, the undifferentiated gonad develops into two compartments: the testicular cords and the interstitial tissue (**1**). These compartments host the Sertoli and the Leydig cells, respectively. However, the separation is intrinsically linked to vascularisation development driven by Vascular Endothelial Growth Factor A (VEGF A) and the Platelet-derived Growth Factor B (PDGF B) (**1**). The interplay between these factors drives the formation of the coelomic vessel, an arterial vessel unique to the testis (**13**). Furthermore, during this period, the Sertoli cells start to link together and enclose the germ cells, giving rise to the testicular cords, precursors of the seminiferous tubules (**1**). The interaction of the Sertoli cells and the myoid peritubular cells initiates the formation of the basal membrane, isolating the cells within the testicular cords.

Early studies in rabbits (**14**) demonstrated that substances produced by the testes were necessary for the development of the male phenotype, since castrated male fetuses developed as female. At least three testicular factors have been reported to participate in gonadal differentiation: anti-Müllerian hormone (AMH), testosterone and Insulin-like Factor 3 (ILF-3) (**5**). Anti-Müllerian hormone is one of the earliest factors produced by the pre-Sertoli cells (as mentioned above) and it induces the involution of the Müllerian ducts (**5, 12**). Testosterone and ILF-3 are produced in the Leydig cells (**5, 15**). In fact, steroidogenic enzymes are present during early seminiferous tubules formation (**5**) with testosterone production initiating around 90 days of gestation in humans. Both factors, testosterone and ILF-3, were reported to be necessary for testicular descent to the scrotum in mice (**15**). Testosterone is involved in the development of male-associated structures, apart from the testis, by inducing the development of the Wolffian ducts that originate the epididymis, vas deferens and seminal vesicles (**5, 16**). In addition, testosterone and/or dihydrotestosterone (DHT) induce the formation of the male urethra and prostate from the urogenital sinus, and the formation of the penis and scrotum from the genital tubercule and urethral fold, respectively (**5, 16**). As described in the above information, male sexual development is an "active" process that involves the expression and synthesis of different genes and factors, however ovarian development seems to be blocked once SRY expression occurs which indicated that differentiation is a balance between pro-male and pro-female factors.

15.4 Gonadal Differentiation: Ovary

In the absence of expression of SRY and the factors that it induces, the undifferentiated gonad develops into an ovary (**5**). However, this is not a passive process because several genes are necessary for female differentiation of the somatic cells, such as WNT4, β-catenin, R-spondin 1 (RSPO1) and FOXL2 (**17**). In the undifferentiated gonads, WNT4 and FGF9 are expressed similarly in the mesonephric border and the coelomic surface, respectively (**9**). In the absence of SRY expression, RSPO1 and WNT4 are preferentially expressed stimulating β-catenin and FOXL2 expression and a positive feedback loop is established between these factors (**1**). WNT4/β-catenin and FOXL2 inhibit expression of SOX9 and FGF9, actively blocking the male differentiation pathway and blocking steroidogenic enzymes, such as 3 β hydroxy-steroid dehydrogenase, inhibiting testosterone production (**9, 17**).

Early ovarian formation in humans has two features, the functional differentiation, i.e., oestradiol production, and morphological differentiation, i.e., follicular formation. Around day 60 of pregnancy, most of the characteristic structures of the ovary are present (**18**). Human ovarian development is still under investigation, but it is believed that follows a process similar to that described in ruminant species such as sheep and cattle (**18**).

In cattle and humans, the structures that originate primordial follicles (i.e., ovigerous cords) start to develop in the fetal ovary around day 50–60 of pregnancy (**19**). The ovigerous cords contain pre-granulosa cells recruited from the epithelial surface cells of the early ovary (**18–20**). In cattle, ovigerous cords are separate from the rest of the ovary but open to the surface epithelium until approximately day 150 and are no longer evident at days 190–210 of gestation (**19, 21**). In cattle and humans, these structures contain germ cells (oogonia) that are undergoing rapid proliferation by mitosis (**19, 22**). Germ cells proliferate by mitosis and transform into oogonias. In cattle, the number of germ cells or oogonias was reported to increase from ~16,000 at day 50 to ~2.5 million at day 110 (**23**), while in humans a similar number of oocytes is reported at term (**1**). Around day 70 in humans and day 90 in cattle, oogonias enter meiosis and start recruiting cells to form primordial follicles. Fully formed primordial follicles containing an oocyte arrested in prophase I are visible between 105–110 days of pregnancy in humans and cattle (**18, 19, 24**), which coincides with the onset of apoptosis that dramatically reduces the number of germ cells (**1, 20, 24**). Nevertheless, apoptosis only occurs in germ cells but not in pre-granulosa cells, which associate with the remaining germ cells to form the primordial follicles, as observed in sheep (**20**).

Formation of primordial follicles also coincides with a reduction in the oestradiol concentrations (**19, 21, 25**), processes that are thought to trigger primordial follicle formation (**26, 27**). In cattle, there is an interval of 20–50 days (depending on the study) between the appearance of primordial and primary follicles, which are visible between day 90 and 140 of gestation in the fetal ovary (**21, 24, 25**). In cattle, this delay in the progress from primordial to primary follicle was associated with the stage of meiosis, because primordial follicles containing oocytes in pre-diplotene stage were not able to activate into primary follicles until the oocyte was arrested in the diplotene stage of prophase I (**25**). In addition, steroids have also been implicated in the activation of primordial follicles, since addition of oestrogen and progesterone to *in vitro* cultured fetal ovarian explants blocked the formation and activation of primary follicles in cattle (**25**) and rodents (**27**). After primordial follicles are activated to progress to the primary follicle stage, the latter follicles further differentiate into secondary, preantral and antral follicles following processes similar to those during post-puberty.

It is important to point out that although ovarian differentiation in mice shows similar processes to those described above for humans and cattle, the formation of primordial follicles in this species takes place after birth (Figure 15.1). This is an important research advantage because it allows the exploration and manipulation of the mechanisms involved in primordial follicle formation.

Although granulosa cells from growing follicles in the fetal ovary are able to produce AMH, the amount is lower than that released by the fetal testis. This lower concentration of AMH, allows the proliferation of the Müllerian ducts that give rise to the oviduct, uterus and anterior portion of the vagina in female fetuses (**16**). If fetuses are treated with testosterone during early stages of gonadal development, the presence of male-associated tissues and characteristics were observed in female mice (**5**), sheep (**28**) and cattle (**29, 30**). Therefore, it seems that in the absence of AMH and testosterone, the undifferentiated gonad becomes an ovary and originates the formation of female reproductive organs.

15.5 Hypothalamic Sex Differentiation: GnRH Release

The development of the reproductive axis (i.e., hypothalamus-pituitary-gonadal axis) follows a hierarchic order, this means that the higher level of the axis develops first (**31**). The GnRH neurones arise from the olfactory placode, and during early embryogenesis they migrate along the pathway of the nervus terminalis-vomeronasal complex to their final location in the forebrain, ventral telencephalic and diencephalic areas in the adult animal (**32, 33**). In the mouse, the GnRH-producing neurones are first observed at day 11 of gestation and they begin the migration from the olfactory bulb to the hypothalamus at day 17 to 19 (**31**). At this stage of fetal development, the hypothalamus is sexually undifferentiated.

Similar to the gonadal, hypothalamic sex differentiation (i.e., GnRH release) also occurred during fetal life and involves two complementary processes: masculinization and defeminisation. Masculinisation refers to the organisation of hypothalamic centres to display male reproductive behaviors and the pulsatile release of GnRH, while defeminisation corresponds to the inactivation of female reproductive behaviours and GnRH surge activity (**34, 35**). In humans, hypothalamic differentiation initiates around day 70–90 and remains open until day 160–170 of gestation (**36**). However, brain sexual differentiation can continue postnatally driven by rises in testosterone and oestradiol concentration in boys and girls, respectively, during this period (**36**).

Sexual differentiation occurs in different neuronal hypothalamic nuclei that are central to reproductive regulation in males and females during a specific window of development. In rodents, several regions of the hypothalamus associated to reproductive control (i.e., GnRH release) have been described to differ between male and female individuals such as preoptic area, ventromedial nucleus, arcuate nucleus and spinal nucleus of the bulbocavernosus (**5, 35**). In sheep, it has been proposed that there is a difference in the signals that arrive at the GnRH neurones at the ventromedial nucleus since these cells have twice the number of synaptic contacts in females than in male lambs, and *in utero* testosterone-treated ewe lambs show a reduction in the number of synapses (**37**). Therefore, it is evident that androgens and/or oestrogens cause a differential organisation of the hypothalamic tissue; therefore, incoming information from the body is integrated differently, inducing a different response in female than in male animals (**38**). Most of the information regarding sexual differentiation of the hypothalamic GnRH system has been obtained in rodents and sheep models, whether a similar mechanism occurs in cattle, remains to be elucidated.

High concentrations of testosterone are central to hypothalamic differentiation. Paradoxically, the hormone causing the masculinisation and defeminisation of hypothalamic nuclei is not testosterone, but its metabolite: oestradiol (**36**). Testosterone needs to be transformed into oestradiol by the aromatase enzyme (P450arom) present within the hypothalamic tissue in order to exert its "defeminising" effects (**39, 40**). This was confirmed in sheep where treatment with DHT, a non-aromatizable androgen, failed to "defeminise" the hypothalamus (**28**). Similar to gonadal sex, the control

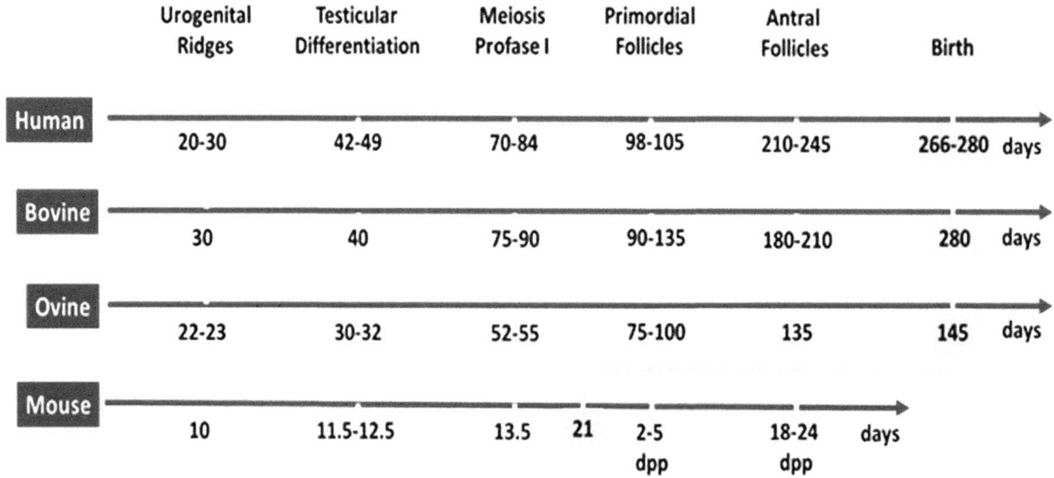

FIGURE 15.1 Some of the events occurring during fetal ovarian development in different model species. (dpp = days postpartum).

of GnRH release is believed to be female by default, because the absence of testosterone or its functional signalling (lack of androgen receptors or aromatase activity) results in feminisation of the hypothalamus, i.e., the establishment of the GnRH surge centre and organisational pathways associated to female reproductive behaviours (**28, 36, 38**). Fetal sheep treated with testosterone during the critical period of hypothalamic differentiation (30–60 days), showed a reduced GnRH/LH pulsatile release in response to oestradiol and altered negative steroidal feedback regulating this release (**41–43**). However, in primates (**44**), recent evidence suggested that oestradiol may not be solely responsible for masculinisation of the hypothalamus, but a direct effect of testosterone may be involved (**36**). Due to restrictions to studying hypothalamic differentiation experimentally in humas, most of the research available has been generated post-mortem, so the basic physiological mechanisms for this process remain to be fully elucidated in this species.

Recent studies, mostly in rodents, have questioned the role of steroids, i.e., testosterone/oestradiol, as unique drivers for sexual differentiation of the hypothalamic nuclei. Thanks to rodent models where SRY has been translocated to somatic chromosomes (**45**) dissociating sex differentiation from sex chromosomes, it has been described that the presence and dose of X and Y chromosomes can cause differential development of certain brain cell populations and regions (**46**). These findings point towards an effect of sex chromosomes on sexual differentiation in early stages of embryo and fetal development, even before gonadal differentiation and steroidal production. This theory does not necessarily contradict the steroid-centric theory but may be complementary to it, because the steroid effects are largely organisational.

15.6 Conclusion

Sex differentiation is not a simple or single process, but a series of concatenated events that culminate in phenotypic and behavioural sex: chromosomal sex determination, gonadal differentiation, reproductive organ differentiation and hypothalamic differentiation. Initial chromosomal sex determination drives the expression of SRY in male fetuses causing a series of events resulting in the formation of the testes and the male-associated reproductive organs. Conversely, ovarian differentiation, although initially thought of as a passive process, it is as complex as testes formation. Moreover, it is clear that gonadal differentiation, and by implication reproductive organ and hypothalamic differentiation, is a balancing act where male and female factors battle to keep each under control to allow the formation of the gonads corresponding to the chromosomal sex. However, the processes mentioned above are not deterministic, when expression of factors occurs at the wrong time or at lower concentrations than those required, sex differentiation can be derailed causing mismatch between the components of the reproductive axis.

Most of the knowledge about sex differentiation has been generate in model species, showing the robustness of this process across species. Although mostly similar to humans, there are still gaps in the knowledge about human sexual differentiation that needs to be investigated before a full picture emerges.

REFERENCES

1. Rey R, Josso N, Racine C. Sexual differentiation. In: Feingold KR, Anawalt B, Boyce A, et al., editors. *Endotext*. South Dartmouth, MA: MDText.com, Inc.; 2020.
2. Lundgaard Riis M, Jorgensen A. Deciphering sex-specific differentiation of human fetal gonads: insight from experimental models. *Front Cell Dev Biol*. 2022;10:902082.
3. Svingen T, Koopman P. Building the mammalian testis: origins, differentiation, and assembly of the component cell populations. *Genes Dev*. 2013;27(22):2409–2426.
4. Kocer A, Reichmann J, Best D, et al. Germ cell sex determination in mammals. *Mol Hum Reprod*. 2009;15(4):205–213.
5. Swain A. Sex determination and differentiation. In: Knobil E, Neill JD, editors. *Knobil and Neill's Physiology of Reproduction, vol. 1*. 3rd Edition. Philadelphia, USA: Academic Press; 2006. pp. 245–260.
6. Koopman P, Gubbay J, Vivian N, et al. Male development of chromosomally female mice transgenic for SRY. *Nature*. 1991;351(6322):117–121.
7. Hacker A, Capel B, Goodfellow P, et al. Expression of SRY, the mouse sex determining gene. *Development*. 1995;121(6):1603–1614.
8. Sekido R, Lovell-Badge R. Sex determination and SRY: down to a wink and a nudge? *Trends Genet*. 2009;25(1):19–29.
9. Kim Y, Kobayashi A, Sekido R, et al. Fgf9 and Wnt4 act as antagonistic signals to regulate mammalian sex determination. *PLoS Biol*. 2006;4(6):e187.
10. Jager RJ, Anvret M, Hall K, et al. A human XY female with a frame shift mutation in the candidate testis-determining gene SRY. *Nature*. 1990;348(6300):452–454.
11. Yao HH, DiNapoli L, Capel B. Meiotic germ cells antagonize mesonephric cell migration and testis cord formation in mouse gonads. *Development*. 2003;130(24):5895–5902.
12. Shen WH, Moore CC, Ikeda Y, et al. Nuclear receptor steroidogenic factor 1 regulates the mullerian inhibiting substance gene: a link to the sex determination cascade. *Cell*. 1994;77(5):651–661.
13. Brennan J, Tilmann C, Capel B. Pdgfr-alpha mediates testis cord organization and fetal Leydig cell development in the XY gonad. *Genes Dev*. 2003;17(6):800–810.
14. Jost A, Perlman S, Magre S. The initial stages of testicular differentiation in the rabbit fetus. *Arch Anat Microsc Morphol Exp*. 1985;74(1):69–75.
15. Zimmermann S, Schottler P, Engel W, et al. Mouse Leydig insulin-like (Ley I-L) gene: structure and expression during testis and ovary development. *Mol Reprod Dev*. 1997;47(1):30–38.
16. Parker KL, Schimmer BP. Embryology and genetics of the mammalian gonads and ducts. In: Knobil E, Neill JD, editors. *Knobil and Neill's Physiology of Reproduction, vol. 1*. 3rd Edition. Philadelphia, USA: Academic Press; 2006. pp. 313–336.
17. Chassot AA, Ranc F, Gregoire EP, et al. Activation of beta-catenin signaling by Rspo1 controls differentiation of the mammalian ovary. *Hum Mol Genet*. 2008;17(9):1264–1277.
18. Nicol B, Estermann MA, Yao HH, et al. Becoming female: ovarian differentiation from an evolutionary perspective. *Front Cell Dev Biol*. 2022;10:944776.
19. Garverick HA, Juengel JL, Smith P, et al. Development of the ovary and ontongeny of mRNA and protein for P450 aromatase (arom) and estrogen receptors (ER) alpha and

beta during early fetal life in cattle. *Anim Reprod Sci.* 2010;117(1–2):24–33.
20. Sawyer HR, Smith P, Heath DA, et al. Formation of ovarian follicles during fetal development in sheep. *Biol Reprod.* 2002;66(4):1134–1150.
21. Burkhart MN, Juengel JL, Smith PR, et al. Morphological development and characterization of aromatase and estrogen receptors alpha and beta in fetal ovaries of cattle from days 110 to 250. *Anim Reprod Sci.* 2010;117(1–2):43–54.
22. Juengel JL, Sawyer HR, Smith PR, et al. Origins of follicular cells and ontogeny of steroidogenesis in ovine fetal ovaries. *Mol Cell Endocrinol.* 2002;191(1):1–10.
23. Erickson BH. Development and senescence of the postnatal bovine ovary. *J Anim Sci.* 1966;25(3):800–805.
24. Tanaka Y, Nakada K, Moriyoshi M, et al. Appearance and number of follicles and change in the concentration of serum FSH in female bovine fetuses. *Reproduction.* 2001;121(5):777–782.
25. Yang MY, Fortune JE. The capacity of primordial follicles in fetal bovine ovaries to initiate growth in vitro develops during mid-gestation and is associated with meiotic arrest of oocytes. *Biol Reprod.* 2008;78(6):1153–1161.
26. McNatty KP, Reader K, Smith P, et al. Control of ovarian follicular development to the gonadotrophin-dependent phase: a 2006 perspective. *Soc Reprod Fertil Suppl.* 2007;64:55–68.
27. Kezele P, Skinner MK. Regulation of ovarian primordial follicle assembly and development by estrogen and progesterone: endocrine model of follicle assembly. *Endocrinology.* 2003;144(8):3329–3337.
28. Robinson J. Prenatal programming of the female reproductive neuroendocrine system by androgens. *Reproduction.* 2006;132(4):539–547.
29. Ford JJ, D'Occhio MJ. Differentiation of sexual behavior in cattle, sheep and swine. *J Anim Sci.* 1989;67(7):1816–1823.
30. Hamernik DL, McFarland SY, de Avila D, et al. Endocrine and body growth traits in heifers exposed to testosterone-propionate during early fetal development. *J Anim Sci.* 1987;64(6):1858–1866.
31. Huhtaniemi I. Molecular aspects of the ontogeny of the pituitary-gonadal axis. *Reprod Fertil Dev.* 1995;7(5):1025–1035.
32. Caldani M, Antoine M, Batailler M, et al. Ontogeny of GnRH systems. *J Reprod Fertil Suppl.* 1995;49:147–162.
33. Brooks AN, Hagan DM, Sheng C, et al. Prenatal gonadotrophins in the sheep. *Anim Reprod Sci.* 1996;42(1):471–481.
34. McCarthy MM. Sexual differentiation of the brain in man and animals: of relevance to Klinefelter syndrome? *Am J Med Genet C Semin Med Genet.* 2013;163C(1):3–15.
35. Schwarz JM. Chapter 10 – sex and the developing brain. In: Shansky RM, editor. *Sex Differences in the Central Nervous System.* 1st Edition. Oxford, UK: Academic Press; 2016. pp. 221–245.
36. Bakker J. The role of steroid hormones in the sexual differentiation of the human brain. *J Neuroendocrinol.* 2022;34(2):e13050.
37. Kim SJ, Foster DL, Wood RI. Prenatal testosterone masculinizes synaptic input to gonadotropin-releasing hormone neurons in sheep. *Biol Reprod.* 1999;61(3):599–605.
38. Foster DL, Jackson LM, Padmanabhan V. Programming of GnRH feedback controls timing puberty and adult reproductive activity. *Mol Cell Endocrinol.* 2006;254–255:109–119.
39. Peruffo A, Cozzi B, Ballarin C. Ontogenesis of brain aromatase P450 expression in the bovine hypothalamus. *Brain Res Bull.* 2008;75(1):60–65.
40. Roselli CE, Resko JA, Stormshak F. Estrogen synthesis in fetal sheep brain: effect of maternal treatment with an aromatase inhibitor. *Biol Reprod.* 2003;68(2):370–374.
41. Herbosa CG, Dahl GE, Evans NP, et al. Sexual differentiation of the surge mode of gonadotropin secretion: prenatal androgens abolish the gonadotropin-releasing hormone surge in the sheep. *J Neuroendocrinol.* 1996;8(8):627–633.
42. Robinson JE, Forsdike RA, Taylor JA. In utero exposure of female lambs to testosterone reduces the sensitivity of the gonadotropin-releasing hormone neuronal network to inhibition by progesterone. *Endocrinology.* 1999;140(12):5797–5805.
43. Sharma TP, Herkimer C, West C, et al. Fetal programming: prenatal androgen disrupts positive feedback actions of estradiol but does not affect timing of puberty in female sheep. *Biol Reprod.* 2002;66(4):924–933.
44. Wallen K. Hormonal influences on sexually differentiated behavior in nonhuman primates. *Front Neuroendocrinol.* 2005;26(1):7–26.
45. Arnold AP. Sexual differentiation of brain and other tissues: five questions for the next 50 years. *Horm Behav.* 2020;120:104691.
46. McCarthy MM. A new view of sexual differentiation of mammalian brain. *J Comp Physiol A Neuroethol Sens Neural Behav Physiol.* 2020;206(3):369–378.

16

Recurrent Implantation Failure and Miscarriage

Yealin Chung

16.1 Definition

16.1.1 Recurrent Implantation Failure (RIF)

RIF may be defined as the repeated implantation failure following transfer of embryos. Taking a couple through an in-vitro fertilisation (IVF) cycle may be viewed as an investigation as well as a treatment, as it allows each step of the treatment pathway to be compartmentalised and inspected. This helps to narrow down the reason behind a couple's subfertility to a specific cause. RIF became as clinically recognised phenomenon following the introduction of IVF where the cause of subfertility is inferred to lie at the implantation stage.

Although a recognised condition, there is no universally accepted diagnostic criteria to define RIF. Currently adopted definition appear to vary depending on the clinic size (<50 to >200 RIF patients treated per year), the types of treatment setting (private, public vs. University-affiliated) and geographical location (European vs. non-European) (**1**). Amongst the research literature, the definition remains diverse; some investigators have based their definition on the number of IVF cycles whereas others have adopted the number of embryos or transfers as the key defining criteria (**2**). The professional societies also fail to agree on a clear definition. The American Society for Reproductive Medicine (ASRM) are yet to publish a specific criterion and the European Society of Human Reproduction and Embryology Preimplantation Genetic Diagnosis (ESHRE PGD) Consortium defines RIF as ">3 embryo transfers with high quality embryos or the transfers of ≥10 embryos in multiple transfers; exact numbers to be determined by each centre" (**3**). An international survey of 735 clinicians suggest that the majority (84%) define RIF based on the number of embryos transferred with the most common threshold adopted being three transfers of fresh or frozen embryos (**1**).

The challenge of defining RIF is a reflection of the extreme complexity that lies behind the implantation process, which largely remains poorly understood. Despite the diversity in the currently adopted definition of RIF, a common theme persists; the consensus that RIF definition and diagnosis should be reserved for those with an abnormally low chance of pregnancy per embryo. The purpose of identifying these couples is to validate the need for further investigation or interventions with the aim of improving treatment outcomes in subsequent embryo transfers.

16.1.2 Miscarriage

Miscarriage is commonly defined as the loss of an intrauterine pregnancy before the viability is reached. There is a wide variation in the method of pregnancy diagnosis, definition of intrauterine pregnancy and viability, which leads to bewildering disparity in how miscarriage may be defined among countries, international organisations and professional societies (**4**). For example, the legal and clinical definition of viability varies from country to country, with lower gestational threshold commonly adopted by the high-income countries where neonatal care for preterm infants is inclined to be more medically advanced, easier to access and effective.

The World Health Organisation (WHO) defines miscarriage as "the expulsion or extraction of a fetus (embryo) weighing less than 500g equivalent to approximately 22 weeks gestation" (**5, 6**). The ASRM defines miscarriage as "a clinical pregnancy loss of less than 20 weeks of gestation" (**7**). Finally, the ESHRE defines miscarriage as "the loss of pregnancy before 22 weeks of gestation" (**8**).

16.2 Prevalence Risk

The criteria used to define RIF and miscarriage are diverse. Therefore, the estimation of their risk and prevalence also varies widely in the currently available literature.

For RIF, the prevalence is estimated to be 15% when defined using the criteria of three failed IVF cycles (**9**). In contrast, if defined following 3 successive euploid transfers in morphologically normal endometrium, the risk falls to <5% (**10**).

For miscarriage, the overall risk for the general population is estimated to be 15.3% (**4**). This estimation was calculated from six prospective cohort studies using self-reported pregnancy outcomes. Female age and the number of previous miscarriages appear to have a significant effect on the miscarriage risk with the lowest miscarriage risk of 12% in the age group of 20–29 years which rises to 65% for those who are equal and above 45 years. In the absence of any prior history of miscarriage, the risk is 11%. This, however, increases by 10% for each additional miscarriages and following 3 or more previous miscarriages, the risk reaches 42% (**4**).

16.3 Aetiology and Management

A successful implantation and maintenance of pregnancy requires a carefully timed dialogue between a competent embryo and the receptive endometrium. Failure in this process may result from one or more factors. In most couples, the cause is likely to be multifactorial and it is unlikely that

DOI: 10.1201/9781003269502-16

treatment or pregnancy failure results from the same factor(s) every time.

RIF and miscarriage are two separate clinical entities; RIF may only be diagnosed in couples who received IVF treatment and miscarriage may occur as a pregnancy complication following any modes of conception. However, both result in the same conclusion of subfertility with a wide overlap of the underlying pathophysiology. Therefore, the aetiology and management of both conditions will be concurrently reviewed.

Broadly, the causes of implantation failure or miscarriage may be divided into 2 categories: 1) embryonic factors, and 2) non-embryonic factors.

16.3.1 Embryonic Factors

- Chromosomal aneuploidy
- Gene mutations
- Methylation

Development of a competent quality embryo must begin with a good quality mature oocyte and spermatozoa. The number and quality of oocyte follow a gradual decline with biological ageing and this appears to accelerate after the age of 37 years (**11**). This age-related decline in oocyte quality is reflected by the strong positive correlation between aneuploidy rates and maternal age. The severity of chromosomal aberration in the resulting oocyte or embryo will determine its reproductive potential, clinically manifest anywhere along the spectrum of reproductive failure; the arrest of embryonic development to implantation failure or miscarriage. For spermatozoa, it is undisputed that abnormal semen parameters are associated with globally poorer treatment outcomes. There is also increasing evidence suggesting higher DNA fragmentation rate may be associated with increased miscarriage risk. In patients undergoing IVF treatment, embryos with major chromosomal anomalies such as autosomal monosomies, haploidy or polyploidy will frequently arrest and do not continue to develop into the blastocyst stage to allow transfer. The clinical significance of segmental aneuploidy or mosaicism, thus their effect on implantation potential is less clear but are commonly associated with increased miscarriage risk. Chromosomal anomalies are the commonest identifiable reason for miscarriage and are found in 60% of miscarried tissue (**12**). It is also likely to be the cause for treatment failure in the majority of couples undergoing IVF. This theory is supported by the latest data from the Human Fertilisation and Embryology Authority (HFEA) which demonstrates that the live birth rates following IVF treatment with donor oocytes are comparable and remain high across all recipient age groups.

Apart from chromosomal euploidy status, gene mutations and alterations in methylation have also been theorised to play a potential role in regulating an embryo's implantation potential. In mice models, specific gene mutations have been associated with implantation failure although such mutations have not been identified in humans (**13, 14**). Epigenetic modification, specifically DNA methylation are essential to healthy embryo development, supported by evidence from animal-based experimental models (**2, 15**). In human observations, methylation alterations have been identified in patients with long-standing infertility, although it is unclear whether the relationship is causal (**16**).

Currently no investigation exists that allow direct measurement of oocyte quality. Sperm Oxidative Stress (SOS) or DNA fragmentation tests are emerging as valuable tools to measure the sperm quality. In recent years, considerable progress has been made to overcome the embryonic factors. These include improved identification of good quality embryos using technology such as embryoscope and semi-automated analysis of morphokinetic data with assistance from artificial intelligence. The use of pre-implantation genetic testing now allows identification and exclusion of genetically abnormal embryos before transfer. Routine parental karyotyping is generally not recommended as does no predict the risk of subsequent miscarriages. However, should be considered in couples with a history of 5 or more miscarriages, strong family history of recurrent miscarriages or genetic anomalies. There has been a gradual shift in clinical practice from cleavage stage to blastocyst stage embryo transfer which allows self-selection of viable embryos. Finally, there is now increasing acceptance among the couples undergoing IVF treatment to use donor gametes. This, possibly, has made the greatest difference thus far in improving treatment success rates in subfertile couples with poor embryo quality.

16.3.2 Non-Embryonic Factors

- Anatomical
- Haematological
- Endocrinological
- Microbiome
- Endometritis/Infection
- Immunological
- Endometrial receptivity
- Lifestyle and environmental

16.3.2.1 Anatomical

Anatomical abnormalities such as fibroids, polyps, congenital uterine anomalies, intrauterine adhesions, and hydrosalpinges may impair implantation and pregnancy establishment.

Fibroids are non-cancerous growths made up of the muscle and connective tissue from the uterine wall. They have been shown to adversely impair implantation and increase miscarriage risk. Possible mechanisms include venous congestion, reduced vascular supply and increase in myometrial contractility (**11**). The severity of impact is closely correlated to its size and location. Subserosal fibroid are not thought to impact reproductive outcome of women undergoing IVF and myomectomy of these lesions makes no difference to the outcome (**17**). For intramural fibroid, the evidence remains uncertain with conflicting evidence. Low quality evidence suggests removal of fibroids that are cavity distorting or more than 2cm in size may improve pregnancy rate (**18–20**). The negative effect of subserosal fibroid on reproductive outcome is clear (**17, 21, 22**) and myomectomy has been shown to double the clinical pregnancy rate (**17**). ASRM advises surgery to be considered on an individual basis depending on its size, risks of surgery and potential for pregnancy complications. In addition, myomectomy for asymptomatic, non-cavity distorting fibroids are not advised (**23**).

Polyps are endometrial overgrowths and the most common uterine lesions that cause implantation failure (**24, 25**). Similar to fibroids, adverse effects are suspected to be linked to increased glycodelin, reduced HOXA10 and IL10 levels (**11**). Hysteroscopic polypectomy has been shown to double the pregnancy rate. However, the exact indication for surgery (size or location) that would outbalance the operative risks remains uncertain.

Congenital uterine anomalies are uterine malformations that develop during fetal life and are common findings in women with a history of subfertility (**26**). Example anomalies include didelphys (double uterus), unicornuate or bicornuate uterus and uterine septum. The aetiology would depend upon the type of anomaly but possible mechanisms include poor vascularisation and placentation, reduced sensitivity to reproductive steroid hormones and uncoordinated uterine contractions (**11**). The majority of evidence is based on observational findings and suggests an association with reduced pregnancy rate, increased risks of miscarriage and obstetric complications (**27**). The only congenital uterine anomaly that is amenable to surgical treatment is the uterine septum. However, the quality of evidence remains low and there is increasing controversy on whether hysteroscopic septoplasty improves reproductive outcomes (**11**). ASRM in their latest guideline concluded that "it may be reasonable to consider septum incision following counselling regarding potential risks and benefits of the procedure" (**28**).

Intrauterine adhesions also called Asherman syndrome are reported in 8% of infertile women (**29**) and 38% of women with miscarriage history (**30**). It usually results as a complication from uterine instrumentation or surgery. The negative reproductive effect is likely to be mechanical disrupting sperm or embryo transport, implantation and placentation. The level of evidence investigating treatment effects is low with no high quality RCTs. However, the findings appear consistent with the existing studies demonstrating increased pregnancy and live birth rate while reducing miscarriage risk (**31–33**).

Finally, hydrosalpinx refers to damaged or dysfunctional fallopian tubes that fill with fluid and remain dilated. The hydrosalpinx fluid is embryo-toxic, impairs endometrial receptivity and may disrupt implantation through mechanical flushing (**34, 35**). The presence of hydrosalpinx reduces implantation, clinical pregnancy and live birth rate by 50% in women undergoing IVF (**36, 37**). Salpingectomy is the gold standard treatment for hydrosalpinx which have been shown to double the clinical pregnancy rate (**38**). Alternative treatment options include tubal occlusion, when compared to salpingectomy, have comparable outcomes. Aspiration and sclerotherapy have also been explored but the evidence is limited with the quality of existing evidence low (**11**). ASRM recommends "salpingectomy or proximal tubal occlusion in women with hydrosalpinges undergoing IVF" (**39**).

16.3.2.2 Haematological

Successful implantation and pregnancy development requires a series of complex events including vascular remodelling and haemodynamic changes. Thrombophilia has been linked with many adverse reproductive outcomes and its association with miscarriage risk is well established (**40**). However its effect on implantation potential is less certain with conflicting results from existing evidence (**11**). ESHRE recommends "the use of low dose aspirin and heparin in women with antiphospholipid syndrome" to reduce miscarriage risk (**8**). However, there is no evidence to support empirical use of anti-coagulant therapy in women with inherited thrombophilia or no thrombophilia diagnosis. Empirical use may, in reverse, cause harm with evidence suggesting increased miscarriage risk with aspirin use in women who do not have thrombophilia (**41**).

16.3.2.3 Endocrinological

Thyroid hormones play an important role in regulating all stage of reproduction from ovarian function to pregnancy development. Therefore, normal thyroid function is essential for optimum reproductive function and as such, hypo- and hyperthyroidism should be screened, identified and treated before starting any fertility treatment. The clinical uncertainty lies in how to manage those patients in the early stages of thyroid dysfunction such as subclinical hypothyroidism or presence of thyroid antibodies in the absence of any thyroid dysfunction. Subclinical hypothyroidism is defined by high serum thyroid stimulating hormone outside the laboratory reference range, alongside normal concentration of circulating thyroid hormones. Evidence suggests levothyroxine treatment of patients with subclinical hypothyroidism may result in increased implantation rate and reduced miscarriage risk (**42**). Presence of thyroid antibodies are more common in women with history of subfertility (**43**). However, there is insufficient evidence to confirm that the presence of thyroid antibodies alone impairs implantation. In contrast, the evidence on miscarriage risk is consistent and suggests presence of thyroid antibodies are associated with increased miscarriage risk (**44**). ESHRE states that the treatment of women with subclinical hypothyroidism may reduce the miscarriage risk but the potential benefit of treatment should be balanced against the risks and recommends the treatment is only initiated pre-conception or during pregnancy where the diagnosis of subclinical hypothyroidism is made based on TSH levels (**8**).

Metabolic disorders such as polycystic ovarian syndrome (PCOS) or obesity have strong association with poor reproductive outcomes. Multiple pathways have been linked (**11**). Impaired progesterone signalling due to hyperinsulinemia and insulin resistance and alteration of uterine receptivity, markers of decidualisation and implantation. Endometrial receptors may be dysregulated, glucose transport and utilisation may be impaired leading to a state of heightened chronic inflammation. Uterine vascularity and immune modulation may be adversely altered and abnormal endometrial gene expression may be induced (**45**). The most effective treatment, if indicated, is weight loss to a healthy range with the aim of reducing the insulin resistance. There is also some evidence to suggest that miscarriage risk may be reduced in patients with metformin treatment (**46**).

16.3.2.4 Microbiome

Microbiome refers to the complex community of microbes that inhabit a specific site on the body. It is known that the female reproductive tract is not a sterile environment. Thus, research into the role of the microbiome and its effect on reproductive function is gaining increasing attention. The microbiome may exert a diversity of functions through metabolic, epigenetic and immunological effects (**47–49**) and are thought to be essential to maintaining a healthy environment. It is acknowledged that microbial dysbiosis may impair fertility (**11**). However, the uterine microbiota is underexplored and poorly understood due to the invasive nature of sampling procedures. Therefore, healthy uterine and endometrial microbial compositions, and their role in reproduction are yet to be established.

16.3.2.5 Endometritis/Infection

Endometritis i.e., endometrial inflammation is a recognised cause of subfertility. Most of the acute endometritis is caused by infection with bacteria. They tend to be short lasting, responds well to antibiotic therapy and usually resolve without any long-term reproductive sequelae. In contrast, chronic endometritis may be caused by a variety of pathogens and is difficult to diagnose with no typical clinical or ultrasound findings. Diagnosis of chronic endometritis can be made following the histological assessment of endometrial biopsy and findings of plasma cell infiltration in the endometrial stroma (**50, 51**). The prevalence rate of chronic endometritis has been reported to be as high as 42% in women with RIF (**52**) and 58% in women with history of recurrent miscarriages of 3 or more (**53**). Chronic endometritis is thought to impair fertility by disrupting the endometrial receptivity (**54–56**) and up to a threefold reduction in implantation rates have been reported (**57, 58**). Ideally, women with chronic endometritis should receive targeted antibiotic therapy following the isolation of the responsible pathogen from the endometrial culture. However, not all pathogens responsible are culturable. Therefore, this leads to a clinical quandary on how best to manage these patients with non-specific chronic endometritis. A broad-spectrum antibiotic therapy has the potential to harm, specifically when the offending pathogen is resistant to the treatment, by causing further microbial imbalance and disruption to the microbial composition within the reproductive tract. This likely explains the conflicting results from studies assessing the benefit of antibiotic treatment in improving reproductive outcomes (**54, 55, 58–60**).

16.3.2.6 Immunological

Under the influence of ovarian sex steroid hormones, the endometrial leukocytes undergo a cyclical change every menstrual cycle. Of these leukocytes, one that has gained much attention in recent years is uterine natural killer (uNK) cells. During the follicular phase, uNK cells are almost absent in the endometrial decidua. Following the ovulation, uNK cell numbers rapidly rise in response to the increasing progesterone level and eventually peak to constitute 70% of the leukocyte population within the decidualised endometrium. uNK cells modulate vascular growth and fetal trophoblast invasion and their presence has been established as crucial to successful implantation and placenta development (**61**). Few studies observed uNK cell levels may be raised in women with RIF or recurrent miscarriages (**62–67**), although it is unclear whether this association is causal. Extrapolating on these findings, many investigators started to explore treatment with an array of immune-modulating drugs in the absence of clear evidence demonstrating treatment benefit (**68**).

Aside from uNK cell testing, other immune aspects that have been explored in women with history of RIF or recurrent miscarriages is the measurement of Type 1 (Th1) and Type 2 (Th2) T helper cell ratio. They regulate the delicate balance of pro and anti-inflammatory cytokines and control the maternal immune response to the embryo. A high Th1/Th2 cell ratio has been linked to RIF and recurrent miscarriages (**69**). However, as other tests for immune markers, the evidence to date have shown conflicting results and the clinical implications remain uncertain.

To date, several treatment modalities have been explored to modulate various aspects of immune system. These include steroids, intravenous immunoglobulin, tumour necrosis factor-alpha blocking drugs and intralipid infusions. The quality of evidence for these treatments is very low and there is insufficient evidence to support the use of immunotherapy to reduce RIF and miscarriage risk.

Adenomyosis is a condition where endometrium-like cells are deposited within the myometrium. Endometriosis is defined when these cells are found outside the uterus. There is emerging evidence linking the presence of these conditions as a risk factor for poor reproductive outcomes. Indeed, it is accepted that the prevalence of endometriosis is increased in the subfertile population when compared to those with normal fertility (**70**). The mechanism of adverse effects is likely to be multifactorial but overall suspected to impair immune modulation. To support this theory, uNK cell dysfunction has been reported in women with adenomyosis and reduced implantation rate (**71**). These conditions are also thought to induce a pro-inflammatory state which then may act as a pathogenic mechanism for implantation failure or pregnancy loss. Unlike other anatomical conditions that were reviewed earlier in this chapter, endometriosis or adenomyosis are not easily amenable to surgical treatment. Indeed, no surgical treatment has been shown to improve RIF or miscarriage risk. Alternative down-regulation protocols have been explored to investigate whether fertility treatment outcomes may be improved. There is a suggestion that the GnRH agonist ultra-long protocol may benefit and improve the clinical pregnancy rate (**72**). However, more evidence is needed to better guide the clinical practice.

16.3.2.7 Endometrial Receptivity

During the luteal phase of a normal menstrual cycle, the endometrium undergoes a transformative change to become receptive. This process is driven by progesterone secreted from the corpus luteum. Luteal phase deficiency (LPD) occurs when progesterone exposure is insufficient to maintain the endometrium and the pregnancy. For women undergoing ART, the majority will develop LPD as a result of ovarian stimulation. The degree of pituitary suppression causing LPD is patient specific. Nevertheless, in the absence of predictive markers which accurately identify those at risk of LPD, all women undergoing ART are given luteal phase support. It is accepted that luteal phase support improves ART outcomes but there is no consensus on which regimen is the most effective with the least side effects. In women with a history of recurrent miscarriages, there is increasing evidence to support the use of progesterone supplementation (**46**). Despite being first described several decades ago, LPS remains difficult to diagnose. The traditional diagnosis is based on histological assessment which is invasive and not sufficiently reliable or reproducible. Assessment of gene expression signatures from endometrial sampling have now emerged as valuable diagnostic tool for use in couples undergoing IVF treatment. Of these, endometrial receptivity analysis (ERA) test is perhaps the most widely known in the commercial market (**73, 74**). The test classifies the endometrial sample in relation to the receptive window and provides individualised suggestion on the best time to schedule the embryo transfer.

16.3.2.8 Lifestyle and Environmental

The following lifestyle choices have been associated with adverse reproductive outcomes: smoking, high alcohol intake, use of recreational drugs or gym supplements, high caffeine consumption, micronutrient deficiencies and extremes of weight (under- or over-weight) (**25**). Other factors such as stress and cortisol levels have also been shown to be associated with increased implantation failure and miscarriage risk. Many of these factors do not have clear evidence of a causal relationship. However, implementation of positive lifestyle choices is simple, easy and effective to optimise the reproductive health of a subfertile couple and generate the sense of self-empowerment for the couple during their fertility journey.

16.4 Conclusion

A coordinated dialogue between a competent embryo and a receptive endometrium is required for a successful implantation of an embryo and for maintenance of a pregnancy. As discussed, there are various causes or factors that can lead to failure in treatment and pregnancy, and those factors are not necessarily the same every time. There is a wide overlap of the underlying pathophysiology of repeated implantation failure (RIF) and recurrent miscarriage (RM), and therefore, further investigation or interventions of couples suspected with RIF and RIM are often needed in order to improve treatment outcomes in subsequent embryo transfers.

REFERENCES

1. Cimadomo D, Craciunas L, Vermeulen N, et al. Definition, diagnostic and therapeutic options in recurrent implantation failure: an international survey of clinicians and embryologists. *Hum Reprod Oxf Engl.* 2021 Jan 25;36(2):305–317.
2. Garneau AS, Young SL. Defining recurrent implantation failure: a profusion of confusion or simply an illusion? *Fertil Steril.* 2021 Dec;116(6):1432–1435.
3. Thornhill AR, deDie-Smulders CE, Geraedts JP, et al. ESHRE PGD consortium 'best practice guidelines for clinical preimplantation genetic diagnosis (PGD) and preimplantation genetic screening (PGS)'. *Hum Reprod Oxf Engl.* 2005 Jan;20(1):35–48.
4. Quenby S, Gallos ID, Dhillon-Smith RK, et al. Miscarriage matters: the epidemiological, physical, psychological, and economic costs of early pregnancy loss. *Lancet.* 2021 May;397(10285):1658–1667.
5. Ugurlu EN, Ozaksit G, Karaer A, et al. The value of vascular endothelial growth factor, pregnancy-associated plasma protein-A, and progesterone for early differentiation of ectopic pregnancies, normal intrauterine pregnancies, and spontaneous miscarriages. *Fertil Steril.* 2009 May;91(5):1657–1661.
6. World Health Organization. *World Health Organization & International Conference for the Ninth Revision of the International Classification of Diseases (1975: Geneva), (1977).* In: Manual of the International Statistical Classification of Diseases, Injuries, and Causes of Death: Based on the Recommendations of the Ninth Revision Conference, 1975, and Adopted by the Twenty-Ninth World Health Assembly, 1975 revision. 1977. Available from: https://apps.who.int/iris/handle/10665/40492.
7. Practice Committee of the American Society for Reproductive Medicine. Evaluation and treatment of recurrent pregnancy loss: a committee opinion. *Fertil Steril.* 2012 Nov;98(5):1103–1111.
8. ESHRE Guideline Group on RPL, et al. ESHRE guideline: recurrent pregnancy loss. *Hum Reprod Open.* 2018;2018(2):hoy004.
9. Busnelli A, Reschini M, Cardellicchio L, et al. How common is real repeated implantation failure? An indirect estimate of the prevalence. *Reprod Biomed Online.* 2020 Jan;40(1):91–97.
10. Pirtea P, Scott RT, de Ziegler D, et al. Recurrent implantation failure: how common is it? *Curr Opin Obstet Gynecol.* 2021 Jun 1;33(3):207–212.
11. Franasiak JM, Alecsandru D, Forman EJ, et al. A review of the pathophysiology of recurrent implantation failure. *Fertil Steril.* 2021 Dec;116(6):1436–1448.
12. Hardy K, Hardy PJ, Jacobs PA, et al. Temporal changes in chromosome abnormalities in human spontaneous abortions: results of 40 years of analysis. *Am J Med Genet A.* 2016 Oct;170(10):2671–2680.
13. Gao F, Bian F, Ma X, et al. Control of regional decidualization in implantation: role of FoxM1 downstream of Hoxa10 and cyclin D3. *Sci Rep.* 2015 Sep 9;5:13863.
14. Pawar S, Starosvetsky E, Orvis GD, et al. STAT3 regulates uterine epithelial remodeling and epithelial-stromal crosstalk during implantation. *Mol Endocrinol Baltim Md.* 2013 Dec;27(12):1996–2012.
15. Razin A, Shemer R. DNA methylation in early development. *Hum Mol Genet.* 1995;4 Spec No:1751–1755.
16. Denomme MM, Haywood ME, McCallie BR, et al. The prolonged disease state of infertility is associated with embryonic epigenetic dysregulation. *Fertil Steril.* 2021 Aug;116(2):309–318.
17. Pritts EA, Parker WH, Olive DL. Fibroids and infertility: an updated systematic review of the evidence. *Fertil Steril.* 2009 Apr;91(4):1215–1223.

18. Yan L, Yu Q, Zhang YN, et al. Effect of type 3 intramural fibroids on in vitro fertilization-intracytoplasmic sperm injection outcomes: a retrospective cohort study. *Fertil Steril.* 2018 May;109(5):817–822. e2.
19. Bulletti C, Coccia ME, Battistoni S, et al. Endometriosis and infertility. *J Assist Reprod Genet.* 2010 Aug;27(8):441–447.
20. Casini ML, Rossi F, Agostini R, et al. Effects of the position of fibroids on fertility. *Gynecol Endocrinol.* 2006 Feb;22(2):106–109.
21. Somigliana E, Vercellini P, Daguati R, et al. Fibroids and female reproduction: a critical analysis of the evidence. *Hum Reprod Update.* 2007 Oct;13(5):465–476.
22. Klatsky PC, Tran ND, Caughey AB, et al. Fibroids and reproductive outcomes: a systematic literature review from conception to delivery. *Am J Obstet Gynecol.* 2008 Apr;198(4):357–366.
23. Practice Committee of the American Society for Reproductive Medicine. Removal of myomas in asymptomatic patients to improve fertility and/or reduce miscarriage rate: a guideline. *Fertil Steril.* 2017 Sep;108(3):416–425. ASRM@asrm.org.
24. Fatemi HM, Kasius JC, Timmermans A, et al. Prevalence of unsuspected uterine cavity abnormalities diagnosed by office hysteroscopy prior to in vitro fertilization. *Hum Reprod Oxf Engl.* 2010 Aug;25(8):1959–1965.
25. Bashiri A, Halper KI, Orvieto R. Recurrent implantation failure-update overview on etiology, diagnosis, treatment and future directions. *Reprod Biol Endocrinol.* 2018 Dec 5;16(1):121.
26. Grimbizis GF, Camus M, Tarlatzis BC, et al. Clinical implications of uterine malformations and hysteroscopic treatment results. *Hum Reprod Update.* 2001 Apr;7(2):161–174.
27. Chan YY, Jayaprakasan K, Tan A, et al. Reproductive outcomes in women with congenital uterine anomalies: a systematic review. *Ultrasound Obstet Gynecol.* 2011 Oct;38(4):371–382.
28. Practice Committee of the American Society for Reproductive Medicine. Uterine septum: a guideline. *Fertil Steril.* 2016 Sep 1;106(3):530–540. ASRM@asrm.org.
29. Wang XY, Li Z, NI AY, et al. Hysteroscopy for early abortion after IVF-ET: clinical analysis of 84 cases. *Zhonghua Nan Ke Xue Natl J Androl.* 2011 Jan;17(1):52–54.
30. Thomson AJM, Abbott JA, Deans R, et al. The management of intrauterine synechiae. *Curr Opin Obstet Gynecol.* 2009 Aug;21(4):335–341.
31. Yu D, Wong YM, Cheong Y, et al. Asherman syndrome – one century later. *Fertil Steril.* 2008 Apr;89(4):759–779.
32. Katz Z, Ben-Arie A, Lurie S, et al. Reproductive outcome following hysteroscopic adhesiolysis in Asherman's syndrome. *Int J Fertil Menopausal Stud.* 1996 Oct;41(5):462–465.
33. Deans R, Abbott J. Review of intrauterine adhesions. *J Minim Invasive Gynecol.* 2010 Oct;17(5):555–569.
34. Savaris RF, Pedrini JL, Flores R, et al. Expression of alpha 1 and beta 3 integrins subunits in the endometrium of patients with tubal phimosis or hydrosalpinx. *Fertil Steril.* 2006 Jan;85(1):188–192.
35. Mukherjee T, Copperman AB, McCaffrey C, et al. Hydrosalpinx fluid has embryotoxic effects on murine embryogenesis: a case for prophylactic salpingectomy. *Fertil Steril.* 1996 Nov;66(5):851–853.
36. Zeyneloglu HB, Arici A, Olive DL. Adverse effects of hydrosalpinx on pregnancy rates after in vitro fertilization-embryo transfer. *Fertil Steril.* 1998 Sep;70(3):492–499.
37. Camus E, Poncelet C, Goffinet F, et al. Pregnancy rates after in-vitro fertilization in cases of tubal infertility with and without hydrosalpinx: a meta-analysis of published comparative studies. *Hum Reprod Oxf Engl.* 1999 May;14(5):1243–1249.
38. Melo P, Georgiou EX, Johnson N, et al. Surgical treatment for tubal disease in women due to undergo in vitro fertilisation. *Cochrane Database Syst Rev.* 2020 Oct 22;10:CD002125.
39. Practice Committee of the American Society for Reproductive Medicine. Role of tubal surgery in the era of assisted reproductive technology: a committee opinion. *Fertil Steril.* 2015 Jun;103(6):e37–e43.
40. Brenner B. Inherited thrombophilia and fetal loss. *Curr Opin Hematol.* 2000 Sep;7(5):290–295.
41. Zhang T, Ye X, Zhu T, et al. Antithrombotic treatment for recurrent miscarriage: Bayesian network meta-analysis and systematic review. *Medicine (Baltimore).* 2015 Nov;94(45):e1732.
42. Velkeniers B, Van Meerhaeghe A, Poppe K, et al. Levothyroxine treatment and pregnancy outcome in women with subclinical hypothyroidism undergoing assisted reproduction technologies: systematic review and meta-analysis of RCTs. *Hum Reprod Update.* 2013 Jun;19(3):251–258.
43. Poppe K, Glinoer D, Van Steirteghem A, et al. Thyroid dysfunction and autoimmunity in infertile women. *Thyroid.* 2002 Nov;12(11):997–1001.
44. Dhillon-Smith RK, Boelaert K, Jeve YB, et al. Subclinical hypothyroidism and antithyroid autoantibodies in women with subfertility or recurrent pregnancy loss: scientific impact paper no. 70 June 2022. *BJOG.* 2022 Nov;129(12):e75–e88.
45. Palomba S, Piltonen TT, Giudice LC. Endometrial function in women with polycystic ovary syndrome: a comprehensive review. *Hum Reprod Update.* 2021 Apr 21;27(3):584–618.
46. Coomarasamy A, Dhillon-Smith RK, Papadopoulou A, et al. Recurrent miscarriage: evidence to accelerate action. *Lancet Lond Engl.* 2021 May 1;397(10285):1675–1682.
47. Maranduba CM da C, De Castro SBR, de Souza GT, et al. Intestinal microbiota as modulators of the immune system and neuroimmune system: impact on the host health and homeostasis. *J Immunol Res.* 2015;2015:931574.
48. Belkaid Y, Harrison OJ. Homeostatic immunity and the microbiota. *Immunity.* 2017 Apr 18;46(4):562–576.
49. Flint HJ, Scott KP, Louis P, et al. The role of the gut microbiota in nutrition and health. *Nat Rev Gastroenterol Hepatol.* 2012 Oct;9(10):577–589.
50. Kitaya K, Yasuo T. Immunohistochemistrical and clinicopathological characterization of chronic endometritis. *Am J Reprod Immunol* (N Y N 1989). 2011 Nov;66(5):410–415.
51. Kasius JC, Fatemi HM, Bourgain C, et al. The impact of chronic endometritis on reproductive outcome. *Fertil Steril.* 2011 Dec;96(6):1451–1456.
52. Romero R, Espinoza J, Mazor M. Can endometrial infection/inflammation explain implantation failure, spontaneous abortion, and preterm birth after in vitro fertilization? *Fertil Steril.* 2004 Oct;82(4):799–804.

53. Zolghadri J, Momtahan M, Aminian K, et al. The value of hysteroscopy in diagnosis of chronic endometritis in patients with unexplained recurrent spontaneous abortion. *Eur J Obstet Gynecol Reprod Biol.* 2011 Apr;155(2):217–220.
54. Kitaya K, Matsubayashi H, Takaya Y, et al. Live birth rate following oral antibiotic treatment for chronic endometritis in infertile women with repeated implantation failure. *Am J Reprod Immunol* (N Y N 1989). 2017 Nov;78(5).
55. Cicinelli E, Matteo M, Tinelli R, et al. Prevalence of chronic endometritis in repeated unexplained implantation failure and the IVF success rate after antibiotic therapy. *Hum Reprod Oxf Engl.* 2015 Feb;30(2):323–330.
56. Buzzaccarini G, Vitagliano A, Andrisani A, et al. Chronic endometritis and altered embryo implantation: a unified pathophysiological theory from a literature systematic review. *J Assist Reprod Genet.* 2020 Dec;37(12):2897–2911.
57. Johnson N, van Voorst S, Sowter MC, et al. Surgical treatment for tubal disease in women due to undergo in vitro fertilisation. *Cochrane Database Syst Rev.* 2010 Jan 20;(1):CD002125.
58. Johnston-MacAnanny EB, Hartnett J, Engmann LL, et al. Chronic endometritis is a frequent finding in women with recurrent implantation failure after in vitro fertilization. *Fertil Steril.* 2010 Feb;93(2):437–441.
59. Tersoglio AE, Salatino DR, Reinchisi G, et al. Repeated implantation failure in oocyte donation. What to do to improve the endometrial receptivity? *JBRA Assist Reprod.* 2015 May 1;19(2):44–52.
60. Yang R, Du X, Wang Y, et al. The hysteroscopy and histological diagnosis and treatment value of chronic endometritis in recurrent implantation failure patients. *Arch Gynecol Obstet.* 2014 Jun;289(6):1363–1369.
61. Moffett-King A. Natural killer cells and pregnancy. *Nat Rev Immunol.* 2002 Sep 1;2(9):656–663.
62. Bulmer JN, Lash GE. Uterine natural killer cells: time for a re-appraisal? *F1000Research.* 2019;8:F1000 Faculty Rev-999.
63. Vacca P, Vitale C, Munari E, et al. Human innate lymphoid cells: their functional and cellular interactions in decidua. *Front Immunol.* 2018;9:1897.
64. Timeva T, Shterev A, Kyurkchiev S. Recurrent implantation failure: the role of the endometrium. *J Reprod Infertil.* 2014 Oct;15(4):173–183.
65. Lédée-Bataille N, Bonnet-Chea K, Hosny G, et al. Role of the endometrial tripod interleukin-18, -15, and -12 in inadequate uterine receptivity in patients with a history of repeated in vitro fertilization-embryo transfer failure. *Fertil Steril.* 2005 Mar;83(3):598–605.
66. Laird SM, Tuckerman EM, Li TC. Cytokine expression in the endometrium of women with implantation failure and recurrent miscarriage. *Reprod Biomed Online.* 2006 Jul;13(1):13–23.
67. Quenby S, Farquharson R. Uterine natural killer cells, implantation failure and recurrent miscarriage. *Reprod Biomed Online.* 2006 Jul;13(1):24–28.
68. Moffett A, Regan L, Braude P. Natural killer cells, miscarriage, and infertility. *BMJ.* 2004 Nov 27;329(7477): 1283–1285.
69. Kuroda K, Nakagawa K, Horikawa T, et al. Increasing number of implantation failures and pregnancy losses associated with elevated Th1/Th2 cell ratio. *Am J Reprod Immunol* (N Y N 1989). 2021 Sep;86(3):e13429.
70. D'Hooghe TM, Kyama C, Debrock S, et al. Future directions in endometriosis research. *Ann N Y Acad Sci.* 2004 Dec;1034:316–325.
71. Horton J, Sterrenburg M, Lane S, et al. Reproductive, obstetric, and perinatal outcomes of women with adenomyosis and endometriosis: a systematic review and meta-analysis. *Hum Reprod Update.* 2019 Sep 11;25(5):592–632.
72. Cao X, Chang HY, Xu JY, et al. The effectiveness of different down-regulating protocols on in vitro fertilization-embryo transfer in endometriosis: a meta-analysis. *Reprod Biol Endocrinol.* 2020 Feb 29;18(1):16.
73. Díaz-Gimeno P, Horcajadas JA, Martínez-Conejero JA, et al. A genomic diagnostic tool for human endometrial receptivity based on the transcriptomic signature. *Fertil Steril.* 2011;95(1):50–60. e15.
74. Ruiz-Alonso M, Valbuena D, Gomez C, et al. Endometrial Receptivity Analysis (ERA): data versus opinions. *Hum Reprod Open.* 2021;2021(2):hoab011.

17

Infertility: Definition, Referral, and Initial Consultation

Charlotte Palmer

Infertility is defined as the inability of a couple to conceive after having regular unprotected intercourse for 12 months. This definition can be further sub classified into ***primary infertility,*** in which no previous pregnancies have been achieved, or ***secondary infertility*** in which there has been at least one prior pregnancy, although not necessarily resulting in a live birth. Finally, **fecundability** is the probability of achieving a pregnancy within one menstrual cycle.

Very few couples have absolute infertility (sterility) which can be the result of congenital or acquired irreversible loss of functional gametes (oocytes or spermatozoa), or the absence of a uterus in a female (**1**). According to this principle, a large majority of couples would be able to conceive spontaneously with time, however because of known or unidentifiable causes, their fecundability is low and warrants medical intervention.

When couples are concerned about their chances of conception, it is often helpful to discuss cumulative probabilities of conceiving, by the number of menstrual cycles (**2**).

A prospective fecundability study published in 2004, demonstrated that infertility increases with couples' age (**1**); however, 80% of couples under 40 will conceive within the first 12 months of trying and 90% within the first 2 years (general population). (See further Table 17.1.)

It is estimated that infertility affects 10–15% of couples, and it is often appropriate to offer further clinical assessment and investigation to those concerned by these delays.

Care provided by a primary practitioner should include initial advice regarding lifestyle factors that can influence fertility, and an enquiry about sexual history. Table 17.2 details the main lifestyle factors that should be addressed and optimised.

TABLE 17.1

Cumulative Probability of Conceiving a Clinical Pregnancy by the Number of Menstrual Cycles in Different Age Categories (this Assumes Vaginal Intercourse Twice per Week) (Data from [**3**, **4**])

Age category (years)	Pregnant after 1 year (12 cycles) %	Pregnant after 2 years (24 cycles) %
19–26	92	98
27–29	87	95
30–34	86	94
35–39	82	90

TABLE 17.2

Lifestyle Factors That Should Be Discussed with Couples Concerned Regarding Their Fertility

Lifestyle Factor	Advice
Weight – body mass index (BMI)	**Aim for BMI 19–30** **Women** with a BMI> 30 are likely to take longer to conceive. A BMI <19 could affect menstruation regularity. **Men** with a BMI >30 are likely to have reduced fertility
Alcohol	**Women** should keep intake to a minimum and aim to keep below 4 units per week. **Men** should be aware that excessive alcohol intake is detrimental to semen quality. Intake within the recommended daily intake is unlikely to affect semen quality.
Smoking	**Women** who smoke are likely to reduce their fertility and should be offered smoking cessation support. Passive smoking is also likely to affect chances of conception. **Men** should aim to stop smoking for their overall health and know there is an association between smoking and reduced semen quality. The use of electronic cigarettes (e-cigarettes) or commonly termed 'vaping' is generally viewed as less harmful than conventional smoking, nonetheless animal models have shown detrimental effects on spermatogenesis (**5–7**), and negative effects on implantation success. Whilst there are so many unknowns with regards to vaping and fertility in humans, this should be advised against and encouraged to give up.
Recreational Drugs	Recreational drugs interfere with male and female fertility and support should be offered for cessation.
Tight underwear	**Men** should be informed that there is an association between elevated scrotal temperature and reduced semen quality (**8**).
Occupational hazards	Some occupational exposures can reduce female and male fertility and a specific enquiry about this should be made.

DOI: 10.1201/9781003269502-17

After further exploration of history, referral to a fertility specialist may be indicated early if

- the female is > 36 years, or
- there is a known or a suspected history of a condition that predisposes to infertility. Examples of such conditions include Turner's syndrome, endocrine dysfunction, Endometriosis, previous pelvic inflammatory disease or abdominal sepsis, uterine anomalies, cystic fibrosis (this list is not exhaustive).

17.1 Referral to a Fertility Specialist

The initial encounter with a fertility specialist is arguably the most important as it sets the tone for subsequent evaluation and treatment. This ideally should be with both partners present to facilitate a thorough assessment of their clinical histories, and to offer the opportunity to ask questions.

It is important that the couple feel they are both involved in decision-making and that the clinician is receptive to both of their concerns. The attitude and behaviour of the health care professional should be supportive, communicative, and empathetic and help create a 'safe' environment to discuss very sensitive issues.

This first consultation is also a good opportunity to explore the emotional impact of infertility on the couple. The psychological burden may already be considerable and further intimate and invasive investigations may exacerbate stress and anxiety. Discussions surrounding psychological support that is available are crucial and may include onward referral to counselling services or signposting to fertility support groups.

17.2 History Taking

When a fertility practitioner is taking a detailed history with a couple, they are trying to ascertain where potential problems could be within the reproductive tracts or in the process of fertilisation and implantation.

A systematic approach is often helpful to ensure lines of enquiry are not missed. Table 17.3 details important information required from all fertility histories.

TABLE 17.3

Fertility History Taking

History Feature	Features	Reason for enquiry
Menstrual cycle	• Regularity • Cycle length • Number of days of bleeding • Associated symptoms • Any climacteric symptoms • Any intermenstrual bleeding	• Trying to establish if likely to have regular ovulatory cycles • Exploring signs and symptoms of ovulatory disorders and ovarian insufficiency • Screening for symptoms of pathology
Contraceptive history	• History of all contraceptive methods used including long acting reversible contraceptives (LARCs) and intrauterine devices (IUDs) • Explore any problems or complications with these	• Understand previous exposure to hormonal therapy: explore any side effects • Establish if potentially fertility problems have existed for longer
Pregnancy history	• Any previous positive pregnancy tests • Dates and details of any US scan findings • Management of any miscarriages – conservative, medical, surgical • History of any terminations and details of these • Details of any deliveries: gestation and mode of delivery • Any complications during pregnancy	• Determine if primary or secondary infertility • Explore history of recurrent miscarriage and possibility of Antiphospholipid syndrome (APS) • Understand if any previous problems in pregnancy that may need further risk assessment and optimisation • Previous ectopic pregnancy could be indicative of tubal damage
Smear history	• Up to date with screening? • Any abnormal smears and outcomes of further treatment • Any surgical procedures on cervix	• Important for opportunistic health surveillance • Explore possible difficulties with speculum or pelvic examinations and surrounding anxieties • Assess potential for difficulties accessing uterus for other investigations or treatment • Understand if there are risk factors for cervical incompetence that may need further review prior to planning a pregnancy.
Sexual history	• Frequency • Timing: Knowledge of fertile time of cycle/ovulation testing • Physical difficulties • Pre-existing conditions that affect intercourse • Previous sexually transmitted infections and management • Any psychosexual issues • Any previous history of sexual abuse	• Ascertain if the couple are having intercourse frequently enough • Enquiry about erectile dysfunction, ejaculatory problems and dyspareunia may highlight the need for further investigation or referral to alternative specialists. • Identification of social and psychological factors that may need further support

(Continued)

TABLE 17.3 ***(Continued)***

Fertility History Taking

History Feature	Features	Reason for enquiry
Medical and surgical History	• List any pre-existing medical conditions and if any specialist involvement. • Explore previous conditions that may have been cured/ treated but still have implications i.e. previous cancer treatment, previous infections • Document any previous surgeries and any anaesthetic issues. • Any possible events in life that could have caused harm or damage to reproductive organs i.e. testicular injury, mumps, severe infections/hypoperfusion, radiotherapy/ chemotherapy • Any previous fertility treatment or assessment	• Assess the need for further specialist input prior to planning a pregnancy • Are all pre-existing conditions well managed and optimised? • Consideration for effects of treatment and pregnancy on conditions • Consideration of any previous surgeries and whether these could affect gamete production or accessibility of ovaries for treatment. • Particularly important surgical procedures: undescended tests, orchidopexy, hernia repair, testicular torsion, vasectomy, reversal of vasectomy, • Do either of the couple have a genetic condition that may need genetic counselling consideration before embarking on a pregnancy? • Obtain all details of previous fertility treatment and response, to help plan future options.
Family History	• Explore if any fertility issues within the family e.g. premature ovarian failure, endometriosis, polycystic ovarian syndrome • Any genetic conditions that need to be considered	• Consider the need for screening for genetic or familial conditions. • Understand potential risk factors in the family i.e. clotting disorders, autoimmune
Social History	• Occupation • Weight • Alcohol • Smoking • Exercise frequency and intensity • Recreational drugs • Diet	• Assess the potential for any occupational hazards that may affect fertility e.g. exposure to ionising radiation, pesticides, aniline dyes, lead, chronic heat exposure. • Evaluate if any lifestyle factors that can be modified to improve chances of conception • Always consider if anything within the history raises concerns with safeguarding and consideration of welfare of the child.
Medication	• All prescriptions – details of doses, preparations, and frequency • Any over the counter medication taken • Other supplements/vitamins • Any allergies or sensitivities to medication	• Ensure all medical problems have been accounted for in the medical history • Assess if on any medications that are teratogenic or should be avoided whilst trying to conceive • Explore if any supplements could be detrimental to fertility health • Understand what further supplements could be advised to take

Problems with delayed conception may be multi-factorial and can come from either or both partners (**2**). It is therefore vital to explore both partners' histories in detail and follow up with history specific investigations that may run in parallel with other routine baseline investigations. A fertility assessment should also include physical examination of both partners as this may pick up possible clinical signs or a new diagnosis of a condition not revealed within history taking (**9**). Boxes 17.1 and 17.2 describe aspects of the Female and Male examination that are important, together with findings terminology that may be included in medical documentation.

BOX 17.1 FEMALE PHYSICAL EXAMINATION

- Record height, weight and calculate BMI
- Observe for any signs of thyroid dysfunction, hyperandrogenism and galactorrhoea and note hair distribution.
- Perform an abdominal palpation to assess for any abdominal masses
- Inspect the pubic region for any discharge, inflammation, atrophy, ulceration or abnormalities of the Bartholin's gland.
- Inspect for any signs of pelvic organ prolapse or urinary leakage on coughing or straining down.
- Perform a speculum examination to identify the cervix and note its appearance including any ectropion, polyps, abnormal or suspicious lesions.
- Consider swabs or a cervical smear if due.
- Note down any observed difficulties with the examination such as vulvodynia or extreme discomfort.
- Consider a bimanual examination

EXAMINATION TERMINOLOGY

Vaginal atrophy is the thinning, drying and inflammation of the vaginal mucosa that may occur when the body is exposed to lower concentrations of oestrogen (mainly evident post menopause).

Cervical ectropion (previously termed erosion) is the appearance of a red, velvet like and often raw looking area on the outer surface of the cervix. This is a benign finding and a variation of normal. It is caused by the delicate columnar cells that line the cervical canal, migrating onto the outside surface of the cervix in response to hormonal fluctuations.

Vulvodynia refers to persistent pain within the vulva,

Cervicitis

Vaginitis is inflammation of the vagina and may be indicative of infection, dietary deficiency or poor hygiene.

Vaginismus is the sudden and painful contraction of the muscles surrounding the vagina usually in response to the vulva or vagina being touched.

Cervical motion tenderness (excitation) describes the discomfort displayed by a patient upon palpation or movement of the cervix. This is often a sign of pelvic pathology, most commonly pelvic infection.

Vaginal septum is a partition within the vagina that could be partial or full

Galactorrhoea describes the discharge of a milky substance from the nipples unrelated to normal milk production in breastfeeding.

Hyperandrogenism refers to an excessive secretion of androgens in women. This can lead to clinical signs and symptoms such as acne, hirsutism, menstrual disturbances.

BOX 17.2 MALE PHYSICAL EXAMINATION

- Observe for any signs of decreased body hair or gynaecomastia suggestive of androgen insufficiency
- Record height, weight and calculate BMI
- Inspect the groin, perineum, penis and scrotal skin for any redness, rashes, swelling, or ulceration. Observe with the patient standing to see if any visible varicocele.
- Palpate the penis and note any abnormal curvature, pigmentation, discharge, nodules or masses. Retract the prepuce (foreskin) to check for phimosis or adhesions.
- Palpate the scrotum and check the size of the testes using an orchidometer for volume estimation. A mean volume of 20ml in the adult is considered normal.
- Assess the testes consistency, noting any nodules or irregularities. The testes should be soft and smooth and may be slightly different sizes.
- Palpate the distribution of the epididymis. This should barely be palpable in its normal state and should not be tender.
- If any abnormal symptoms of discharge or dysuria, consider whether a urethral swab is indicated.
- Abnormalities in the male genital examination often warrant referral to a Urologist for further assessment.

EXAMINATION TERMINOLOGY (SEE ALSO FIGURES 17.1, 17.2)

Hydroceles are common and are an accumulation of fluid in the tunica vaginalis.

Spermatoceles are smaller cysts of the epididymis.

Varicoceles are a collection of dilated veins in the spermatic cord, more commonly affecting the left side of the scrotum. They are sometimes described as 'a bag of worms' in the scrotum. They are usually asymptomatic, but can cause an occasional aching discomfort. In some cases, varicoceles are associated with a reduced semen parameters.

Epididymitis is inflammation of the epididymis usually caused by sexually transmitted infections, urinary tract pathogens or non-gonococcal urethritis.

Orchitis is painful inflammation and swelling of the testis and is often associated with epididymitis and less commonly mumps or syphilis infection. This may affect one or both testes. The pain is often deep and accompanied with nausea.

Unilateral testicular atrophy may result from mumps infection, vascular compromise after inguinal hernia repair or following later orchidopexy for undescended testes.

Bilateral testicular atrophy suggests primary or secondary hypogonadism. Correlate with signs of secondary sexual characteristics and signs of anabolic steroid use.

Orchidopexy is the name given to the surgical procedure in which undescended testes in the groin is mobilised and fixed in the scrotum. This operation should be performed well before puberty to allow the testis every chance of normal development.

Phimosis is the inability to retract the foreskin.

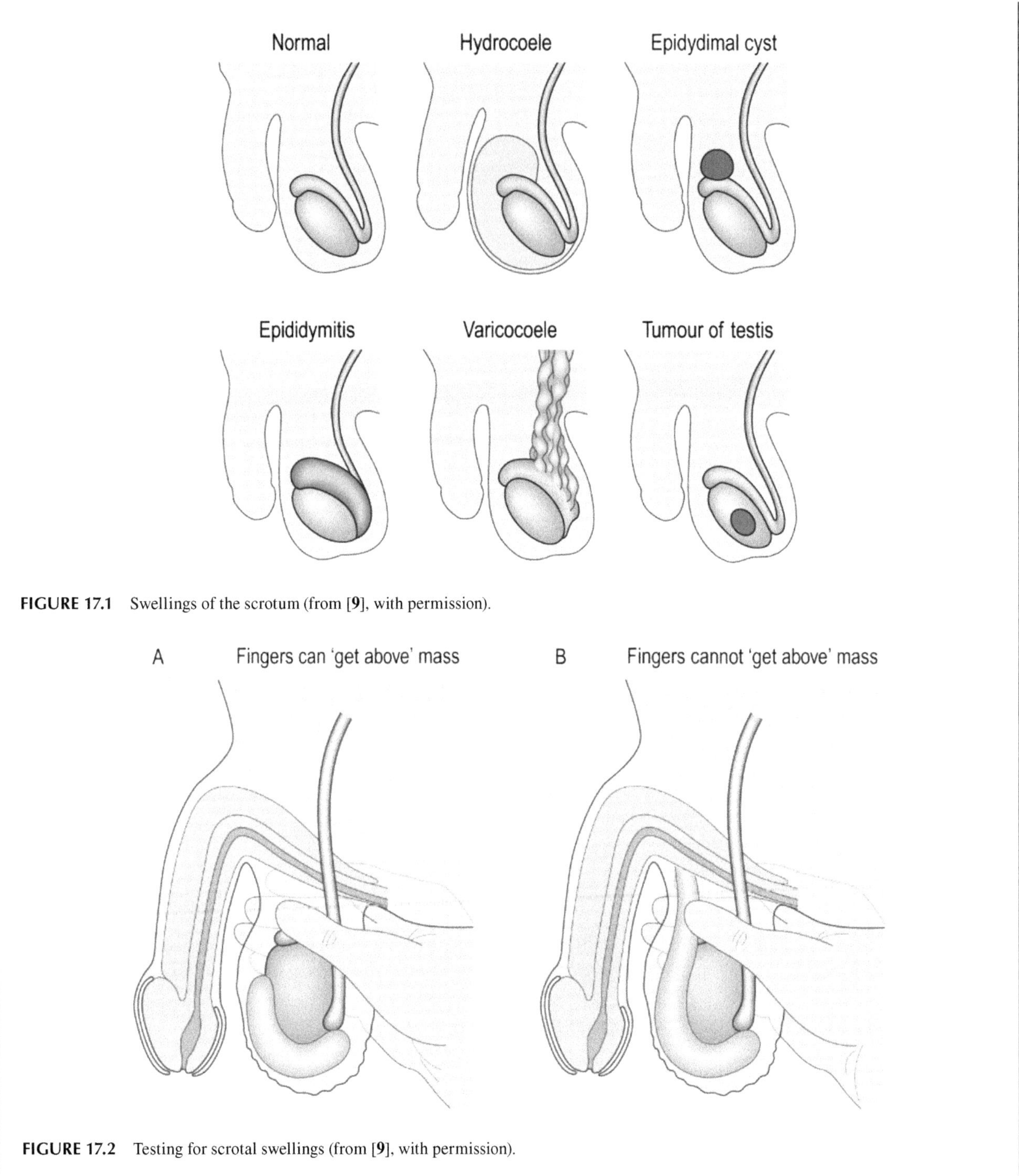

FIGURE 17.1 Swellings of the scrotum (from [**9**], with permission).

FIGURE 17.2 Testing for scrotal swellings (from [**9**], with permission).

17.3 Baseline Investigations

Before any treatment plan is devised, four basic investigations should ideally be performed and reviewed (Figure 17.3):

- Ovarian reserve
- Ovulation confirmation
- Tubal patency
- Semen analysis

Whilst this is good medical practice, if patients or clinicians already know there are features in the history that necessitate ART, or if it is the couple's choice to go straight for empirical treatment with IVF, then testing of the fallopian tubes may be academic with no implications for treatment.

17.3.1 Testing for Ovarian Reserve

Ovarian reserve testing provides an indirect estimate of a woman's remaining follicular pool (**10**). It is well known that

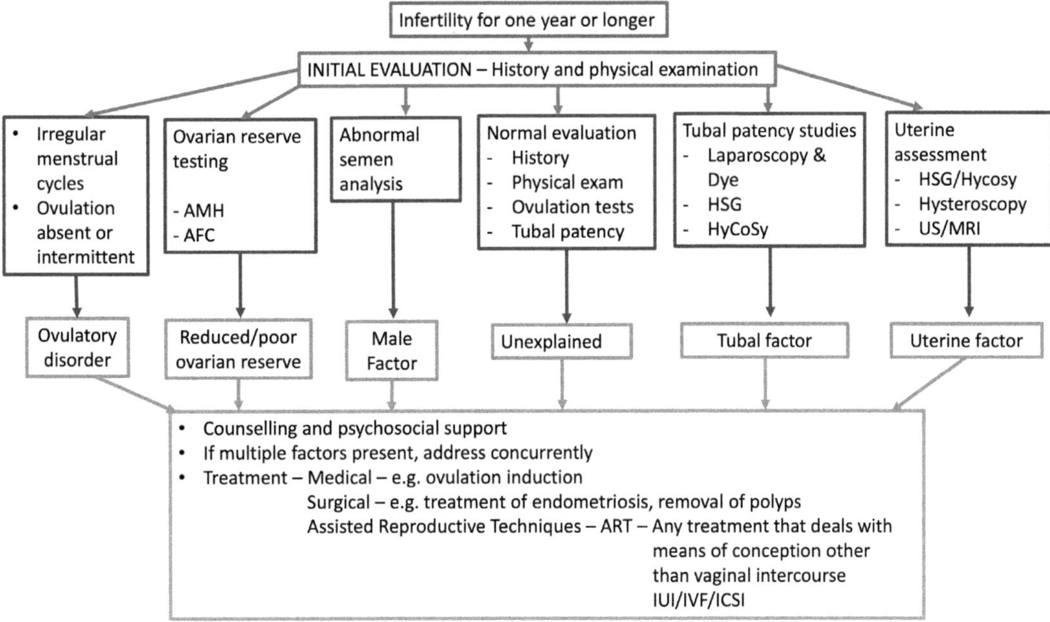

FIGURE 17.3 Key baseline investigations and potential causes of conception delay (adapted from [**20**]).

reproductive capacity is related to chronological age, however ovarian reserve is not always equivalent to chronological age and therefore this relationship is not absolute, for example a woman in her mid-20s could potentially have a very low ovarian reserve and display signs and symptoms of premature ovarian insufficiency (**11**).

There are various investigations that have been employed to evaluate a woman's ovarian reserve including serum markers, (basal FSH, AMH, inhibin B, basal oestradiol), ultrasound markers (AFC and ovarian volume) and less commonly used, challenge tests (Clomiphene citrate challenge test, exogenous FSH ovarian reserve test, GnRH agonist stimulation test).

The presence of so many different markers demonstrates that none of these tests are ideal, with relative merits and limitations (**12**). The three more commonly used tests will be considered here; basal FSH, AMH and AFC.

17.3.2 Basal FSH

Basal FSH testing refers to the serum level of FSH during the early follicular phase between day 2 and 5 of a woman's menstrual cycle. An FSH level of >10u/L at this time of the woman's cycle indicates a reduced ovarian reserve.

17.3.3 AMH

In the female, AMH is initially expressed by the granulosa cells in the ovary from as early as 36 weeks gestation (in utero). Its production continues until menopause (see Box 17.3).

> **BOX 17.3 UNDERSTANDING MENOPAUSE TERMINOLOGY (13)**
>
> ***Menopause*** is defined as the time period following 12 months of amenorrhoea (no periods). The terms *menopause* and *post-menopause* are often used interchangeably to describe the phase of a woman's life from this point (**13**).
>
> The ***perimenopause*** comprises the time from a woman's 'mature reproductive state' at the point when she begins to experience variability in the length of her menstrual cycle, or characteristic symptoms of the menopausal transition (climacteric), to the year following her final menstrual period.
>
> ***Climacteric*** symptoms include vasomotor (hot flashes or night sweats), urogenital (vaginal dryness and irritation, pelvic organ prolapse, urinary frequency, urgency and incontinence, increased risk of urinary tract infections), psychological (depression, irritability, poor concentration, memory loss) and other physical symptoms such as sleep disturbance, restless leg syndrome, lethargy and menorrhagia.

AMH is a dimeric glycoprotein belonging to the growth factor family. It is exclusively produced by the granulosa cells of preantral (primary and secondary) and small antral follicles in the ovary, therefore being a good indicator of the size of the ovarian antral follicle pool (**11**).

Its production first begins following transition of a primordial follicle into the primary stage and continues until follicles reach the antral stage with diameters between 2 and 6mm. Its main physiological function is to inhibit the recruitment of further primordial follicles into the antral follicle pool, thereby creating a negative feedback loop to prevent wastage. It also reduces the sensitivity of the growing follicles to FSH (**11**).

AMH can reliably be measured at any stage during the menstrual cycle due to its negligible intracycle and inter-cycle variation (**14**). This makes it a much more favourable and reproducible marker but also avoids menstrual timing of the test. The lower a woman's AMH, the smaller her antral follicle pool and consequently ovarian reserve. High levels of AMH are suggestive of polycystic ovaries (**11**).

AMH can also be used to predict a quantitative response to ovarian stimulation in ART (**15, 16**). This makes it useful in individualising stimulation protocols and trying to prevent Ovarian Hyperstimulation Syndrome (OHSS) (**15**).

17.3.4 AFC

Antral follicle count (AFC) is defined as the total number of follicles measuring between 2mm and 10mm in greatest diameter (from both ovaries) identified on ultrasound. A total antral follicle count of less than or equal to 4 indicates a predicted low response to stimulation (low reserve), whereas an AFC greater than 16 predicts a high response (high reserve) (**2**). AFC is comparable to AMH in predicting ovarian reserve (**11, 16**).

17.3.5 Investigating Ovulation

Women with regular menstrual cycles are likely to be ovulating (**2**). This can be confirmed by either commercial ovulation testing kits or by testing the progesterone in the middle of the luteal phase (day 21 in a regular 28-day cycle).

This can be problematic in patients with oligomenorrhoea and should be adjusted according to the patient's individual cycle length where known.

17.3.6 Tubal Patency Studies

Assessment of the fallopian tubes for potential obstruction or blockage can be achieved by various means including hysterosalpingography (HSG), hysterosalpingo-contrast-ultrasonography (HyCoSy) or a laparoscopy and dye test (**17**). In order to reduce the risk of iatrogenic introduction of infection, patients should have a pre-procedure vaginal swab performed and reviewed. If any infection is identified this should be treated prior to any tubal patency studies.

17.3.7 HSG

HSG evaluates the shape and patency of the fallopian tubes by using X rays to capture movement of a contrast dye that is injected through the cervical canal. If the fallopian tubes are patent then subsequent radiological images can display the dye moving through the uterus, into the fallopian tubes and out the fimbrial ends, so called 'fill and spill'. It is a relatively cheap and accessible test (**17**) and therefore has a large pool of evidence to support its use with a high specificity of 87% (a negative test correctly identifies patent tubes in 87% of cases) (**18**). Occasionally false positives can be created due to spasm of the fallopian tube appearing like a blockage, or due to the presence of debris that may cause an intermittent obstruction (**17**).

The radiation exposure should also be considered as this is significantly higher than a standard chest X ray (**19**).

17.3.8 HyCoSy

HyCoSy uses vaginal ultrasound to track the dissipation of a water-soluble contrast medium injected into the uterine cavity. It avoids the use of radiation and is usually performed in an outpatient setting similar to HSG. On a comparative basis, HyCoSy is more sensitive and specific than HSG and is usually very well tolerated (**17**).

17.3.9 Laparoscopy and Dye

A laparoscopy is a surgical procedure employed to visualise the internal abdominal and pelvic organs. It is a much more invasive tubal patency procedure usually requiring a general anaesthetic. In addition to providing direct visualisation of the entire length of the fallopian tubes, if a patient has a history suggestive of previous infection or endometriosis, this can also be assessed. There is also the possibility of opportunistic treatment of mild endometriosis or peri-adnexal adhesions which could confer a significant therapeutic benefit (**17**).

17.3.10 Semen Analysis

Further detail of this has been provided in Chapter 20, however see Box 17.4 for the WHO classification criteria and diagnostic terminology.

BOX 17.4 SEMEN REFERENCE RANGES AND REPORT TERMINOLOGY (2)

Parameter	Reference limit
Semen volume (ml)	1.5
Sperm concentration (10^6/ml)	15.0
Total number (106/ejaculate)	39.0
Total motility (PR + NP, %)	40.0
Progressive motility (PR, %)	32.0
Normal forms (%)	4
Vitality (%)	58

NP = Non-Progressive Motility PR = Progressive Motility

Oligozoospermia: low numbers of sperm within the ejaculate (reduced sperm count).

Teratozoospermia: high numbers of abnormal sperm within the ejaculate

Asthenozoospermia: sperm with poor motility

Oligo-asthenoteratozoospermia (OATS): low numbers, reduced motility and abnormality of the sperm shape in the ejaculated sample

Azoospermia: complete absence of sperm in the ejaculate

Motile forms: sperm with a heightened ability to swim

As is often the case in medicine, if a good relationship is built with the couple from the start, they will divulge the vast majority of information you need to understand the potential fertility problems.

REFERENCES

1. Novak E. *Berek & Novak's Gynecology*. Philadelphia, PA: Lippincott Williams & Wilkins; 2007.
2. Karavolos S, Panagiotopoulou N, Alahwany H, et al. An update on the management of male infertility. *Obstet Gynaecol*. 2020;22(4):267–274.
3. NICE. *Fertility Problems: Assessment and Treatment*. Clinical Guideline, National Institute for Health and Care Excellence, 2013. Available from: www.nice.org.uk/guideline/cg156.
4. Dunson DB, Baird DD, Colombo B. Increased infertility with age in men and women. *Obstet Gynecol*. 2004; 103(1):51–56.
5. Wetendorf M, Randall LT, Lemma MT, et al. E-cigarette exposure delays implantation and causes reduced weight gain in female offspring exposed in utero. *J Endocrine Soc*. 2019;3(10):1907–1916.
6. Rahali D, Jrad-Lamine A, Dallagi Y, et al. Semen parameter alteration, histological changes and role of oxidative stress in adult rat epididymis on exposure to electronic cigarette refill liquid. *Chin J Physiol*. 2018;61(2):75–84.
7. El Golli N, Rahali D, Jrad-Lamine A, et al. Impact of electronic-cigarette refill liquid on rat testis. *Toxicol Mech Methods*. 2016;26(6):417–424.
8. Karavolos S, Stewart J, Evbuomwan I, et al. Assessment of the infertile male. *Obstet Gynecol*. 2013;15(1):1–9.
9. Douglas G, Nicol F, Robertson C. *Macleod's Clinical Examination*. Amsterdam, The Netherlands: Elsevier Health Sciences; 2005.
10. Jirge PR. Ovarian reserve tests. *J Hum Reprod Sci*. 2011;4(3):108.
11. Bhide P, Shah A, Gudi A, et al. The role of anti-müllerian hormone as a predictor of ovarian function. *Obstet Gynecol*. 2012;14(3):161–166.
12. Nandi A, Homburg R. Unexplained subfertility: diagnosis and management. *Obstet Gynecol*. 2016;18(2):107–115.
13. Panay N, Briggs P, Kovacs G. *Managing the Menopause 21st Century Solutions, P. No 289*. Cambridge, UK: Cambridge University Press; 2015. p. 291.
14. La Marca A, Stabile G, Artenisio AC, et al. Serum anti-Mullerian hormone throughout the human menstrual cycle. *Hum Reprod*. 2006;21(12):3103–3107.
15. Broer S, Dólleman M, Opmeer B, et al. AMH and AFC as predictors of excessive response in controlled ovarian hyperstimulation: a meta-analysis. *Hum Reprod Update*. 2011;17(1):46–54.
16. La Marca A, Sighinolfi G, Radi D, et al. Anti-Müllerian hormone (AMH) as a predictive marker in assisted reproductive technology (ART). *Hum Reprod Update*. 2010;16(2):113–130.
17. Suresh YN, Narvekar NN. The role of tubal patency tests and tubal surgery in the era of assisted reproductive techniques. *Obstet Gynecol*. 2014;16(1):37–45.
18. Broeze KA, Opmeer BC, Van Geloven N, et al. Are patient characteristics associated with the accuracy of hysterosalpingography in diagnosing tubal pathology? An individual patient data meta-analysis. *Hum Reprod Update*. 2011;17(3):293–300.
19. Hart D, Hillier M, Wall B. National reference doses for common radiographic, fluoroscopic and dental X-ray examinations in the UK. *Br J Radiol*. 2009;82(973):1–12.
20. Yao M. *Clinical Management of Infertility*. Washington, DC: The Advisory Board; 2000.

18

Ovarian Stimulation Protocols

Pedro Melo

18.1 Introduction

Ovarian stimulation constitutes one of the pillars of medically assisted conception. It involves administering oral or injectable drugs that promote follicle development and ovulation. Ovarian stimulation can be used to treat a range of conditions, including anovulation due to polycystic ovary syndrome and hypogonadotrophic hypogonadism. In addition, in women undergoing in vitro fertilisation, ovarian stimulation is often performed concomitantly with pituitary suppression to prevent untimely ovulation; this is termed controlled ovarian stimulation (COS). This chapter describes the principles underlying ovarian stimulation, the pharmacology of exogenous gonadotrophins, and commonly used stimulation protocols.

18.2 Physiology of Ovarian Stimulation

The ovarian cycle comprises three main stages: the follicular phase, marked by the development of several antral follicles, of which one usually becomes dominant under the influence of follicle-stimulating hormone (FSH); ovulation, during which the dominant follicle releases an oocyte into the fallopian tube after a surge in serum luteinising hormone (LH) levels; and the luteal phase, where progesterone, synthesised by the corpus luteum, induces the secretory activity of the endometrium and facilitates embryo implantation (**1**).

Follicle development depends on the coordinated actions of granulosa and theca cells. Under the influence of LH, the theca interna cells convert cholesterol into androgens; these, in turn, undergo conversion into oestrogens by the enzyme aromatase in granulosa cells. The granulosa cells of antral follicles contain apical surface receptors that are responsive to FSH. In the follicular phase, FSH activity results in follicle growth and oestrogen synthesis from theca-derived androgen precursors (**2**). As antral follicles grow and reach a diameter above 10 mm, the granulosa cells also begin expressing LH receptors, thus becoming sensitised to the LH surge just before ovulation (**3**). FSH and LH are essential to follicle development in the natural ovarian cycle. In cycles stimulated with exogenous gonadotrophins, however, it remains unclear whether adding LH to FSH preparations towards the end of the follicular phase improves treatment outcomes (**4**).

Ovarian stimulation treatment requires oral tablets or gonadotrophin injections to obtain one or more ovulatory follicles containing mature eggs. It is essential to distinguish ovulation induction, which usually involves ovarian stimulation in the absence of pituitary suppression, from COS, which requires downregulation of the pituitary gland to prevent premature ovulation and allow clinicians to schedule oocyte retrieval procedures in IVF.

In women with anovulatory subfertility, ovulation induction can be performed with oral agents (e.g., clomifene citrate and letrozole) or gonadotrophin injections (e.g., urinary or recombinant FSH), followed by timed intercourse or intrauterine insemination (IUI). However, if timed intercourse or IUI fail, or where additional pathology underlies a couple's subfertility (e.g., tubal or male factor), COS may be required. This usually involves gonadotrophin injections, administered to induce the growth of multiple follicles, in addition to preventing premature ovulation by suppressing the hypothalamic-hypophyseal axis (e.g., with gonadotrophin-releasing hormone analogues or progestogens).

18.3 Oral Agents for Ovulation Induction

Ovulation induction is usually administered to women with World Health Organisation type II anovulation, of which polycystic ovary syndrome (PCOS) accounts for over 80% of cases (**5**). The Rotterdam criteria, set by an international consensus in 2003, establish that a diagnosis of PCOS should be made where at least two of the following features are present: polycystic ovary morphology on transvaginal ultrasound (12 or more follicles per ovary measuring 2–9 mm, or an ovarian volume above 10 ml); irregular menstrual cycles (shorter than 21 days or longer than 35 days, or fewer than eight cycles per year); and clinical or biochemical evidence of hyperandrogenism (hirsutism, acne, alopecia; and high free testosterone or high free androgen index) (**6**). The diagnostic criteria for PCOS have since evolved to reflect improvements in ultrasound technology; for example, the latest international guidance suggests that the threshold for polycystic ovary morphology should be an antral follicle count of ≥20 and/or an ovarian volume ≥ 10 ml (**7**).

Three main oral agents are used for ovulation induction: clomifene citrate, letrozole and metformin.

18.3.1 Clomifene Citrate

Clomifene citrate has been used in ovulation induction since the early 1960s (**8**). It is a selective oestrogen receptor modulator exhibiting agonist and antagonist activity depending on

DOI: 10.1201/9781003269502-18

endogenous oestrogen levels. Clomifene exerts antagonistic effects upon oestrogen receptors mainly in the hypothalamus, and to a lesser extent the pituitary gland (**9**). Its central blockage of oestrogen receptors disrupts the negative feedback loop exerted by circulating oestradiol levels, resulting in increased FSH secretion by the pituitary. Rising circulating FSH levels, in turn, act on the granulosa cells in the ovary and promote follicle growth and a rise in oestradiol levels. This results in a substantial increase in ovulation rates, with as many as 4 in 5 anovulatory women with an intact hypothalamic-hypophyseal-ovarian axis experiencing ovulation resumption after clomifene citrate (**10**). Cumulatively, the live birth rate with clomifene treatment can be as high as 60% after six cycles, in the absence of additional pathology contributing to an individual's subfertility (**11**).

Clomifene is administered initially at a dose of 50 mg once daily for five days in the early follicular phase (from days 2 to 6, or from days 3 to 7) (**12, 13**). In women who remain anovulatory, as detected by an absent LH surge on urine testing or an absent corpus luteum on transvaginal ultrasound in the luteal phase, the dose can be up titrated monthly by 50 mg increments up to a total of 150 mg once daily. In the United Kingdom, The National Institute for Health and Care Excellence (NICE) recommends no more than six consecutive cycles of clomifene treatment before considering second-line oral therapies (e.g., metformin or gonadotrophins) or in vitro fertilisation, because any additional cycles of clomifene are unlikely to be effective (**14**). It is estimated that up to 20% of anovulatory women are resistant to clomifene citrate, although the reason for this remains unclear (**15**).

Albeit usually well tolerated, clomifene citrate treatment may result in significant adverse events, including hot flushes, gastrointestinal disturbances, ovarian cysts, and visual disturbances which can range from reversible reduction in acuity to permanent optic neuropathy (**16, 17**). Importantly, from a reproductive standpoint, clomifene has been associated with thinning of the endometrium and a high rate of multiple pregnancies (6–8%), usually twins (**18, 19**). For this reason, fertility specialists recommend cycle cancellation and avoidance of unprotected intercourse where more than two dominant follicles are seen on ultrasound during the follicular phase of clomifene-treated menstrual cycles. Lastly, moderate and severe OHSS cases are rare in clomifene citrate cycles (**20**).

18.3.2 Letrozole

Letrozole inhibits the enzyme aromatase, responsible for the conversion of androgens into oestrogens in the granulosa cells of ovarian follicles. This reduces the levels of circulating estradiol, largely eliminating its negative feedback upon the pituitary gland, whose secretion of FSH hence increases (**21**). Like clomifene citrate, letrozole is usually administered for five days in the beginning of the menstrual cycle, in doses ranging between 2.5 and 7.5 mg once daily, titrated according to response (**22, 23**). A seminal randomised controlled trial including more than 700 participants identified evidence that letrozole improves the live birth rate and reduces the risk of multiple pregnancy in comparison to clomifene citrate in women undergoing OI for PCOS-associated subfertility (**24**). The side effects associated with letrozole include hot flushes and night sweats, although they are rarely severe. In a recent network meta-analysis investigating treatment strategies for ovulation induction, the authors confidently identified a reduction in multiple pregnancy rates associated with letrozole in comparison to clomifene (odds ratio [OR] 0.46, 95% confidence interval [CI] 0.23 to 0.92) (**25**).

Based on the existing evidence, the 2018 International Evidence-Based Guideline for the Assessment and Management of Polycystic Ovary Syndrome recommends letrozole as the first-line treatment for OI in PCOS-associated subfertility (**7**).

18.3.3 Metformin

Metformin is a biguanide that acts by improving insulin sensitivity. While it is mostly used as a treatment for type 2 diabetes mellitus, the association between insulin resistance and PCOS has led researchers to investigate the use of metformin in ovulation induction. There is a paucity of high-certainty evidence on the effectiveness of metformin for WHO type II anovulatory women, but a recent Cochrane review found evidence that when used in isolation, metformin may improve live birth rates compared with placebo (OR 1.59, 95% CI 1.00 to 2.51) (**26**). The aforementioned 2018 guideline recommends that clinicians should consider metformin as a second-line treatment for anovulatory PCOS, alone or in combination with letrozole or clomifene, mainly for its metabolic properties (**7**).

18.4 Gonadotrophins for Ovarian Stimulation

Exogenous gonadotrophins remain the most commonly used drugs in ovarian stimulation. In women undergoing ovulation induction because of WHO type I anovulation (e.g., hypogonadotrophic hypogonadism), gonadotrophins constitute the first-line stimulation drugs, whereas in cases of WHO type II anovulation they are usually administered as second-line agents after oral agents have failed. In COS for IVF/ICSI, exogenous gonadotrophins are almost universally used to induce multifollicular growth, although some authors suggest that oral agents may have a role in women with predicted low response, either alone or in combination with gonadotrophins (**13, 22, 23**).

There are various types of gonadotrophins, differing in source, molecular composition, purity and administration route.

18.4.1 Urinary Gonadotrophins

Urinary gonadotrophins are derived from the urine of postmenopausal women, who excrete high levels of FSH and LH; and pregnant women, whose urine contains high levels of human chorionic gonadotrophin (hCG) (**27**). These drugs have been commercially available since the 1960s, and were initially used exclusively for the purposes of ovulation induction in women with anovulation. A decade later, the advent of IVF brought about the routine use of gonadotrophins for ovarian stimulation before oocyte retrieval. Since these gonadotrophins were extracted from the urine of postmenopausal women, the combination of FSH and LH was called human menopausal gonadotrophin (hMG) (**28**). Such preparations contained both FSH and LH in a 1:1 ratio, yet the presence of other urinary protein compounds reduced their purity. Thus, the first generation of hMG drugs featured high inter-batch variation, in addition to substantial immunogenicity requiring intramuscular administration (**29**). It is also important to note that the need to obtain urine from human volunteers renders hMG a potentially finite resource.

As extraction methods improved, pharmaceutical companies developed highly purified hMG preparations, with the first product introduced in Europe in the year 2000 (**30**). Although the ratio of FSH to LH remained 1:1, these refined formulations contained a reduced amount of contaminants and were therefore suitable for subcutaneous administration, lowering the risk of allergic reactions and increasing patient tolerability to daily injections (**27, 29**).

In view of evidence demonstrating the predominant effect of FSH upon initial follicle recruitment and development, as well as concerns about the potentially deleterious effect of LH upon endometrial receptivity, preparations containing purified urinary FSH (uFSH) were also introduced in the 1980s (**27**). Historically these contained varying degrees of LH activity, whereas today highly purified uFSH drugs hold fewer than 0.1 international units (IU) of LH per 1 IU of FSH (**29**). In addition, urinary FSH preparations are usually more acidic than recombinant forms, due to differences in glycosylation patterns (**27**).

18.4.2 Recombinant Gonadotrophins

In the 1990s, the massification of recombinant DNA technology led to the development of recombinant gonadotrophin formulations, whose manufacturing was possible in industrial amounts using Chinese Hamster Ovary (CHO) cells. Pharmaceutical companies have since released a plethora of recombinant forms, including rFSH, rLH and rhCG. These offer improved accessibility, large scale manufacturing, minimal batch-to-batch variability and low immunogenicity. They are also administered subcutaneously, resulting in less pain and fewer adverse reactions compared with some intramuscular urinary preparations (**27, 29**).

Multiple FSH preparations exist across the world, yet not all FSH drugs are the same. This is because there are many FSH isoforms, which despite featuring a similar core structure, possess varying biochemical properties resulting from different post-translational modifications within the FSH molecules, including glycosylation and the addition of sialic acid residues (**31**). The first rFSH formulation, introduced in 1995, was named follitrophin alpha, and there have since been various additional preparations including follitrophin beta and follitrophin delta, whose biochemical structure varies slightly (**32**). Follitrophin alpha and beta are synthesised in CHO cells, however follitrophin delta is unique in that its manufacturing requires human fetal retinal cells (**33**). Additional biochemical modifications affect the pharmacokinetics of rFSH preparations; for example, corifollitrophin alpha is a type of rFSH whose long half-life allows the effect of a single injection to last for seven days, thus requiring much fewer injections for stimulation and improving patient tolerability to treatment (**27, 29**).

In the past decade, following the expiration of the original follitrophin alpha patent, pharmaceutical companies have developed biosimilar drugs containing a version of the active compound whose effectiveness and safety should in principle be equivalent to those of the original follitrophin alpha. The evidence from randomised controlled trials (RCTs) comparing the reference drug to the newly developed biosimilars is scarce, however, and largely underpowered to detect differences in live birth rates, focusing instead on oocyte numbers (**27, 34**).

18.4.3 Effectiveness and Safety of Exogenous Gonadotrophins

The most recent Cochrane review investigating urinary versus recombinant gonadotrophins was published in 2011 (**35**). In it, the authors compared rFSH with the main types of urinary gonadotrophins (i.e., hMG and uFSH). Among 42 trials including 9,606 couples, the evidence showed a small-to-moderate reduction in live births using rFSH in comparison with hMG (OR 0.84, 95% CI 0.72 to 0.99), but no evidence of a difference when rFSH was compared with uFSH. However, existing systematic reviews have largely failed to report on subgroups of women according to predicted ovarian response to stimulation, which may result in inaccurate generalisations about the effectiveness and safety of stimulation protocols. Based on the existing evidence, the most recent guideline on ovarian stimulation by the European Society of Human Reproduction and Embryology states that the use of rFSH and hMG for ovarian stimulation is equally recommended (**36**).

A recent systematic review evaluated five RCTs comparing biosimilar alpha rFSH preparations to the original drug (**34**). The investigators found evidence of a 17% mean reduction in live birth with biosimilar drugs (risk ratio [RR] 0.83, 95% confidence interval (CI) 0.71 to 0.97; moderate-quality evidence). This result was mimicked by those of secondary out comes, including clinical pregnancy (RR 0.82, 95% CI 0.72 to 0.94) and ongoing pregnancy (RR 0.81, 95% CI 0.68 to 0.96). Contrary to these findings, however, the meta-analysis confidently demonstrated an increase in oocyte number when all biosimilar preparations were compared to follitrophin alpha (mean difference [MD] 1.95, 95% CI 1.78 to 2.12), although there was high statistical heterogeneity (I^2 = 88%). These results require further corroboration, specifically by conducting adequately powered studies to investigate the effect of biosimilar drugs on frozen embryo numbers and cumulative live birth rates.

18.5 Gonadotrophin-Releasing Hormone and Analogue Drugs

Gonadotrophin-releasing hormone is a tropic peptide hormone synthesised and released from hypothalamic GnRH neurons in a pulsatile fashion. Once synthesised, GnRH is secreted into the portal blood vessels and carried to the pituitary gland, where it acts on G-coupled receptors on the apical surface of anterior pituitary cells (**37, 38**). Binding of GnRH to these receptors induces the release of gonadotrophins (FSH, LH), whose synthesis otherwise occurs in periods of absent GnRH binding. The secretion of FSH and LH will then regulate the follicular and luteal phases of the menstrual cycle (**39**).

Gonadotrophin-releasing hormone analogues, including agonists and antagonists, are structurally similar to endogenous GnRH.

18.5.1 GnRH Agonists

Gonadotrophin-releasing hormone agonists were the first drugs used for pituitary suppression in COS prior to IVF. Like endogenous GnRH, GnRH agonists are decapeptide molecules. However, changes in the amino acid sequence (specifically positions 6 and 10) result in improved affinity towards GnRH receptors in the pituitary and a prolonged half-life compared to the natural GnRH hormone (**40**). Once administered, GnRH agonists exert a transient flare effect, increasing FSH secretion. Yet, continued agonist administration desensitises the GnRH receptors, resulting in pituitary downregulation after 10–14 days (**41**). This prevents a premature endogenous LH surge, thus allowing assisted conception practitioners to appropriately time ovulation triggering and oocyte retrieval.

Examples of GnRH agonist drugs include buserelin, triptorelin, leuprorelin, nafarelin, deslorelin and goserelin. They vary according to route (subcutaneous, intramuscular, nasal), dose, and frequency of administration (depot injection, daily injection or nasal administration several times a day) (**42**). Prolonged administration of GnRH agonists may result in a profoundly hypoestrogenic state, which often manifests through menopause-like symptoms including hot flushes, lethargy, low libido and vaginal dryness. These symptoms may persist after discontinuation of the GnRH agonist drug, but usually resolve within 2–4 weeks (**41, 43**).

18.5.2 GnRH Antagonists

The use of GnRH antagonists is akin to performing chemical hypophysectomy. Antagonist molecules contain ten amino acids, of which positions 1, 2, 3, 6 and 10 differ from those of endogenous GnRH (**44, 45**). They exhibit medium affinity (i.e., higher than that of natural GnRH, but lower than that of GnRH agonists) towards GnRH receptors and have an immediate onset of action (**46**).

Examples of GnRH antagonists include cetrorelix and ganirelix. Because they are administered for a short period of time and only after the onset of ovarian stimulation with gonadotrophins, GnRH antagonists rarely induce pituitary hormone withdrawal symptoms and are well tolerated. In addition, once these drugs are discontinued pituitary function resumes as normal (**47**).

18.6 Controlled Ovarian Stimulation Protocols

Stimulation protocols historically involved the use of gonadotrophin drugs in the menstrual cycle, followed by an ovulation trigger injection and oocyte retrieval 36–40 hours later. Premature ovulation was common in such protocols, resulting in high cancellation rates and failure to collect oocytes. In the 1980s, clinicians started using GnRH agonists for pituitary downregulation prior to ovarian stimulation with gonadotrophins (**48**). Since then, various protocol variations have been introduced into clinical practice, including the administration of GnRH antagonists instead of agonist drugs.

18.6.1 Long GnRH Agonist Protocols

Long agonist protocols involve the administration of GnRH agonist drugs for pituitary downregulation prior to ovarian stimulation. There are various regimens to achieve downregulation with GnRH agonists. They differ in the type of agonist used (e.g., buserelin, triptorelin, leuprorelin, nafarelin) and frequency of administration (e.g., nasal administration multiple times a day, daily subcutaneous injection, or a single intramuscular depot injection in the midluteal phase of the preceding menstrual cycle). Further, there have been trials investigating midluteal versus follicular initiation of GnRH agonists (**49**). Irrespective of the type, initiation timing and administration frequency of these drugs, their use aims to downregulate the pituitary before starting ovarian stimulation with exogenous gonadotrophins. Approximately one to two weeks after commencement of the agonist drug, or when patients experience menstrual bleeding, downregulation is usually confirmed by visualising quiescent ovaries (with all follicles measuring <10 mm) and a thin endometrial lining (<4–6 mm) on transvaginal ultrasound (**50**). Once downregulation has been established, gonadotrophin injections are usually started. In their latest Ovarian Stimulation guideline, ESHRE recommends a starting dose of 150–225 IU of gonadotrophins (**36**). Once stimulation begins, clinicians monitor ovarian response by performing regular ultrasound scans and recording the number and size of growing follicles on folliculogram charts. These measurements inform dose changes where required, with up or down titration of the stimulation drugs according to follicle numbers and development. Where a dose increase is required for low ovarian response during stimulation, the evidence suggests that total daily amounts of gonadotrophins beyond 300 IU are unlikely to accrue substantial benefit (**36**). The total duration of gonadotrophin administration varies according to the pace of follicle growth (usually 1–2 mm per day), with most women requiring 10 to 12 days of stimulation prior to ovulation triggering (**51**).

Long agonist protocols have remained the mainstay of COS regimens for years. In addition to substantially reducing the risk of cycle cancellation due to untimely ovulation, these protocols are associated with a more synchronous growth of ovarian follicles during stimulation and a higher oocyte yield, particularly in low-responding women (**52**). However, the advent of GnRH antagonists for pituitary suppression brought about a change in paradigm in favour of these newer drugs because of their improved safety and non-inferior effectiveness, as demonstrated by reduced OHSS and equivalent live birth rates to those of women having long agonist protocols (**47**).

18.6.2 Short GnRH Antagonist Protocols

Unlike long GnRH agonist protocols, where pituitary downregulation precedes the administration of gonadotrophins, in short antagonist protocols women commence exogenous gonadotrophins shortly after menstruation. Gonadotrophin-releasing hormone antagonists (e.g., cetrorelix or ganirelix) are then started to prevent premature ovulation, although there is no consensus on the optimal initiation timing of GnRH antagonist. There are various regimens, including a flexible-start protocol where clinicians make the decision to start antagonist injections once the leading follicle reaches a certain size (usually ≥14 mm), and a fixed-start protocol, in which women initiate the GnRH antagonist on days 5 or 6 of ovarian stimulation (**53**). To date, existing trials have not confidently identified a difference between the flexible and fixed initiation times (**54**).

An important benefit of GnRH antagonist protocols is that ovulation trigger may be administered both in the form of hCG or GnRH agonist. In women at high risk of OHSS (e.g., due to a history of PCOS or high serum anti-Müllerian hormone), a GnRH agonist trigger is preferred, as it temporarily displaces the antagonist drug from the pituitary GnRH receptors, thus inducing an endogenous LH surge required for oocyte maturation. While this reduces the risk of OHSS, the endogenous LH in cycles triggered with GnRH agonists is also insufficient for adequate luteal phase support. For this reason, ESHRE guidance recommends a freeze-all strategy in women undergoing short antagonist cycles with a GnRH agonist trigger. In long agonist cycles, it is not possible to trigger ovulation using GnRH agonists as this would only further suppress the pituitary. Instead, a reduced dose of hCG (usually 5,000 international units) should be considered in women at high risk of OHSS (**36**).

Meta-analysis data suggest that short antagonist protocols result in a lower oocyte yield when compared with long agonist regimens in an unselected population (**47**). This may be partly explained by a more asynchronous follicle growth in antagonist protocols, whereas in long agonist protocols, studies suggest a more homogenous growth of follicle cohorts once ovarian stimulation commences. Historically there have also been systematic reviews of RCT data suggesting that the clinical pregnancy rate per woman may be lower in people undergoing short antagonist protocols in comparison with long agonist protocols (**55**), yet recent meta-analyses have disputed such data by presenting moderate-certainty evidence that short antagonist protocols probably result in little to no difference in live birth rates (**47, 54**).

Importantly, however, there is a lack of data on long-term outcomes, including the number of frozen embryos and cumulative live birth rates per stimulation cycle. For example, it would be important to ascertain whether the improved oocyte yield obtained with long agonist protocols translates into a tangible difference in cumulative live birth rates. Existing studies have largely reported on the live birth rate following the first embryo transfer rather than cumulatively.

18.6.3 GnRH Agonist Flare Short Protocols

The administration of GnRH agonist drugs results in an initial flare effect due to a rise in FSH levels which lasts a few days, followed by pituitary suppression due to receptor desensitisation. In agonist flare short protocols, the GnRH agonist is started concurrently with gonadotrophins on day 2 of the menstrual cycle, and continued until the day of trigger injection to prevent premature ovulation. It has been suggested that low-responding women may benefit from such a protocol in view of the flare effect, enhanced synthesis of endogenous FSH and reduced duration of downregulation, although this may result in the development of fewer oocytes and impair endometrial function. Nonetheless, existing meta-analyses have not confidently identified a difference in live birth rates compared with long agonist protocols. Additionally, the latter have been shown to yield a higher oocyte number than agonist flare protocols (**41**).

18.6.4 GnRH Agonist Flare Ultrashort Protocols

In agonist flare ultrashort protocols, GnRH agonists are initiated concomitantly with gonadotrophins and continued for only a few days (usually 3), beyond which women continue gonadotrophin injections only. Authors who support such a protocol defend its flare effect and the absence of subsequent pituitary suppression as strategies to improve oocyte yield. However, meta-analysis data have not confidently identified a benefit in effectiveness in low-responding women (**41**; see Figure 18.1).

Figure 18.1 shows examples of commonly used COS protocols.

18.6.5 Relative Effectiveness and Safety of COS Protocols

The findings of a Cochrane systematic review and network meta-analysis investigating the effect of different COS protocols according to predicted ovarian response (high, normal or low) are currently awaited (**56**). Network meta-analysis (NMA; Figure 18.2) differs from standard pairwise comparisons in that it uses advanced statistical methodology to infer indirect evidence from existing direct comparisons. Provided that there are RCTs comparing one intervention and any other within one network, it is possible to calculate a weighted estimate using direct and indirect evidence, so that the final effect size corresponds to the network estimate. This allows researchers to compare interventions that may not have been investigated head-to-head in existing RCTs. Further, when enough network evidence exists, it is possible to use NMA to rank all the interventions in one network according to their effectiveness and safety (**57**).

The investigators leading the aforementioned Cochrane NMA on COS have recently reported their preliminary findings, including over 300 RCTs. The evidence showed that short antagonist protocols probably reduce OHSS rates by as much as 52% in predicted high-responding women, and 32% in predicted normal-responding women, without evidence of a reduction in live birth rates for all groups of women (predicted normal-, high-, and low-responding). Further, in women with predicted high response undergoing short-antagonist protocols, there was moderate-certainty evidence of a reduction in OHSS when performing COS with hMG compared with rFSH (**58**).

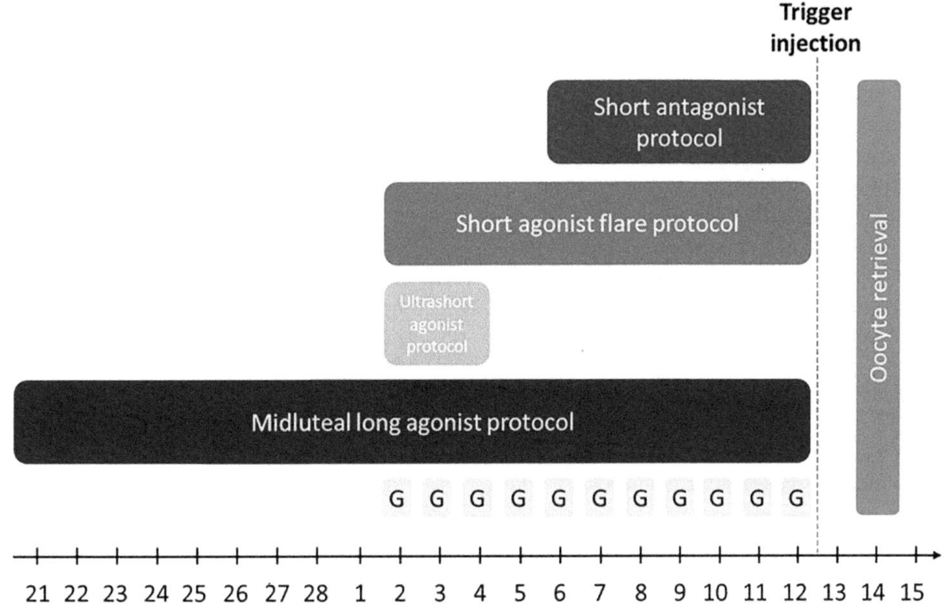

FIGURE 18.1 Examples of controlled ovarian stimulation protocols. The horizontal axis represents the days of the menstrual cycle. G, gonadotrophin injection.

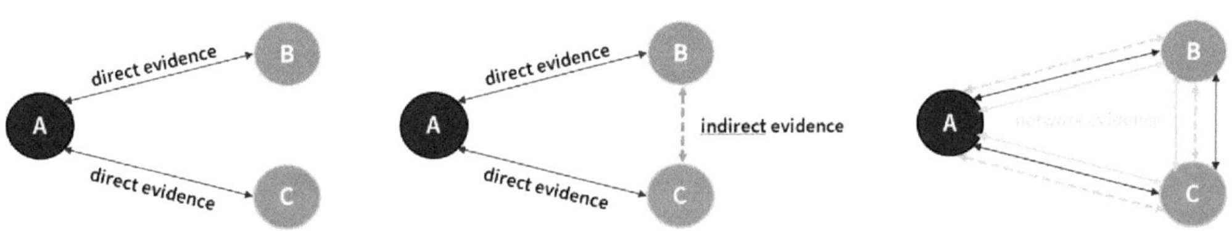

FIGURE 18.2 Network meta-analysis. Left: network diagram illustrating direct RCT evidence between treatments A vs. B, and A vs. C. Middle: inference of the B vs. C comparison is possible because of common comparator (treatment A). Right: the weighing of direct and indirect comparisons between all three treatments results in network estimates and ranking of all three treatments according to effectiveness and safety. RCT, randomised controlled trial.

18.7 Conclusion and Future Perspectives

Controlled ovarian stimulation is a fundamental step in fresh IVF cycles. There have been various combinations of gonadotrophin and pituitary suppression drugs, and multiple RCTs comparing these protocols to one another. Yet existing systematic reviews have failed to categorically identify a regimen with superior effectiveness and safety in comparison to all others. This stems partly from a lack of subgroup analyses according to predicted response to COS. However, the evidence suggests that short antagonist protocols reduce the rates of OHSS in normal- and high-responding women; it is important to take this in consideration when counselling patients about which protocol to choose. Finally, while it may be logistically difficult for RCTs to report on cumulative live birth rates per stimulation cycle initiated due to the long follow-up time, researchers should endeavour to collect such data (for example, by conducting secondary analyses), as well as reporting on proxy markers such as the number of frozen embryos per participant.

REFERENCES

1. Baerwald AR, Adams GP, Pierson RA. Ovarian antral folliculogenesis during the human menstrual cycle: a review. *Hum Reprod Update.* 2012;18(1):73–91.
2. Hillier SG, Whitelaw PF, Smyth CD. Follicular oestrogen synthesis: the 'two-cell, two-gonadotrophin' model revisited. *Mol Cell Endocrinol.* 1994;100(1–2):51–54.
3. Jeppesen JV, Kristensen SG, Nielsen ME, et al. LH-receptor gene expression in human granulosa and cumulus cells from antral and preovulatory follicles. *J Clin Endocrinol Metab.* 2012;97(8):E1524–E1531.
4. Mochtar MH, Danhof NA, Ayeleke RO, et al. Recombinant luteinising hormone (rLH) and recombinant follicle stimulating hormone (rFSH) for ovarian stimulation in IVF/ICSI cycles. *Cochrane Database Syst Rev.* 2017;5(5):Cd005070.
5. Balen AH, Morley LC, Misso M, et al. The management of anovulatory infertility in women with polycystic ovary syndrome: an analysis of the evidence to support the development of global WHO guidance. *Hum Reprod Update.* 2016;22(6):687–708.

6. Wang R, Mol BW. The Rotterdam criteria for polycystic ovary syndrome: evidence-based criteria? *Hum Reprod.* 2017;32(2):261–264.
7. Teede HJ, Misso ML, Costello MF, et al. Recommendations from the international evidence-based guideline for the assessment and management of polycystic ovary syndrome. *Hum Reprod.* 2018;33(9):1602–1618.
8. Dickey RP, Holtkamp DE. Development, pharmacology and clinical experience with clomifene citrate. *Hum Reprod Update.* 1996;2(6):483–506.
9. Brown J, Farquhar C. Clomifene and other antioestrogens for ovulation induction in polycystic ovarian syndrome. *Cochrane Database Syst Rev.* 2016;12(12):CD002249.
10. Steiner AZ, Terplan M, Paulson RJ. Comparison of tamoxifen and clomifene citrate for ovulation induction: a meta-analysis. *Hum Reprod.* 2005;20(6):1511–1515.
11. Messinis IE. Ovulation induction: a mini review. *Hum Reprod.* 2005;20(10):2688–2697.
12. Lin YH, Hwang JL, Seow KM, et al. Comparison of outcome of clomifene citrate/human menopausal gonadotropin/cetrorelix protocol and buserelin long protocol – a randomised study. *Gynecol Endocrinol.* 2006;22(6):297–302.
13. Revelli A, Chiadò A, Dalmasso P, et al. "Mild" vs. "long" protocol for controlled ovarian hyperstimulation in patients with expected poor ovarian responsiveness undergoing in vitro fertilisation (IVF): a large prospective randomised trial. *J Assist Reprod Genet.* 2014;31(7):809–815.
14. NICE. *Fertility Problems: Assessment and Treatment: Clinical Guideline.* London, UK: National Institute for Health and Care Excellence; 2013.
15. Overbeek A, Kuijper EAM, Hendriks ML, et al. Clomifene citrate resistance in relation to follicle-stimulating hormone receptor Ser680Ser-polymorphism in polycystic ovary syndrome. *Hum Reprod.* 2009;24(8):2007–2013.
16. Viola MI, Meyer D, Kruger T. Association between clomifene citrate and visual disturbances with special emphasis on central retinal vein occlusion: a review. *Gynecol Obstet Invest.* 2011;71(2):73–76.
17. Frattarelli JL, Dempsey MS. Characteristics of baseline ovarian cysts in clomifene citrate ovulation cycles. *Fertil Steril.* 2004;82(4):979–981.
18. Quintero RB, Urban R, Lathi RB, et al. A comparison of letrozole to gonadotropins for ovulation induction, in subjects who failed to conceive with clomifene citrate. *Fertil Steril.* 2007;88(4):879–885.
19. Hawkins Bressler L, Fritz MA, Wu SP, et al. Poor Endometrial proliferation after clomifene is associated with altered estrogen action. *J Clin Endocrinol Metab.* 2021;106(9):2547–2565.
20. Delvigne A, Rozenberg S. Epidemiology and prevention of ovarian hyperstimulation syndrome (OHSS): a review. *Hum Reprod Update.* 2002;8(6):559–577.
21. Requena A, Herrero J, Landeras J, et al. Use of letrozole in assisted reproduction: a systematic review and meta-analysis. *Hum Reprod Update.* 2008;14(6):571–582.
22. Goswami SK, Das T, Chattopadhyay R, et al. A randomised single-blind controlled trial of letrozole as a low-cost IVF protocol in women with poor ovarian response: a preliminary report. *Hum Reprod.* 2004;19(9):2031–2035.
23. Bülow NS, Skouby SO, Warzecha AK, et al. Impact of letrozole co-treatment during ovarian stimulation with gonadotrophins for IVF: a multicentre, randomised, double-blinded placebo-controlled trial. *Hum Reprod.* 2022;37(2):309–321.
24. Legro RS, Brzyski RG, Diamond MP, et al. Letrozole versus clomifene for Infertility in the polycystic ovary syndrome. *N Engl J Med.* 2014;371(2):119–129.
25. Wang R, Kim BV, van Wely M, et al. Treatment strategies for women with WHO group II anovulation: systematic review and network meta-analysis. *BMJ.* 2017;356:j138.
26. Sharpe A, Morley LC, Tang T, et al. Metformin for ovulation induction (excluding gonadotrophins) in women with polycystic ovary syndrome. *Cochrane Database Syst Rev.* 2019;12(12):CD013505.
27. Bergandi L, Canosa S, Carosso AR, et al. Human recombinant FSH and its biosimilars: clinical efficacy, safety, and cost-effectiveness in controlled ovarian stimulation for in vitro fertilization. *Pharmaceuticals (Basel).* 2020;13(7).
28. Schwartz M, Jewelewicz R, Dyrenfurth I, et al. The use of human menopausal and chorionic gonadotropins for induction of ovulation. Sixteen years' experience at the Sloane Hospital for Women. *Am J Obstet Gynecol.* 1980;138(7 Pt 1):801–807.
29. Lunenfeld B, Bilger W, Longobardi S, et al. The development of gonadotropins for clinical use in the treatment of infertility. *Front Endocrinol (Lausanne).* 2019;10:429.
30. Zwart-van Rijkom JEF, Broekmans FJ, Leufkens HGM. From HMG through purified urinary FSH preparations to recombinant FSH: a substitution study. *Hum Reprod.* 2002;17(4):857–865.
31. Andersen CY. Effect of FSH and its different isoforms on maturation of oocytes from pre-ovulatory follicles. *Reprod Biomed Online.* 2002;5(3):232–239.
32. Welcker JT, Nawroth F, Bilger W. Patient evaluation of the use of follitropin alfa in a prefilled ready-to-use injection pen in assisted reproductive technology: an observational study. *Reprod Biol Endocrinol.* 2010;8:111.
33. Haakman O, Liang T, Murray K, et al. In vitro fertilisation cycles stimulated with follitropin delta result in similar embryo development and quality when compared with cycles stimulated with follitropin alfa or follitropin beta. *F&S Rep.* 2021;2(1):30–35.
34. Chua SJ, Mol BW, Longobardi S, et al. Biosimilar recombinant follitropin alfa preparations versus the reference product (Gonal-F®) in couples undergoing assisted reproductive technology treatment: a systematic review and meta-analysis. *Reprod Biol Endocrinol.* 2021;19(1):51.
35. van Wely M, Kwan I, Burt AL, et al. Recombinant versus urinary gonadotrophin for ovarian stimulation in assisted reproductive technology cycles. *Cochrane Database Syst Rev.* 2011;2011(2):Cd005354.
36. ESHRE Guideline Group On Ovarian Stimulation, et al. ESHRE guideline: ovarian stimulation for IVF/ICSI(†). *Hum Reprod Open.* 2020;2020(2):hoaa009.
37. Conn PM, Crowley WF, Jr. Gonadotropin-releasing hormone and its analogs. *Annu Rev Med.* 1994;45:391–405.
38. Flanagan CA, Manilall A. Gonadotropin-releasing hormone (GnRH) receptor structure and GnRH binding. *Front Endocrinol.* 2017;8.
39. Constantin S. Physiology of the gonadotrophin-releasing hormone (GnRH) neurone: studies from embryonic GnRH neurones. *J Neuroendocrinol.* 2011;23(6):542–553.

40. Loumaye E, Naor Z, Catt KJ. Binding affinity and biological activity of gonadotropin releasing hormone agonists in isolated pituitary cells. *Endocrinology.* 1982;111(3):730–736.
41. Siristatidis CS, Gibreel A, Basios G, et al. Gonadotrophin-releasing hormone agonist protocols for pituitary suppression in assisted reproduction. *Cochrane Database Syst Rev.* 2015(11):Cd006919.
42. Georgiou EX, Melo P, Baker PE, et al. Long-term GnRH agonist therapy before in vitro fertilisation (IVF) for improving fertility outcomes in women with endometriosis. *Cochrane Database Syst Rev.* 2019;2019(11).
43. Tarlatzis BC, Bili H. Safety of GnRH agonists and antagonists. *Expert Opin Drug Saf.* 2004;3(1):39–46.
44. Hodgen GD. GnRH analogs in reproductive medicine. *Keio J Med.* 1991;40(1):25–32.
45. Hayden C. GnRH analogues: applications in assisted reproductive techniques. *Eur J Endocrinol.* 2008;159(Suppl. 1):S17–S25.
46. Clayton RN, Catt KJ. Receptor-binding affinity of gonadotropin-releasing hormone analogs: analysis by radioligand-receptor assay. *Endocrinology.* 1980;106(4):1154–1159.
47. Lambalk CB, Banga FR, Huirne JA, et al. GnRH antagonist versus long agonist protocols in IVF: a systematic review and meta-analysis accounting for patient type. *Hum Reprod Update.* 2017;23(5):560–579.
48. Jing M, Lin C, Zhu W, et al. Cost-effectiveness analysis of GnRH-agonist long-protocol and GnRH-antagonist protocol for in vitro fertilisation. *Sci Rep.* 2020;10(1):8732.
49. Ron-El R, Herman A, Golan A, et al. The comparison of early follicular and midluteal administration of long-acting gonadotropin-releasing hormone agonist. *Fertil Steril.* 1990;54(2):233–237.
50. Barash A, Weissman A, Manor M, et al. Prospective evaluation of endometrial thickness as a predictor of pituitary down-regulation after gonadotropin-releasing hormone analogue administration in an in vitro fertilisation program. *Fertil Steril.* 1998;69(3):496–499.
51. Abbara A, Vuong LN, Ho VNA, et al. Follicle size on day of trigger most likely to yield a mature oocyte. *Front Endocrinol (Lausanne).* 2018;9:193.
52. Ou J, Xing W, Li Y, et al. Short versus long gonadotropin-releasing hormone analogue suppression protocols in IVF/ICSI cycles in patients of various age ranges. *PLoS One.* 2015;10(7):e0133887.
53. Lainas T, Zorzovilis J, Petsas G, et al. In a flexible antagonist protocol, earlier, criteria-based initiation of GnRH antagonist is associated with increased pregnancy rates in IVF. *Hum Reprod.* 2005;20(9):2426–2433.
54. Al-Inany HG, Youssef MA, Ayeleke RO, et al. Gonadotrophin-releasing hormone antagonists for assisted reproductive technology. *Cochrane Database Syst Rev.* 2016;4(4):CD001750.
55. Al-Inany H, Aboulghar M. GnRH antagonist in assisted reproduction: a Cochrane review. *Hum Reprod.* 2002;17(4):874–885.
56. Gallos ID, Eapen A, Price MJ, et al. Controlled ovarian stimulation protocols for assisted reproduction: a network meta-analysis. *Cochrane Database Syst Rev.* 2017;37(1):009.
57. Wang R, Seidler AL, Askie L, et al. Network meta-analyses in reproductive medicine: challenges and opportunities. *Hum Reprod.* 2020;35(8):1723–1731.
58. Melo PEA, Chung Y, Jeve Y, et al. *Controlled Ovarian Stimulation Protocols for Assisted Reproduction: A Cochrane Systematic Review Network Meta-Analysis.* Milan: European Society of Human Reproduction and Embryology; 2022.

19

Oocyte Retrieval and Evaluation

Bryony Swift

19.1 Development of Modern-Day Techniques

Clinical practice has evolved significantly since the pioneering work of Steptoe, Edwards and Purdy, which led to the birth of Louise Brown in 1978; the first successful birth following human *in vitro* fertilisation. During the early days of IVF, laparoscopic techniques were employed to allow minimally invasive access to the ovaries. With this method, the patient would require a general anaesthesia. Utilising the laparoscope, the inner abdomen was made visible and the fluid-filled maturing follicle could be visualised protruding from the surface of the ovary. Aspiration of the follicular fluid to obtain the preovulatory oocyte was originally achieved via a syringe, and a thin hollow needle penetrating the abdominal wall. This method was superseded by the development of a bypass valve that permitted controlled suction of the contents of the follicle (**1**).

Subsequent developments focused on identifying the optimum timing of oocyte retrieval (to recover oocytes just prior to ovulation), and harvesting multiple oocytes (to increase the patient's chance of success). At the time, unstimulated cycles of IVF (monofollicular development) yielded approximately 0.7 oocytes per retrieval (**2**). The introduction of ovarian stimulation to initiate multifollicular development was pivotal in increasing pregnancy rates following IVF (from 6% per cycle from unstimulated IVF, to 30% per oocyte retrieval in 1983 (**3**)).

Improvements in ultrasound technology revolutionised the practice of oocyte retrieval. First reported in the early 1980s (**4**), transabdominal ultrasound imaging provided guidance for numerous modes of oocyte recovery, including transvesical, transurethral and transvaginal follicular aspiration.

Additional advancements in ultrasound transducers resulted in further modernisation of the technique, enabling transvaginal imaging to guide transvaginal follicle aspiration. Transvaginal sonography enabled superior visualisation and greater accuracy when tracking the needle tip throughout the procedure, particularly with the availability of needles supplemented with echogenic tips (**2**).

Sonographically-guided transvaginal puncture and follicle aspiration offers numerous advantages in comparison to laparoscopic methods. This surgical technique can be performed with a local anaesthetic, or under conscious sedation. Consequently, it dramatically reduces both the recovery time for the patient and the procedural time itself, whilst carrying a reduced surgical risk, and a reduced expense, compared with general anaesthesia (**5**).

19.2 Procedural Timing

Following a course of controlled ovarian stimulation and ultrasound monitoring of follicular growth, a patient will receive instructions to administer a 'trigger' injection around 36 hours prior to the time of their scheduled oocyte retrieval. In the menstrual cycle, luteinising hormone (LH) has a dual function; it triggers ovulation and follicular rupture 36 hours post-surge, and causes the resumption of oocyte meiotic maturation. Human chorionic gonadotrophin (hCG) is capable of binding to LH receptors and is therefore an effective substitute for the naturally occurring LH surge to trigger ovulation. To prevent the introduction of additional exogenous hCG in patients at risk of ovarian hyperstimulation syndrome (OHSS), the 'flare effect' of a gonadotrophin-releasing hormone agonist trigger can be utilised to trigger ovulation, but is only effective alongside antagonist stimulation protocols (**6**).

Timing of oocyte retrieval is crucial, to ensure that the patient does not undergo ovulation before the oocytes can be recovered surgically, and to give sufficient time for oocyte maturation to occur. The time of the procedure is dictated by the 'trigger' time, and must commence close to 36 hours post-injection. Commonly, each procedure is allocated 30–45 minutes, and it is important for theatre lists to run to plan to ensure successive patients are not impacted by delays.

19.3 Oocyte Retrieval

19.3.1 Theatre Equipment

When the patient arrives to theatre for the procedure, it is mandatory for the theatre team and embryologist to perform an identity check. The patient will then receive either a local or general anaesthetic to prepare for the surgical procedure, or more commonly in current practice, be administered with a conscious sedation.

Guided by a transvaginal ultrasound probe, a needle is inserted through the vaginal wall, and used to puncture antral follicles from each ovary. The needle is connected to a suction pump, which functions by creating a negative pressure to aspirate follicular fluid from each follicle. Aspiration pressures will vary depending upon the diameter of the needle employed and needle manufacturer guidelines, and range from 100–200mmHg. The narrower the diameter, the greater

DOI: 10.1201/9781003269502-19

the pressure necessary to maintain flow rate. Perception that a higher aspiration pressure would increase the risk of damage to oocytes is not necessarily accurate, providing that the flow rate remains stable, as turbulent flow can be responsible for mechanical stress being exerted on the oocyte (**7**).

Two types of needles can be utilised for the procedure; single or double lumen needles, each with slightly different functionality. Single lumen needles are the current standard, and will penetrate and aspirate the fluid within the follicle. Alternatively, a double lumen needle possesses two channels. One allows for the extraction of fluid, whilst the other introduces medium to 'flush' the follicle; with the aim to detach any oocytes still tethered to the follicle wall, or 'trapped' within a collapsed follicle. A double lumen needle can preferentially be selected by the operator, often for poor responders, or patients with a low ovarian reserve. However, studies show little to no benefit of follicle flushing when comparing oocyte recovery rates between the two types, and is not recommended according to NICE Guidelines (**8, 9**). Needle diameter can also vary; thinner needles have been linked to a significant reduction in patient discomfort, immediately after and in the days following oocyte recovery (**10**).

Flushing medium may be supplemented with heparin, a naturally occurring glycosaminoglycan acting as an anticoagulant to minimise blood clot formation that could impede oocyte identification (**11**). Prior to the procedure, flushing medium must be prewarmed in an incubator. Throughout the retrieval, it can be kept at physiological temperatures of 37°C in a heated block to prevent the detrimental effects of temperature change on the oocytes.

19.3.2 Laboratory Equipment

Once extracted, collection vials or tubes of follicular fluid can be passed from the theatre to the laboratory and temporarily held within a heat-controlled warmer/block, to maintain the fluid at the optimal temperature of 37°C. Aspirates should carefully be poured into sterile, pre-warmed dishes, on a heated stage to maintain the temperature at 37°C, inside a Class II Biological Safety Cabinet. This type of workstation is equipped with HEPA filters, simulating laminar airflow within the hood. This protects both the samples and the embryologist from exposure to biohazardous agents, and maintains the quality of the air that the samples are held within. Sterility is also maintained through the use of aseptic technique and gloves when handling bodily fluids and sterile consumables.

Oocytes can be identified within the drained fluid, inside a mass of cumulus cells, known as the cumulus-oocyte complex (COC). A stereomicroscope provides adequate magnification to visualise COCs (typically 10x magnification). The embryologist can also expect to identify granulosa cells deriving from the antral follicle wall.

Following identification, COCs should be washed to remove residual follicular fluid. Best practice dictates that oocytes should not be exposed to follicular fluid for a prolonged period of time, and exposure to light should also be minimal (**12**). COCs should be thoroughly washed and collected into dishes containing prewarmed medium that is typically buffered with either MOPS or HEPES, or else maintained in a gas mix to sustain pH. These buffering agents maintain a stable pH in atmospheric conditions, to protect oocytes from fluctuations in extracellular pH. Upon completion of the procedure, once adequately washed, COCs can be transferred into bicarbonate-buffered media that supports fertilisation and is optimal within the controlled CO_2 environment of a gassed incubator. Oocytes can be returned to *in vitro* culture prior to insemination. See further Video 19.1. (Access the videos at www.routledge.com/9781032216577).

Video 19.1 The Oocyte Retrieval Procedure, from Both Laboratory and Theatre Perspectives, Including Set-Up of the Laboratory Work Area.

19.3.3 Ovarian Reserve and Yield

Oocyte yield per retrieval is variable and related to the individual's ovarian reserve, in addition to the mode of ovarian stimulation. Studies suggest that the optimal number of oocytes collected to result in a live birth lies between 6 and 15 (**13, 14**). Lower numbers may compromise treatment outcomes due to a direct reduction in the number of oocytes available for insemination, leading to a smaller cohort of embryos. To the contrary, some reports suggest that overstimulation of the ovaries may be of detriment to the quality of oocytes retrieved, although this could arguably originate from the prevalence of patients with polycystic ovaries falling into this category (**15, 16**).

19.3.4 Ovarian Cysts

Ovarian cysts may be aspirated during oocyte collection. Whilst similar in appearance on ultrasound imaging, the drained fluid has characteristic features to distinguish its presence from regular follicular fluid.

Endometriomas are fluid-filled sacs that develop on the ovaries, containing endometrial fluid that is dark brown in appearance. This type of cyst is commonly observed in patients diagnosed with endometriosis, and they can be referred to as 'chocolate cysts'.

Functional ovarian cysts can arise spontaneously during the menstrual cycle, but also during pituitary downregulation and ovarian stimulation (**17**). These follicular cysts contain straw-coloured fluid, often granular in appearance, and more frequently observed than endometriomas.

19.4 Oocyte Handling and Maintaining Gamete Viability

It is essential to control both the laboratory environment and the culture conditions of oocytes to optimise viability. The following factors are pivotal in maintaining gamete viability:

19.4.1 Temperature

Oocyte spindles have a pivotal role in the alignment and segregation of chromosomes during meiotic divisions and fertilisation. It is well documented that fluctuations in temperature can impact on spindle integrity, thus initiating irregular distribution of chromosomes and increasing the risk of abnormal fertilisation.

Studies have revealed that the cooling of oocytes to 33°C for 10 minutes is sufficient to cause complete spindle disassembly, occurring in as little as 5 minutes when cooled to 25°C or 28°C. The ability of spindles to recover from lower temperatures is determined by how severely the temperature declines and the duration of exposure. Those cooled to 33°C appeared to undergo a full recovery, whereas spindles in oocytes cooled to 25°C did not reassemble. However, a further observation of decreased microtubule density following the rewarming of oocytes implies that spindles do not fully repolymerise, and therefore brief exposures to suboptimal conditions may have lasting effects on spindle dynamics (**18**). As such, it is crucial for embryologists to work efficiently during oocyte recovery. Working in a controlled but timely manner will reduce the risk of oocyte exposure to temperatures below 37°C and subsequent disruption to meiotic spindles.

19.4.2 pH

Many biological processes are sensitive to pH and therefore dysregulation of intracellular pH (pH_i) can be of detriment to cellular function and growth. Ion transport mechanisms within the oocyte that regulate pH_i undergo inactivation during meiotic maturation, and resume following successful fertilisation (**19**). Hence, oocytes at the time of retrieval are particularly susceptible to alterations in their surrounding pH. This could arise due to increased time outside of a controlled incubator, and through changes in temperature.

The pH_i of an oocyte is around 7.4. Whilst oocytes have the capacity to recover from exposure to an alkaline environment, they are unable to recover from acidosis, even after being returned to neutral pH conditions. It is only upon blastocyst formation that acid-buffering mechanisms develop within the embryo to enable the regulation of H+ ions across the membrane (**20**). Consequently, it is essential to provide an extracellular environment of neutral, stable pH to support homeostasis and metabolic control of the oocyte. This can be achieved through adequate warming and gas exchange of dishes containing buffered medium prior to exposure (ideally overnight), choosing the correct buffer for the procedure in question i.e. MOPS or HEPES for procedures of increased exposure to atmospheric conditions, oil overlay to prevent rapid changes to pH from CO_2 loss, and working quickly; to minimise exposure outside of optimum incubator conditions.

19.4.3 Osmolality

Oocytes are susceptible to changes in osmolality. Evidence suggests that perturbations in osmotic conditions result in the disruption of oocyte meiotic spindles (**21**). The inclusion of amino acids in culture media offers some protection from changes in osmolality, but it has its limits. Working quickly lessens the risk of evaporation of culture medium arising from increased air movement over the work surface within flowhoods.

Also, avoiding very small, microdrop volumes of medium, and using an oil overlay on dishes containing gametes helps to minimise evaporation that could elicit osmotic changes affecting cell volume, leading to oocyte shrinking or swelling.

Additional benefits from oil overlay include a reduction in potential heat loss from warmed medium, reduced gaseous exchange with the environment leading to pH alterations, and a layer of protection from outside contaminants. Maintaining aseptic technique application throughout the procedure is also imperative to prevent the contamination of dishes with microbial infections; which could be of detriment to gamete and embryo development.

19.5 In Vitro Culture and Preparation for Insemination

Conventional IVF involves the direct addition of prepared semen to dishes or drops containing COCs. Once inseminated, proteolytic enzymes released from the spermatozoan acrosome will digest the proteins embedded in the extracellular matrix to break down the cumulus mass (**22**). As such, the maturity and quality of IVF-inseminated oocytes remains unknown until the point of fertilisation check when external cells are removed.

Conversely, for ICSI, cumulus and corona radiata cells must be removed from the oocyte prior to insemination, to determine maturity and subsequent suitability for intracytoplasmic sperm injection. Denudation of the oocytes is achieved mechanically by moving the COCs through a series of micropipettes of decreasing diameter, to loosen and shed the cells. This process is assisted by brief exposure to hyaluronidase, an enzyme that specifically catalyses the breakdown of hyaluronan, which is abundant in the cumulus extracellular matrix.

19.6 Oocyte Evaluation

19.6.1 Cumulus-Oocyte Complex

Morphological assessment of COCs can provide some insight into oocyte maturity. Typically, a mature preovulatory COC is characterised by radiating coronal cells, and a loose expanded mass of outer cumulus cells. Dense corona radiata, with compact, unexpanded cumulus cells are more commonly associated with immature oocytes (**23**). One morphological abnormality associated with a reduction in oocyte quality is the presence of blood clots within the cumulus mass (**24**).

19.7 Oocyte Maturity

Oocyte cytoplasmic maturation affords the oocyte with the developmental competence required for subsequent embryo development post-fertilisation, and is essential for structural rearrangement of organelles and biochemical alterations, occurring synchronously with nuclear maturation and the resumption of meiosis (**25**).

An assessment of maturity can be performed using a stereomicroscope at the time of mechanical denudation for ICSI, and an indication of quality may be determined at the time of ICSI using the higher magnification microscope connected to micromanipulation equipment (200–400x magnification).

19.7.1 Germinal Vesicle

In a cohort of oocytes recovered following ovarian stimulation, approximately 10% will be classified as germinal vesicle (GV) stage. The GV is a nucleus located within the ooplasm featuring a prominent nucleolus. An intact GV is displayed in oocytes that are arrested at the diplotene stage of meiosis prophase.

19.7.2 Metaphase II

It is anticipated that 85% of retrieved oocytes will be at the Metaphase II stage (MII) and deemed mature. In response to the LH surge (or exogenous administration of hCG/GnRH-agonist), meiosis resumes and the nuclear envelope of the GV breaks down (GVBD). The first meiotic division takes place, and one set of chromosomes is extruded via the first polar body (PB1) in a process of reductional division. The PB is visible in the

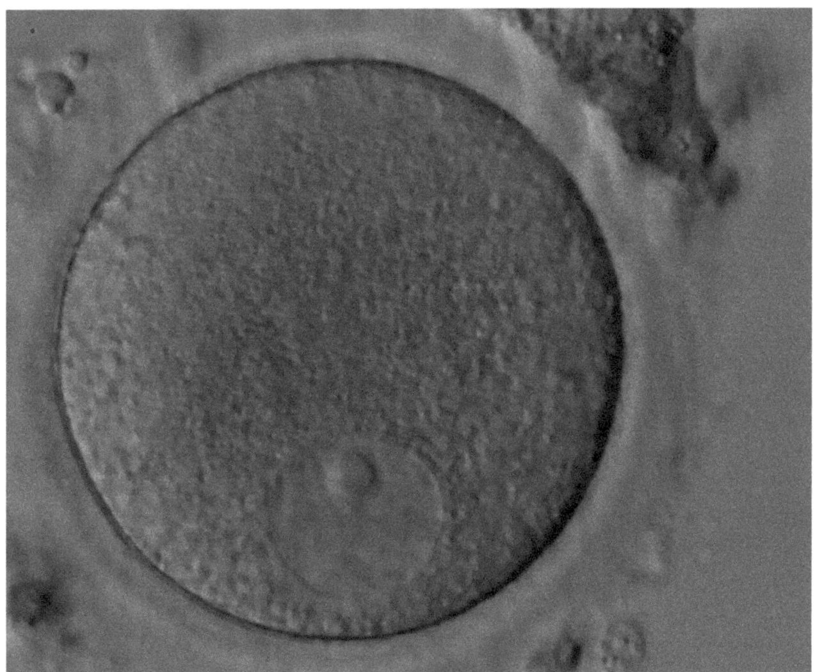

FIGURE 19.1 A denuded germinal-vesicle stage human oocyte, magnified 400x (from ref 26 with permission).

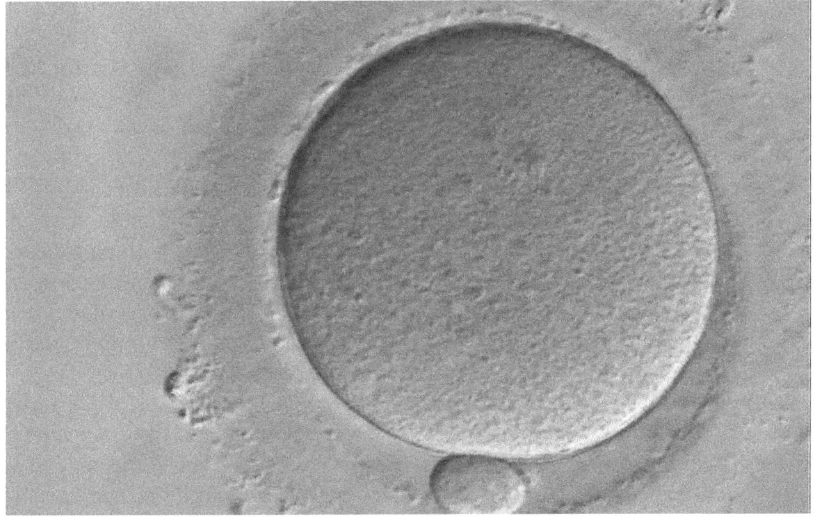

FIGURE 19.2 A denuded mature oocyte at the MII stage, displaying a visible polar body at approximately '6 o'clock' within the PVS (from ref 26 with permission).

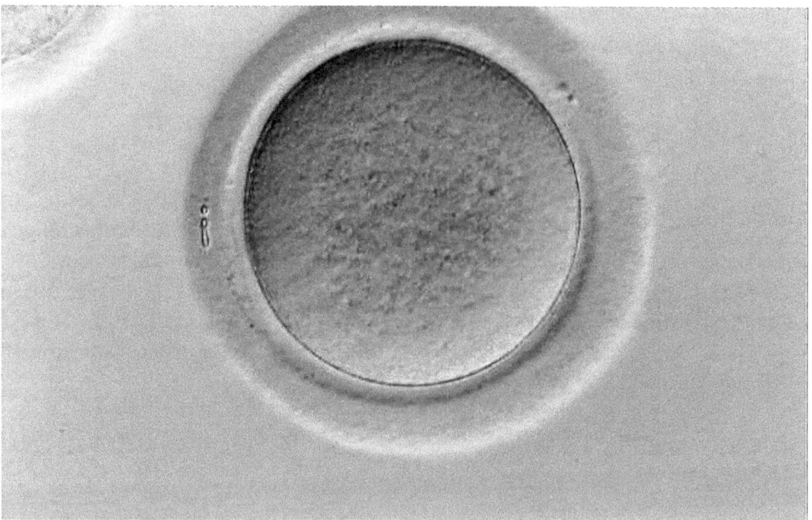

FIGURE 19.3 A denuded MI oocyte, with no visible PB or GV (from ref 26 with permission).

perivitelline space (PVS). One set of chromosomes is retained within the oocyte. Sister chromatids assemble on the metaphase II spindle, in preparation for fertilisation and the resumption of the final meiotic division, as fertilisation occurs (**26**).

The presence of the first extruded PB is imperative, as it defines the mature egg and the point at which oocytes have reached nuclear maturation. It is at MII that oocytes have the capacity to fertilise (**27**).

19.7.3 Metaphase I

The final 5% is accounted for by oocytes that display neither a polar body, nor a visible GV. They are defined as Metaphase I (MI) oocytes. At MI, homologous chromosomes are aligned on the metaphase plate in preparation for the first meiotic division.

In vitro maturation can occur, with the late release of PB1 observed in MI oocytes prior to the ICSI insemination taking place. Late maturing oocytes can be injected, but embryos deriving from these have reduced implantation potential (**26, 28**).

19.8 Oocyte Quality

The higher magnification of an inverted microscope utilised for ICSI provides greater visibility of oocyte quality; including cytoplasmic appearance, the zona pellucida (ZP) and the perivitelline space (PVS).

19.8.1 Shape

A regular oocyte is spherical in shape, surrounded by a rounded ZP; an extracellular matrix consisting of glycoproteins which surrounds the mammalian egg. On occasion, elongated, ovoid shaped oocytes can be observed, either with both an ovoid shaped ZP and ooplasm, or an abnormally shaped ZP containing a regular shaped oocyte. The latter may be explained by the presence of a septate ZP, or segregation or duplication of the ZP inner layers.

19.8.1.1 Giant Oocytes

There is a marked difference in size when comparing a normal oocyte to a giant, with giant oocytes characterised as being >130–200μm in diameter. Cytogenetic analysis on giant oocytes has revealed an increased incidence of diploid chromosome complements, leading to the development of digynic triploid embryos upon fertilisation with haploid spermatozoa (**29, 30**). Giant oocytes may potentially arise via meiotic errors during oogenesis, and they are not recommended for use in treatment.

19.8.2 Zona Pellucida

The role of the ZP is crucial throughout oocyte growth and embryonic development, including embryo hatching. This glycoprotein coat not only presents a block to polyspermy, it is essential for sperm-oocyte binding to facilitate fertilisation, and encloses and protects the preimplantation embryo throughout development (**30–32**).

A normal ZP is homogenous in colour and thickness, and uniform in shape. Whilst darkness or increased thickness do not appear to be of detriment to fertilisation and embryo development, oocytes with an exceptionally thin ZP may be at increased risk of degeneration upon injection at ICSI (**33**). Alternatively, elevated ZP thickness or hardening present an obstacle to embryo hatching and therefore may influence implantation potential (**34**).

Alterations in ZP shape could impact the pattern of embryonic divisions and the arrangement of blastomeres. Close associations between blastomeres may be significant in facilitating cell signalling, and be of particular importance when establishing cell-cell contact during compaction. As such, embryos with an irregular shaped ZP, with less compact cells, will have reduced contact for extracellular communication to occur and potentially delayed development pre- and post-compaction (**33**).

19.8.2.1 Empty Zona Pellucida

One phenomenon observed following oocyte retrieval, or oocyte denudation, is the presence of empty zona pellucida. Namely, when a ZP is visible with no discernible ooplasm inside. This may occur due to mechanical stress exertion on the oocyte itself, leading to a breach in the structural integrity of the ZP and subsequent loss of the oocyte membrane and cytoplasmic contents. Empty ZP are not suitable for insemination.

One causal factor is the application of high pressure when aspirating follicles during oocyte retrieval, or the utilisation of a small diameter needle for aspiration. Damage can also occur due to the use of narrow diameter denudation micropipettes when removing coronal cells prior to ICSI. A pipette of similar diameter to that of the oocyte itself (approximately 110µm), may cause stress and ultimately a breach in the ZP wall (**29, 30**). On occasion, fragments of ooplasm or 'zona-free' oocytes can be observed in close proximity to the empty zona at denudation. In some instances, the ooplasm may have undergone the process of degeneration, potentially via cell apoptosis (**30**).

19.8.3 Polar Body

The predictive prognostic value of the first extruded polar body (PB1) is controversial. A normal PB is intact and has a smooth appearance. Morphological anomalies include the presence of a fragmented PB, being enlarged or irregular in size, or possessing a rough surface. Numerous studies have found no significant difference in clinical outcomes with the presence of fragmented PBs, but evidence does suggest that an enlarged PB is associated with lower fertilisation and cleavage rates, and a reduction in the number of good quality embryos (**35, 36**). The larger the PB, the greater the quantity of cytoplasm extruded alongside the haploid set of chromosomes during metaphase II. Therefore, it is postulated that oocytes exhibiting a much larger PB are of reduced viability (**37**).

19.8.4 Dark Cytoplasm or Granularity

Cytoplasm is deemed normal if homogeneous and light-coloured in appearance. Deviations from the norm include the presence of granular cytoplasm. Heterogeneous cytoplasm is commonplace amongst a cohort of retrieved oocytes, but the severity (defined by depth and diameter) and location of the granulation can be of significant prognostic value (**38**). Granularity can be diffuse or present across the whole cytoplasm, or less commonly, can be a condensed centrally located area with a clear border; which is of greater concern as it suggests organelle clustering and thus a reduction in implantation potential (**38–40**). Oocytes with fine granules are documented to have better outcomes in terms of pregnancy and live birth in comparison to those with dispersed granulation across the entirety of the ooplasm (**41**). Occasionally observed in human oocytes is the presence of refractile bodies, which are comprised of dense granule material and lipids. Some evidence suggests a deleterious effect of refractile bodies on fertilisation rates with conventional IVF, but this appears to be bypassed with the use of ICSI (**42, 43**).

19.8.5 Smooth Endoplasmic Reticulum Discs

Smooth endoplasmic reticulum (SER) is an organelle with an essential role in storing and redistributing calcium within the ooplasm. However, if SER aggregates to form SER clusters or discs, this has an adverse impact on the calcium functionality of the cell, including calcium oscillations essential to the fertilisation process. This cytoplasmic dysmorphism is associated with a significant reduction in fertilisation and blastocyst formation rates, in addition to decreased embryo quality. By appearance, these structures are translucent, flat discs approximately 10–18µm in diameter and visible by phase-contrast microscopy (**44**). Past publications have indicated that oocytes containing SER clusters should not be injected due to the occurrence of chromosomal abnormalities. However, expert consensus was changed recently, due to lack of evidence to support avoiding their use (**45**).

19.8.6 Vacuoles

Vacuoles are membrane-bound structures filled with fluid, and a common observation in human oocytes. Larger vacuoles have increased potential to disrupt biological processes, by displacing cytoskeletal elements of the oocyte. Vacuoles >14µm in size are associated with failure to fertilise, whereas smaller vacuoles 5–10µm are less likely to interfere with fertilisation and development (**39, 46, 47**).

19.8.7 Perivitelline Space

The size of the PVS is linked to the stage of oocyte maturity. The gap enlarges and will reach full size upon completion of oocyte maturation to MII. One commonly observed extracytoplasmic anomaly is the presence of a large PVS, suggested to be a consequence of 'over-mature' eggs. Another dysmorphism is the incidence of coarse dark granules within the PVS. Both factors have been associated with a reduction in implantation when observed across an entire cohort of retrieved oocytes (**48, 49**) although the literature is conflicting and many studies did not solely assess PVS anomalies, but evaluated outcomes based on multiple factors (**50**). Oocytes with a large degree of cellular debris within the PVS, in addition to a fragmented PB, can sometimes obscure identification of the PB and therefore are not favourable.

19.8.8 Membrane Behaviour at ICSI

High resistance to the penetration of injection needles during ICSI may be linked to rigidity of the oocyte membrane. Increased oolemma resistance, or conversely, little resistance before oolemma breakage, can be an influencing factor on fertilisation and later embryonic development and quality (**38, 51**).

19.8.9 Aneuploidy

Ploidy refers to the number of complete sets of chromosomes present within a cell. Aneuploidy, (containing the incorrect number of chromosomes), is relatively frequent within human oocytes and its incidence increases with advancing maternal age. Oocytes are intrinsically susceptible to errors in chromosome segregation, with an estimated 10–25% of oocytes aneuploid in women aged 30, increasing to >50% in women >40 and rapidly rising to ~80% by the age of 42. Meiotic aneuploidy can arise in oocytes during meiotic divisions due to chromosomal segregation errors, such as failure to segregate (nondisjunction) or premature sister chromatid separation (**52, 53,** 54).

Upon fertilisation, such oocytes can give rise to aneuploid embryos which ultimately result in implantation failure, miscarriage, or less commonly, offspring with chromosomal disorders, such as Trisomy 18 (Edward Syndrome), or Monosomy X (Turner Syndrome) (**53**). Aneuploid oocytes that fertilise can develop into transferrable blastocysts, but cannot be distinguished by normal methods of embryo morphological assessment. Oocytes and embryos may appear morphologically normal, but this does not necessarily reflect quality when considering the underlying genetics. One potential method to evaluate these embryos would be using pre-implantation genetic testing for aneuploidy (PGT-A), which will be discussed in another chapter of this book.

19.9 Conclusion

A number of developments in aspiration needle types and quality to improve patient comfort and successful retrieval of cumulus oocyte complexes have been introduced since the early 1980s. Further improvements have also been introduced in terms of control of temperature and other environmental conditions to maintain the viability of oocytes in preparation for *in vitro* fertilisation.

REFERENCES

1. Johnson MH. A short history of *in vitro* fertilization (IVF). *Int J Dev Biol.* 2019;63:83–92.
2. Wang J, Sauer MV. In vitro fertilization (IVF): a review of 3 decades of clinical innovation and technological advancement. *Ther Clin Risk Manag.* 2006;2(4):355–364.
3. Edwards RG, Steptoe PC. Current status of in-vitro fertilisation and implantation of human embryos. *Lancet.* 1983;2:1265–1269.
4. Gleicher N, Friberg J, Fullan N, et al. Egg retrieval for in vitro fertilisation by sonographically controlled vaginal culdocentesis. *Lancet.* 1983;2:508–509.
5. Cohen J, Debache C, Pez JP, et al. Transvaginal sonographically controlled ovarian puncture for oocyte retrieval for in vitro fertilization. *J In Vitro Fertil Embryo Trans.* 1986;3:309–313.
6. Smitz J, Platteau P. Influence of human chorionic gonadotrophin during ovarian stimulation: an overview. *Reprod Biol Endocrinol.* 2020;18:80.
7. The ESHRE Working Group on Ultrasound in ART, et al. Recommendations for good practice in ultrasound: oocyte pick up. *Hum Reprod Open.* 2019;2019(4):hoz025.
8. Georgiou EX, Melo P, Brown J, et al. Follicular flushing during oocyte retrieval in assisted reproductive techniques. *Cochrane Database Syst Rev.* 2018;2018(4):CD004634.
9. National Institution for Health and Care Excellence. *Fertility Problems: Assessment and Treatment [Internet].* London: NICE; 2013 [updated 2017 Sep; cited 2022 Aug 18]. (Clinical guideline [CG156]). Available from: www.nice.org.uk/guidance/cg156/chapter/Recommendations#procedures-used-during-ivf-treatment.
10. Buisman ETIA, de Bruin, JP, Braat DDM, et al. Effect of needle diameter on pain during oocyte retrieval – a randomized controlled trial. *Fertil Steril.* 2021;115(3):683–691.
11. Weidenbaum E, Shaw J, McCaffrey C, et al. Heparin, to clot or not? Is it needed in oocyte retrieval flush media? *Fertil Steril.* 2021;116(1):E14.
12. ESHRE Guideline Group on Good Practice in IVF Labs, et al. Revised guidelines for good practice in IVF laboratories (2015). *Hum Reprod.* 2016;31(4):685–686.
13. Ji J, Liu Y, Tong XH, et al. The optimum number of oocytes in IVF treatment: an analysis of 2455 cycles in China. *Hum Reprod.* 2013;28(10):2728–2734.
14. Gaast MH, Eijkemans MJC, Net JB, et al. Optimum number of oocytes for a successful first IVF treatment cycle. *Reprod Biomed Online.* 2006;13(4):476–480.
15. Akagbosu F, Marcus S, Abusheikha N, et al. Does ovarian hyperstimulation syndrome affect the quality of oocytes? *Hum Reprod.* 1998;13(9):2583–2584.
16. Aboulghar MA, Mansour RT, Serour GI, et al. Oocyte quality in patients with severe ovarian hyperstimulation syndrome. *Fertil Steril.* 1997;68(6):1017–1021.
17. Ron-El R, Herman A, Golan A, et al. Follicle cyst formation following long-acting gonadotropin-releasing hormone analog administration. *Fertil Steril.* 1989;52(6):1063–1066.
18. Wang WH, Meng L, Hackett RJ, et al. Limited recovery of meiotic spindles in living human oocytes after cooling-rewarming observed using polarized light microscopy. *Hum Reprod.* 2001;16(11):2374–2378.
19. Fitzharris G, Baltz JM. Regulation of intracellular pH during oocyte growth and maturation in mammals. *Reproduction.* 2009;138:619–627.
20. Dale B, Menezo Y, Cohen J, et al. Intracellular pH regulation in the human oocyte. *Hum Reprod.* 1998;13(4):964–970.
21. Mullen SF, Agca Y, Broermann DC, et al. The effect of osmotic stress on the metaphase II spindle of human oocytes, and the relevance to cryopreservation. *Hum Reprod.* 2004;19(5):1148–1154.
22. Hall JE, Hall ME. Reproductive and hormonal functions of the male (and function of the Pineal gland). In: Hall JE, Hall ME, editors. *Guyton and Hall Textbook of Medical Physiology.* 14th Edition. Philadelphia: Elsevier; 2020. Chapter 81. pp. 1011–1025.
23. Wynn P, Picton HM, Krapez JA, et al. Pretreatment with follicle stimulating hormone promotes the numbers of human oocytes reaching metaphase II by in-vitro maturation. *Hum Reprod.* 1998;13(11):3132–3138.
24. Ebner T, Moser M, Shebl O, et al. Blood clots in the cumulus-oocyte complex predict poor oocyte quality and post-fertilization development. *Reprod Biomed Online.* 2008;16(6):801–807.
25. Trebichalská Z, Kyjovská D, Kloudová S, et al. Cytoplasmic maturation in human oocytes: an ultrastructural study. *Biol Reprod.* 2021;104(1):106–116.

26. Rienzi L, Balaban B, Ebner T, et al. The oocyte. *Hum Reprod*. 2012;27(Suppl. 1):i2–i21.
27. Yang Q, Zhu L, Wang M, et al. Analysis of maturation dynamics and developmental competence of in vitro matured oocytes under time-lapse monitoring. *Reprod Biol Endocrinol*. 2021;19(183).
28. Vellez LT, Brogliato C, Berton CZ, et al. ICSI in late matured oocytes, is it worth it? Study with laboratory, clinical and genetic evaluation results. *JBRA Assist Reprod*. 2020;24(2):173–174.
29. Kitasaka H, Konuma Y, Tokoro M, et al. Oocyte cytoplasmic diameter of ≥130µm can be used to determine human giant oocytes. *F&S Sci*. 2022;3(1):10–17.
30. Siristatidis C, Tzanakaki D, Simopoulou, et al. Empty Zona Pellucida only case: a critical review of the literature. *Int J Environ Res Publich Health*. 2021;18(17):9409.
31. Zhou Z, Ni C, Wu L, et al. Novel mutations in *ZP1*, *ZP2* and *ZP3* cause female infertility due to abnormal zona pellucida formation. *Hum Genet*. 2019;138:327–337.
32. Gupta SK. Human zona pellucida glycoproteins: binding characteristics with human spermatozoa and induction of acrosome reaction. *Front Cell Dev Biol*. 2021;11(9):619868.
33. Ebner T, Shebl O, Moser M, et al. Developmental fate of ovoid oocytes. *Hum Reprod*. 2008;23(1):62–66.
34. Wang Y, Chen C, Liang J, et al. A comparison of the clinical effects of thinning and drilling on laser-assisted hatching. *Lasers Med Sci*. 2022;37:1–9.
35. Navarro PA, de Araújo MM, de Araújo CM, et al. Relationship between first polar body morphology before intracytoplasmic sperm injection and fertilization rate, cleavage rate and embryo quality. *Int J Gynaecol Obstet*. 2009;104(3):226–229.
36. Ebner T, Yaman C, Moser M, et al. Prognostic value of first polar body morphology on fertilization rate and embryo quality in intracytoplasmic sperm injection. *Hum Reprod*. 2000;15(2):427–430.
37. Fancsovits P, Tóthné ZG, Murber Á, et al. Correlation between first polar body morphology and further embryo development. *Act Biologica Hungarica*. 2006;57:331–338.
38. Rienzi L, Vajta G, Ubaldi F. Predictive value of oocyte morphology in human IVF: systematic review of the literature. *Hum Reprod Update*. 2011;17(1):34–45.
39. Alpha Scientists in Reproductive Medicine and ESHRE Special Interest Group of Embryology. The Istanbul consensus workshop on embryo assessment: proceedings of nan expert meeting. *Hum Reprod*. 26(6):1270–1283.
40. Kahraman S, Yakın K, Dönmez E, et al. Relationship between granular cytoplasm of oocytes and pregnancy outcome following intracytoplasmic sperm injection. *Hum Reprod*. 2000;15(11):2390–2393.
41. Hu J, Molinari E, Darmon S, et al. Predictive value of cytoplasmic granulation patterns during in vitro fertilization in metaphase II oocytes: part I, poor-prognosis patients. *Fertil Steril*. 2021;116(2):431–443.
42. Otsuki J, Nagai Y, Chiba K. Lipofuscin bodies in human oocytes as an indicator of oocyte quality. *J Assist Reprod Genet*. 2007;24(7):263–270.
43. Takahashi H, Otsuki J, Yamamoto M, et al. Clinical outcomes of MII oocytes with refractile bodies in patients undergoing ICSI and single frozen embryo transfer. *Reprod Med Biol*. 2020;19(1):75–81.
44. Wang X, Xiao Y, Sun Z, et al. Smooth endoplasmic reticulum clusters in oocytes from patients who received intracytoplasmic sperm injections negatively affect blastocyst quality and speed of blastocyst development. *Front Physiol*. 2021;12:732547.
45. ESHRE Special Interest Group of Embryology and Alpha Scientists in Reproductive Medicine. The Vienna consensus: report of an expert meeting on the development of art laboratory performance indicators. *Hum Reprod Open*. 2017;35(5):494–510.
46. Wallbutton S, Kasraie J. Vacuolated oocytes: fertilization and embryonic arrest following intracytoplasmic sperm injection in a patient exhibiting persistent oocyte macro vacuolization – case report. *J Assist Reprod Genet*. 2010;27(4):183–188.
47. Ebner T, Moser M, Sommergruber M, et al. Occurrence and developmental consequences of vacuoles throughout preimplantation development. *Fertil Steril*. 2005;83(6):1635–1640.
48. Miao Y, Ma S, Liu X, et al. Fate of the first polar bodies in mouse oocytes. *Mol Reprod Dev*. 2004;69(1):66–76.
49. Ferrarini ZB, de Almeida FBDP, Souza SA, et al. Is perivitelline space morphology of the oocyte associated with pregnancy outcome in intracytoplasmic sperm injection cycles? *Eur J Obstet Gynaecol*. 2018;231:225–229.
50. Hassa H, Aydın Y, Taplamacıoğlu F. The role of perivitelline space abnormalities of oocytes in the developmental potential of embryos. *J Turk Ger Gynecol Assoc*. 2014;15(3):161–163.
51. Maziotis E, Sfakianoudis K, Giannelou P, et al. Evaluating the value of day 0 of an ICSI cycle on indicating laboratory outcome. *Sci Rep*. 2020;10:19325.
52. Thomas C, Cavazza T, Schuh M. Aneuploidy in human eggs: contributions of the meiotic spindle. *Biochem Soc Trans*. 2021;49(1):107–118.
53. Mikwar M, MacFarlane AJ, Marchetti F. Mechanisms of oocyte aneuploidy associated with advanced maternal age. *Mutat Res Rev Mutat Res*. 2020;785:108320.
54. Capalbo A, Hoffman ER, Cimadomo D, et al. Human female meiosis revised: new insights into the mechanisms of chromosome segregation and aneuploidies from advanced genomics and time-lapse imaging. *Hum Reprod Update*. 2017;23(6):706–722.

20

Semen Analysis, Preparation, and Selection

Sue Montgomery

20.1 Semen Analysis

The assessment of the male partner plays a key role in diagnosing infertility and managing treatment decisions for the infertile couple. The guidelines for diagnostic semen analysis are clearly outlined in the WHO manual for semen analysis – edition 6 (**1**). Semen analysis falls into two main components, macroscopic evaluation, and microscopic assessment of the sample. Some of the processes are time dependent, for example the motility must be assessed within 60 minutes of sample production, or the motility may begin to decline (**1**). Therefore, this must be prioritised above other parts of the test that are not time dependent, in practice in the laboratory.

20.1.1 Critical Patient Information

There are multiple clinical and patient factors that can affect the outcome of the semen analysis test (**2, 3**), and therefore to aid the interpretation of the results, it is vital that the following information is collected from the patient at the time the sample is produced:

a) Abstinence period (a period of 2–7 days prior to producing a sample for analysis is recommended)
b) Time of production. The sample must be received by the laboratory within 60 minutes of production, or the motility may be affected before the analysis can be completed
c) Whether the sample collected into the non-toxic container supplied by the clinic
d) Whether any lubricants were used
e) Whether the entire sample was collected
f) If the patient is taking steroids or any form of medication prescribed by a doctor

20.2 Macroscopic Evaluation

Macroscopic evaluation includes the following assessments:

a) Liquefaction

Upon production the seminal fluid is a coagulated mass, which liquefies (becomes watery) within 15–60 minutes post production at room temperature. The coagulum which traps the sperm is liquefied by the action of prostatic proteases. For the analysis, to aid this process the sample is placed in the small incubator/warming cabinet at 37°C until liquefied. If liquefaction is not complete by 45 minutes after production, then preparation should proceed regardless, with this information recorded on the final report. Normal liquefied semen samples may contain jelly-like granules (gelatinous bodies) which fail to liquefy but these do not appear to have any clinical significance.

Liquefaction, is assessed by swirling the sample in the container as well as by later examination under the microscope. The sample should appear homogenous. If liquefaction is delayed or incomplete the sample will appear as a semi-solid coagulated mass. Incomplete liquefaction will affect the motility of the sample and the ability of the sperm to progress through the female reproductive tract (**4, 5**).

In some cases, the liquefaction may be delayed and there is a strong association between delayed liquefaction and chronic prostatitis (**6**). In such cases it may be necessary to aid liquefaction. The use of α-Chymotrypsin is generally avoided in the fertility laboratory and the preferred method is by mechanical breakdown of the viscous sample by forcing the semen through the narrow opening of an 18-gauge blunt needle, fitted to a sterile 5ml syringe with a rubber-free plunger. The semen should then be very thoroughly mixed by repeated pipetting before analysis. In extreme cases of delayed liquefaction, the addition of an equal volume of culture media may be required together with repeated pipetting. The quantity of media added is then taken into consideration for the final calculation of sperm concentration and pH should be measured prior to the addition of the media.

b) Viscosity

The viscosity of a semen sample is assessed by drawing a small volume of the semen into a Pasteur pipette and dropping it back into the sample pot drop by drop. If the viscosity is normal, it will fall back into the pot in discrete drops, however, if it is viscous, it will form a thread, several centimetres long. Abnormal viscosity can be an indication of enzymatic problems, hypofunction of the prostate or seminal vesicles, or infection, which increases the

DOI: 10.1201/9781003269502-20

number of leucocytes present in the sample (**5**). More recently, increased viscosity of the seminal plasma has also been linked to oxidative stress, which may compromise the quality of the sample. It has been suggested that anti-oxidants may be beneficial in these cases (**7**).

c) Appearance

Normal semen samples can vary a little in colour, however a normal sample is usually described as slightly off-grey and opaque. Any observed colour changes can be an indication of other pathologies that may need further investigation. For example:

Red/pink may indicate the presence of blood.

Yellow may indicate urine contamination and/or infection.

Brown may indicate occluded blood.

Green may indicate an infection.

It is very important to record and report any colour change in the semen sample, so that it can be further investigated, as it can be a marker of a more serious issue and require medical follow-up (**1**).

d) Volume

The volume of the sample is estimated by weight. This is achieved by pre weighing the container and subsequently re weighing the container including the sample. The weight of the empty container can then be subtracted, to give the weight of just the sample. It is assumed that the density of semen is 1g/ml (**8**). The normal reference range for volume is 1.4 millilitres or above (**1**). Any volume above 6 millilitres is considered abnormal and could be indicative of other conditions. This is known as hyperspermia. A volume below 1.4 millilitres is known as hypospermia (**1**). A low volume may indicate an absence of the vas deferens, an ejaculatory duct obstruction or abnormality, or collection problems (**3**).

e) Semen pH

The pH of the semen sample is measured by spreading a drop of semen evenly onto pH paper. It is necessary to wait a few seconds for the colour of the impregnated zone to become uniform. The observed colour can then be compared to the colour on the calibration strip for the pH papers, to read the pH. The normal range is a pH of >7.2. The pH can be a good indicator of blockages and/or genetic conditions. By knowing the pH you can isolate the origins of the components of the ejaculate (as shown in Table 20.1). this may indicate congenital absence of the vas deferens or ejaculatory duct obstruction and should be further investigated (**9**).

TABLE 20.1

The Components of Seminal Plasma and Their Corresponding pH

	% of Volume	pH
Seminal Plasma		
Seminal vesicle fluid	65–75	7.2
Prostatic fluid	25–30	6.1–6.5
Epididymal plasma	5	6.2
Bulbourethral gland	1	7.2

20.3 Microscopic Evaluation

The microscopic evaluation of a semen sample includes assessment of the number of sperm present (concentration), how well they swim (motility) and the shape of the sperm (morphology). The assessment should also record the presence of any round cells in the sample (**1**).

20.3.1 Calculating the Concentration

Many chambers are available for determining the concentration of spermatozoa in the sample, but the most reliable option, as recommended by the WHO is the Improved Neubauer chamber (**1**). This chamber is a fixed depth chamber of 0.1mm, with a glass cover slip that is placed on top of the chamber so that a seal is formed. The sample is then taken by capillary action under the cover glass and fills the chamber with a precise and reproducible volume on each occasion. For use with this chamber, the sample must be diluted and mixed carefully, depending on the concentration of the sample. The assessment is carried out in the following manner:

a) Initial evaluation of the ejaculate is required to select the appropriate dilution factor for preparation of two replicate dilutions. Aliquot 10µl of well mixed semen onto a clean glass slide and cover with a clean 22mm x 22mm coverslip. Examine at x400 magnification and count the number of sperm present in an average field of view and select an appropriate dilution ratio using Table 20.2 as a guide. This can be performed using the slides prepared for motility assessment.
b) Label two microfuge tubes A and B together with corresponding patient details. Prepare two replicates of the chosen appropriate semen dilution. Use an air displacement pipette to add the required volume of diluent (water) to each tube. Using a positive

TABLE 20.2

Appropriate Dilutions for Sperm Handling for Sperm Concentration Assessment Using the Improved Neubauer Counting Chamber (from [1]with Permission)

Spermatozoa per x400 field	Dilution ratio required	Semen (µl)	Diluent (µl)
>200	1: 50 (1 + 49)	50	2450
40–200	1: 20 (1 + 19)	50	950
16–40	1: 10 (1 + 9)	50	450
2–15	1: 5 (1 + 4)	50	200
<2	1: 2 (1 + 1)	100	100

displacement pipette, aspirate the appropriate volume of well mixed semen into each of the two microfuge tubes containing the diluent.

c) Prepare the Neubauer chamber by fixing the coverslip to the chamber. This is achieved by making the surface of the Neubauer slightly damp by breathing on it and then securing the coverslip by sliding it on and pressing firmly onto the chamber pillars until Newton's rings are visible.

Close the caps and vortex both tubes for at least 10 seconds at the maximum speed to mix sample thoroughly. Immediately proceed to loading the Neubauer chamber before the spermatozoa have time to settle out of suspension.

To load the chamber, take an air displacement pipette and add 10µl of the diluent/semen mixture from the first tube and slowly depress the plunger with the tip resting at the V-shaped groove at the edge of the Neubauer, allowing capillary action to flood the chamber. The chamber should not be overfilled as this may lift the coverslip whilst being loaded, or under filled as this may result in air getting into the chamber.

Remove 10µl from the second tube to load the second chamber of the Neubauer as detailed above.

d) Place the Neubauer haemocytometer in a humidified chamber to settle for 5–10 minutes at room temperature to allow the cells to sediment onto the grid. The chamber should be assessed within 10–15 minutes following preparation, after which evaporation has noticeable effects on sperm position within the chamber.

e) Focusing on the central grid (grid C) (see Figure 20.1) of the first side of the Neubauer chamber, start counting sperm in the top left-hand side square and tally using a laboratory counter. The number of round cells can be counted at the same time The middle line of the three lines at the edge of the square defines the square's boundary and all spermatozoa within this boundary should be counted. Therefore, all sperm with their heads on the inner line will be counted but those with their heads on the outer lines will not. If sperms are lying on middle line, only count the sperms which are present on the lower and left-hand side line. Those present on the middle lines of the top and right-hand side lines are NOT included.

f) Count across the five squares of the top row and if fewer than 200 sperms have been seen, move to the next row below and continue counting whole rows of 5 squares until 200 or more sperm have been reached. This may necessitate counting the whole grid of 5 rows (25 squares). When more than 200 sperm have been reached in whole rows, stop counting and make a note of the number of sperm and the number of rows counted on the first grid. DO NOT STOP COUNTING MID-ROW. If 200 sperm are not seen after counting the whole grid of 25 squares, then a lower dilution should be prepared. If a 1 in 2 dilution has been prepared and there are still fewer than 200 sperm on the whole grid, this should be recorded.

g) Move to the second grid on the Neubauer chamber and count the same number of rows as the first grid. If 200 sperm are counted on the second grid in fewer rows than on the first grid, it is still imperative that the same number of rows is counted as on the first chamber. The counts from both grids should be close enough for the difference to be accepted. This is based on the maximum difference between counts that could be expected to occur in 95% of samples due to sampling error alone (95% confidence interval) and the acceptable differences are shown in Table 20.3.

If the limit difference between the counts is less than or equal to the value given in Table 20.3 then the counts are accepted, and concentration can be calculated based on their mean. If the difference is greater, then this is either suggestive of miscounting, pipetting errors or failure to mix the sample thoroughly resulting in a non-random distribution of sperm on the grid. When the difference exceeds the acceptable limit then the dilutions should be discarded, and two fresh dilutions made and re-counted. Where the number of sperms counted are small, an indication of uncertainty in the final result should be reported.

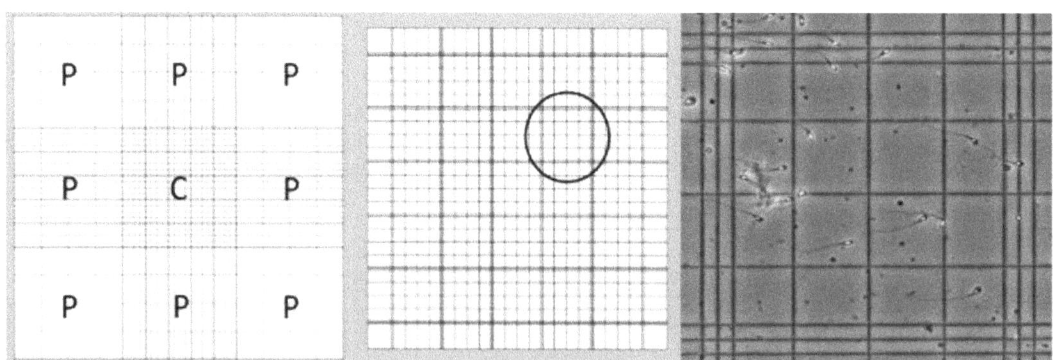

FIGURE 20.1 The improved Neubauer showing all nine grids of the Neubauer (left), the central grid (C) and eight peripheral grids (P). The central grid consists of 25 squares, each of these squares has 16 smaller squares (right) (graphics and micrograph by courtesy of Lars Björndahl).

TABLE 20.3

Comparison of Difference between Replicate Counts and Relation to Uncertainty of Result (from [1] with Permission)

Range of Sum	Limit difference	Error of final result based on number of observations (%)
969–1000	61	3.2%
938–968	60	3.3%
907–937	59	3.3%
876–906	58	3.4%
846–875	57	3.4%
817–845	56	3.5%
788–816	55	3.6%
760–787	54	3.6%
732–759	53	3.7%
704–731	52	3.8%
678–703	51	3.8%
651–677	50	3.9%
625–650	49	4.0%
600–624	48	4.1%
576–599	47	4.2%
551–575	46	4.3%
528–550	45	4.4%
504–527	44	4.5%
482–503	43	4.6%
460–481	42	4.7%
438–459	41	4.8%
417–437	40	4.9%
396–416	39	5%
376–395	38	5.2%
357–375	37	5.3%
338–356	36	5.4%
319–337	35	5.6%
301–318	34	5.8%
284–300	33	5.9%
267–283	32	6.1%
251–266	31	6.3%
235–250	30	6.5%
219–234	29	6.8%
206–218	28	7.0%
190–205	27	7.3%
176–189	26	7.5%
163–175	25	7.8%
150–162	24	8.2%
138–149	23	8.5%
126–137	22	8.9%
115–125	21	9.3%
105–114	20	9.8%
94–104	19	10.3%
85–93	18	10.8%
76–84	17	11.5%
67–75	16	12.2%
59–66	15	13.0%
52–58	14	13.9%
44–51	13	15.1%
38–43	12	16.2%
32–37	11	17.7%
27–31	10	19.2%
22–36	9	21.3%
17–21	8	24.3%
13–16	7	27.7%
10–12	6	31.6%
7–9	5	37.8%
5–6	4	44.7%
3–4	3	57.7%
2	2	70.7%
1	1	100%

h) The calculation for determining the concentration of sperm requires a correction factor, which is dependent on the dilution used and the number of rows counted, shown in Table 20.4.

The concentration is calculated as follows:

$$\textbf{Concentration of sperm (M/ml)} = \frac{\text{Number of sperms on grid 1 + number of sperms on grid 2}}{\text{Correction factor}}$$

Some examples of the calculation to determine concentration follow.

Example 1

1:5 dilution used

Grid 1: 201 sperms counted in 2 rows,

Grid 2: 210 sperms counted in 2 rows

Difference = 9

Acceptable difference for 411 sperm counted is 39, therefore a difference of 9 is acceptable

Correction factor for 2 rows (per replicate) of 1:5 dilution = 16

Therefore, 411/16 = $\mathbf{25.7\ x10^6\ ml^{-1}}$

Example 2

1:5 dilution used

Grid 1: 91 sperms counted in 5 rows,

Grid 2: 106 sperms counted in 5 rows

Fewer than 400 sperm have been counted therefore a new dilution of 1:2 should be prepared and a fresh counting chamber loaded.

1:2 dilution used

Grid 1: 189 sperms counted in 5 rows,

Grid 2: 216 sperms counted in 5 rows

Acceptable difference for 405 sperm counted is 39, therefore a difference of 27 is acceptable

Correction factor for 5 rows (per replicate) of 1:2 dilution = 100

Therefore, 405/100 = $\mathbf{4.1\ x10^6\ ml^{-1}}$

TABLE 20.4

Correction Factor for Calculating Sperm Concentration

Dilution	Number of counted rows (on each side of the chamber)				
	5 rows each side (10 rows total)	4 rows each side (8 rows total	3 rows each side (6 rows total)	2 rows each side (4 rows total)	1 row each side (2 rows total)
1:2	100	80	60	40	20
1:5	40	32	24	16	8
1:10	20	16	12	8	4
1:20	10	8	6	4	2
1:50	4	3.2	2.4	1.6	0.8

Example 3

1:20 dilution

Grid 1: 189 sperms counted in 5 rows,

Grid 2: 216 sperms counted in 5 row s

Acceptable difference for 405 sperm counted is 39, therefore a difference of 27 is acceptable

Correction factor for 10 rows of 1:20 dilution = 10

Therefore, 405/10 = ***40.5 x10⁶ ml⁻¹***

i) The total number of spermatozoa in the ejaculate is calculated by multiplying the concentration in millions/ml by the ejaculate volume in ml.

20.3.2 Suspected Azoospermia

If no sperm are seen upon an initial microscopic assessment of a 10µl aliquot, then the sample should be assessed using a Large Volume Fixed Depth (LVFD) slide, as described below.

a) Using a positive displacement pipette, take a 25µl aliquot of the semen and gently add to the entrance area (labelled "add 25 µl") in chamber A of the slide. The chamber will fill by capillary action. Repeat for chamber B then place the LVFD slide in a humidified chamber in the incubator for at least 15 minutes to allow any non-motile sperm to settle.

b) Examine the whole of chamber A using a phase-contrast microscope at x200 or x400 in a systematic grid pattern, ensuring the whole chamber is assessed, and tally the number of motile and immotile sperm seen. Repeat for chamber B.

c) Express count as total number of sperm seen in 50µl (25µl aliquot in each chamber) and multiply by 20 to give the sperm concentration in number of sperm per millilitre, together with an assessment of the percentage of progressive and non-progressive motility. The report should clearly state that this count is individual sperm per millilitre and not a count in millions per millilitre, to avoid any clinical misinterpretation of the result. To express the finding in millions of sperm/ml, divide the result by 1 million.

d) The absence of spermatozoa suggests azoospermia. If this classification is given for an initial semen analysis, then it should be reported as 'suspected azoospermia.' Azoospermia should be confirmed via a repeat analysis after 3 months.

20.3.3 Assessing the Motility

Sperm motility should be assessed as soon as possible after liquefaction and within 60 minutes of sample production to prevent changes due to temperature or pH variation. Motility assessment should be done twice (using two separate aliquots of 10µl and counting 200 sperm each time) in order to increase the accuracy and should be carried out at 37°C which is achieved by the use of a heated stage warmer, as follows:

Place 10µl of semen on a glass slide and place a cover slip on top. The weight of the coverslip spreads the sample but take care to try and avoid the formation of air bubbles. Place the slide at 37°C, wait approximately 60 seconds for the sample to stop drifting then assess the motility of 200 spermatozoa on for each replicate according to the WHO criteria (see below) using a phase contrast microscope at either x200 or x400. Assess sperm which are at least 5mm in from the edge of the coverslip to avoid any areas of drying.

Scan the slide in a systematic way to avoid viewing the same area. Change the field often and in a random fashion so that at least 5 fields are assessed. Tally the different grades using a counter as described below.

20.3.4 Categories of Sperm Motility

The WHO 2021 manual categorises spermatozoa motility into four groups, this classification has changed from three groups since clinical data has demonstrated the importance of the number of 'progressive sperm'. The four grades of sperm motility classification are described below:

- Rapid progression (Grade A) – (25µm/s) sperm moving actively, either linearly nor in a large circle, covering a distance, from the starting point to the end point, of at least 25 µm (or ½ tail length) in one second.
- Slow progression (Grade B) – (5 to < 25 µm/s) spermatozoa moving actively, either linearly or in a large circle, covering a distance, from the starting point to the end point, of 5 to < 25 µm (or at least one head length to less than ½ tail length) in one second.
- Non-progressive (Grade C) (< 5 µm/s) all other patterns of active tail movements with an absence of progression i.e. swimming in small circles, the flagellar force displacing the head less than 5 µm (one head length), from the starting point to the end point.
- Immotile (Grade D) – no active tail movements.

Calculate the percentage of sperm with A, B, C and D motility in each replicate. Using the Acceptable Difference Table (Table 20.5), determine if the difference seen in the most

TABLE 20.5

Acceptable Difference Table for Motility (from [1] with Permission)

Average (%)	Acceptable % Difference*	Average (%)	Acceptable % Difference*
1	2	56–72	9
2–3	3	73–80	8
4–6	4	81–86	7
7–9	5	87–90	6
10–13	6	91–93	5
14–19	7	94–96	4
20–27	8	97–98	3
28–44	9	99	2
45–55	10	100	1

* *based on the rounded 95% confidence interval*

common category could have occurred by chance; if so, the averages (rounded to the nearest whole number) are accepted. If the difference is greater than the acceptable limit, two fresh aliquots are prepared, and the sperm motility re-assessed. In cases of severe oligozoospermia it may not be possible to assess at least 200 sperm for the motility assessment. If <200 sperm are assessed, then a note is made in the report, indicating how many sperm were actually assessed along with whether motile sperm were observed or not.

Example 1

Category	*1st replicate*	*2nd replicate*	*Average*	*Difference*
PR	*30%*	*50%*		
NP	*5%*	*15%*		
IM	*65%*	*35%*	*50%*	*30%*

The most common category is immotile sperm with an average of 50% for which we would expect a difference of 10% to occur by chance alone (see table 20.5, average 35–65). As the difference exceeds this limit, the results are discarded, and two fresh motility slides are prepared and re-assessed.

Example 2

Category	*1st replicate*	*2nd replicate*	*Average*	*Difference*
PR	*37%*	*28%*	*32%*	
NP	*3%*	*6%*	*4%*	
IM	*60%*	*66%*	*63%*	*6%*

The most common category is immotile sperm with an average of 63% for which we would expect a difference of 9% to occur by chance alone (see table 20.5, average 35–65). As the difference is within this limit, the results are accepted, and the mean values reported.

20.3.5 Assessing the Morphology

There is evidence that sperm morphology can have an impact on fertility (**10**), however, due to the variety of different methods and interpretation of the value of 'normal,' the assessment of morphology remains controversial. Pre-stained morphology slides are used to stain sperm for morphology assessment, which compare favourably to the recommended smear preparation and Diff Quick staining described in the WHO manual.

a) Dispense 5µl of semen onto a pre-stained slide for morphological assessment and cover with coverslip. Using the back of your finger, apply gentle pressure on the coverslip through the flat part of your fingernail to spread the semen evenly over the slide. Care should be taken not to push down too hard and risk breaking the coverslip. The slide is left for approximately 15–30 minutes for the sperm to become immotile.

b) Examination is performed using the x100 oil-immersion bright field objective lens and immersion oil of a refractive index of 1.50–1.55. The phase ring is turned to phase 3 for the x100 objective. An eyepiece graticule is present in order to aid assessment of morphology where one small division = 1µm.

c) Sperm morphology is assessed by evaluating 200 sperm and tallying the number of normal and abnormal sperm, as well as where the defects in abnormal sperm occur (see Table 20.6). These are tallied during the assessment as; head, neck and midpiece, tail and excessive residual cytoplasm defects. This is carried out by grading normal and abnormal forms then holding the clicker for abnormal down and tallying where the defects are at the same time. This is recorded as %H, %N, %M, %T and %C.

Only sperm where the three regions (head, neck and midpiece and tail) can be observed fully should be assessed and therefore agglutinated clumps should not be analysed. Assessment of sperm should be made in different, systematically selected areas of the slide in order to prevent biased selection of particular sperm.

For a spermatozoon to be scored as normal, the head, midpiece, and tail should all be normal according to the following criteria:

Head: Oval in shape, smooth and regularly contoured. A well-defined acrosome region comprising of 40–70% of the head area (**11**). There should be an absence of vacuoles within the post-acrosomal region, however, up to two small vacuoles within the acrosomal region (not more than 20% of the sperm head) is acceptable. Dimensions of the head should be 4.0–5.0µm in length with a width of 2.5–3.5µm.

Midpiece: This region, immediately behind the head, should be slender and regular. Residual cytoplasm (cytoplasmic droplets) may be present in normal

TABLE 20.6

Examples of sperm morphology defects

Head	Neck and Midpiece	Tail
Large	Bent	Absent tail
Small	Distended	Short
Tapering	Irregular	Multiple
Pyriform	Thin (no mitochondrial sheath)	Hairpin
Amorphous	Cytoplasmic droplets	Broken
Vacuolated (>20% head area)		Irregular width
Multiple heads		Coiled
Headless (pinhead)		Presence of terminal droplets

sperm, however, if they exceed 1/3 of the sperm head size the sperm should be classified as abnormal (**12**). Dimensions of the midpiece should be approximately 1–1.5x the length as the head and less than 1.0μm in width.

Tail: The tail should be thinner than the midpiece and have a uniform calibre along its length. Only a single tail should be present. The length should be approximately 10x the head length (approximately 45μm). The tail may be looped back on itself but should not contain any sharp angles which would indicate a flagellum break.

Any sperm not fulfilling these criteria, including 'borderline forms' should be classed as abnormal.

4. The teratozoospermia index (TZI) is then calculated using the formula:

20.4 Sum of All Abnormalities/ Number of Abnormal Sperm

The result should be between 1.00 and 4.00 (recorded to two decimal places).

Example of calculating the TZI

Normal forms 12/200 = 6%

Abnormal heads 184/200 = 91%

Abnormal neck/midpieces 102/200 = 51%

Abnormal tail 30/200 = 15%

Percentage with excess residual cytoplasm 44/200 = 22%

TZI (184 + 102 + 30 + 44)/188 = 1.91

20.4.1 Round Cells

The presence of round cells in the ejaculate should be reported in millions per ml and are counted alongside the sperm concentration using the Neubauer chamber, in a diluted sample, applying the appropriate calculation for the respective dilution factor used. Clinical interpretation must be provided by the referring clinician.

20.4.2 Reporting and Interpreting the Results

The normal reference ranges for a semen sample are shown in Table 20.7 (**1**).

The recommended terms for classification of a semen sample are shown in Table 20.8.

The results from the analysis are reported back to the referring clinician, who will explain the findings to the patient and arrange any further investigations deemed necessary.

TABLE 20.7

Reference Ranges (Compiled from [**1**])

Parameter	References ranges
Count	Lower limit $16x10^6$ ml^{-1}
Total sperm number	Lower limit $39x10^6$ ml^{-1}
Progressive motility	Lower limit 30%
Total motility	Lower limit 42%
Morphology	Lower limit 4% normal
pH	Lower limit 7.2
Volume	Lower limit 1.4ml
Round cells	Lower limit $1.0x10^6$ ml^{-1}

TABLE 20.8

WHO Classification Terms (as Compiled from [**1**]).

Normozoospermia	Normal ejaculate
Haemospermia	Presence of red blood cells
Cryptozoospermia	Very few sperm seen in the ejaculate (only after concentrating sample)
Asthenozoospermia	Reduced sperm motility
Oligozoospermia	Reduced sperm count
Teratozoospermia	Reduced sperm morphology
Asthenoteratozoospermia	Reduced sperm motility and morphology
Oligoasthenozoospermia	Reduced sperm count and motility
Oligoteratozoospermia	Reduced sperm count and morphology
Oligoasthenoteratozoospermia	Reduced sperm count, motility, and morphology
Suspected azoospermia	Absence of sperm
Aspermia	Absence of ejaculate

20.5 Preparation of Semen for Treatment

The principle of sperm preparation for treatment is to separate the motile sperm in the sample from the immotile sperm, cellular debris and seminal fluid. This is generally achieved via the use of centrifugation. Prior to preparation, the sample must be analysed to determine the number of sperm in the sample, what percentage are motile and how many have a normal morphology. This is carried out to ensure that the sample is suitable for the proposed treatment and also so that the appropriate preparation technique can be used, depending on the quality of the sample. To make this assessment an overall picture of the quality of the sample is required and so a method is used that assesses both the concentration and the motility together, the Makler chamber. This method of assessment is not as reliable or reproducible as the method described above for semen analysis (using the Improved Neubauer chamber), it is only suitable for pre-preparation assessment, where a decision on the best preparation method that suits the sample quality, is required. The grid on the chamber consists of 100 squares (10 x 10). All of the sperm that fall in one column (of 10 squares) are counted, to give the sperm count in millions per millilitre of semen (see Figure 20.2). Using this grid, the percentage motile can also be assessed, using the same four categories as described above. The percentage with normal morphology is also assessed on a pre-stained slide as described in detail above.

In the UK, there is an HFEA witnessing requirement that must be applied throughout the semen preparation process. The HFEA Act states that every time sperm is moved between receptacles (such as the pot, or centrifugation tubes), the step

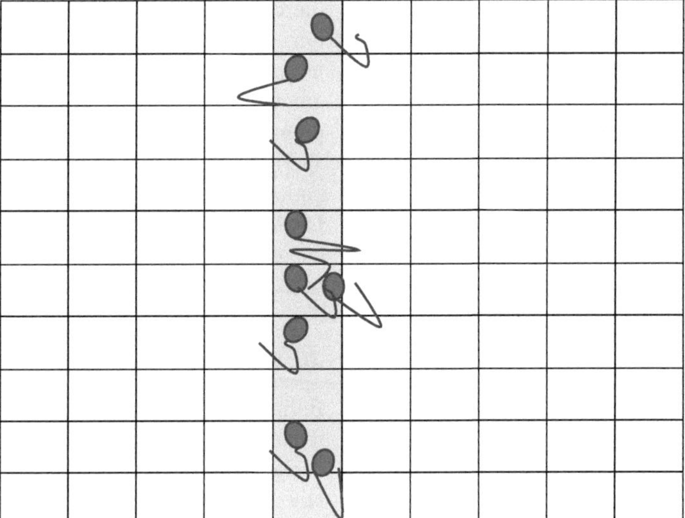

FIGURE 20.2 Close-up view of the grid on a Makler chamber; sperm that fall in one whole column (of 10 squares) are equivalent to that number in millions per millilitre.

must be witnessed, to ensure that the labelling (with three identifiers) is the same and matches the initial pot on each receptacle. This witnessing can be carried out using an electronic witnessing system, or with a second person providing a manual witness.

There are three main methods that are used to prepare sperm for fertility treatment, which are based on methods described in the early days of IVF and still used today (**13, 14**). These main techniques are the wash, the swim-up and the density gradient, although often two may be used together. For example (as described below) a density gradient may be performed on the sample first, followed by a washing step, to ensure a very clean sample is available for the proposed treatment.

20.5.1 Wash

If the number of sperm in the sample is very low and/or the motility is very poor on initial inspection, then a simple wash procedure is performed. This reduces the risk of losing all of the spermatozoa, as any sperm that are present will be concentrated down into a pellet, conserving the sperm, whilst effectively removing the seminal plasma. This technique is most often used for surgically retrieved samples, or severe oligozoospermic samples (**13, 14**). The wash is carried out a follows:

a) Two to 3 millilitres of sperm wash media is added to the sample in a centrifuge tube and mixed thoroughly by repeatedly pipetting.
b) The tube is centrifuged for 5–10 minutes (depending on the total volume) at 320G/1600rpm. The resulting pellet is resuspended in 0.5–1.0 millilitres of fresh sperm preparation media.

Samples of this quality are only suitable for use in ICSI treatment and can be added to a large media drop in the ICSI dish. This will allow the motile sperm present to swim to the edge of the drop, where they can be harvested using an injection pipette and transferred to a drop of PVP for immobilisation and injection.

20.5.2 Swim Up

After the wash procedure above has been completed, if the pellet contains a reasonable amount of motile sperm, then the highly motile sperm can be separated further by performing a "swim-up" on the pellet, in the following manner:

a) Remove the supernatant using a Pasteur pipette, leaving a small volume above the pellet.
b) Loosen the pellet by agitation and carefully add a layer of fresh sperm washing medium on top of the pellet, being careful not to disturb the pellet whilst doing this.
c) Leave the tube at 37°C for 20–60 minutes (tilting the tube at an angle to increase the surface area will improve the yield of motile sperm).
d) Using a Pasteur pipette, remove the supernatant without disturbing the pellet and place in a 5ml tube.
e) Leave tubes at room temperature, tight-capped, until use.

This technique is very effective in producing a clean preparation of sperm with excellent motility and is able to select the best sperm from the sample for treatment, similar to the selection that semen would undergo in the female reproductive tract (**13, 14**).

20.5.3 Density Gradient

As performing the swim-up is quite time consuming, a density gradient is often used in the clinical setting as an alternative method of separating the motile sperm. In addition, this technique can be used if the motility is slower or less abundant and also when the percentage of immotile sperm and debris is high. However, it is important that the concentration and motility are adequate to result in an appropriate recovery for the intended treatment. If this is not likely, then the wash technique described above, to pellet the sperm should be used (**13, 14**).

As mature, morphologically normal sperm have a density of >1.12g/ml, compared to the Immature and/or abnormal sperm that have densities between 1.06 and 1.09 g/ml, they can be separated by how far they can travel through a density gradient. This technique relies on the fact that particles of specific density sediment until they reach the point where their density is the same as the gradient media. A gradient is set up in a tube using layers of different density, a 40–45% solution and an 80–90%, as follows:

a) Using a glass Pasteur pipette, layer 1millilitre upper 40–45% gradient over 1millilitre of the lower 80–90% gradient in a conical tube.
b) Using a Pasteur pipette, layer up to 2ml semen onto the gradient.
c) Spin for 10 minutes at 320G/1600rpm. After centrifugation, a pellet will be visible at the bottom of the conical tube.
d) Using a Pasteur pipette, take the pellet from the bottom of the gradient and place into a wash tube containing 3ml of sperm washing medium. Spin for 5 minutes at 320G/1600rpm.

For IVF, take the final pellet and place into the IVF dilution tube and calculate the final insemination volume (μl). The final concentration should be between 5–20M/ml giving an insemination volume between 10–40μl for insemination (see Chapter 21).

For ICSI, using a Pasteur pipette remove the supernatant and resuspend in an appropriate volume of clean medium.

Leave the tubes tight-capped at room temperature until the injection procedure for ICSI or the incubation time prior to insemination, IVF or IUI.

20.5.4 The Future of Sperm Selection and Preparation for Treatment

In recent years, research has focused on improving the sperm selection methods that we use today, in order to refine the approach. Ideally, we would like to be able to select sperm not just based on their motility, but also on other factors that may contribute to their function and ability to produce a competent embryo that is capable of implanting, such as maturity and absence of DNA fragmentation. Sperm DNA fragmentation is thought to contribute to recurrent miscarriage and recurrent implantation failure, via its effect on embryo quality and development (**15–17**). The precise mechanisms of DNA fragmentation in sperm are not known, but there is an association with some life style factors, such as smoking, alcohol, diet and exercise, as well as potential genetic factors. Unfortunately, the centrifugation techniques that are currently employed in our sperm preparation methodologies, may also be contributing to DNA fragmentation of the sperm by increasing the amount of oxygen free radicals in the semen sample during the preparation process. Therefore, current research focusses on sperm preparation techniques that no longer require centrifugation, but can also actively select mature sperm with intact DNA, for use in treatment. The two main approaches that are currently being considered are microfluidics and hyaluronan binding (**18**).

20.5.4.1 Microfluidics

In this technique the motile sperm are separated by their ability to swim through a series of channels, or pores, that are designed to only allow those with a normal shape and density through (**19, 20**). This helps to minimise any further DNA damage from occurring, but also selects the sperm in the cohort that are less likely to be damaged in the first place. Studies have shown these techniques are effective in selecting sperm with very low levels of DNA fragmentation (**19**). There is also evidence that microfluidic devices can improve IVF success rates, when used to select sperm for patients experiencing male infertility (**21**). However, several reviews of the use of microfluidics for sperm selection have concluded that there is no improvement in clinical outcomes such as fertilisation and pregnancy rates when this technique is used across the entire patient population (**22, 23**).

20.5.4.2 Hyaluronan Binding

This technique is based on the theory that the presence of hyaluronic acid binding sites on the sperm plasma membrane are indicative of sperm maturity and can select a sperm that is structurally normal and less likely to contain DNA damage. This is carried out using dishes that contain hyaluronan plaques. When motile sperm are added to the dish, the normal, mature sperm will bind to the plaques and can then be dislodged with an ICSI pipette and used for injection However, results with this technique are varied and there are several studies that show that this does not improve clinical results in all patient groups (**24, 25**).

20.6 Conclusion

Semen analysis remains an important factor in the decision regarding the fertilisation method that will be recommended and performed as part of the patient treatment. It is therefore imperative that the methods are quality-managed to ensure reliability of the results. Novel methods of sperm preparation and selection for insemination and fertilisation have been developed, but further research and clinical validation are needed to assess which specific patient groups, if any, can benefit from such approaches; as well as any other novel methods which may be introduced.

REFERENCES

1. *WHO Laboratory Manual for the Examination and Processing of Human Semen [Internet].* Who.int. World Health Organization; 2021 [cited 2023 May 2]. Available from: www.who.int/publications/i/item/9789240030787
2. Agarwal A, Baskaran S, Parekh N, et al. Male infertility. *Lancet [Internet].* 2021 [cited 2023 May 2];397 (10271):319–333.
3. Andrade-Rocha FT. Semen analysis in laboratory practice: an overview of routine tests. *J Clin Lab Anal [Internet].* 2003 [cited 2023 May 2];17(6):247–258.
4. Anamthathmakula P, Winuthayanon W. Mechanism of semen liquefaction and its potential for a novel non-hormonal contraception. *Biol Reprod [Internet].* 2020 [cited 2023 May 2];103(2):411–426.
5. Agarwal A. Semen hyperviscosity causes consequences and cures. *Front Biosci (Elite Ed) [Internet].* 2013 [cited 2023 May 2];E5(1):224–231.
6. Zhang Y-F, Liang C-Z. Progress in the studies of semen delayed liquefaction from chronic prostatitis. *Zhonghua Nan Ke Xue [Internet].* 2007 [cited 2023 May 4];13(1):53–56.
7. Barbagallo F, La Vignera S, Cannarella R, et al. The relationship between seminal fluid hyperviscosity and oxidative stress: a systematic review. *Antioxidants (Basel) [Internet].* 2021 [cited 2023 May 4];10(3):356.
8. Matson PL, Myssonski K, Yovich S, et al. The density of human semen and the validation of weight as an indicator of volume: a multicentre study. *Reprod Biol [Internet].* 2010 [cited 2023 May 4];10(2):141–153.
9. Sharma A, Minhas S, Dhillo WS, et al. Male infertility due to testicular disorders. *J Clin Endocrinol Metab [Internet].* 2021 [cited 2023 May 4];106(2):e442–e459.
10. Danis RB, Samplaski MK. Sperm morphology: history, challenges, and impact on natural and assisted fertility. *Curr Urol Rep [Internet].* 2019 [cited 2023 May 4];20(8):43.
11. Menkveld R, Holleboom CAG, Rhemrev JPT. Measurement and significance of sperm morphology. *Asian J Androl [Internet].* 2011 [cited 2023 May 4];13(1):59–68.
12. Mortimer D, Menkveld R. Sperm morphology assessment – historical perspectives and current opinions. *J Androl.* 2001;22(2):192–205.
13. Mortimer D, Mortimer ST. Methods of sperm preparation for assisted reproduction. *Ann Acad Med Singapore [Internet].* 1992 [cited 2023 May 4];21(4):517–524.
14. Henkel RR, Schill W-B. Sperm preparation for ART. *Reprod Biol Endocrinol [Internet].* 2003 [cited 2023 May 4];1(1):108.
15. Agarwal A, Majzoub A, Baskaran S, et al. Sperm DNA fragmentation: a new guideline for clinicians. *World J Mens Health [Internet].* 2020 [cited 2023 May 4];38(4):412–471.
16. Simon L, Emery B, Carrell DT. Sperm DNA fragmentation: consequences for reproduction. *Adv Exp Med Biol [Internet].* 2019 [cited 2023 May 4];1166:87–105.
17. McQueen DB, Zhang J, Robins JC. Sperm DNA fragmentation and recurrent pregnancy loss: a systematic review and meta-analysis. *Fertil Steril [Internet].* 2019 [cited 2023 May 4];112(1):54–60. e3.
18. Vaughan DA, Sakkas D. Sperm selection methods in the 21st century. *Biol Reprod [Internet].* 2019 [cited 2023 May 4];101(6):1076–1082.
19. Quinn MM, Jalalian L, Ribeiro S, et al. Microfluidic sorting selects sperm for clinical use with reduced DNA damage compared to density gradient centrifugation with swim-up in split semen samples. *Hum Reprod [Internet].* 2018 [cited 2023 May 4];33(8):1388–1393.
20. Samuel R, Feng H, Jafek A, et al. Microfluidic-based sperm sorting & analysis for treatment of male infertility. *Transl Androl Urol [Internet].* 2018 [cited 2023 May 4];7(Suppl. 3):S336–S347.
21. Ozcan P, Takmaz T, Yazici MGK, et al. Does the use of microfluidic sperm sorting for the sperm selection improve in vitro fertilization success rates in male factor infertility? *J Obstet Gynaecol Res [Internet].* 2021 [cited 2023 May 4];47(1):382–388.
22. Olatunji O, More A. A review of the impact of microfluidics technology on sperm selection technique. *Cureus [Internet].* 2022 [cited 2023 May 4];14(7):e27369.
23. Alias AB, Huang H-Y, Yao D-J. A review on microfluidics: an aid to assisted reproductive technology. *Molecules [Internet].* 2021 [cited 2023 May 4];26(14):4354.
24. Beck-Fruchter R, Shalev E, Weiss A. Clinical benefit using sperm hyaluronic acid binding technique in ICSI cycles: a systematic review and meta-analysis. *Reprod Biomed Online [Internet].* 2016 [cited 2023 May 4];32(3):286–298.
25. Avalos-Durán G, Cañedo-Del Ángel AME, Rivero-Murillo J, et al. Physiological ICSI (PICSI) vs. Conventional ICSI in couples with male factor: a systematic review. *JBRA Assist Reprod [Internet].* 2018 [cited 2023 May 4];22(2):139–147.

21

Fertilisation Methods

Sue Montgomery and Ruth Arnesen

21.1 Introduction

The aim of this chapter is to provide some insight into the fertilisation methods that may be employed in a fertility clinic. The choice of method will depend on a variety of factors including male and female parameters that will be assessed when the patient(s) first attend the clinic, during consultation. Once the outcome of any required tests is known, the consultant will select the most appropriate treatment and this decision will dictate the method of fertilisation to be used. There are 3 main methods of fertilisation, namely intrauterine insemination (IUI), in vitro fertilisation (IVF) and intracytoplasmic sperm injection (ICSI). These methods are described below.

21.2 Intrauterine Insemination (IUI)

The principle of IUI treatment is to facilitate the meeting of the oocyte and a motile sperm sample that has been prepared in the laboratory, in the body, so that the process of fertilisation can take place *in vivo* (**1**). To achieve this, the development of follicles in the egg provider must be monitored, so that sperm can be inseminated into the uterus around the time of ovulation. This can be via a natural cycle, where a single follicle will be tracked and monitored until it reaches around 18mm. Or, with the use of mild gonadotrophin stimulation to encourage two or three follicles to develop (**2, 3**). This increases the chances of successful fertilisation and therefore implantation taking place, but carries with it a risk of multiple follicular development. For this reason, it is vital that these cycles are monitored closely using ultrasound scanning to identify the number of follicles developing. Any treatment cycle producing more than three follicles must either be abandoned, or converted to a cycle of IVF, due to the risk of high order multiple pregnancies if treatment proceeds.

For IUI to be an option for the patient, the ovulated oocyte and the motile sperm must be able to meet *in vivo* and so this treatment is only suitable for patients with demonstrated patent tubes. This can be confirmed from a diagnostic test such as a HyCoSy or laparoscopy, or is sometimes inferred from the knowledge of a confirmed previous pregnancy. IUI is a first line treatment and is useful where there is no evidence of other infertility factors, such as for single woman, using donor sperm. However, the results with IUI are not as high as they are for IVF and so patients will generally be advised to move on to the next stage of treatment, if they have not been successful within three attempts. This likely due to the minimal information gained from this technique and the inability to ascertain if the oocytes are capable of undergoing fertilisation and if so, what the quality of the developing embryo is like. That coupled with the low number of oocytes available for each cycle, makes this treatment option less successful. This is not a successful treatment for women of advanced reproductive age (**4**).

The nature of IUI treatment dictates that the semen sample must be of good quality, ideally being classified as WHO normal, to give a realistic chance of success. The minimum requirements are a volume greater that 1.5 millilitres, a sperm concentration of 15 million per milliliter (M/ml) and progressive sperm motility (a+b progression) of at least 35%. In addition, the morphology of the sperm must be a minimum of 4%.

In the laboratory the sperm is prepared to separate the motile sperm from the semen, immotile sperm and debris. There are two main methods for doing this, which are the "swim up" and the "density gradient" approach. These methods are both described in full in Chapter 20 on sperm preparation methods. Spermatozoa are hardy cells, but scientists must be mindful that when handling them outside of the body during the preparation process, care must be taken to minimise exposing them to conditions that would not be found *in vivo*. The main risks are the extended exposure to seminal plasma, temperature changes and pH fluctuations. Therefore, laboratory protocols must dictate that the sample is prepared (to separate the motile sperm from the seminal plasma) quickly after production and that all media used has been warmed to room temperature in advance. To minimise pH fluctuations, media may be used that contains a buffer to keep the pH stable. Although, this does not appear to be a necessity, as long as the prepared sample is restored to the correct pH before being inseminated or introduced to oocytes in culture during IVF.

For IUI treatment, after the preparation process of choice, the sample must contain a minimum of 5 million motile sperm, ideally with 100 percent progression. Prior to the insemination procedure, the sperm sample is warmed up to 37°C for 30 minutes. Excessive incubation prior to insemination should be avoided.

21.3 In Vitro Fertilisation (IVF)

The process of IVF was pioneered by Edwards and Steptoe in 1978. This process enables mature oocytes that have been retrieved from the ovary, to be fertilised in a dish in the laboratory and was initially designed for patients where the egg

DOI: 10.1201/9781003269502-21

and oocyte could not meet *in vivo*, specifically women with blocked fallopian tubes. However, it is now also used for other infertility types, where the sperm is good enough quality to attempt the process of fertilisation without the need for micromanipulation techniques. The main difference between IVF and the more invasive technique of intracytoplasmic sperm injection (ICSI) is that with IVF, there is still an element of natural selection, in terms of which sperm are actually able to penetrate the oocyte. It is therefore a more "natural" process than ICSI.

The sperm preparation process for IVF is identical to that of IUI, described in Chapter 20. During IVF and after the sperm preparation process, the washed sperm are added directly to drops of culture media (under oil) in a dish containing the oocyte-cumulus complexes (Figure 21.1). Enough sperm must be added to enable the digestion of the cumulus cells and between 50,000–200,000 sperm per oocyte are required to achieve this.

The actual number of sperm added will vary depending on the size of the culture drop that the oocyte is placed in for insemination. The sperm concentration that we wish to achieve is around 150,000 motile sperm/ml of culture media and so a simple calculation can be carried out to determine what volume of our prepared sperm should be added.

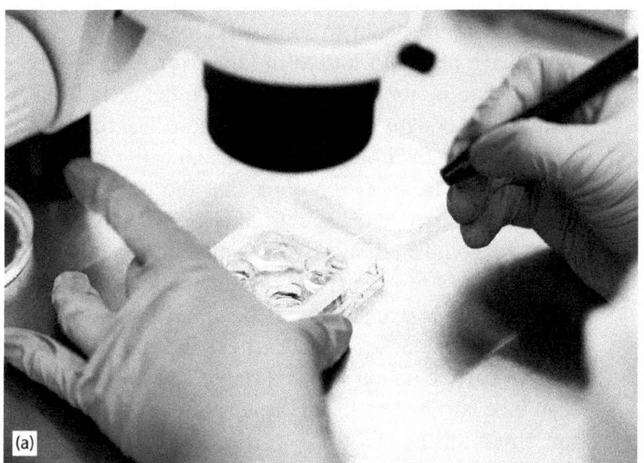

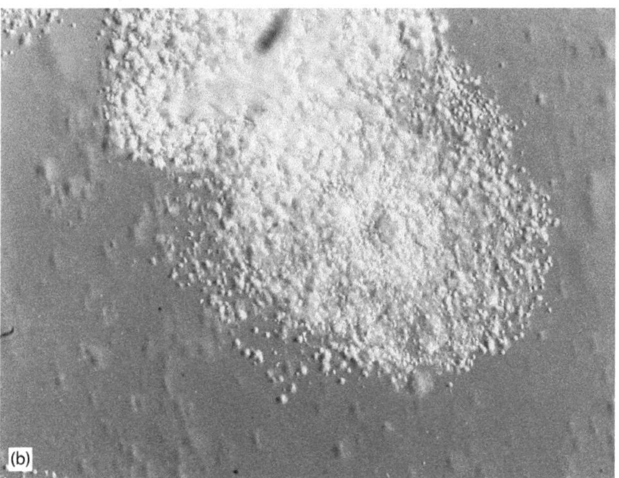

FIGURE 21.1 (a) The process of insemination in IVF (image courtesy of Shutterstock); (b) view of the oocyte-cumulus complexes.

For example:

If the sperm count of the prepared sample is: 10 x 10^6/ml

And the volume that the oocyte is in is: 1.0 ml

Then:

The number of sperm per microlitre is 10 million ÷ 1000 = 10,000

So: 150,000 ÷ 10,000 = 15 microlitres insemination volume.

Usually, fertilization triggers the cortical reaction in the oocytes which prevent polyspermic fertilisation (fertilisation by more than one sperm) (**5**), resulting in abnormal embryos that cannot be transferred. The likelihood of polyspermic fertilization is increased if too many motile sperm are used (**6**).

An additional consideration for IVF is the fact that the washed and prepared spermatozoa are going to be added to culture drops containing the oocyte-cumulus complexes, which are very susceptible to pH and temperature fluctuations. Throughout the process of IVF, oocytes must be maintained in stable culture conditions (**7, 8**). Therefore, before an IVF insemination can take place, the prepared suspension of motile sperm must be equilibrated to the same conditions as the culture drops containing the oocytes. This is usually achieved by incubating the suspension at 37°C for between 30–60 minutes (**9**) in an incubator in an atmosphere of between 5 and 6% CO_2 and 5% oxygen. The media used for the final sperm suspension generally contains a sodium bicarbonate buffer, which under these CO_2 conditions, will maintain the spermatozoa suspension at the required Ph of 7.2–7.3 required by the oocytes. The actual procedure of insemination, where the desired volume of spermatozoa suspension is added to the media droplets containing the oocyte-cumulus complexes via a Gilson pipette, must be carried out quickly, on a heated stage, to minimise temperature, pH and osmotic shock to the oocytes.

Once inseminated, the dishes will be returned to the safe environment of the incubator and left undisturbed until the fertilisation check. In standard culture conditions, without the use of time-lapse, the fertilisation check must be carried between 16–18 hours post insemination, otherwise the time when the pronuclei are visible, may be missed (**10, 7**).

21.3.1 Short Incubation Time

Some authors have suggested that a short insemination time of only two or three hours might be beneficial with IVF, as it reduces the time that the oocytes are exposed to spermatozoa cells and any potentially associated oxygen free radicals that might cause oxidative stress and potential damage. Insemination times of between 30 minutes to 6 hours have been reported and associated with increased clinical pregnancy and live birth rates (**11**). In this method the oocytes are inseminated as normal, but after two or three hours the cumulus oocyte complexes are taken out of the sperm drops and moved to new drops. The evidence suggests that this is sufficient time for enough sperm to have penetrated the cumulus cells and be available for fertilisation. The oocyte incubation is continued, and the fertilisation check is performed as normal, between 16–18 hours post insemination. A recent review found that a short co-incubation time was advantageous to the implantation rate, ongoing pregnancy rate and top-quality embryo rate, however, the live-birth rate displayed no difference between the two in vitro fertilisation methods (**12**).

21.4 Intra Cytoplasmic Sperm Injection

21.4.1 History

Intracytoplasmic sperm injection (ICSI) is a form of micro assisted fertilisation, but it was not the first technique to be attempted to achieve fertilisation in the human, where conventional IVF techniques had failed. Techniques such as zona drilling, partial zona dissection and sub zonal insemination (**13, 14**) were earlier techniques employed to overcome the barrier of fertilisation observed in 5–10% of conventional IVF cases. Eventually live births in the human were reported using the technique of ICSI (**15**) and this quickly became recognized as the most successful approach. There are several key reviews that describe how the development of this groundbreaking technique revolutionized the treatment of male factor infertility in the 90s (**16, 17**).

21.4.2 When to Use ICSI

ICSI is recommended in the following clinical situations in order to improve the chances of achieving successful fertilisation, compared to conventional IVF techniques:

1. In cases of reduced sperm quality: Oligozoospermia, Asthenozoospermia, Teratozoospermia (**18, 19**).
2. When using non-ejaculated sperm: Surgically recovered sperm (**20, 21**), Sperm collected following electroejaculation (**22**), Sperm collected following retrograde ejaculation (**23**).
3. With the following clinical indications: presence of antisperm antibodies (**24**), viral positive patients, patients with high levels of DNA fragmentation (**25**).
4. With the following egg factors: Vitrified oocytes, in vitro matured oocytes, the use of AOA (**26**).
5. Following previous failure of fertilisation with conventional IVF (**18, 19**).

21.4.3 The Equipment Required for ICSI

ICSI is carried out on an inverted microscope, which must be fitted with a heated stage and usually requires some form of anti-vibration control, due to the delicate nature of the process. The inverted microscope will be fitted with a set of micromanipulators on each side (Figure 21.2). The micromanipulators are comprised of a series of joy-sticks (coarse and fine control) that are used to control the tool holders. The joy sticks enable the embryologists hand movements on the joy-sticks to translate to very tiny movements at the end of the tool holders. Glass pipettes are placed in the tool holders and using this system the embryologist can make precise movements under the microscope, via the micromanipulators.

The left-hand tool-holder is fitted with a holding pipette which is a smooth open-ended pipetted that will be used to hold the oocyte in position during the injection process (Figure 21.3). The right-hand tool holder is fitted with a sharp, much thinner injection pipette, which will be used to immobilise and pick up the sperm, before injecting it into the oocyte.

Both of the pipettes can be controlled by gentle suction, as they are attached via tubing to air syringes). Using this set up the holding pipette can be manoeuvred into place under the microcope and gentle suction applied to hold the oocyte in place for the injection process. Similarly, the injection pipette can be manoeuvred in three planes and gentle aspiration and blowing applied via the air syringe at the same time, to collect an immobilised sperm and inject it directly into the oocyte.

21.4.4 Stages in the ICSI Process

1. Oocyte denudation and assessing maturity

   After collection, the oocytes are still surrounded by their cumulus cells, which need to be removed and the eggs assessed for maturity, as only mature oocytes can be injected with a sperm, in order to achieve normal fertilisation. The cumulus cells are removed by incubating in a solution of the enzyme hyaluronidase, followed by gentle aspiration to loosen the cells. This is carried out by adding a maximum of 100µl of hyaluronidase suspension to a holding dish containing the oocytes, for no more than 60 seconds, to allow the enzyme to begin to loosen the cells. Once the cells have begun to loosen in the enzyme a 200µm pipette can be used to gently remove the cells from around the oocyte via gentle aspiration. The remaining cells can then be removed mechanically using a 145µm pipette. It is important that the oocytes are not over exposed to the hyaluronidase, so this process must be completed quickly. It is also important that the oocytes are not exposed to fluctuations in temperature or pH whilst they are being denuded, so the hyaluronidase must be pre-warmed and the manipulations carried out on a heated stage. The pH stability can be controlled by using dishes pre-equilibrated in an environment of $C0_2$, with a sodium bicarbonate buffer, or by using a medium with a Hepes or MOPS buffer, that will maintain the pH outside of the CO_2 environment. The ICSI procedure must be performed within two hours if cumulus removal.

   Dish set up

   Particular dishes are used for the ICSI procedure, which have shallow sides, to allow room for the injection pipettes to come in at an angle and be arranged parallel with the bottom of the dish. The injection dishes are made no more than 2 hours prior to use, but must also be given enough time to warm to 37°C before use. The time taken to achieve this will vary depending on the selected dish, the volume of the drops and the oil overlay. Independent validation of this warming time must be completed by each laboratory, to ensure the oocytes are not subjected to an unfavorable environment during the process. The drops that will contain the oocytes must be made from a media containing a pH buffer

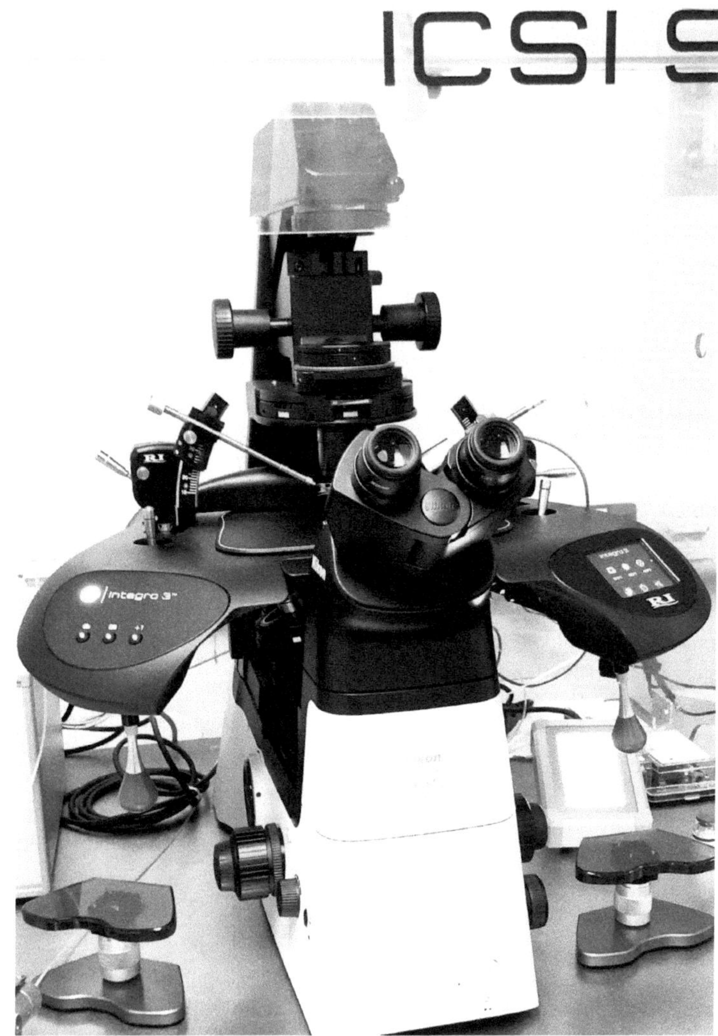

FIGURE 21.2 An inverted microscope fitted with a set of manipulators. The movement of the manipulators in three directions is achieved using the coarse x,y lever and the fine x,y,z lever as shown. There is a pipette tool holder in each arm of the manipulators. An air syringe on each side is connected via tubing to each pipette tool holder, to achieve gentle aspiration and blowing through the pipette in the pipette tool holder.

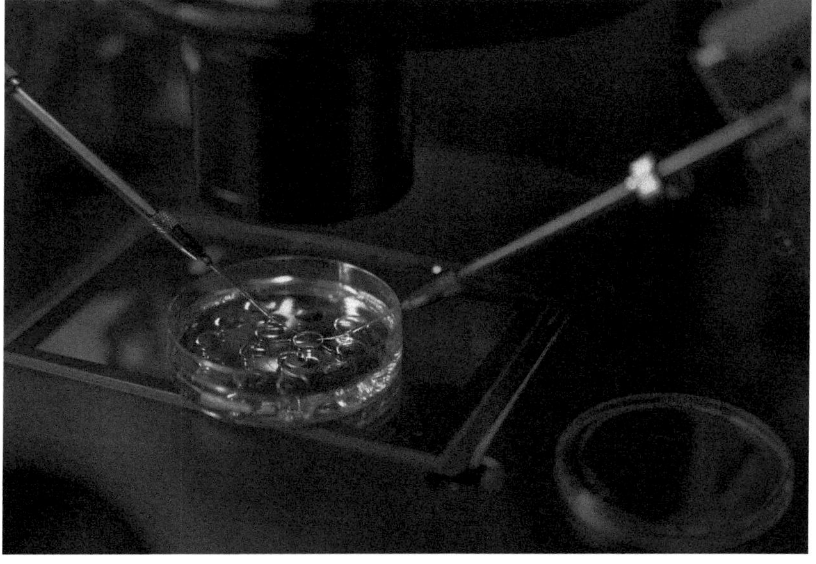

FIGURE 21.3 Closeup of micromanipulator during the fertilization process.

that is suitable for use outside of a CO_2 incubator, such as MOPS or Hepes. The sperm will be placed in drops of a sperm slowing medium, such as PVP or hyaluronan. It is important to remember that when placing the drops in the dish, each drop must be accessible with both pipettes. Due to the angle that the pipettes enter the dish, the perimeter of the dish may not be a suitable place for the drops. Again, this must be validated individually by the laboratory, depending on the consumables and equipment used. The drops must be covered with an oil overlay, to provide further protection from heat loss, pH changes and debris.

The volume of sperm suspension added to the PVP/hyaluronan can vary up to 20 percent of the final drop volume. If a lot of debris is present in the preparation, add sperm directly into the centre of the sperm drop and wait for any motile sperm to swim to the edge.

2. Tools

   An injection pipette and a holding pipette are positioned in the tool holders as described above. They are placed so that they can be raised above the level of the dish and so that they are parallel with the bottom of the dish. Once in place, they are equilibrated in a drop of medium, by aspirating some medium inside and then breaking the pressure by pressing the screw actuated syringe (SAS) release valves, allowing the pipettes to reach a state of equilibrium without any movement by capillary action. This is important to maintain complete control of sperm movement in the pipetted, during the injection process.

3. Sperm selection and immobilisation

   With the sperm in the PVP drop, select a sperm that is morphologically normal (according to WHO criteria). Use the injection pipette to cut across the tail with the injection pipette. The sperm must be completely immotile at this stage with a damaged tail. Take care not to damage the sperm head or the midpiece during this procedure. Aspirate the immobilised sperm into the injection needle, tail first, ensuring that it moves freely up and down in the needle, without sticking. If it does not move freely select another sperm.

4. Oocyte Injection

   a. Using gentle suction from the holding pipette, rotate the oocyte in order to hold it with its polar body at approximately 12 or 6 o'clock.
   b. Bring the injection pipette into focus.
   c. Ensure the oolemma and injection pipette are in focus so that the injection needle enters the centre of the oocyte when injection takes place.
   d. Approach the zona from the 3 to 9 o'clock position (depending on which side the injection needle is); this ensures that you will enter the oocyte in the centre.
   e. Position the sperm at the needle tip and push the needle into the cytoplasm in one straight, controlled push.
   f. To ensure that the oolemma is broken before injecting the sperm, aspirate to draw the membrane back into the needle and await the cytoplasmic rush. If necessary, a short stab will break the membrane.
   g. Gently release the aspirated cytoplasm and the sperm into the ooplasm.
   h. Slowly withdraw the needle. Take care not to vibrate or cause the needle to be moved in any other axis than the horizontal plane as this can irreparably damage the oolemma causing lysis.
   i. To avoid incidental re injection of an oocyte, a position should be defined by the practitioner that indicates that the oocyte has been injected i.e. moving the oocyte to the top of the drop.
   j. Once all the oocytes in the dish have been injected, witness the injection dish and the new culture dish using manual witnessing or electronic witnessing.
   k. Moving in small groups and no more than half of the total, wash the oocytes through the top row of drops of the culture dish (standard incubation) or the designated wash drops in time-lapse dishes (time-lapse culture).
   l. Place each washed oocyte into single culture wells, taking care to note the correct well number for each item.
   m. Complete the insemination details, the embryology notes and sign for the procedure on the embryology checklist, as appropriate.

Major causes of damage

- Touching the opposing membrane with the injection needle; do not push the injection needle much further than half way.
- Injection of mineral oil; care must be taken when aspirating sperm from the edge of the microdrop.
- Excessive vibration or movement.

Causes of fertilisation failure

- Sperm tail not sufficiently broken.
- Oocyte membrane not penetrated.
- Sperm deposited in vacuoles.
- Excess medium transferred with sperm.

21.5 Conclusion

There are a number of developments in ICSI including novel selection methods by intracytoplasmic morphologically selected sperm injection (IMSI) and physiological ICSI (PICSI) which will be discussed further in Chapter 33. In order to maintain good results and to also improve them, optimisation of laboratory conditions, staff training and competency, controlling the equipment and monitoring of key performance indicators (KPIs) are among the most important factors.

REFERENCES

1. Kandavel V, Cheong Y. Does intra-uterine insemination have a place in modern ART practice? *Best Pract Res Clin Obstet Gynaecol.* 2018 [cited 2023 Apr 24];53:3–10.
2. Wessel JA, Danhof NA, van Eekelen R, et al. Ovarian stimulation strategies for intrauterine insemination in couples with unexplained infertility: a systematic review and individual participant data meta-analysis. *Hum Reprod Update.* 2022 [cited 2023 Apr 25];28(5):733–746.
3. Kuru Pekcan M, Tokmak A, Ulubasoglu H, et al. The importance of infertility duration and follicle size according to pregnancy success in women undergoing ovulation induction with gonadotropins and intrauterine insemination. *J Obstet Gynaecol.* 2023 [cited 2023 Apr 25];43(1):2173058.
4. Nesbit CB, Blanchette-Porter M, Esfandiari N. Ovulation induction and intrauterine insemination in women of advanced reproductive age: a systematic review of the literature. *J Assist Reprod Genet.* 2022 [cited 2023 Apr 25];39(7):1445–1491.
5. Rojas J, Hinostroza F, Vergara S, et al. Knockin' on egg's door: maternal control of egg activation that influences cortical granule exocytosis in animal species. *Front Cell Dev Biol.* 2021 [cited 2023 Apr 24];9:704867.
6. Siu KK, Serrão VHB, Ziyyat A, et al. The cell biology of fertilization: gamete attachment and fusion. *J Cell Biol.* 2021 [cited 2023 Apr 24];220(10).
7. Anagnostopoulou C, Maldonado Rosas I, Singh N, et al. Oocyte quality and embryo selection strategies: a review for the embryologists, by the embryologists. *Panminerva Med [Internet].* 2022 [cited 2023 Apr 24];64(2):171–184.
8. Gatimel N, Moreau J, Parinaud J, et al. Need for choosing the ideal pH value for IVF culture media. *J Assist Reprod Genet.* 2020 [cited 2023 Apr 24];37(5):1019–1028.
9. Agarwal A, Maldonado Rosas I, Anagnostopoulou C, et al. Oxidative stress and assisted reproduction: a comprehensive review of its pathophysiological role and strategies for optimizing embryo culture environment. *Antioxidants (Basel).* 2022 [cited 2023 Apr 24];11(3):477.
10. Coticchio G, Borini A, Zacà C, et al. Fertilization signatures as biomarkers of embryo quality. *Hum Reprod.* 2022 [cited 2023 Apr 25];37(8):1704–1711.
11. Huang Z, Li J, Wang L, et al. Brief co-incubation of sperm and oocytes for in vitro fertilization techniques. *Cochrane Database Syst Rev.* 2013 [cited 2023 Apr 25];(4):CD009391.
12. Fan Y, Wu Z, Peng F, et al. Brief and long co-incubation of sperm and oocytes for in vitro fertilization: a meta-analysis of randomized controlled trials. *BMC Pregnancy Childbirth.* 2023 [cited 2023 Apr 25];23(1):200.
13. Sathananthan AH, Ng SC, Trounson A, et al. Human micro-insemination by injection of single or multiple sperm: ultrastructure. *Hum Reprod.* 1989 [cited 2023 Apr 25]; 4(5):574–583.
14. Fishel S, Dowell K, Lisi F, et al. Subzonal insemination and zona breaching techniques for assisting conception in vitro. *Baillieres Clin Obstet Gynaecol.* 1994 [cited 2023 Apr 25]; 8(1):65–84.
15. Palermo G, Joris H, Devroey P, et al. Pregnancies after intracytoplasmic injection of single spermatozoon into an oocyte. *Lancet.* 1992 [cited 2023 Apr 25];340(8810):17–18.
16. Palermo GD, Neri QV, Takeuchi T, et al. ICSI: where we have been and where we are going. *Semin Reprod Med.* 2009 [cited 2023 Apr 25];27(2):191–201.
17. Rosenwaks Z, Pereira N. The pioneering of intracytoplasmic sperm injection: historical perspectives. *J Reprod Fertil.* 2017 [cited 2023 Apr 24];154(6):F71–F77.
18. Palermo GD, O'Neill CL, Chow S, et al. Intracytoplasmic sperm injection: state of the art in humans. *J Reprod Fertil.* 2017 [cited 2023 Apr 25];154(6):F93–F110.
19. Devroey P, Van Steirteghem A. A review of ten years' experience of ICSI. *Hum Reprod Update.* 2004 [cited 2023 Apr 25];10(1):19–28.
20. Arshad MA, Majzoub A, Esteves SC. Predictors of surgical sperm retrieval in non-obstructive azoospermia: summary of current literature. *Int Urol Nephrol.* 2020 [cited 2023 Apr 25];52(11):2015–2038.
21. Gao S, Yang X, Xiao X, et al. Outcomes and affecting factors for ICSI and microTESE treatments in nonobstructive azoospermia patients with different etiologies: a retrospective analysis. *Front Endocrinol (Lausanne).* 2022 [cited 2023 Apr 25];13:1006208. Avail.
22. Schatte EC, Orejuela FJ, Lipshultz LI, et al. Treatment of infertility due to anejaculation in the male with electroejaculation and intracytoplasmic sperm injection. *J Urol.* 2000 [cited 2023 Apr 25];163(6):1717–1720.
23. Fedder J, Carlsen E, Jørgensen N, et al. Treatment of male infertility. *Ugeskr Laeg.* 2021 [cited 2023 Apr 25];183(48).
24. Lu S-M, Li X, Wang S-L, et al. Success rates of in vitro fertilization versus intracytoplasmic sperm injection in men with serum anti-sperm antibodies: a consecutive cohort study. *Asian J Androl.* 2019 [cited 2023 Apr 25];21(5): 473–477.
25. Khalafalla K, Majzoub A, Elbardisi H, et al. The effect of sperm DNA fragmentation on intracytoplasmic sperm injection outcome. *Andrologia.* 2021 [cited 2023 Apr 25]; 53(10):e14180.
26. Borges E, Jr, de Almeida Ferreira Braga DP, de Sousa Bonetti TC, et al. Artificial oocyte activation with calcium ionophore A23187 in intracytoplasmic sperm injection cycles using surgically retrieved spermatozoa. *Fertil Steril.* 2009 [cited 2023 Apr 25];92(1):131–136.

22

Embryo Culture Methods and Metabolic Requirements

Rachel Smith

It is clear that high quality embryo culture is imperative to successful embryo development, successful implantation and potentially the ongoing health and wellbeing of children born as a result of in vitro culture (**1–3**). Understanding the changing needs of the embryo and the impact the culture environment can have on development will help to ensure you avoid possible hazards and maximise the embryos potential (**4**).

Within this chapter we will consider the evolution of embryo culture to where it stands today, focusing on the metabolic requirements of the oocyte and embryo over its time in culture. The impact of the type of culture medium, its composition, the introduction of commercialisation and quality assessment including European regulation to aid standardisation. Single step or sequential culture medium systems, for use with single embryo or group culture, the pros and cons when considering these different approaches. The importance of environmental conditions for successful embryo culture; the effects of temperature, pH, osmolality and volatile organic compounds, the decisions on consumables and incubator types including timelapse image capture and the potential of undisturbed culture for standard incubation. With multiple options for the practical application of embryo culture within laboratories; effective monitoring, troubleshooting and problem solving against known key performance indicators will ensure a stress-free culture environment. Looking ahead to microfluidics, automation and AI: what will embryo culture look like in the future?

The goal of in-vitro embryo culture is to provide conditions that will lead to the production of embryos that have the same developmental potential as the embryos that develop in vivo (**4**). To be able to support embryo development the culture media needs to support the changing needs of the embryo as it develops.

22.1 Metabolic Requirements

The fundamentals of basic embryo metabolism are well established, with the use of animal models it has been possible to monitor embryos developing in vivo, these models provide the basis for in vitro embryo culture to ensure the dynamic requirements of the oocyte and embryo are met by the embryo culture environment, to maximise viability and avoid stress. The culture media is one aspect of the culture system that supports the changing requirements of the embryo.

22.1.1 Energy Source

Pyruvate, glucose and lactate are most commonly added to culture media. There are two main pathways for Adenosine triphosphate (ATP) generation necessary for embryo metabolism (Figure 22.1), aerobic glycolysis or Krebs cycle (TCA) and anaerobic glycolysis, by the Embden-Meyerhof pathway (**5**). The requirements of the embryo are stage specific, prior to embryo genomic activation the levels of biosynthesis and metabolism are less, therefore the energy requirement is low. This 'quieter' metabolism gives rise to higher levels of ATP which in turn regulates or blocks the glycolysis pathway. Carboxylic acid-based metabolism predominates during the cleavage stage where pyruvate and lactate are the embryo's main source of energy.

22.1.2 Pyruvate

From fertilisation and through early cleavage, pyruvate is the metabolite transported to the mitochondria, converted to Acetyl-Co A entering the Krebs cycle (TCA) to create ATP to support development by oxidative phosphorylation. Nutrients such as amino acids, lactate, and endogenous fatty acids derived from triglyceride, have overlapping metabolic roles, providing embryos with potential energy sources when combined with pyruvate in early embryo development and beyond compaction to blastocyst formation.

22.1.3 Lactate

During early embryo development pyruvate and lactate are regularly interchanged, lactate dehydrogenase (LDH) interconverts both pyruvate and lactate based on relative concentrations (**6**). Following embryo compaction lactate is produced by anaerobic glycolysis, the culture environment requires a lower lactate concentration at this stage of development to promote blastocyst derived lactate to facilitate implantation (**6**).

22.1.4 Glucose

Before embryo compaction the uptake of glucose is low, although it is required during early development for signalling purposes and a potential energy substrate. Following 3 days of embryo development following embryonic activation, a shift in the energy production mechanisms occurs from mitochondrial to cytoplasmic glucose metabolism, anaerobic glycolysis is the

DOI: 10.1201/9781003269502-22

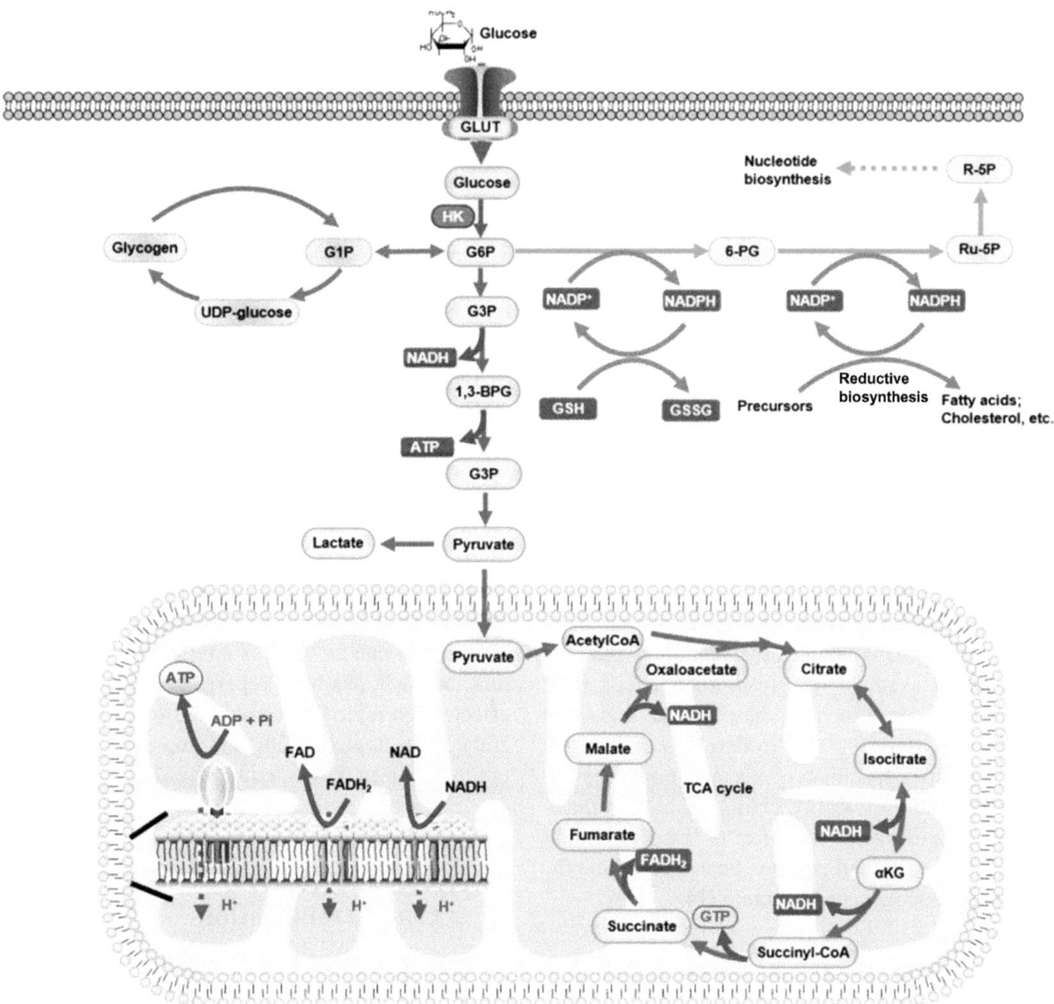

FIGURE 22.1 The two main pathways for ATP generation (from Han R, Liang J, Zhou B. Glucose metabolic dysfunction in neurodegenerative diseases – new mechanistic insights and the potential of hypoxia as a prospective therapy targeting metabolic reprogramming. *Int J Mol Sci.* 2021;22:5887, under Creative Commons licence).

preferred pathway generating pyruvate which is taken up by the mitochondria, producing lactate. Rather than being considered a waste product, lactate is considered a signalling molecule, involved in three major aspects of implantation- invasion, angiogenesis and immune modulation (**7**). The blastocyst produces significant quantities of lactate and consequently low pH which are used to facilitate implantation. Recent evidence has suggested that the ICM and the trophectoderm manufacture energy in different ways; the ICM using glycolysis and the trophectoderm using the TCA cycle in mitochondria (**8**).

There has been much debate over the toxic effect of glucose, as a high amount of glucose for embryos in their early stages has been attributed to reduced production of ATP and embryo arrest. Glucose is present in tubal fluid (**9**), and has since been determined as essential (**10**) and not harmful to the early embryo development with uptake pre compaction controlled by the inclusion of amino acids and EDTA, this combination is thought to regulate the reactive oxygen species and overcome the 2-cell block. Many studies have been performed comparing varying concentrations of glucose within media for embryo culture, confirming 1.0–2.0mmol/l which is reflective of concentrations in the human oviduct, can support blastocyst development when used from fertilisation and does not affect embryo quality (**11**).

22.1.5 Amino Acids

After pyruvate and lactate, amino acids are recognised as the preferred energy source over glucose (**12**). Now added routinely to culture media, AAs are essential for translation of stored polyadenylated mRNAs for new protein synthesis during the period following fertilisation but also have essential roles as pH buffers, antioxidants and metabolism regulators. There have been some concerns over the toxic effect of ammonia on the embryo, a single human embryo, along with the incubation of the culture medium at 37°C, can produce 100uM of ammonium over 4 days of culture with further accumulation through the deamination reaction of L glutamine considered an essential component of culture media. The accumulation of ammonia is thought to be less critical when controlling for pH and temperature within incubator environments of lowered O2 concentration. Many commercial culture media have included a more stable dipeptide glutamine as standard.

Ethylenediaminetetraacetic acid (EDTA) is generally included in culture media, post fertilisation, it has the role of a chelating agent against toxic metal ions and offers protection against oxidative stress as free radical scavenger. It has a further role in glucose metabolism in early embryo development. Some evidence suggests that EDTA at a high concentration causes a reduced cell count in the ICM of the mouse suggesting a sequential approach is required but lower concentrations in a continuous media of 0.01mmol/l does not affect implantation and removes the possible deleterious effect.

Protein importance is recognized in culture media, with early culture media using human serum predominantly, the variable nature of human serum and potential health risks mean it is no longer used. Human serum albumin (HSA) or synthetic serum (SS) in combinations of 5–20% is the main source but the recombinant form recHSA is also available. HSA is the only protein listed as present in commercially available media but studies have revealed that many more proteins are present in commercially available medias such as alpha and beta globulins, dextran for example with recommendations from users for these protein supplements to have greater definition (**13**). Proteins are necessary for embryo development and the uptake and degradation of specific proteins may provide essential information on embryo viability, clarity on protein inclusion has important ramifications for safety of the offspring as a correlation has been identified between birth weight and the source or the time of supplementing protein (**14**).

22.1.6 Other Micronutrients and Antioxidants

Vitamins are sometimes added to IVF culture media, folic acid and vit B12 are necessary for methylation processes whilst other vitamins C and E act as redox regulators. Due to the nature of multiple manipulation of gametes and embryos under atmospheric oxygen, and the extended embryo culture systems, and a result of endogenous triggers to the gametes and embryos, the accumulation of reactive oxygen species (ROS) is common problem in the IVF laboratory (**15**). The addition of single or combinations of antioxidants such as acetyl-L-carnitine, N-acetyl-cysteine and α-lipoic acid have been reported to improve embryo development and clinical outcomes (**16, 17**).

22.1.7 Antibiotics

The inclusion of antibiotics is standard practice in culture media to reduce the possible introduction of microbial infection, the concentration of the antibiotic can vary between media types. Penicillin streptomycin combination or gentamicin are the most commonly used antibiotics in culture media, with concentrations based on toxicity studies (**18**).

22.1.8 Buffers

Sodium Bicarbonate for use under CO_2 controlled environment to maintain pH within the media is necessary for important cell functions and is more important for embryos, pre compaction that rely on environmental pH to a greater degree than post compaction embryos to maintain intracellular pH (pHi). When handling oocytes or embryos outside of the controlled incubator environment, two buffers are regularly used in these 'handling' medias, HEPES and MOPS, both have a pKa value of 7.2 closest to pHi of embryos of 7.12.

22.1.9 Macromolecules

Granulocyte-macrophage colony – stimulating factor (GM-CSF) is an essential cytokine which plays an important role in preimplantation embryo development as it is present in the oviduct and uterine epithelium. A Cochrane review considering studies up to 2019 showed that the evidence of improvement in live birth outcome was of low quality (**19**). Recombinant GM-CSF is limited to one media type currently and this limits its wide spread use so a clinical assessment is premature.

Hyaluronan is a macromolecule that is present in high concentrations in the reproductive tract, and it has also been demonstrated to have a positive role in embryo culture media. Although it can be used as a replacement for albumin in culture media, it has been reported to have the most significant effect when added in combination with albumin to improve embryo development (**20**), and improved survival and implantation of frozen thawed embryos (**21**).

22.2 Embryo Culture/History and Commercialisation

Prior to the availability of commercially produced media, media was often made in house with very little quality control to ensure consistency. The first concept for human embryo culture, known as B2, was described by Menezo et al. (1984) by adding serum albumin as a source of amino acids, whilst the first media to mimic the in vivo environment was Human Tubal Fluid (HTF) with balanced salt solutions. Both B2 and HTF became the basis and gold standard for commercial human embryo culture (**1**). In the last 40 years, the commercial media market has expanded with many available 'ready to use' options.

All culture media contain the basic requirements of salts, energy substrates, serum supplements, AAs, buffer solutions, antibiotics, vitamins, nucleotides, GFs, and other reagents such as trace elements, nuclease inhibitors, etc but it is unclear what the function of all these reagents are (**1**). Manufacturers supply detailed information for the correct use and storage on their websites and on their information for use (IFU). Within the EU and UK, the culture media is defined as a high-risk class III medical device, therefore manufacturers are required to communicate and justify changes to media composition to users and provide evidence of long-term studies and efficacy.

Sunde et al. (**22**) completed a literature review regarding the composition of media and concluded that greater transparency is needed from the manufacturer, currently there is full disclosure for constituents but not the concentrations of these within the media. A review of six commercial culture media focusing on HSA added to IVF media revealed that HSA contained many other proteins and that the amount varied from batch-to-batch (**13**). More transparency from the manufacturers is required before we can understand the secretome of the embryo to examine potential markers of good and poor development from the spent culture media.

22.3 Types of Media

22.3.1 Single Step

The single step media or continuous culture media use increased with the advent of timelapse incubation where embryos are cultured in an undisturbed environment. The media supplies all components within the acceptable ranges and the embryo utilises what is required. The embryos are cultured from either day 0 or day 1 without a media change until the day of transfer. The concern with extended culture over time is the build-up of ammonia which is toxic to embryos (Figure 22.2).

22.3.2 Sequential Media

Designed to cater for the changing metabolic needs of the embryo as it develops with a reduction in the harmful effects of ammonia which accumulates over time (Figure 22.2). The two-step media requires a media and dish change, generally on day 3, this has the potential to introduce an additional risk of damage and stress as the embryos are required to be handled and moved to a new dish. The first media reflects the oviduct environment with the second media responds to the increase in metabolic activity of the embryos as it develops to a blastocyst.

There have been a number of meta-analysis on outcomes following sequential or continuous culture, Sfontouris et al. (**23**) did not observe any difference between single continuous and sequential media in the ongoing pregnancy rate or in miscarriage rate, although some results indicated better blastocyst rates in continuous media. While Dieamant et al. (**24**) considered the pregnancy rate and found a similar result with not significantly different ongoing pregnancy and miscarriage rate when comparing continuous and sequential media.

22.3.3 Suites of Media Tailored to a Specific Process

Consider the process design and the media requirements – will the process require handling of the media outside the incubator, will the process need the media to be stable for pH in atmospheric air and ambient temperature and when cultured inside an incubator at 5–6% CO2 environment and 37°C. There are media available tailored to sperm preparation, oocyte holding following egg collection, fertilisation and embryo culture.

Understanding the composition of this media, the complexity of use, the cost of implication and the known outcomes will help to drive the decisions on the media for use in the laboratory.

The composition of embryo culture media has raised a common question of whether humans derived from assisted reproduction are heathy? Some studies have revealed susceptibility during the pre-implantation to epigenetic changes that may not be apparent at birth but may develop later in childhood or early adulthood. Early development is considered the area of greatest concern as embryos are more sensitive to environmental stress during these early stages. Follow up studies of individuals born as a result of IVF are of great importance to answer these questions over the potential adverse effects specific to embryo culture media.

Deciding which culture media may therefore be the single most important decision and should only be considered following a thorough review of the current evidence in publications alongside the manufacturers evidence of validation studies. Although all commercial media is quality assured continuous monitoring of known markers of successful outcome including fertilisation, utilisation and clinical pregnancy outcome is advised to ensure ongoing performance. However, it is important to remember that embryo culture medium is only one of many factors in the IVF laboratory that might affect the outcome of any given cycle (**25**).

22.4 Incubation

The incubator has a vital role in the success of embryo culture and is a critical piece of equipment. Consideration needs to

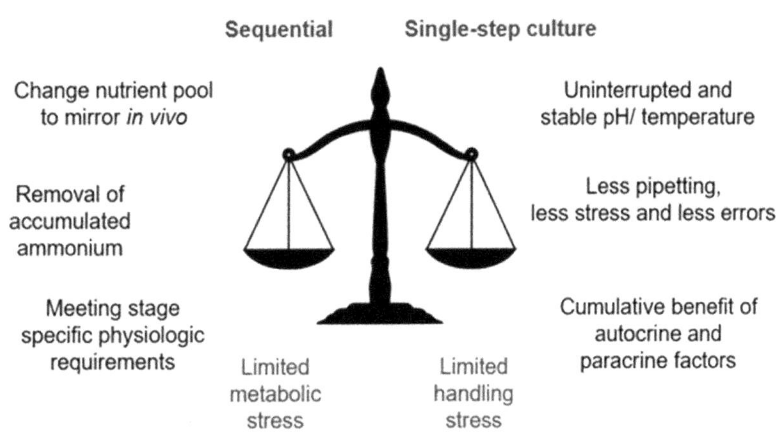

FIGURE 22.2 Balance of stresses between sequential and single-step culture media.

be made for the overall capacity or volume of the incubator in comparison to the potential workload, the environmental conditions how they are monitored and the rate of recovery following access and overall reliability. This is the work horse of the laboratory, responsible for controlling multiple environmental variables of temperature, gas regulation and humidity to ensure the conditions for embryo culture are ideal. See chapter on equipment within the laboratory for further details.

22.4.1 Temperature

Controlling the temperature is imperative as culture media is designed for use at 37°c, it is well known that changes in temperature can affect meiotic spindle stability (**26**) and have been indicated to affect metabolism (**3**). Understanding changes in temperature under conditions of use can be accomplished by using adapted and validated temperature mapping equipment. Focus on the temperature of the media surrounding the oocyte or embryo not only the set temperature of the equipment (**27**). Both within the incubator or on heated stages, determine temperature hotspots or temperature gradients, recovery times and the correct working ranges, with consideration for working at maximal laboratory capacity. Data logging and recording these temperature measurements, with regular review will to ensure stability of temperature over diverse heated equipment.

22.4.2 CO_2/O_2 Gas Regulation and pH

CO_2 is imperative for maintaining the physiological pH within the media, generally a CO_2 concentration of 5%-6% will maintain the environmental pH (pHe) at between 7.2 and 7.4 (**28**). The relationship between the CO_2 and factors such as altitude, ambient temperature and media constituents will affect the environmental pHe. Regular testing of the pH of the culture media is recommended, with a calibrated blood gas analyser often performed by a professional to ensure accurate resulting on all incubation environments and on all culture media types in use to ensure all are within the correct pHe range.

22.4.3 Oxygen Concentration

The concentration of O_2 in the incubator is important for the regulation of metabolism, O_2 is present in ambient air at ~ 21%, incubator culture can be maintained at ambient O_2 levels or reduced to a lower level of 5% to mimic the physiological conditions within the female reproductive tract. Many studies have investigated the effects of atmospheric O_2 on the developing embryo, during cleavage stages in the mouse embryo 20% O_2 increases AA uptake and pyruvate uptake, in contrast after compaction the glucose uptake is reduced along with AA turnover (**29**). Glucose uptake following compaction is known to increase dramatically as a marker of embryo viability, possibly explaining why no studies have shown a positive effect of culture at this O_2 concentration, leading to the Cairo consensus (**4**) suggesting culture of human embryos at atmospheric levels of O_2 is unethical as it constitutes exposure to a known embryo toxin.

22.4.4 Air Quality

In vivo there is protection offered to the developing embryo to reduced exposure to volatile organic compounds through management within the kidneys, liver and lungs (**4**). The exposure of the embryos in vitro should therefore be kept to a minimum as poor air quality has been observed to have detrimental effects on pregnancy outcomes (**30**), for full details see Chapter 2.

22.4.5 Humidity

Humidification within incubators is often attained by passive evaporation by the presence of a water reservoir or flask. The water should be changed regularly as this can be a source of contamination within a warm, moist environment. Humidity is not required for embryo culture but in a non-humidified incubator and with the majority of laboratories moving to extended embryo culture with single step media, there is an increased chance of evaporation of water from the culture media increasing the osmolality. Osmolality is the measure of solute within a solution and should normally reside between 255–295 mOsm/kg, osmolality, outside of this range may impair embryo development.

Increasing the oil overlay has been suggested to prevent the loss from the culture media in a non-humidified incubation system. Fawzy et al. (**31**) completed a randomised controlled trial comparing a humidified to a dry incubator revealing a significantly lower clinical pregnancy and implantation rate in the non- humidified environment with the same oil overlay. However, interpretation of such RCT should be analysed in the context of incubator and study design as those vary between clinics.

The presence of an oil overlay may therefore not be adequate to prevent the loss of water from the media over prolonged culture or in extremely low relative atmospheric humidity of 15–30% conditions where normal relative humidity is in the range of 30–50%. Understanding changing osmolality overtime within a culture system may be alleviated by switching to higher viscosity (heavy) oils (**32**), or the inclusion of a dish refresh on day 3 or day 5, but the potential benefit may be offset by the manual handling of the dish (**33**). A comparison of evaporation of commercially available time-lapse dishes of unique designs, each prepared according to the manufacturer's instructions, has concluded that certain designs have a significant effect on stability of osmolality (**34**). Whether an incubator is humidified or non-humidified is often dictated by the incubator manufacturer so understanding the effects on the embryo environment in relation to changes to osmolality and pH, within the laboratory may dictate the choice of incubation and embryo culture systems.

The rapid recovery of environmental conditions within the incubator should be a consideration when choosing incubation equipment but despite advancements and design changes there is a move towards an alternative approach to culture to remove the potential environmental changes. Following assessment of fertilisation, the embryos remain undisturbed until the day of transfer, this is already the system of culture within timelapse incubation (TL) but not the general approach for standard incubation (SI). SI, traditionally involves the removal of the embryo from the incubator to observe the daily development events and assess the morphological grade. This creates a series of snapshot static observations documented on the days prior to the embryo transfer, used, in some cases, to inform the day of transfer and to a greater of lesser extent for selection of an embryo from within a cohort, for transfer. Alhelou et al. (**35**) reported a significant improvement during uninterrupted culture in time-lapse non-humidified incubation compared to humidified standard incubation, removing the daily assessment of embryos of standard incubation, has the potential to reduce environmental change during embryo culture with the additional benefits of removal of the risks associated with handling dishes, alongside accumulation of positive paracrine and autocrine factors, as well as reducing the workflow within the laboratory. These potential benefits should be weighed against the prolonged exposure of the media to factors such as evaporation and associated osmolality and pH increases, as well as oil peroxidation or VOC accumulation, which could offset any advantage of reduced dish and embryo handling (**28**).

22.5 Media Storage

Quality assured dish preparation is essential for a robust embryo culture system, this process starts with the chain of delivery and correct storage of the media prior to use. The media manufacturers have strict guidelines for the safe delivery and storage of media with the main considerations for temperature and light exposure. It is good practice to monitor the mean kinetic temperature of the delivery container whilst in transit, if this is not possible to measure the temperature at delivery as both extremes of heat and cold can have detrimental effects. Any temperatures outside of the expected range should be raised with the manufacturer and the media not used until the impact on the media quality is known.

On delivery the media is stored according to the manufacturer's instructions, if using refrigeration equipment, it is strongly advised to monitor the temperature using an external thermometer at least daily. Specific instructions for medias in relation to exposure to ambient light or sunlight should be followed to prevent exposure, which can lead to peroxidation (**36**).

22.6 Dish Preparation

Media handling should be completed in a clean laminar flow-hood cabinet, using aseptic techniques. All media is checked to be within the expiry date for safe use and traceable for each batch to each patient.

The dish preparation should be completed in advance of use following advised equilibration times from the manufacturer, preparation is normally completed at ambient temperature, it is advised to consider the ambient humidity when preparing dishes especially for small volumes (<50ul) for potential risk of evaporation. All dish preparation should be completed as quickly as possible.

Appropriate training, competency assessment and continuous monitoring of the dish preparation process are needed to ensure adherence to the standard operating procedures.

Auditing is essential part of quality assurance consider questions for practitioners: -

- Does the scientist have records of training and competency for the task?
- Did the scientist preparing the dishes/tubes wash their hands before starting?
- Were the dishes/tubes prepared in a laminar flow cabinet which had been on for at least 10 minutes?
- Was the surface of the preparation area at ambient temperature, and not heated?
- Was the surface of the laminar flow cabinet wiped down before starting?
- Was the cabinet area that was used for dish preparation free from any clutter that might disrupt the air flow?
- Before using any media, was the expiry date checked?
- If a new batch was opened was this logged for traceability?
- Was aseptic technique used throughout? (no touching of the tops of bottles, placing lids upside-down, not touching the ends of pipettes etc)

22.6.1 Dishes and the Microenvironment

The choice of dish is often driven by the incubator – time-lapse incubation will have specific dishes to ensure accurate image capture. These will likely be single welled to allow traceability of the embryo. Dishes have to withstand temperature and humidity within the laboratory, whilst ensuring the ideal media environment is maintained, imperative to this is the design, and more importantly the material composition to ensure no toxic effects change the media.

22.7 Developing Areas of Embryo Culture

The static culture platforms are a current area of focus with a movement towards culture in reduced media volumes (<5ul) to increase embryo density and maximise the potential beneficial effects through the secretion of trophic autocrine/paracrine factors (**37**). Reducing the volume of the media and culture large numbers of embryos in close proximity needs close attention to pH and osmolality as these smaller volumes will be more susceptible to environmental changes. Studies to date have been inconclusive to the benefits of this type of culture combining group culture and concentration of trophic autocrine/paracrine factors with reduced embryo spacing. These culture platforms if developed successfully could be a key development to facilitating concentration of secreted markers of development for analysis.

Dynamic culture systems are an exciting area of new development including microfluidics, a culture device that engineers a flow of culture media over commonly adopted static culture which is not truly static due to convection and movements of the dish.

Microfluidic systems serve to handle gametes, mature oocytes, culture embryos, and perform other basic procedures in a microenvironment that closely imitates conditions in vivo (**38**). These systems are complex, potentially expensive, with no current understanding of the true benefits, for wide spread adoption they need to be cost effective and operate safely and efficiently, as the current culture dish system is proven to be relatively cheap and easy to use.

Already commercial microfluidic devices are available for sperm sorting aiming to reduce DNA damage associated with centrifugation–Zymot chip. Other devices to sort oocytes and to successfully add vitrification media prior too rapid cooling are in development. Many more devices are in development and have been used in animal models, it is an exciting emerging area of science meets engineering. They have the capacity to reduce risk through minimal need for intervention and introduction of contamination with the further advantage of potentially improving the outcomes for patients.

Controlled fluid flow or perfusion devices have the potential to offer a changing environment in line with the changing needs of the developing embryo, constantly removing waste products, without the need to disturb or manipulate the embryo outside of the incubator. This provides an advantage over sequential media, which currently has not been proven to benefit embryo development to date. Real time subtle changes to culture media can be introduced, gradually without the sharp contrast experienced when moving an embryo in a two-step system with potential of undue stress on the embryo. Creating a 'smart' culture environment is the final goal where the individual embryo dictates the changing needs of the culture environment.

These microfluidic platforms have the potential to combine other technologies of timelapse imaging for assessment of morphology and morphokinetics, real time analysis of known biomarkers related to embryo viability by non-invasive analysis including oxygen consumption, AA turnover and energy metabolism and detection of cell free DNA within the spent culture media for non-invasive PGT. These devices will revolutionise the laboratory workflow and time management with the potential for improved outcomes but with the challenges of making the devices affordable and safe for its widespread application.

For successful application, these culture platforms will need to utilise new technologies of engineering, artificial intelligence and modern materials, requiring scrutiny of the perceived advantages prior to commercialisation, exciting future but still many considerations before we see these devices commonly used in laboratories.

22.8 Conclusion

Embryo culture is a dynamic process reliant on numerous factors that require quality assessment and continuous monitoring to ensure that each part is functioning as expected to support the development of the embryo. The process starts with understanding the metabolic requirements of the embryo, with consideration for the laboratory work flow and equipment that will determine the type of media or suites of media for use. There are limitations to published analysis of different culture systems due to diverse culture; from equipment, consumables and operation, future studies require control of variables for adequate comparation. The safe delivery, storage and batch assessment of the media are integral parts of the quality management system to assures optimal outcomes. Temperature and pH maintenance at each step in the culture process is crucial with oxygen concentration advised to 5% concentration compared to atmospheric within the incubator environment. Key performance indicators should be devised to ensure that system performance is maintained and any change or introduction should be validated prior to adoption in line with good laboratory and assessment practice.

New technologies such as culture platforms and microfluidics are emerging and have the potential to radically change embryo culture with potential leaps in outcomes promised due to standardisation, customisation and continuous monitoring to reduce the environmental stresses on the embryo and improve known outcomes of blastocyst formation and clinical pregnancy. These will need to be proven to be safe, effective and cost saving for wide spread adoption and will call on expertise from many different disciplines.

REFERENCES

1. Chronopoulou E, Harper JC. IVF culture media: past, present and future. *Hum Reprod Update.* 2015;21(1):39–55.
2. Leese HJ. Metabolism of the preimplantation embryo: 40 years on. *Reproduction.* 2012;143(4):417.
3. Brison DR, Roberts SA, Kimber SJ. How should we assess the safety of IVF technologies? *Reprod Biomed Online.* 2013;27(6):710–721.
4. CairoConsensusGroup. There is only one thing that is truly important in an IVF laboratory: everything, Cairo consensus guidelines on IVF culture conditions. *Reprod Biomed Online.* 2020;40(1):33–60.
5. Botros L, Sakkas D, Seli E. Metabolomics and its application for non-invasive embryo assessment in IVF. *Mol Hum Reprod.* 2008;14(12):679–690.
6. Lane M, Gardner DK. Lactate regulates pyruvate uptake and metabolism in the preimplantation mouse embryo. *Biol Reprod.* 2000;62(1):16–22.
7. Gardner DK. Lactate production by the mammalian blastocyst: manipulating the microenvironment for uterine implantation and invasion? *Bioessays.* 2015;37(4):364–371.
8. Chi F, Sharpley MS, Nagaraj R, et al. Glycolysis-independent glucose metabolism distinguishes TE from ICM fate during mammalian embryogenesis. *Dev Cell.* 2020;53(1):9–26. e4.
9. Dickens C, Maguiness S, Comer M, et al. Physiology: human tubal fluid: formation and composition during vascular perfusion of the fallopian tube. *Hum Reprod.* 1995;10(3):505–508.
10. Ludwig TE, Lane M, Bavister BD. Differential effect of hexoses on hamster embryo development in culture. *Biol Reprod.* 2001;64(5):1366–1374.
11. Macklon N, Pieters M, Hassan M, et al. A prospective randomized comparison of sequential versus monoculture systems for in-vitro human blastocyst development. *Hum Reprod.* 2002;17(10):2700–2705.

12. Biggers J, Whittingham D, Donahue R. The pattern of energy metabolism in the mouse oöcyte and zygote. *Proc Natl Acad Sci*. 1967;58(2):560–567.
13. Dyrlund TF, Kirkegaard K, Poulsen ET, et al. Unconditioned commercial embryo culture media contain a large variety of non-declared proteins: a comprehensive proteomics analysis. *Hum Reprod*. 2014;29(11):2421–2430.
14. Zhu J, Li M, Chen L, et al. The protein source in embryo culture media influences birthweight: a comparative study between G1 v5 and G1-PLUS v5. *Hum Reprod*. 2014;29(7):1387–1392.
15. Guérin P, El Mouatassim S, Ménézo Y. Oxidative stress and protection against reactive oxygen species in the preimplantation embryo and its surroundings. *Human Reprod*. 2001;7(2):175–189.
16. Truong TT, Soh YM, Gardner DK. Antioxidants improve mouse preimplantation embryo development and viability. *Human Reprod*. 2016;31(7):1445–1554.
17. Gardner DK, Kuramoto T, Tanaka M, et al. Prospective randomized multicentre comparison on sibling oocytes comparing G-series media system with antioxidants versus standard G-series media system. *Reprod Biomed Online*. 2020;40(5):637–644.
18. Mehta RH. Growth of human preimplantation embryos in vitro. *Reprod Biomed Online*. 2001;2(2):113–119.
19. Armstrong S, MacKenzie J, Woodward B, et al. GM-CSF (granulocyte macrophage colony-stimulating factor) supplementation in culture media for women undergoing assisted reproduction. *Cochrane Database Syst Rev*. 2020;7(7):CD013497.
20. Lane M, Gardner DK. Embryo culture medium: which is the best? *Best Pract Res Clin Obstet Gynaecol*. 2007;21(1):83–100.
21. Stojkovic M, Kolle S, Peinl S, et al. Effects of high concentrations of hyaluronan in culture medium on development and survival rates of fresh and frozen-thawed bovine embryos produced in vitro. *Reproduction (Cambridge)*. 2002;124(1):141–153.
22. Sunde A, Brison D, Dumoulin J, et al. Time to take human embryo culture seriously. *Hum Reprod*. 2016;31(10):2174–2182.
23. Sfontouris IA, Kolibianakis EM, Lainas GT, et al. Blastocyst development in a single medium compared to sequential media: a prospective study with sibling oocytes. *Reprod Sci*. 2017;24:1312–1318.
24. Dieamant F, Petersen CG, Mauri AL, et al. Single versus sequential culture medium: which is better at improving ongoing pregnancy rates? A systematic review and meta-analysis. *JBRA Assist Reprod*. 2017;21(3):240.
25. Pool TB, Schoolfield J, Han D. Human embryo culture media comparisons. *Embryo Cult: Methods Protoc*. 2012: 367–386.
26. Wang W-H, Meng L, Hackett RJ, et al. Rigorous thermal control during intracytoplasmic sperm injection stabilizes the meiotic spindle and improves fertilization and pregnancy rates. *Fertil Steril*. 2002;77(6):1274–1277.
27. Lane M, Mitchell M, Cashman KS, et al. To QC or not to QC: the key to a consistent laboratory? *Reprod Fertil Dev*. 2007;20(1):23–32.
28. Swain JE. Media composition: pH and buffers. *Embryo Cult: Methods Protoc*. 2012:161–175.
29. Wale PL, Gardner DK. Oxygen regulates amino acid turnover and carbohydrate uptake during the preimplantation period of mouse embryo development. *Biol Reprod*. 2012;87(1):24, 1–8.
30. Khoudja RY, Xu Y, Li T, et al. Better IVF outcomes following improvements in laboratory air quality. *J Assist Reprod Genet*. 2013;30:69–76.
31. Fawzy M, AbdelRahman MY, Zidan MH, et al. Humid versus dry incubator: a prospective, randomized, controlled trial. *Fertil Steril*. 2017;108(2):277–283.
32. Mestres E, Matia-Algué Q, Villamar A, et al. Characterization and comparison of commercial oils used for human embryo culture. *Hum Reprod*. 2022;37(2):212–225.
33. Bartolacci A, Borini A, Cimadomo D, et al. Humidified atmosphere in a time-lapse embryo culture system does not improve ongoing pregnancy rate: a retrospective propensity score model study derived from 496 first ICSI cycles. *J Assist Reprod Genet*. 2023;1–7.
34. Mestres E, García-Jiménez M, Casals A, et al. Factors of the human embryo culture system that may affect media evaporation and osmolality. *Hum Reprod*. 2021;36(3):605–613.
35. Alhelou Y, Adenan NAM, Ali J. Embryo culture conditions are significantly improved during uninterrupted incubation: a randomized controlled trial. *Reprod Biol*. 2018;18(1):40–45.
36. Pomeroy KO, Reed ML. The effect of light on embryos and embryo culture. *J Reprod Stem Cell Biotechnol*. 2012;3(2):46–54.
37. Swain J, Smith G. Advances in embryo culture platforms: novel approaches to improve preimplantation embryo development through modifications of the microenvironment. *Hum Reprod Update*. 2011;17(4):541–557.
38. Wheeler MB, Rubessa M. Integration of microfluidics in animal in vitro embryo production. *MHR: Basic Sci Reprod Med*. 2017;23(4):248–256.

23

Ethics and the Law in Embryology

Gillian Lockwood

23.1 Introduction

Jean Purdy was the embryologist and nurse whose contribution with Steptoe and Edwards to the world's first IVF birth was unacknowledged for too long. Louise Brown's birth in 1978 was initially hailed not just with admiration and joy but with hostility. Critics pointed to the 'low' success rates (105 embryo transfers before a healthy birth), and many commented on the high cost (which would inevitably limit access to the wealthy few in the richer countries). Some religious authorities forbad its use for their adherents, claiming that it was 'unnatural' and morally repugnant. Some social commentators considered it to mark another potential slip down the 'slope' that could lead to the commodification and commercialisation of human reproduction. Latest estimates suggest that over 10 million 'test-tube' babies have been born worldwide and their contribution to the sum of human happiness cannot be overestimated.

Scientists working in the field of fertility are still confronted by opposition and misunderstanding, and the media frequently misrepresent what has been achieved or may be possible in the future. It is therefore vital that embryologists have a solid grasp of the ethical basis of their work and can explain and justify what they do with conviction.

Since Beauchamp and Childress published the first edition of their seminal book on biomedical ethics (**1**) in 1979, it has become almost conventional wisdom to analyse medical ethical problems in terms of their 'Four Principles' namely autonomy, beneficence (the promotion of good), the avoidance of harm (non-maleficence), and justice. Patient autonomy is considered to be the most important that effectively trumps the other three (Figure 23.1). However, medical and scientific practice must operate within a society that is subject not just to statute law but also to social acceptance.

The potential for modern fertility treatment to offer the chance of biological parenthood to otherwise infertile couples, in an environment where patients have expectations of achieving all their goals, inevitably raises questions about both the entitlement to treatment and the nature of that provision. Embryologists should never consider themselves as merely 'technicians' even if robotics and artificial intelligence (AI) may come to replace some of the skilled tasks currently performed in the IVF laboratory.

23.2 Embryology and the Law in the UK

The Human Fertilisation and Embryology Act 1990 is the primary legislation governing embryology in the UK. The Act was passed to regulate the use of in vitro fertilisation (IVF) and other assisted reproduction techniques (ART). The Act established the Human Fertilisation and Embryology Authority (HFEA) as the regulatory body responsible for overseeing the use of ART in the UK. The HFEA has the power to grant licences to clinics that offer ART services.

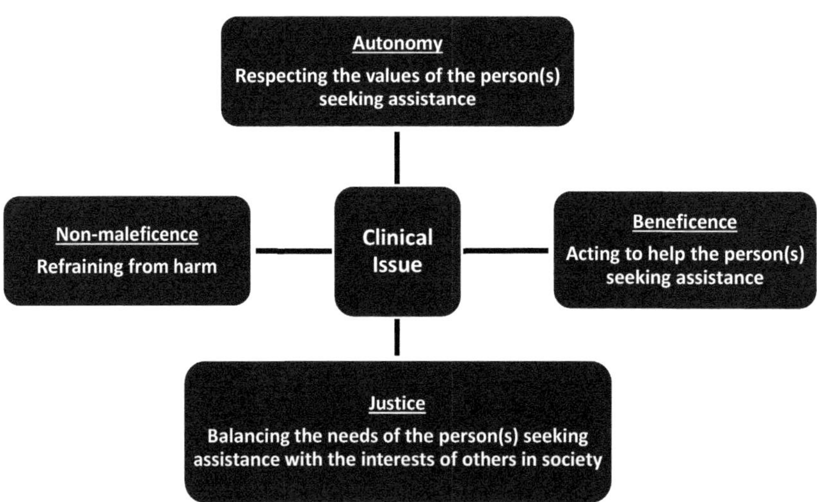

FIGURE 23.1 Ethical principles in reproductive medicine (see further [**1**])

DOI: 10.1201/9781003269502-23

The Human Fertilisation and Embryology Act 1990 was amended by the Human Fertilisation and Embryology Act 2008. The 2008 Act updated the legal framework for the use of ART in the UK. The 2008 Act extended the regulation of ART to cover a wider range of techniques, including the use of human-animal hybrids, and the use of techniques such as pre-implantation genetic diagnosis (PGD) and mitochondrial donation.

In addition to regulating the use of ART, UK law also governs the use of embryos for scientific research. The Human Fertilisation and Embryology Act 1990 permits the use of embryos for research purposes, subject to certain conditions. The HFEA has the power to grant licences for the use of embryos in research. The HFEA only grants licences for research that is deemed to be necessary and beneficial. The HFEA also ensures that embryos used for research are destroyed after a certain period of time.

23.3 Why Is Fertility Medicine Different?

Fertility treatment differs from other branches of medicine in two fundamental respects. First the fertility patient is not 'ill' in any conventional sense even though their infertility may have a pathological basis. Infertility may be a source of significant morbidity causing depression and social dysfunction, and in some cultures, childlessness (which is still seen as a predominantly female 'problem') is a huge social stigma. Second, infertility treatment is perceived as being generally 'unsuccessful' and is compared unfavourably with other treatments of acute conditions in surgery or therapeutics. This widespread perception is clearly mistaken as modern fertility treatments offer cumulative success rates over several cycles of treatment that compare favourably with those of a normally fertile couple trying to conceive naturally.

Even in cases in which extraordinary procedures are required such as ovum donation for premature ovarian failure (POF) or percutaneous epididymal sperm aspiration (PESA) with intracytoplasmic sperm injection (ICSI) for obstructive azoospermia the eventual outcome of treatment is likely to be influenced more by lack of resources to provide the treatments required than by deficiencies in the techniques available.

Opponents of IVF often claim that the successful delivery of a baby is not a 'cure' for infertility because the couple remain infertile as long as they rely on technology to assist them to procreate. This is sheer sophistry; a baby is a cure of infertility in exactly the same way as a beta blocker is a cure for hypertension. There may be some psychological benefits for the ultimately unsuccessful couple in just undertaking fertility treatment in that they may feel that at least their needs have been recognised and they have taken the opportunity to challenge their fate. However, one significant disadvantage of fertility treatment is that the desired outcome, the safe delivery of a healthy baby is an 'all or nothing' event. Unsuccessful treatment can rarely offer palliation or therapeutic benefit in the way that a less than wholly successful operation may offer an acceptable if sub-optimal outcome. Indeed a 'biochemical' pregnancy or early miscarriage following treatment may be perceived as 'worse' than a negative test.

Long-term follow-up studies of couples who embarked on fertility treatment but were ultimately unable to achieve a successful pregnancy, have shown that they do suffer significantly initially in terms of depression and regret, but that over time (5–7 years) they return to levels of life satisfaction that compare favourably with those who did succeed with fertility treatment and with the spontaneously fertile. As would be expected, individuals who make a 'positive' decision to abandon further fertility treatment after repeated failures fare better than those who wished to continue but could not undertake further treatment because of age or resource allocation.

In clinical terms, the decision to offer fertility treatment has significantly different implications from all other (successful) clinical interventions. In treating other medical problems, successful end results clearly affect the patients, their relatives and to some extent the wider society, but a successful fertility treatment involves an additional party in the child that is born. This individual's very existence inevitably has significant influence on all other social and family relationships, indeed the arrival of the child may create the family.

23.4 Considering Possible People

To what extent the scientist needs to consider the potential existence of this, as yet, un-conceived child is a complex philosophical issue. The interests of people who may be born as a result of fertility treatment clearly are not as tangible as those of existing people, but legislation governing the application of the new reproductive technologies sets great store by the interests of the (possible) child. The Human Fertilisation and Embryology act (1991) states that 'centres considering treatment must take into account the welfare of any child that may be born'. From that standpoint it would seem difficult to justify restricting availability or access to treatments except in the limiting case where the expected quality of life of the child is so low that the child might realistically wish that it had never been born. All other children born as a result of fertility treatment (1.5% of all babies born in the UK and 10 million world-wide since 1987 following IVF) represent a significant addition to the sum of human happiness, and this is so even if we ignore the happiness of their parents and relations.

It may seem that adding the interests of the 'potential person' to an equation for setting medical priorities in therapies that include fertility treatment involves a significant problem of incommensurability: how do we weigh the interests of 'potential' against those of 'actual' people? £5000 could 'buy' an IVF cycle for a young couple who, with fresh and subsequent, frozen embryo transfers, could realistically achieve the birth of at least one healthy child. That same £5000 would make very little contribution to the cost of providing gene therapy for toddlers with rare neurodegenerative disease currently costing £3 million.

The inevitable conclusion must be that withholding fertility treatment on the grounds of the interest of the 'welfare of the child' is a philosophically unsustainable position. Whether this is equivalent to claiming that we have a positive duty to 'make more' happy people is equally contentious. Perhaps this is a political rather than an ethical decision. Many governments have promoted pro-natalist policies because of concern about declining populations and falling birth rates, and in the era of ART, some governments are actively supporting state-funded fertility treatment as a way of ensuring that their citizens (usually the educated, professional classes who are most likely to be childless) are encouraged and helped to have children.

23.5 Ethical Approaches

23.5.1 Consequentialism

Conventional medical ethics theory tends to be divided into consequentialist doctrines that try to evaluate the outcome of clinical decisions in terms of consequences, good or bad, and rights- or rule- based systems that judge clinical decisions and outcomes in terms of the extent to which a 'right' is advanced or a 'good' rule applied. In the simplest case, a single successful cycle of IVF for a childless couple resulting in the birth of a healthy baby seems to be a purely positive outcome. On the basis of a cost-benefit analysis, the financial costs are modest (even allowing for the opportunity cost of diverting scarce resources to fertility treatment) and the foreseeable medium- and long-term consequences are equally positive.

Some potential negative consequences may be foreseen. For example the child may be neglected or abused, or the couple's relationship may founder under the psychological stress of even a successful cycle but these are rare cases. As a society we recognise that a significant proportion of births are unplanned and accidental (50% according to some surveys,) yet we would be horrified at the prospect of spontaneously fertile people being required to fulfil the criteria of 'suitability to parent' that some treatment centres impose on their patients in the name of equity or the 'interests of the child'. One in five babies born in the UK grow up in a household with no father, but single women seeking to become mothers in a safe and lawful way face significant obstacles in accessing treatment and the financial burden for them is high.

23.5.2 Comparisons with Adoption

Consider the analogy that is often drawn between allocating access to fertility treatment and the authorities 'choosing' the best possible adoptive parents for a baby that has been given up at birth by its mother. Given the 'shortage' of healthy newborns available for adoption in the UK, and the large number of couples who would like to adopt a baby, it is generally accepted that the authorities must 'choose' the 'best' possible would-be parents for that child. However a large number of children are taken into our Care Homes, and their life outcomes are recognised to be very compromised. Should we then accept that possibly 'lower' standards of potential parenting may be acceptable for prospective adoptive parents in these cases? Caring and half-competent parenting is infinitely preferable for 'looked after' children who have been rescued from neglect and abuse to them remaining in Institutions.

This is clearly a false analogy to make with decisions about the provision of fertility treatment. The child that may, or even will, be born as the result of successful fertility treatment can only be born to the would-be parents who came to the fertility clinic. They may not be, potentially, the 'best' parents, but they are the only parents that this, as yet un-conceived, child can have.

23.5.3 Rights-Based Systems of Ethics

Rights-based systems are ethically even more contentious. Article 12 of the European Convention on Human Rights does protect the right to 'found a family', but this legislation was drawn up at a time when an individual's right not to be compulsorily sterilised was the issue at stake, and in the era before assisted reproductive technology was even envisaged. There can be no right to have a child, in the sense that somebody, possibly Society, has a corresponding duty to provide successful fertility treatment. Demand for medical treatment, including fertility treatment, is theoretically unlimited since even in wealthy countries there will always be a disparity between what individuals could theoretically benefit from and what Society can afford to provide. For this reason the concept of rationing in healthcare, including fertility treatment, is accepted and the issue becomes one of ensuring justice, equity of distribution or simply rationing 'fairly'.

23.5.4 Fairness

In an acute or progressive clinical situation, the condition itself generates its own therapeutic agenda. Responsible clinicians treat the life threatening and rapidly deteriorating conditions before the mild and stable, and little or no consideration is given either to the cost of the intervention, the responsibility of the patients for their condition or even the likelihood of a successful outcome. A computer algorithm that could predict the outcome of admission of a patient to ITU with 98% accuracy (and therefore save the pain, anguish and expense) of often a prolonged and ultimately futile time spent in intensive care) was condemned as inhumane. Yet, decisions about access to funded (or even private) fertility treatment are made on criteria with much less statistical rigour such as AMH levels or BMI.

However infertility patients are generally not perceived to be in this position, however great their distress. The condition itself does not deteriorate except in the sense that advancing female age may eventually make it less likely to succeed. Funding Commissioners may feel entitled to consider the issue of desert and responsibility in the field of infertility treatment when they would not in any other medical arena. Diabetics who smoke or transplant patients who do not comply with their medication will still be treated, unlike fertility patients who are often held to be 'responsible' for their childlessness. Patients report, through tears, of being asked, 'Why didn't you start trying for a baby when you were younger?' or 'How do you think you got the Chlamydia that has blocked your tubes?'! Even when the needs of all infertile people are recognised, allocation of resources is often made on the basis of personal desert or utility. A 30-year-old childless married woman with tubal blockage due to peritonitis will be offered IVF on the NHS whereas a 36-year-old, previously sterilised, mother of two cannot get the treatment she needs to have a baby with her new partner. When discussing questions of need in this context, the issue is one of how to allocate limited resources so that utility is maximised and injustice is minimised. The sheer complexity of human motivation is such that the calculation of needs and deserts are fraught with difficulty, and that is assuming that we can answer the fundamental question of whether the fertile five-sixth of the population or the decision makers (that is the clinicians or commissioners who control access to treatment) are entitled to make judgments about the lifestyles, needs and deserts of the one sixth of the population who cannot reproduce spontaneously.

Some authorities have claimed that if guidelines for access to fertility treatments can be agreed, then justice demands only that the guidelines are applied impartially: that is the content of the guidelines is relatively unimportant. This type of 'procedural' justice is exemplified by the 'post-code lottery' that has prevailed in England and Wales notwithstanding the NICE guideline of 2004 which recommended 3 'full' (including frozen embryo transfers) for all eligible childless couples.

23.6 The Legal and Moral Status of the Human Embryo

The original Human Fertilisation and Embryology Act (1990) and its subsequent iterations accords a special status to human embryos generated *in vitro* and this has resulted in strict limitations on the nature and extent of embryo research and fertility treatment that can be carried out in the UK. This special status derives from the embryo's recognised **potential** to become a human being and seems to be in stark contrast to other UK legislation that permits termination of pregnancy at much more advanced gestations.

The Act provides that embryos are subject to a range of legal controls, including the requirement that they be stored and used only for specified purposes. For example, the Act stipulates that embryos must be used for the treatment of infertility, or for the purposes of research, but not for any other purpose (s. 3(1)). The Act also prohibits the sale of embryos, and makes it an offence to create an embryo for any purpose other than those specified in the Act.

In addition, the guidelines stipulate that the embryos must not be allowed to develop beyond 14 days, and that the cells derived from them must not be used to create a complete human being. The guidelines also require that the donors of the embryos give informed consent, and that they be given the option to withdraw their consent at any time.

Notwithstanding different religious perspectives on the point at which 'life' begins (fertilisation, implantation, 'quickening', viability, delivery), it is reasonable to consider at what point in the development of the human organism a creature with a 'right to life' has come into being. If we accept that potential personhood is taken to confer a serious right to life, then the only grounds on which a termination of pregnancy could be defended would be the need to protect the life or health of the mother or the presence in the fetus of an incurable defect that would make its life, if it were to survive, not worth living.

However, we must recognise the political and societal environment in which the field of ART evolved. In 1967, David Steel's Abortion Act permitted termination of pregnancy on a wide number of grounds up to 28 weeks gestation in Great Britain (but not Northern Ireland). The HFEA Act of 1990 reduced the time limit from 28 to 24 weeks (in the light of developments in neo-natal intensive care) and subsequent attempts to reduce the time limit to 22 and 20 weeks have been resisted in Parliament. The implementation of the Steel Act in 1968 occurred just 10 years before Louise Brown's birth and it is clear that attempts to make significant alterations to the HFEA Act risk re-opening the highly politically contentious area of termination of pregnancy.

As the embryologist studies the images of the microscopic cluster of cells which is the blastocyst, they are fully aware that this can progress by an uncertain but inexorable process from the Petri dish to the cradle.

For successful IVF parents the leap of imagination required to envisage their embryo as a child is very difficult. After successful delivery however, the supernumerary frozen embryos that represent potential siblings hold a huge, and often painful, emotional significance if the couple do not wish to have further children but feel they cannot donate 'their' children to be brought up by other parents or let 'them' be allowed to perish.

23.7 Ethical Considerations Around Embryonic Stem Cells

Embryonic stem cells are derived from embryos that are usually surplus to requirements following IVF treatment. These cells have the potential to develop into any type of cell in the body, and therefore have enormous potential for use in medical treatments. However, the use of embryonic stem cells raises a range of ethical issues, particularly with regard to the destruction of embryos and the possibility that embryos could be created purely to provide specific 'matched' stem cells.

The UK has taken a relatively liberal approach to the use of embryonic stem cells, and in 2001 the HFEA issued guidelines allowing the use of surplus embryos for research purposes, subject to strict ethical guidelines. These guidelines require that the creation and use of embryos for research must be justified on scientific grounds, and that the research must be carried out with the aim of improving human health (**2**; HFEA, 2023).

23.8 Confidentiality and Infertility

Confidentiality is central to the doctor-patient relationship in all branches of medicine, but it is especially so in fertility practice, where patients often feel a sense of shame or guilt about their status. The legislation specifies the care that must be taken not to communicate anything about a patient's fertility care, even that they are having IVF, without their express permission and consent. History taking in fertility consultations is rife with danger. There may be emerging secrets: previous unacknowledged paternity, adoption, termination of pregnancy even sterilization or gender reassignment may all have enormous impact on the prospects for treatment outcome and the couple's ongoing relationship. Embryologists are increasingly encouraged to involve themselves with the clinical care of patients. They are, after all, best placed to explain the implications of the types of abnormality they see in gametes and embryos. Patients too see the embryologist as having a special 'relationship with 'their' embryos, describing them as being 'looked after' or 'chosen' by their embryologist.

The fertility doctor and the embryologist have a special duty to enhance patient autonomy by communicating sensitively and effectively so the decision about undertaking fertility treatment and the responsibility for it is shared. It is vital to recognise the limits to accuracy and effectiveness of many diagnostic and therapeutic procedures in fertility practice (and that the patient may have a different perspective).

Some of the basic principles of behavioural economics can assist with managing patient expectations, in that it is vital to recognise that under situations of stress and anxiety people often make apparently 'irrational' decisions and, when faced with complex scenarios, may be incapable of choosing. Fertility treatment is so often expressed in terms of percentages that it is easy to lose sight that percentages apply to populations and not to an individual couple's 'chances' of a baby. Where female age and ovarian reserve indicate a less than 10% chance of a live birth, then donor eggs may seem the obvious 'solution'. But for the couple with a 15-year history of primary infertility, even a 10% 'chance' is an option they may wish to consider taking.

23.9 Ethical Dilemmas Arising from the Cryopreservation of Gametes

Since the development in the 1950s of successful sperm cryopreservation it has been possible to separate both temporally and spatially the act of gamete production from that of fertilisation and conception. Technologies of ICSI and TESE allied with cryopreservation of sperm, oocytes and embryos have revolutionised the way in which society looks at reproductive behaviour and relationships.

Ethical dilemmas can arise from a new found ability to manipulate our reproductive life span to such an extent that old age and even death are no longer seen as a barrier to having children. It is well recognised that natural fertility and fecundity start to decline quite markedly from the mid-thirties in most women with normal reproductive function, and for women in their forties the chance of achieving a healthy pregnancy with their own eggs, even with IVF, is quite small

23.9.1 Posthumous Reproduction and the Cryopreservation of Gametes

Many societies question whether it is acceptable or appropriate for a widow to use frozen embryos that were created with her late husband to give birth to a posthumous child. In the UK, so long as the correct consent forms have been signed, such treatment is available and the deceased father can have his name put on the baby's birth certificate. In contrast, in France creation of the embryo is viewed as a joint 'project' which ceases to have a purpose on the death of one of the project's originators. In the United States, the uniform anatomical gift act (UAGA) which is in effect in every state gives the next of kin, in designated order of closeness, the right to make material gifts of the deceased's body without limiting the uses that can be made of the gift. Does this authority extend to retrieving gametes to be used by the next of kin for their own reproductive purposes or that of others? Similarly contentious there is the use of cryopreserved sperm from a deceased partner to impregnate or otherwise achieve pregnancy in the surviving spouse.

As a society we may wish to consider whether there is any legal or moral distinction in the status of a child who was conceived spontaneously the week before his father's untimely death or that of the child conceived using ART and stored gametes or sperm acquired peri-mortem. Where the degree of medical involvement in the three processes is clearly different, nevertheless the child's existence and rights are identical. Clinicians often wish to make a distinction between acts of procreation in which they have had no or only minimal involvement (prescribing clomiphene or advising on the 'fertile period' for example) and identically motivated acts which require high levels of medical and technological input. It could be argued that the existence of the resulting child is just as much or as little the responsibility of the clinician irrespective of their level of involvement.

The Warnock report of 1984, which gave rise to the Human Fertilisation and Embryology act of 1990, considered the issue of the post-mortem use of gametes and expressed grave misgivings because this use may 'give rise to profound psychological problems for the child and the mother'. However, the report made no direct recommendation for action, stating instead that 'Posthumous use of gametes is a practice which we feel should be actively discouraged'. The Act did not prohibit the retrieval and storage of gametes but required the consent of the source of gametes before they could be stored. It was this aspect of the law that in 1998 prevented Diane Blood being treated in the UK with sperm that had been illegally obtained from her dying husband, and equally illegally stored. The European Court allowed the 'export' of the sperm to Belgium where she was successfully treated and gave birth to two sons.

Issues that arise in the area of posthumous reproduction focus on intention and consent. When there is known intention and legal consent matters may be straight forward, although the requirement for other parties, including the ART team to be involved, raises the possibility that individuals could be frustrated in their intention by other parties' reluctance to co-operate. When intention is merely implied or the only evidence of the deceased's intention is the testimony of a third party with an interest in the outcome, then the issue is more difficult.

23.9.2 Posthumous Children

In general, the law does suggest that the interests of the deceased may be considered to end with their death. It would allow a man, while still alive, to veto extraction of his sperm post-mortem so that his widow could use it in an ICSI cycle she planned to undertake. However as a society we place enormous emphasis on a legal and moral duty to respect the expressed or even implied wishes of deceased individuals.

I may feel very strongly that my uncle was mistaken in leaving his fortune to his local donkey sanctuary, but unless I can show that undue influence was brought to bear on him, I have no chance in law of overturning his will. Similarly, there was a case of a widow who, because her late husband had stipulated so in his will, felt morally obliged to have the frozen embryos that she had generated with him transferred to her womb even though she really did not wish to become pregnant, let alone posthumously so.

However, much importance we may attach to a deceased persons wishes, I would contend that society does not usually expect them to be allowed to trump the wishes of those who are still alive. We effectively give next of kin the right to have all the transplantable bits of the departed (or departing) loved one donated for altruistic reasons because we are ready to accept the next of kin's claim the person associated with the brain-dead body in question was in favour of organ donation.

However, when the issue is one of harvesting gametes it is not at all clear that the wishes of the next of kin carry such authority. We may be deeply sympathetic to the childless widow who wants her late husband's sperm to be retrieved for her future use, but could other family members have claims too? An only child could feel very strongly that he didn't want some posthumous siblings created with whom he would have to share both his mother and his inheritance.

Appeal is often made to the 'welfare of the child' as the means of deciding whether a proposed course of action using ART techniques is valid and appropriate. The welfare of the child who may be born as a result of treatment is regarded by many as the central and most important tenet expressed in the Human Fertilisation and Embryology act. However, this appeal to the welfare of the posthumous child who may be born if the treatment is successful in achieving a healthy pregnancy is philosophically untenable. A posthumous child may certainly wish that he had been conceived in a more conventional way and he had a father to play football with, but unless his distress at his origins is so great that he genuinely wished to have never been born, he surely has a strong retrospective interest in the application of the technology that engineered his birth.

Society of course also has legitimate interest in this issue and may rightly be charged with a responsibility of ensuring that human beings are not created merely to satisfy the sad cravings of lonely widows or to fulfil the dynastic ambitions of dead tyrants. Clinicians and scientists working in the field of ART should similarly be concerned with judgements that have implications for the allocation of scarce resources. In the UK, in which public funding of ART is severely and inequitably limited and where all health resources are subject to rationing, the right of access to specialist techniques to achieve posthumous reproduction appears to enjoy appropriately low priority. We may need to consider whether this judgment should be made in an NHS or private medical context. Nevertheless, as long as it continues to be true that many spontaneous conceptions are either unplanned or initially unwanted it seems difficult to justify placing insurmountable legal obstacles in the way of those who actually wish to conceive and have legitimate access to gametes.

23.9.3 Controversies in 'Social' or 'Elective' Egg Freezing

Women who wish to freeze their eggs for their own future use face many hurdles, financial, physical and emotional. The technique is either presented as being relatively unsuccessful or it is 'oversold' to a vulnerable group of young women. With vitrification of oocytes and the experience of frozen donor egg banks it is clear that 'young' frozen eggs have a similar reproductive potential to 'fresh' eggs when thawed, fertilised with ICSI and transferred as blastocysts. The optimum time for 'social' egg freezing is the early 30s, but the average age of egg freezers in the UK is 38 and this helps to explain the relatively poor outcomes.

Many recent surveys have shown that women who seek 'social' egg freezing are not doing so because they have other life goals and wish to delay motherhood, but because they have a highly conventional view of parenting and they want to have the opportunity to become a mother in a supportive, long-term relationship. It is important that 'social' freezing is not presented as a 'guaranteed' insurance against age-related infertility, but for women who want the chance to be 'genetic' mothers, it may represent an option that they wish to take.

'Social' egg freezing developed from work to preserve the fertility of young women undergoing potentially sterilising chemotherapy, surgery or radiotherapy. In practice, the distinction between 'social' and medical freezing is increasingly difficult to maintain as significant gynaecological pathologies such as endometriosis or a strong family history of premature menopause may also represent a compelling argument for oocyte freezing for fertility preservation. In the UK, women diagnosed with premature and irreversible infertility may have their eggs frozen for 55 years. The passage of time is just as destructive as chemotherapy to a woman's fertility prospects. Since 2022 the legislation for 'social' freezers in the UK, permits the storage period of their eggs to 55 years but consent for storage must be renewed every 10 years.

There is sparse evidence about the 'usage' rate of socially frozen eggs as most data sets do not distinguish between the various different reasons for which the eggs have been frozen. It is, however, the experience of UK centres that have pioneered 'social' egg freezing, that women either return within a few years to use their eggs (often with donor sperm), or never return at all because, presumably they have achieved a natural pregnancy, had successful conventional fertility treatment or they have never met a suitable partner to parent with.

'Social' egg freezers represent a particularly challenging group of patients, partly because they are often facing severe disappointment that they are not in a position to start a family in a conventional relationship and they are understandably anxious about undergoing a medical procedure that carries no guarantees of a successful outcome. Supportive counselling is absolutely vital at all stages of their treatment cycle.

23.10 Donor Gametes: Ethical Issues for Donors, Recipients and Their Offspring

Donor gametes (eggs and sperm) clearly have an equal genetic contribution to make to the creation of an embryo and hence to a potential person, but the very different problems of procurement should not be allowed to overshadow the fact that the ethical issues for donors and recipients are identical.

Until the end of donor anonymity was enacted in law in 2005, gamete donors were guaranteed lifelong anonymity in the UK and this was thought to be a factor in encouraging young men to become sperm donors. This decision to end anonymity followed a prolonged period of review and public consultation. When fertility clinics were consulted, the majority were opposed because of concerns that it would deter donors at a time when there was already a shortage of donor sperm, and that the removal of anonymity would have no effect on secrecy as many parents never tell their children that a donor was involved in their conception. This is not to underestimate the distress of donor-conceived people who know of their origins but are unable to find out any useful, let alone identifiable, information about their genetic parent.

The incidence of non-paternity (where a child is not the offspring of its putative father) has been estimated as being between 2 and 12% in the general population and as high as 25% where paternity testing is undertaken because suspicions have been raised. An MP on the Select Committee of Science and Technology that reviewed the legislation actually suggested that all new-borns should be DNA fingerprinted to ensure that everyone could exercise their fundamental **right** to know their true genetic identity.

One aspect of the ending of anonymity that was inherent in the new legislation was the degree of asymmetry in available information introduced between donor's 'own' children and their 'biological' siblings and half siblings.

Donor sperm, egg or embryo conceived individuals can apply to the HFEA 'Opening the Register' team for identifiable information about their donors, **if** they know they are donor conceived, at the age of 18, or earlier if they are considering marriage and wish to confirm they are not related to their intended partner. This enquiry will also supply information about siblings and half-siblings if any. However, although donors can be told the outcome of their donations (restricted to number, year of birth and gender), they cannot have any further information for their own children. If they tell their children that they have half-siblings (or in the case of embryo donation, full siblings) and those donor conceived offspring never try to establish contact, then these young people may be left with a 'gap' in their genetic record which was part of the reason why anonymity was ended. However, if the donor does not reveal their donation history to their own children and the family is informed that one or more 18-year-olds is wanting to make contact, that could have harmful repercussions in terms of family trust.

Modern technology in the form of direct-to-consumer (DTC) DNA testing and ancestry tracing may already be undermining the theoretical guarantees of anonymity that donors were offered prior to 2004. People may buy DTC tests for a variety of purposes, but may discover that they are donor conceived and there are DNA-based voluntary contact registers that may allow them to identify both their donor and any siblings.

The current advice is that clinical teams should provide support, guidance and information on the availability and implications of genetic ancestry testing and the lack of control over identity that an individual may have if a blood relation undergoes testing.

23.10.1 Surrogacy

Surrogacy, or at least 'straight' surrogacy, where the birth mother is also the genetic mother, may claim to be one of the oldest forms of fertility treatment as it has been practiced since Biblical times. However, most surrogacy arrangements in the UK involve 'host' or 'gestational' surrogacy where the surrogate mother has no direct genetic link to the child who will be born and will become the legal offspring of the genetic or 'intended parents' (IPs) who have provided the gametes in an IVF treatment.

There are many reasons why IPs turn to surrogacy:

- recurrent miscarriage
- repeated failure of IVF treatment
- premature menopause, often as a result of cancer treatment
- a hysterectomy or an absent or abnormal uterus
- a serious risk to health that may result from pregnancy
- LGBT+ parents wanting to create a family

Britain was in advance of many other jurisdictions in legislating to legalise surrogacy, mainly as a result of a media and professional outcry in the 1980s following the 'Baby Cotton' case in which Kim Cotton admitted to being paid to bear babies for other women. Many European countries outlaw surrogacy, believing that it encourages 'child abandonment' and the establishment of 'baby farms' in developing countries, where poor women act as host surrogates for Western couples, has rightly raised issues of exploitation and the commodification of reproduction.

Straight surrogacy (also known as full or traditional) surrogacy is when the surrogate provides her own eggs to achieve the pregnancy. The intended father, in either a heterosexual or male same-sex relationship, provides a sperm sample for conception through either self-insemination at home or artificial insemination with the help of a fertility clinic. If either the surrogate or intended father has fertility issues, then embryos may also be created in vitro and transferred into the uterus of the surrogate.

Although surrogacy is legal in the UK, surrogacy arrangements are not enforceable in law. The Surrogacy Arrangements Act 1985 makes it clear that it is an offence to advertise that you are seeking a surrogate or are a potential surrogate looking for IPs. It is also an offence under that Act to arrange or negotiate a surrogacy arrangement as a commercial enterprise, however, there are a number of non-profit organisations (also known as 'altruistic') that lawfully assist potential surrogates and IPs to navigate their surrogacy.

The surrogate (and, if she is married or in a civil partnership, her consenting spouse or civil partner) will be the legal parents of the child at birth. Following the birth, there is a legal process – the parental order process – to transfer legal parenthood from the surrogate to the IPs. In order to apply for a parental order and transfer legal parenthood, at least one of the IPs must be genetically related to the baby. Since 2019 Single people have been able to apply for parental orders in surrogacy cases again with the proviso that they are genetically linked to the baby.

The Parental order criteria are strict and indicate the level of anxiety that surrounds the whole area. There have been cases where mothers of women who need a surrogate have effectively 'given birth to their own grandchild' by having an embryo created from their daughter and son-in-law's gametes transferred to their uterus. It is possible that the developing success of 'womb transplants' from both cadaveric and living-related donors may reduce the demand for surrogacy, but there is little evidence at present.

As with all issues arising in Assisted Conception, the Welfare of the Child who may be born (or a child who may be affected by that birth) is pre-eminent. In surrogacy arrangements, it is particularly clear that the information imparted to the child may be vital. The inevitably close relationship that develops between IPs and the surrogate mother (and partner) should encourage an open and honest explanation of the child's origins, but some IPs come to see the process as a form of 'pre-implantation adoption' and do not wish to accord their surrogate a role beyond birth.

In ethical terms it is difficult to justify a distinction between the role of the 'straight' or the 'host' surrogate. It is possible that a host surrogate mother may feel less 'attached' to her newborn if she has no genetic link, but IPs should be sensitive to the needs of their surrogate and her children (who may perceive that they have lost a potential sibling).

23.11 'Designing Babies': Balancing Autonomy with Welfare of the Child

In the developed world, the greatest cause of early death and disability is genetic disease and so it is clearly tempting to consider the application of pre-implantation genetic diagnosis (PGD) as an adjunct to contemporary fertility treatment. PGD is a procedure used prior to embryo implantation to identify genetic defects within embryos. These could be 'expected' where PGD is being carried out because the prospective parents are aware that they carry deleterious genes (i.e. both are CF carriers) or because there is an increased risk of aneuploidy due to advanced maternal age or history of recurrent miscarriage. A procedure which allows prospective parents to embark on a pregnancy confident that their baby will not be affected by a lethal genetic disease or that the normally high age – related risk of miscarriage due to aneuploidy has been significantly reduced would seem to be universally acceptable.

One could even envisage couples who do not **need** IVF to conceive choosing to undergo ART so that their potential children could be 'screened' for rare genetic diseases. Some diseases have variable penetrance and some only generate symptoms in middle or older age. Many would perceive the use of PGD for sex-selection as an unacceptable application of the PGD technology, but gender-based selective termination is widely practised and would seem even less ethically acceptable.

A significant ethical issue in embryo screening and embryo selection relates to decisions about what qualifies as a sufficiently serious or likely genetic anomaly that it is acceptable to screen for it and not transfer affected embryos. Some communities such as those with congenital deafness or achondroplastic dwarfism have claimed a right to screen **for** genetic characteristics that many would consider to be deleterious.

Often described as a 'slippery slope', it is very likely that many physical and even intellectual characteristics may soon be identifiable in PGD screening and then it may prove impossible to put this eugenic genie back in the bottle. We accept as a society that parents can choose to enhance their child's musical, academic or sporting prospects by providing intensive coaching from an early age. if it were possible to use PGD technology to select a 'musical' or 'sporty' 'gene complex would this diminish society's appreciation of exceptional achievement?

23.12 Conclusion

The field of assisted reproduction remains one of the most rapidly evolving branches of medicine and perhaps, what is most remarkable – and the source of its most contentious ethical dilemmas – is that it involves arguably more significant outcomes than any other branches. In ART we are not just saving lives (the pinnacle of oncology therapy or transplant surgery), we are actually **creating** lives with all the implications that entails for the individual, the family and Society.

Developments like CRISPR, cadaveric womb transplants for transgender women and pre-pubescent testicular xeno-transplants for boys requiring sterilising chemotherapies have moved our field from the realm of science fiction to the theoretically and actually possible. It is vital that philosophers who speculate on the ethical challenges of our field are very well informed about what we can and are doing, and it is equally important that doctors and scientists consider the potential ethical implications of their work. As with the (near) universal ban on human cloning, we don't need to do something just because we can. By informing the wider public and explaining our work to our patients, our colleagues and our legislators we can stay out in front of public opinion – but just not too far.

UK Law and Embryology:

The Human Fertilisation and Embryology Act 1990 is the primary legislation governing embryology in the UK. The Act was passed to regulate the use of in vitro fertilisation (IVF) and other assisted reproduction techniques (ART). The Act established the Human Fertilisation and Embryology Authority (HFEA) as the regulatory body responsible for overseeing the use of ART in the UK. The HFEA has the power to grant licences to clinics that offer ART services.

The Human Fertilisation and Embryology Act 1990 was amended by the Human Fertilisation and Embryology Act 2008. The 2008 Act updated the legal framework for the use of ART in the UK. The 2008 Act extended the regulation of ART to cover a wider range of techniques, including the use of human-animal hybrids, and the use of techniques such as pre-implantation genetic diagnosis (PGD) and mitochondrial donation.

In addition to regulating the use of ART, UK law also governs the use of embryos for scientific research. The Human Fertilisation and Embryology Act 1990 permits the use of embryos for research purposes, subject to certain conditions. The HFEA has the power to grant licences for the use of embryos in research. The HFEA only grants licences for research that is deemed to be necessary and beneficial. The HFEA also ensures that embryos used for research are destroyed after a certain period of time.

The law also regulates the creation of embryos for research purposes. The creation of embryos for research purposes is permitted under UK law, subject to certain conditions. The HFEA has the power to grant licences for the creation of embryos for research purposes. The HFEA only grants licences for the creation of embryos for research purposes where there is no alternative method of obtaining the necessary information.

The use of embryonic stem cells for research is also regulated by UK law. Embryonic stem cells are obtained from embryos that are less than 14 days old. The use of embryonic stem cells for research purposes is permitted under UK law, subject to certain conditions. The HFEA has the power to grant licences for the use of embryonic stem cells in research. The HFEA only grants licences for the use of embryonic stem cells where there is no alternative method of obtaining the necessary information.

Ethical Issues:

Assisted reproductive technologies (ARTs) are medical interventions that aim to facilitate pregnancy in cases where natural conception is not possible. In the UK, ARTs are regulated by the Human Fertilisation and Embryology Authority (HFEA), which was established by the Human Fertilisation and Embryology Act 1990. The HFEA is responsible for licensing clinics that provide ARTs, and for ensuring that these clinics comply with the relevant legal and ethical guidelines.

One of the most controversial forms of ART is in vitro fertilisation (IVF), which involves the fertilisation of an egg by sperm outside the body, followed by the transfer of the resulting embryo to the woman's uterus. The use of IVF raises a number of legal and ethical issues, particularly with regard to the status of the embryos created.

Summary of the UK HFEA Act:

The UK HFEA Act (Human Fertilisation and Embryology Act) is a law that governs the use of human embryos and certain assisted reproduction techniques in the UK. The Act sets out regulations for the creation, storage, and use of human embryos and prohibits certain activities, such as human cloning. It also establishes the Human Fertilisation and Embryology Authority (HFEA), a regulatory body responsible for overseeing and enforcing the provisions of the Act. The HFEA has the power to issue licenses for certain activities related to assisted reproduction and to monitor compliance with the Act's regulations.

REFERENCES

1. Beauchamp TL, Childress JF. *Principles of Biomedical Ethics*. 7th Edition. Oxford: OUP; 2013,
2. HFEA. *Code of Practice 2023*. 9th Edition. London, UK: Human Fertilisation and Embryology Authority; 2023.

24

The Patient Experience through an IVF Treatment Cycle

Charmian Short

There are many paths to parenthood. Patients come to the clinic to start a family and clinics should do everything they can to give as many people as possible the chance to have a family. In order to do so, they should aim to get to know the patients to understand their needs, enabling them to provide an individualised treatment plan. A "one size fits all" approach is often less desirable, and patients should always be given the very best chance of success.

In the UK, CARE Fertility group for instance offers a wide range of treatments such as: fertility assessments, fertility preservation, in vitro fertilisation (IVF), intracytoplasmic sperm injection (ICSI), intrauterine insemination (IUI), egg or sperm donation and surrogacy. Specialist genetic services including Pre-implantation Genetic Testing (PGT-A), Pre-implantation Genetic Testing for monogenic diseases (PGT-M) and chromosomal structure rearrangements (PGT-SR) can also offered as part of the embryo evaluation and selection. Patients can also have access to a wide range of diagnostic tests and embryology treatments such as CAREmaps and Zymot and new AI technology.

24.1 How Do Patients Select a Fertility Clinic?

Patients choose a clinic for many reasons:

Research – Patients often research clinics and treatments long before they initially get in touch. It is a very personal journey and can take a lot of courage to make that first call. The HFEA website has a great tool which gives the opportunity to compare clinics across the UK.

Success Rates – There is no denying the importance of success rates when choosing a fertility clinic. Fertility patients can have very different needs and success can vary depending on many factors including age. A fertility doctor should provide predicted success rate ranges based on patient medical history and treatment needs.

Reputation – This could be reputation in the sector or recommendation from a family member, friend or work colleague. Both key to providing the patient with confidence they are making the right decision.

The people and service – Patients expect a dedicated team and personalised service to guide them through treatment and look for a clinic which shows these qualities from the very first contact. Patients may look at what a clinic offers that another doesn't and will routinely seek access to the very latest in medical advances and state of the art equipment.

24.2 Getting Started

Patients' individual needs can vary, they may wish to test their fertility, start a family, grow their family or simply explore their options. To get started, they need to make contact with a chosen fertility treatment provider should be as easy as possible as clinics understand making that very first phone call or initiating that first step is significant for them so they can have the opportunity to ask their questions, discuss costs and arrange suitable investigations and consultations at a time to suit the patient.

Before the first consultation it is recommended that new patients have some investigations so the results are ready for their doctor to review at their appointment. This provides important information to enable the doctor to propose the right treatment plan for them. Clinical staff regularly meet to share best practice and are dedicated in identifying and overcoming some of the most complex fertility problems.

Commonly recommended investigations before first consultation may include:

Transvaginal Scan with an Antral Follicle Count. This checks the health of the uterus and provides a way of counting follicles.

Anti-Mullerian Hormone Blood Test. Along with the scan gives provides a good picture of ovarian reserve and this can help the doctor decide on the most suitable treatment plan.

Diagnostic Semen Analysis. A fertility clinic should offer a full diagnostic semen analysis looking at numerous parameters including volume, number, motility and morphology.

(Before the semen analysis appointment, it is often recommended patients abstain from ejaculation for 3–5 days and avoid alcohol to get the most accurate test result).

Routinely clinics should accept test results dated within a suitable time frame from other clinics or hospitals. The doctor can review these at the consultation. If a patient has had previous treatment elsewhere, it would be beneficial to provide copy notes to their new clinic.

DOI: 10.1201/9781003269502-24

24.3 Modes of Communication with Patients

Once registered at their chosen clinic they will receive correspondence confirming the appointments. Pre-consultation paperwork, complete the medical history questionnaire online, pay invoices and upload of any previous test results or fertility clinic notes direct to their clinic for the doctor to view should be facilitated to allow the clinic to discuss the best course or courses of treatment.

As an overview, patient portals may be used to:

- Complete initial medical questionnaires
- View appointments
- Pay bills
- View account or request copies
- Receive information notifications
- Set notification preferences and partner access
- Receive Embryoscope videos
- Watch Injection Teach videos
- View documents
- Online forms
- Important messaging
- Upload files

24.4 Funding Treatment

Fertility treatment can be expensive and patients will need to consider what the best option for them would be. Some clinics can provide fertility treatment for patients who are eligible for NHS funding or have insurance policies. Alternatively, patients can pay for private treatment or use specialist IVF treatment packages, and some clinics offer an element of refund if treatment is unsuccessful.

24.5 During IVF Treatment

Medical practitioners will provide a treatment plan after the patient has signed their treatment consents. These are signed electronically after viewing some education modules online.

Medication can be ordered and often delivered to the patient's home address on a time and day that suits them best or the patient may choose a private prescription so they can source medications themselves.

Day 1 is normally the first day of the patient's menstrual cycle. Nursing teams will help show the patient how to safely administer their medication and ensure they feel confident with their proposed treatment plan.

For IVF, ovarian stimulant is performed through medications to maximise the number of eggs produced. This phase is closely monitored and reviewed through trans vaginal scans and normally lasts between 3–7 days but this can vary depending on the individual. The nurse will give instruction to the patient to administer an injection of a hormone called human chorionic gonadotrophin (HCG) that helps the egg to mature. This instruction will give the patient a very specific time on when to administer it. The eggs will be collected 36 hours after this medication.

Patients may be given sedation or anaesthesia to make sure the procedure is as comfortable as possible and eggs are routinely collected vaginally. The whole procedure takes less than 30 minutes and involves a small needle being passed through the vagina under ultrasound guidance. Eggs are extracted from the ovarian follicles and passed directly to an embryologist who will look after the eggs from this point. They are placed in a special culture medium. 8–14 are the average number of eggs collected. The patient will be looked after in a quiet day ward to recover. There are always plenty of tea and biscuits! Patients can go home the same day with supervision for 24 hours post sedation.

Behind the scenes, in the laboratory the eggs are mixed with the partners sperm or donor sperm to fertilise and then placed into specialist incubators. Patients can choose to access adjuvant treatments such as time lapse embryo imaging, this provides embryologists with far more information to help the selection process. An embryologist will continue to keep the patient informed of the development of their embryos which can unsurprisingly be a tense time in their treatment.

Embryo transfer is typically arranged on either day 3 or day 5. This is a straightforward procedure taking approximately 15 minutes with no need for sedation. A speculum (similar to the one used in routine smear tests) and a fine catheter containing the embryo is placed through the vagina and cervix and into the womb. The embryo is injected and the catheter removed. A check is done under microscope of the catheter to check the transfer was successful. The patient is advised to rest in the day ward post transfer and discharged same day.

24.6 The Two-Week Wait

This is often described as the hardest part of the IVF journey. It can be a very challenging and anxious time as patients wait before they can test to find out the outcome of their treatment. Patients are provided with a specific date to test on and it is strongly advised they do not test earlier than this date. Patients may require support during these difficult weeks – for example, a patient forum where patients can talk to others at the same stage of treatment.

Test result days are full of emotion and many staff report to have cried with patients in both joy and sadness. It can be the toughest moment for both parties as the clinical wants treatments to be successful for all their patients, whilst some patients will have the devastating moments when the results of the treatment were not what they hoped for.

If the biochemical test result after embryo transfer is positive an ultrasound scan will be booked for approximately 4 weeks later where a nurse sonographer can check for that amazing heartbeat – undoubtedly the best moment ever for patients at this stage. On the other hand, if the test is negative or the pregnancy is not ongoing the clinic offer counselling appointments and further support. A consultation with their fertility doctor is also offered when the patient is ready to review their treatment and discuss potential next steps. Some patients prefer to have some time and space but others wish to see their doctor as soon as possible. Clinics should let patients guide them on this and the clinic should do everything they can to accommodate their patient's needs during this difficult time.

24.7 Patient Support

The fertility treatment journey can be emotionally and physically challenging but also very personal. Whilst some patients choose to lean on friends and families for support, many patients who for different reasons decide to keep their treatment private. Many therefore, look to their own fertility clinic for support. An excellent support networks for patients will sometimes set clinics apart from others. Nobody undergoing treatment should feel alone or isolated.

Some great examples of patient support;

24.7.1 Fertility Support Events

Informal events accessible to all patients regardless of their stage of treatment. These are hosted online with occasionally some extra special events in person called "walk and talks" to provide face to face meetings.

24.7.2 Buddy Systems

Patients can be matched at a similar stage of treatment to share stories and provide friendship.

24.7.3 Forums

A safe space providing love and support, reminding each other of their amazing strength and helping people through their darkest times but also celebrating great success. These forums are free to join, hugely popular and can be a very special place.

Talking to people going through a similar treatment offers more than friends or loved ones can provide as the forum is full of likeminded people who can relate to each other.

24.7.4 Support Counselling

Every journey is different, it is important to ensure every patient has access to an experienced counsellor if and when they need them. This service is usually free of charge and unlimited. This form of therapy can be a great way to understand and process emotions.

Counselling is a talking therapy which allows sharing feelings in a confidential and safe environment. It can help people through the ups and downs of fertility treatment, providing support at critical times.

Patients may also reach out for guidance on adapting to parenthood. After struggling to conceive, a much longed for baby can be a huge change to their life. Sometimes patients make the difficult decision to stop their treatment, either to take a break, continue life childless or explore other paths to parenthood. Specialist fertility counsellors can help through all stages of fertility treatment and decisions.

Every session is completely confidential, unless:

- There are any concerns about the welfare of any children that might be born as a result of treatment, in which case the counsellor will speak to a member of the medical team with consent
- The counsellor has reason to believe there might be a risk of harm to the patient or others
- It's a clinic requirement as part of surrogacy or known donation treatment (this applies to implication counselling only)

24.8 Concluding Thoughts on Creating Families

Anybody who works in the IVF world or anyone who has a friend, relative or work colleague who has had treatment will appreciate the rollercoaster each patient will go through to enable them to become a parent. Whilst many are successful, with 1000's of babies born through IVF every year there will be many who despite the very best efforts of their clinic will not get the precious outcome they have tried so desperately to create. Fertility clinics worldwide continue and strive to obtain the very best success rates for their patients through continued research and best practice.

25

Non-Invasive Markers of Gamete and Embryo Quality

Catherine Pretty

25.1 Introduction

The main goal of any embryologist is to create and select the embryo for treatment which has the very best potential for implantation and success. The ability to choose this embryo without the need for invasive techniques is a gold standard in patient care, with the ability to maximise implantation potential without risking damage to the embryo itself. Selection and use of the best gametes to create this embryo will naturally lead to increased success rates and shorten the time to pregnancy for patients.

Usually, the prediction of success from individual oocytes is likely to be less clinically useful than selection of the most competent spermatozoon, since common clinical practice is to utilize all available oocytes, yet in the majority of cycles there will be some ability to select for the highest quality sperm to be used. Despite this, there is strong interest in prediction of success from both gametes as well as early embryo development, both for clinical decision-making during the course of treatment, and to aid appropriate counselling and to manage expectations of the patient.

In this chapter, those tools in the embryologist's arsenal which do not involve direct manipulation or sampling of the embryo will be explored. These include traditional methods of embryo selection such as observation of morphology, and more recent techniques such as timelapse imaging, secretomics, and non-invasive genetic testing of embryos.

Techniques can be broadly grouped into those involving advances in microscopy; those involving developments in machine learning and artificial intelligence (AI) to analyse existing data; techniques analysing the biochemical activity of the embryo; and attempts to determine the genetic profile of the embryo without removing cells from the embryo itself.

25.2 Traditional and Timelapse Observations

For many years the main selection criteria for embryos was the morphological grade of that embryo at specific timepoints, during early cleavage or at the point of blastocyst development. Clear, regular cellular division occurring on the expected day of development, without the presence of fragmentation, is a positive indicator of embryo quality. Likewise, a high-quality blastocyst with a high probability of implantation will have many contiguous cells in the trophectoderm, and a clearly defined, cohesive, inner cell mass.

More recently, timelapse imaging of embryos has developed into a routinely used technique, where the benefits of stable culture conditions are combined with the ability to observe the developing embryo in minute detail. The advance of embryo morphokinetics and the ability to "timestamp" points of development to predict implantation potential make this a very powerful tool (**1**). Both of these techniques can be considered "noninvasive", but are covered extensively elsewhere in this book so will only briefly be discussed in this chapter.

The main advantages of these techniques are that they are both well established. They can be easily and quickly measured, recorded and communicated to patients. In the case of standard morphology grading there are no expensive or specific equipment requirements.

One significant downside of both of these tools is that they look only at the outward appearance of the embryo, there is little or no information on the functional ability of that embryo. In the case of morphology grading at the cleavage stage, the correlation between grade and implantation potential is limited. In the case of blastocysts, the advent of genetic testing shows us that many morphologically high-quality blastocysts are aneuploid or mosaic, with very low implantation potential. Conversely, most experienced embryologists will be aware of healthy live births from embryos that have been transferred with very poor morphology and where the patient has been counselled that the embryo is unlikely to result in a pregnancy.

Despite the best efforts of the embryology community, both morphology grading and even morphokinetic grade remain subjective. Practitioner to practitioner variation continues to be a challenge, and variation in development profiles in the different culture conditions present in different laboratories hampers the standardisation of these techniques. The more recent development of machine learning and use of AI to perform morphokinetic grading may be a way to reduce or even remove bias, and to standardise and improve the outcomes of this technology.

25.3 Use of Machine Learning and Artificial Intelligence

The use of AI has permeated many branches of modern medicine, and assisted reproduction is no exception. The use of machine learning to observe large datasets and to predict outcomes is doubtless one of the fastest developing branches of reproductive technology at present (**2**).

DOI: 10.1201/9781003269502-25

To develop an AI tool, the computer is typically trained with data of known values, followed by a validation process using unseen data. There is huge potential for the use of AI in assisted reproduction, but there may be many potential pitfalls in this process, and the quality of the model developed will depend on the size and quality of the original data, which should be unbiased and based on balanced data from a variety of scenarios. When AI tools are optimized, they have the potential to remove operator bias, to speed up decision-making and to improve patient outcomes.

There are examples of AI tools being used in almost all aspects of the fertility journey from initial prognosis (**3**); management of ovarian stimulation (**4**); selection of sperm for ICSI (**5**); determination of oocyte maturity and to predict ICSI injection location (**6**) and classification of fertilisation (**7**). Assessment of early embryonic development and prediction of blastocyst formation may be improved by the use of AI instead of traditional manual observations of the embryo (**8, 9**). Embryo ranking by AI is being developed in several different respects, including auto annotation of time lapse images, grading embryos based on static images, and prediction of ploidy status based on images of the embryo (**10**).

Many of these applications are still in their infancy, but there can be little doubt that routine embryology procedures and quality control processes will be enhanced in many ways by the use of AI in the future (**11**).

25.4 Microscopic Advances

The use of bright field and polarized microscopes has long been routine in assisted reproduction. These techniques are fundamental for their ability to observe living cells while preserving their viability for treatment. Newer developments in microscopy include technologies such as polarised microscopy, holographic microscopy and inverted light-sheet microscopy.

Polarised microscopy allows the visualization of structures that are not accessible using standard microscopic techniques. It has been used for many years to increase our understanding of intracellular structures and processes, while more recently it has been used specifically to observe human gametes (**12**). The ability of polarised microscopy to visualise the spindle within the human oocyte allows the observer an insight into the timing of the cell cycle (**13**) and the location of the spindle in relation to the extruded polar body (**14**). The impact of the presence and location of the spindle in relation to clinical outcomes is controversial, but a 2009 meta-analysis of the literature concluded that overall, the presence of a detectable spindle was a positive prognostic indicator for treatment outcome (**15**).

There have been several studies using polarising microscopy to observe the zona pellucida for birefringence properties in an attempt to predict potential for blastulation and ultimately clinical outcome, but further studies are required to determine whether this will become a valuable clinical tool (**12**). Similarly, studies have suggested that the selection of sperm showing birefringence under polarised microscopy may allow for selection of the best sperm for ICSI (**16**) although further work will be needed before this becomes part of clinical practice.

There are other forms of label-free microscopy available to the reproductive scientist (**17**) including confocal Raman spectroscopy (CRS); fluorescence lifetime imaging (FLIM) and gradient light interference microscopy (GLIM). The FLIM technique is able to observe the natural fluorescence of molecules within the cell in order to evaluate the metabolic competence of the cell. Using GLIM the authors hope to visualise intracellular structures within the living oocyte or embryo (**18**). Both of these techniques show promise in understanding the early development of the embryo, and may have clinical purpose in the future.

The technique of light-sheet microscopy is particularly suited to observation of the embryo due to the low light doses required for the technique. Using this method, a three-dimensional time-lapse image may be generated of the embryo through different stages of development (**19**). Following mouse embryos from zygote to blastocyst has allowed these authors to track all cells and construct a lineage tree of the pre-implantation development.

The main advantages of these novel microscopy techniques will be the insight that they give the embryologist into the internal structure and viability of the gametes and embryos that they culture. However, these techniques may require expensive equipment and specialist training that may not be available to the standard clinical IVF laboratory. Further work will doubtless occur to determine which aspects of these techniques have the potential to become a routine tool in the life of a clinical embryologist.

25.5 Intracytoplasmic Morphologically Selected Sperm Injection (IMSI)

The technique of IMSI is a promising method of selecting sperm to use for intracytoplasmic sperm injection (ICSI). IMSI involves a process known as motile sperm organelle morphology examination (MSOME) which allows the scientist to evaluate the morphology of the sperm with a high level of detail in real time (**20**) before using that sperm for treatment. In standard ICSI techniques, sperm will typically be examined at up to x400 magnification, while in contrast using MSOME the sperm are magnified up to x6600 allowing the embryologists to select sperm showing good morphology and in particular those with an intact nucleus (**21**).

Technical advantages of the IMSI technique are clear, the embryologist is able to see with great detail the sperm nucleus, presence or absence of vacuoles in the sperm head, and can observe the general morphology of the sperm with confidence and precision. However, the clinical advantage of this technique has proved rather more controversial. In the general population of male-factor patients there is limited evidence for an increased rate of clinical pregnancy when using IMSI rather than standard ICSI (**22, 23**).

There may be sub-groups of the patient population where IMSI may potentially be of more benefit, these may include patients with at least two previous failed cycles of ICSI (**24**), patients with high levels of sperm DNA fragmentation (**25**), those with azoospermia (**26**) or those with advanced paternal age (**27**). There are suggestions that the percentage of euploid blastocysts created with IMSI may be higher than that created by conventional ICSI (**28**) while another study found little difference in this parameter despite improvements in other laboratory and clinical outcomes (**29**). Other studies have shown little difference in clinical outcome for patients in these categories (**30**) and the role for IMSI in improving clinical pregnancy rates remains controversial (**31**).

Two clear downsides of the technique of IMSI remain the specialist equipment required to enlarge the image of the sperm up to the required x6600 magnification, and the time taken to analyse and process the sample. All aspects of clinical embryology are time-dependent and ICSI is no exception. There may be additional challenges to both the embryology work force and to the cultured oocytes caused by the time taken to analyse a sperm sample for IMSI. Finally, due to the time-intensive nature of the technique, there will usually be an increased cost to the patient paying for their treatment.

The HFEA (the regulatory body of the fertility sector in the UK) has given IMSI an overall traffic light rating of "red", stating that there is no evidence from randomized control trials to show that it is effective at improving the chances of having a baby for most fertility patients.

25.6 Analysis of Spent Culture Media

The potential to obtain information from the spent culture media (SCM) surrounding the developing blastocyst is a fascinating one. Differentiating between two blastocysts of similar grade is one of the recurrent challenges of the clinical embryologist so any additional information may be extremely valuable.

By studying the nutrients taken up by the developing embryo, or the secretions of that embryo, researchers hope to provide a quantitative measure able to predict the implantation potential of that embryo. By testing the culture media after a period of embryo development, the risk of stress or damage to any developing embryo is minimised. By studying the metabolic activity of the embryo, genetic, epigenetic and environment aspects of development may all be included in the assessment of the embryo, taking this field further than the analysis provided by pre-implantation genetic testing of chromosomes alone.

Of course, any assessment of spent culture media would require individual embryo culture, (which may require additional consumable and equipment resources than embryo co-culture), and technology able to interpret the data thus generated. However, many laboratories consider this to be a standard culture method for embryos in order to allow tracking of development so this should not prove a barrier to adopting these techniques if they should become clinically proven.

The study of extra-embryonic compounds in the SCM is known as the field of secretomics, and includes a number of "-omic" sub-fields. Studying aspects of the embryo through from the genetic control of the cell through to the metabolic fingerprint of that cell, these fields include genomics (the study of the genome); transcriptomics (study of mRNA and non-coding RNAs); proteomics (the study of the enzymes and other proteins secreted by the embryo) and metabolomics (the study of metabolites secreted by the embryo).

The use of high-throughput technology to assay a multitude of factors, and to do so during the timeframe required for fresh embryo transfer, may be a valuable adjunct to morphological assessment alone. A number of biomarkers have been assessed for their potential to predict clinical outcomes, but evidence is yet unclear and further work is required (**32**). The assessment of spent culture media generally falls into two categories, the identification and measurement of specific biomarkers, or the analysis of the overall spectral pattern in comparison to a gold-standard scenario.

Some studies have been promising in their suggestion that implantation potential may be predicted by these techniques. As an example, one study using high-performance liquid chromatography (HPLC) to study the amino acid profile of embryo culture medium was able to differentiate embryos that later implanted from those that did not, with high accuracy (**33**) Other markers may include soluble human leukocyte antigen G (sHLA-G) which may be at a higher concentration in the culture media of embryos destined for implantation (**34**). Additional studies looked at the presence and concentration of proteins such as interleukin 6 (IL 6) together with timelapse analysis of the developing embryo to develop a hierarchic model with different categories relating to increasing implantation potential (**35**).

In contrast to these studies of individual substances, wider assays covering the metabolome or proteome are not restricted to specific biomarkers. Although these studies may be in their infancy, with improvements in computational technology and the ability to process large quantities of data quickly, these may yet prove extremely valuable (**32, 36**). Of course, hurdles to this technology include the variability in composition of commercial culture media and differences in laboratory conditions which may affect both the embryo and the assay itself (**37**). However, these promising early studies on small numbers of embryos show the potential of this field of research, although there is clearly further work to be done before the full potential of secretomics is realised.

25.7 Non-Invasive PGT-A

Pre-implantation genetic testing (PGT) of embryos can reveal their chromosomal number and test for certain severe genetic conditions, improving clinical success rates and supporting the development of a healthy pregnancy. However, in order to perform these tests, a biopsy must be removed from the trophectoderm of the developing blastocyst to be tested for ploidy or genetic status. Although this biopsy typically contains just 3–5 cells, the procedure is necessarily invasive and, in some cases, may stress the blastocyst, or even compromise embryo viability. If reliable genetic testing could be performed without need to manipulate the blastocyst, it would open up the field of reproductive genetics further and with less risk or expense. The need for advanced and expensive equipment and for highly trained biopsy practitioners is a significant factor in the access to (and pricing of) PGT in assisted reproduction.

The concept of non-invasive pre-implantation genetic testing (niPGT) is a relatively new field of study, but the appeal is clear. If quantities of extra-embryonic DNA can be obtained for testing, this could provide valuable information regarding the ploidy status of the embryo. Of course, as with secretomics, this method would require single embryo culture, but again this is routine in many clinical IVF laboratories, and if not, could be implemented relatively easily. As well as the reduced price and the decreased need for training and equipment for niPGT, there may be less practitioner-to-practitioner variation when sampling extra-embryonic DNA in comparison to performing an embryo biopsy.

Traditional methods of embryo biopsy such as polar body removal or cleavage-stage biopsy have now typically been replaced by the removal of a group of trophectoderm cells at the blastocyst stage. This allows a greater yield of genetic material while removing a much lower percentage of the total cell number from within the embryo. In turn, this reduces the risk of failure of DNA amplification (and the risk that no result will be obtained) in comparison to testing one or two cells at the cleavage stage, while retaining the implantation potential of the remaining embryo. Another significant advantage of this testing of multiple cells is the reduction in the effect of possible mosaicism on the quality of the results obtained. It is now well understood that there may be different populations of cells with different ploidy states within the developing blastocyst, and that this may be a normal part of embryo development. By testing multiple cells, the ability to detect mosaicism, while avoiding discarding embryos as aneuploid when euploid cells are also present, is greatly increased.

Conversely, when too many cells are removed, we may increase the accuracy of the genetic testing at the cost of causing stress and potential damage to the remaining embryo, decreasing overall implantation rate (**38**). If it was possible to test the overall genetic complement of the blastocyst in its entirety, without the need for taking any biopsied cells, this would truly be the best of both worlds.

A second major advantage of niPGT over traditional methods of biopsy would be that even poorer grade blastocysts could be included in analysis. Blastocysts with a low grade trophectoderm containing fewer cells may not be suitable for successful trophectoderm biopsy, but may yet be euploid and capable of implantation. If there was a way to safely analyse these then the pool of available embryos for transfer may be increased.

There has been considerable interest in the extra-embryonic DNA found within the blastocoel cavity itself. As the blastocyst develops and expands to fill (and eventually expand) the zona pellucida, the movement of water through transmembrane channels in the trophectoderm leads to the formation of a fluid-filled blastocoel cavity. Among a variety of proteins (**39**) this fluid has also been shown to contain DNA (**40**) which in some cases can be amplified and which may be suitable for genetic testing. Whilst the removal of this fluid (a technique sometimes known as "blastocentesis") is not strictly non-invasive, it is certainly easier and quicker to perform than a traditional biopsy of trophectoderm cells. The method involves inserting an ICSI pipette through the trophectoderm layer (away from the inner cell mass) and aspirating the fluid carefully from within the embryo. This technique may mimic the natural collapse and re-expansion of the blastocyst that is seen during the time prior to the blastocyst hatching (**41**). Indeed, many laboratories may perform this technique routinely, prior to vitrification of the blastocyst in an attempt to maximise post-thaw survival (**42**).

There have been some promising studies looking at the extra-embryonic DNA obtained by blastocentesis. Some studies have been able to obtain DNA from a large proportion of the blastocysts tested, and have shown a high concordance with the result of polar body or blastomere biopsy of the same embryo (**43**). In contrast, other groups have found that not only was it more challenging to obtain results, but that those results did not show acceptable concordance rates with embryo biopsy (**44**). DNA in the blastocoel cavity may already be subject to degradation, making it significantly harder to be amplified and detected (**45**). However, there is also a risk (as with traditional cellular biopsy) that lysis of the cells during the process of blastocentesis may cause the leakage of DNA into the cavity prior to sampling, which may affect the quality of the results.

Rather than piercing the blastocyst to obtain fluid for testing, a truly non-invasive technique would be the testing SCM for the presence of extra-embryonic DNA. Some studies are promising in the percentage of samples that yielded DNA suitable for analysis by this method (**46**) while other groups showed more limited concordance (**47**). There are suggestions that these studies may be limited by sample number and variability of study design as well as challenges in amplification techniques (**45**).

Combining the two techniques of SCM analysis and blastocentesis in one test may give a multi-faceted approach and improve concordance with the results of trophectoderm biopsy (**48**). Ultimately, the success of both blastocoel and SCM analysis of cell-free DNA will only be successful if this DNA is genuinely reflective of the blastocyst preparing for implantation. If DNA has been released from cells through the processes of apoptosis or necrosis, then the results thus obtained may reflect a subset of the cells no longer contained within the viable embryo. It has long been hypothesised that apoptosis may be involved in the elimination of abnormal cells and may play a fundamental part in normal embryo development (**49**). However, successful concordance between traditional biopsy and spent culture medium has been obtained for both euploid and aneuploid embryos (**50, 51**), which indicates that there are alternative sources for this cell-free DNA other than apoptotic cells.

Finally, there are the prospects of maternal contamination of SCM through the secretions of cumulus cells, paternal contamination via the sperm cells, and the possibility of DNA contamination via the labware or culture media (**52**). Excellent controls and confirmation of the source of DNA would be required before any of these tests can become clinically useful. Despite the challenges facing the development of niPGT, with optimization of analysis and further understanding of the source of extra-embryonic DNA this may be a fascinating field of research and a tool for better understanding the developing embryo.

25.8 Summary

In conclusion, there are several promising fields of study for selection of gametes and embryos in a non-invasive manner. Developments in microscopy, technology, artificial intelligence and processing of information have opened up fascinating new fields of study in assisted reproduction. Further study will be required to determine which of these will become routine clinical technologies and which may remain interesting fields of study, but which may not become part of the patient treatment pathway.

REFERENCES

1. Campbell A, Fishel S, Bowman N, et al. Modelling a risk classification of aneuploidy in human embryos using non-invasive morphokinetics. *Reprod Biomed Online*. 2013;26(5):477–485.
2. Curchoe CL, Bormann CL. Artificial intelligence and machine learning for human reproduction and embryology presented at ASRM and ESHRE 2018. *J Assist Reprod Genet*. 2019;36(4):591–600.
3. Liao S, Pan W, Dai WQ, et al. Development of a dynamic diagnosis grading system for infertility using machine learning. *JAMA Netw Open*. 2020;3(11).
4. Letterie G, Mac Donald A. Artificial intelligence in in vitro fertilization: a computer decision support system for day-to-day management of ovarian stimulation during in vitro fertilization. *Fertil Steril*. 2020;114(5):1026–1031.
5. Mendizabal-Ruiz G, Chavez-Badiola A, Figueroa IA, et al. Computer software (SiD) assisted real-time single sperm selection associated with fertilization and blastocyst formation. *Reprod Biomed Online*. 2022;45(4):703–711.
6. Dickinson I, Meyer A, Kelly N, et al. Advancement in the future automation of ICSI: use of deep convolutional neural networks (CNN) to identify precise location to inject sperm in mature human oocytes. *Hum Reprod*. 2020;35:70–71.
7. Dimitriadis I, Bormann CL, Kanakasabapathy MK, et al. Deep convolutional neural networks (CNN) for assessment and selection of normally fertilized human embryos. *Fertil Steril*. 2019;112(3):e272.
8. Coticchio G, Fiorentino G, Nicora G, et al. Cytoplasmic movements of the early human embryo: imaging and artificial intelligence to predict blastocyst development. *Reprod Biomed Online*. 2021 Mar 1;42(3):521–528.
9. Campbell A, Nayot D, Krivoi A, et al. Independent assessment of an artificial intelligence based image analysis tool to predict fertilisation and blastocyst utilisation potential of oocytes, and comparison with ten expert embryologists. *Hum Fertil*. 2021;24(1):46–69.
10. Chavez-Badiola A, Flores-Saiffe-Farías A, Mendizabal-Ruiz G, et al. Embryo ranking intelligent classification algorithm (ERICA): artificial intelligence clinical assistant predicting embryo ploidy and implantation. *Reprod Biomed Online*. 2020;41(4):585–593.
11. Dimitriadis I, Zaninovic N, Badiola AC, et al. Artificial intelligence in the embryology laboratory: a review. *Reprod Biomed Online*. 2022;44(3):435–448.
12. Montag M, Köster M, van der Ven K, et al. Gamete competence assessment by polarizing optics in assisted reproduction. *Hum Reprod Update*. 2011;17(5):654–666.
13. Montag M, Schimming T, van der Ven H. Spindle imaging in human oocytes: the impact of the meiotic cell cycle. *Reprod Biomed Online*. 2006;12(4):442–446.
14. Rienzi L, Ubaldi F, Martinez F, et al. Relationship between meiotic spindle location with regard to the polar body position and oocyte developmental potential after ICSI. *Hum Reprod*. 2003;18(6):1289–1293.
15. Petersen CG, Oliveira JB, Mauri AL, et al. Relationship between visualization of meiotic spindle in human oocytes and ICSI outcomes: a meta-analysis. *Reprod Biomed Online*. 2009;18(2):235–243.
16. Gianaroli L, Magli MC, Ferraretti AP, et al. Birefringence characteristics in sperm heads allow for the selection of reacted spermatozoa for intracytoplasmic sperm injection. *Fertil Steril*. 2010;93(3):807–813.
17. Rubessa M, Wheeler MB. Label-free microscopy: a non-invasive new tool to assess gametes and embryo quality. *Theriogenology*. 2020;150:241–246.
18. Nguyen TH, Kandel ME, Rubessa M, et al. Gradient light interference microscopy for 3D imaging of unlabeled specimens. *Nat Commun*. 2017;8(1):1–9.
19. Strnad P, Gunther S, Reichmann J, et al. Inverted light-sheet microscope for imaging mouse pre-implantation development. *Nat Methods*. 2016;13(2):139–142.
20. Nadalini M, Tarozzi N, Distratis V, et al. Impact of intracytoplasmic morphologically selected sperm injection on assisted reproduction outcome: a review. *Reprod Biomed Online*. 2009;19:45–55.
21. Bartoov B, Berkovitz A, Eltes F. Selection of spermatozoa with normal nuclei to improve the pregnancy rate with intracytoplasmic sperm injection. *NEJM*. 2001;345 (14):1067–1068.
22. He F, Wang MJ, Li SL, et al. IMSI versus ICSI for male factor infertility: a meta-analysis. *Zhonghua nan ke xue [Natl J Androl]*. 2018;24(3):254–262.
23. Leandri RD, Gachet A, Pfeffer J, et al. Is intracytoplasmic morphologically selected sperm injection (IMSI) beneficial in the first ART cycle? a multicentric randomized controlled trial. *Andrology*. 2013;1(5):692–697.
24. Bartoov B, Berkovitz A, Eltes F, et al. Pregnancy rates are higher with intracytoplasmic morphologically selected sperm injection than with conventional intracytoplasmic injection. *Fertil Steril*. 2003;80(6):1413–1419.
25. Hammoud I, Boitrelle F, Ferfouri F, et al. Selection of normal spermatozoa with a vacuole-free head (x6300) improves selection of spermatozoa with intact DNA in patients with high sperm DNA fragmentation rates. *Andrologia*. 2013;45(3):163–170.
26. Ai L, Liu SY, Huang J, et al. Intracytoplasmic morphologically selected sperm injection of testicular sperm: clinical outcome in azoospermia patients. *Zhonghua nan ke xue [Natl J Androl]*. 2010;16(9):826–829.
27. Silva LF, Oliveira JB, Petersen CG, et al. The effects of male age on sperm analysis by motile sperm organelle morphology examination (MSOME). *Reprod Biol Endocrinol*. 2012;10(1):1–10.
28. Rita de Cássia SF, Braga DP, Setti AS, et al. Morphological nuclear integrity of sperm cells is associated with preimplantation genetic aneuploidy screening cycle outcomes. *Fertil Steril*. 2011;95(3):990–993.
29. Luna D, Hilario R, Dueñas-Chacón J, et al. The IMSI procedure improves laboratory and clinical outcomes without

compromising the aneuploidy rate when compared to the classical ICSI procedure. *Clin Med Insights: Reprod Health.* 2015;9:CMRH-S33032.

30. Gatimel N, Parinaud J, Leandri RD. Intracytoplasmic morphologically selected sperm injection (IMSI) does not improve outcome in patients with two successive IVF-ICSI failures. *J Assist Reprod Genet.* 2016;33(3):349–355.
31. Teixeira DM, Miyague AH, Barbosa MA, et al. Regular (ICSI) versus ultra-high magnification (IMSI) sperm selection for assisted reproduction. *Cochrane Database Syst Rev.* 2020;2(2):CD010167.
32. Bracewell-Milnes T, Saso S, Abdalla H, et al. Metabolomics as a tool to identify biomarkers to predict and improve outcomes in reproductive medicine: a systematic review. *Hum Reprod Update.* 2017;23(6):723–736.
33. Huo P, Zhu Y, Liang C, et al. Non-invasive amino acid profiling of embryo culture medium using HPLC correlates with embryo implantation potential in women undergoing in vitro fertilization. *Front Physiol.* 2020;11:405.
34. Díaz RR, Zamora RB, Sánchez RV, et al. Embryo sHLA-G secretion is related to pregnancy rate. *Zygote.* 2019;27(2):78–81.
35. Dominguez F, Meseguer M, Aparicio-Ruiz B, et al. New strategy for diagnosing embryo implantation potential by combining proteomics and time-lapse technologies. *Fertil Steril.* 2015;104(4):908–914.
36. Bori L, Dominguez F, Fernandez EI, et al. An artificial intelligence model based on the proteomic profile of euploid embryos and blastocyst morphology: a preliminary study. *Reprod Biomed Online.* 2021;42(2):340–350.
37. Zmuidinaite R, Sharara FI, Iles RK. Current advancements in noninvasive profiling of the embryo culture media secretome. *Int J Mol Sci.* 2021;22(5):2513.
38. Neal SA, Franasiak JM, Forman EJ, et al. High relative deoxyribonucleic acid content of trophectoderm biopsy adversely affects pregnancy outcomes. *Fertil Steril.* 2017;107(3):731–736.
39. Jensen PL, Beck HC, Petersen J, et al. Proteomic analysis of human blastocoel fluid and blastocyst cells. *Stem cells Dev.* 2013;22(7):1126–1135.
40. Palini S, Galluzzi L, De Stefani S, et al. Genomic DNA in human blastocoele fluid. *Reprod Biomed Online.* 2013;26(6):603–610.
41. Bodri D, Sugimoto T, Serna JY, et al. Blastocyst collapse is not an independent predictor of reduced live birth: a time-lapse study. *Fertil Steril.* 2016;105(6):1476–1483.
42. Desai N, Szeptycki J, Scott M, et al. Artificial collapse of blastocysts before vitrification: mechanical vs. laser technique and effect on survival, cell number, and cell death in early and expanded blastocysts. *Cell Preserv Technol.* 2008;6(3):181–190.
43. Gianaroli L, Magli MC, Pomante A, et al. Blastocentesis: a source of DNA for preimplantation genetic testing. Results from a pilot study. *Fertil Steril.* 2014;102(6):1692–1699.
44. Tobler KJ, Zhao Y, Ross R, et al. Blastocoel fluid from differentiated blastocysts harbors embryonic genomic material capable of a whole-genome deoxyribonucleic acid amplification and comprehensive chromosome microarray analysis. *Fertil Steril.* 2015;104(2):418–425.
45. Leaver M, Wells D. Non-invasive preimplantation genetic testing (niPGT): the next revolution in reproductive genetics? *Hum Reprod Update.* 2020;26(1):16–42.
46. Shamonki MI, Jin H, Haimowitz Z, Liu L. Proof of concept: preimplantation genetic screening without embryo biopsy through analysis of cell-free DNA in spent embryo culture media. *Fertil Steril.* 2016;106(6):1312–1318.
47. Liu W, Liu J, Du H, et al. Non-invasive pre-implantation aneuploidy screening and diagnosis of beta thalassemia IVSII654 mutation using spent embryo culture medium. *Ann Med.* 2017;49(4):319–328.
48. Li P, Song Z, Yao Y, et al. Preimplantation genetic screening with spent culture medium/blastocoel fluid for in vitro fertilization. *Sci Rep.* 2018;8(1):1–10.
49. Hardy K. Apoptosis in the human embryo. *Rev Reprod.* 1999;4:125–134.
50. Vera-Rodriguez M, Diez-Juan A, Jimenez-Almazan J, et al. Origin and composition of cell-free DNA in spent medium from human embryo culture during preimplantation development. *Fertil Steril.* 2018;33(4):745–756.
51. Rubio C, Rienzi L, Navarro-Sanchez L, et al. Origin and composition of cell-free DNA in spent medium from human embryo culture during preimplantation development. *Human Reprod.* 2019;112(3):510–519.
52. Hammond ER, McGillivray BC, Wicker SM, et al. Characterizing nuclear and mitochondrial DNA in spent embryo culture media: genetic contamination identified. *Fertil Steril.* 2017;107(1):220–228.

26

Embryo Transfer Procedures and Decisions

Kathryn Berrisford

Embryo transfer (ET) is the culmination of the IVF process and has remained largely unchanged since the birth of Louise Brown in 1978 by Steptoe and Edwards team. The first successful fertilisation of a human oocyte in vitro was 1969, human embryos were first transferred in 1971 and the first clinical pregnancy was recorded in 1975 (which ended in miscarriage).

The first ET took place on 12 December 1971, by trans-cervical procedure – a 16 cell embryo (80 post OR). 'Passage through the cervix was adopted as the method giving least trouble to the mother; a fine catheter of 2mm diameter was passed through the cervical canal in the uterine cavity and a smaller cannula containing the embryo was threaded through it' (**1–3**). There were a further 112 ETs between 1972 and 1978; of these 5 were via laparoscopy, one via mini-laparotomy. A GIFT (gamete intrafallopian transfer) was recorded in 1972 (gamete intra-fallopian transfer) and approximately 5 more in 1973; it seems that GIFT was considered as an option alongside IVF for a time, before concentrating solely on IVF. Number 81 ET was the transfer of an 8-cell embryo at midnight on 12 November 1977 (**2–4**).

Contained in the Steptoe and Edwards notebooks were a list of challenges to the IVF process and number 10 described the technical aspects of embryo transfer, including route of transfer, medium and timing (**2, 3**). Route of transfer seems to have been the easiest challenge to overcome, as evidence shows that trans-cervical transfer was chosen over laparoscopic (which would have been the chosen route for GIFT). Edwards gave more detail about the ET procedure in 1980 – 'A bi-valve speculum was passed with the patient in a modified lithotomy position . . . no instruments were attached to the cervix . . . the loaded cannula was passed through the cervix so that its end would lie in the body of the uterus about 1 cm from the fundus' (**5**).

The challenges of transfer medium and timing were more complex and even to this day still debated.

26.1 Timing of Embryo Transfer

26.1.1 Blastocyst Transfer

Primarily used in the UK since the HFEA implemented its minimisation of multiple birth strategy and as a consequence elective single ET. It is known from the literature that single blastocyst transfer has decreased the multiple birth rates without decreasing pregnancy rates overall. Additional benefits are higher implantation and live birth rates compared to cleavage-stage embryo transfer in good prognosis patients.

The principles behind the improved rates are two-fold –

1. Improved selection of viable embryos. Approx. 50% of cleavage-stage embryos become blastocysts, as the embryonic genome must be activated during early development (around day 3) for blastocyst development.
2. Improve embryonic and uterine synchronicity. In vivo implantation occurs 7–8 days post insemination and therefore cleavage-stage embryos (transferred to the uterus on day 2–3) will be exposed prematurely to the uterine environment, instead of the fallopian tubes. Blastocyst culture also offers time (minimum 48 hours) for the gonadotrophin induced raise in oestrogen levels after stimulation to subside.

26.1.2 Cleavage Stage Embryo Transfer

There is no robust evidence that blastocyst transfers always result in higher or equal cumulative pregnancy rates compared to cleavage-stage embryo transfers overall. Therefore, in poor prognosis patients' cleavage-stage embryo transfers may result in a higher implantation rate. This is most likely to be to increased cycle cancellation rates overall for blastocyst transfer. It cannot be definitively concluded that embryos that fail to blastulate in vitro, would also do so in vivo.

Further research is required to conclude the debate on ET timings. Areas of interest are looking at epigenetic changes in extended culture, is there an altered sex ratio (males: females) and an increase in preterm birth rates. Evidence of epigenetic changes in blastocyst culture is weak, and babies born after blastocyst transfer have a similar chance of being healthy as those born after cleavage-stage embryo transfer (**6**). However, cleavage-stage embryo transfer remains an option available for patients, particularly when very low number of viable embryos are obtained.

26.1.3 Fresh vs. Frozen

During a fresh stimulated cycle, due to down regulation there is a disruption in natural luteal support and therefore artificial support is required to allow implantation. The over physiological oestrogen levels from multi- follicular development leads to negative feedback on the pituitary to inhibit LH secretion. In vivo LH surge causes ovulation, where the follicle becomes the corpus luteum. LH acts on the granulosa cells to produce progesterone, which acts to aid secretory transformation

DOI: 10.1201/9781003269502-26

of the endometrium. Therefore, lack of LH leads to shorter luteal phase and reduced implantation. After implantation the embryo secretes hCG which acts on the corpus luteum to produce progesterone, until the placenta takes over (8–12 weeks after implantation).

Therefore, is it better to transfer the embryo in a natural cycle, with physiological luteal support? With the introduction of vitrification/warming pushing the embryo survival rates from 70% (with slow freezing embryos) to over 95%, this is a viable proposition. There is evidence to show that in ovulatory women there is an increased LBR when transferring SET (blastocyst) compared to fresh (**7, 8**). A Cochrane review in 2021 found LBR with eFER increased and that cumulative LBR was comparable. The risk of OHSS is decreased in the 'freeze all' category, but the risk of maternal hypertensive disorders of pregnancy and having a higher birth weight birth are higher. Risks of multiple pregnancy and miscarriage are comparable (**9**). Care fertility (own data) have found comparable LBR for fresh and frozen ETs and therefore introduced 'freeze all' strategies for PGT patients and those at risk of OHSS.

26.2 Embryo Assessment, Selection and Decision-Making

The gold standard embryo assessment since the 1970s for 40 plus years was embryo morphology. Daily embryo assessment in standard incubators from day 2 onwards. Many different grading systems were devised, all based around the correct stage of development for the day of culture and the level of fragmentation/cell integrity giving the embryo a grade.

26.2.1 Do Not Disturb (DND)

DND is an optimised standard incubation method where embryos are undisturbed during in vitro embryo culture. With standard incubation, daily assessment during early embryo development provides limited information. The decision as to which embryo to transfer is based most effectively, on the assessment of blastocysts, and not on the appearance of the embryos on preceding days.

The undisturbed incubation which is obtained with time lapse imaging provides a much more stable environment for embryo development. In addition, there is an array of technology (time lapse and algorithms, PGT-A) to select the embryo that gives the patient their very best chance of having a live birth.

26.2.2 Timelapse and CareMaps

Timelapse incubators have integrated cameras in them that capture up to 5000 images per zygote/embryo in single embryo culture compared to standard incubation, with 24 hourly observations (maximum 5). This has led to key timed events being determined by the embryologist and annotated on the image software. These key development events have then been linked to known implantation data (KID) and more recently known live birth outcome data to predict the potential of each embryo to become a live birth. CareMaps is the algorithm of this data that ranks the embryo's potential and has been reported to outperform standard morphology alone (**10, 11**).

26.2.3 PGT-A

Aneuploid blastocysts are indistinguishable from euploid blastocysts via normal embryo morphology. The ET of aneuploid blastocysts will result in implantation failure, miscarriage or much less likely, live births with chromosomal disorders (Trisomy 21 – Downs Syndrome, Trisomy 18 – Edwards Syndrome and Monosomy X – Turner Syndrome). The only way to confirm the ploidy status of a blastocyst is via PGT-A, which is discussed in a separate chapter.

26.2.4 The Future (Artificial Intelligence)

Artificial intelligence is well established in some areas of medicine and is beginning to be incorporated into several of the processes associated with IVF and patient management: AI to optimise ovarian stimulation, to detect sperm with high DNA integrity, to predict embryo viability (**11, 12**).

AI annotation is in development to be used directly by CareMaps to predict the potential of each embryo to become a live birth. CareMaps outperforms embryo selection by morphology alone. When AI annotation can be as good as manual annotation by an experienced embryologist, but it is consistent, without bias and available in seconds (therefore highly efficient and embryology time saving). It also contains deep learning to develop in a data rich environment to outperform manual annotation.

26.3 The Endometrium

Optimal timing for endometrial receptivity is an important part of the embryo transfer process resulting in success. Areas for consideration are the thickness and pattern of the endometrium, greater than 7mm thick and triple line, which have shown to improve implantation rates. There is evidence that progesterone luteal support given following natural cycle FER significantly improves implantation rate and live birth rate (**13, 14**). In addition, endometrial receptivity assays that looks at the gene expression signature of 248 genes in the endometrium so that the embryo transfer can be synchronized with the window of implantation have also been reported to improve clinical outcomes of IVF cycles (**15**). This is discussed in more detail in Chapter 14. Therefore, with all the effort and attention given to creating the best possible embryos, selection of embryo for transfer and creating the most viable endometrial receptivity for implantation of the blastocyst, the ultimate step in the process is the embryo transfer.

26.4 Training and Competency of Embryo Transfer Personnel

Following technical and theoretical training, competency assessment is undertaken prior to unsupervised practice associated with the standard operating procedure (SOP).

The training program for the embryo transfer process starts with observation and understanding of the procedure and why it is done the way it is – the theory behind the practice, followed by performing under close supervision (with the supervisor selecting and moving the embryo into the transfer dish and checking the expelled catheter post transfer). Competency sign off – when the practitioner and supervisor agree and the pregnancy rate is in line with the key performance indicator (KPI).

At this point the practitioner will be performing every step of the process –

Using clinical knowledge to select the most viable embryo for transfer, pipetting the embryo into the transfer dish. Loading the embryo into the catheter, handing and supporting the catheter whilst the clinician positions it in the uterine cavity and then under the clinician's instruction, plunging the syringe to expel the embryo into the cavity. Returning to the transfer dish and checking that the embryo has been expelled.

No unregistered practitioner should undertake clinical work without support and supervision by a fully trained State Registered Embryologist. Therefore, a pre – registrant practitioner can undertake the embryo transfer process once competency has been completed, with supervision provided to select the embryo for transfer (Table 26.1).

TABLE 26.1

Competency Assessment Protocols for Embryo Transfer

Task	**Embryo transfer**	
Description	**Embryologist**	**Evaluator**
Demonstrate effective oral, written, and non-verbal communication skills with colleagues and patients		
Maintain documentation and records		
Demonstrate critical judgment in professional practice		
Evaluate and address issues surrounding equipment application and/or operation. Participate in equipment preventative maintenance programs		
Perform embryo transfer procedure according to protocol		
Demonstrate that procedures are witnessed either manually or electronically at the appropriate steps in the procedure		
Clean and disinfect equipment. Apply infection prevention and control precautions		
Handle and dispose of biohazardous waste		
Use personal protective equipment		

Specific knowledge requirement for embryo transfer	**Evidence**	**Embryologist**	**Evaluator**
Lab SOP Embryo grading and embryo transfer	Read receipt		
Broad shoulders review	Completed proforma and report		

Embryologist and evaluator should initial the above boxes to confirm compliance with the description and knowledge requirements.

It is my opinion that ______________________________ may undertake independent work on this task as they have demonstrated the appropriate knowledge and experience for competency.

THIS COMPETENCY MUST BE REVIEWED IF THERE IS A SUBSTANTIAL CHANGE TO PROTOCOLS OR TASK KNOWLEDGE REQUIREMENTS

Evaluator's name
Signature
Date
Position

26.5 Problematic Embryo Transfers

Experience for live troubleshooting is necessary – common areas being an embryo returning in the catheter, requiring reloading and difficult transfers. Here is a list of tips and tricks to overcome difficult embryo transfers:

- The embryo should not be loaded into the catheter until the practitioner has indicated the embryologist to load – they need to ensure they can visualize the path of the catheter through to the uterine cavity.
- Cleaning of the cervix is an important part of the process, as any blood should be removed. If there is blood in the catheter, then this can introduce contamination into the cavity, which can cause uterine contractions.
- Ultrasound is used to visualise the echogenic ET catheter through the cervix, internal os, into the uterine cavity, so the embryo can be deposited a defined distance from the fundus, allowing uterine size and length of cervix to be taken into account. Touching the fundus with the catheter can cause uterine contractions.
- The practitioner may use a trail catheter or stylet, depending on how open the path is. Both of these have increasingly stiff outer sheaths, that make a more definite path to the cavity.
- This may take time if there is decreased uterine cavity visibility, which could be due to the bladder not being full enough, scarring/polyps or cysts in the uterus or surrounding it.
- If the practitioner is still struggling to enter the cavity once the embryo is loaded into the inner catheter, the embryo should be returned to the transfer dish, as a loaded catheter should not be using during attempts to enter the uterine cavity.
- There is risk to the embryo of being expelled or damaged during the attempts and also it will be losing temperature and therefore should be put back into the incubator.
- If there is mucus in the catheter, then this can introduce contamination into the cavity, which can cause uterine contractions.
- To maximise implantation rates, embryos must be transferred into the uterus in a gentle and controlled manner to minimize uterine contractions. Edwards et al. 1980 used Ritodrine/Indomethacin as a precaution against uterine contractions after the transcervical transfer.

26.5.1 Reloading

If the embryo has returned in the catheter or if the practitioner requires a stylet to gain access return the embryos to the dish whilst access is gained. When practitioner is ready – recharge the catheter with fresh ET media and reload – use a fresh catheter if necessary.

In some circumstance it may not be possible to perform the embryo transfer due to unexpected technical difficulty or if the patient has or is at risk of OHSS or is distressed. All suitable embryos must then be frozen for future use.

26.6 Embryo Transfer Catheters

Little has changed in the manufacturing of the embryo transfer catheter since Harry Wallace designed the original for Robert Edwards half a century ago. Typically, an embryo transfer catheter has two parts: a semi-rigid outer sheath and a more flexible inner sheath. The catheter must be constructed of material which is nontoxic and inert. However, there are a couple of exceptions to the original design which have improved outcomes: for example, embryo transfer catheters need to be narrow enough to negotiate the cervical external/internal os and safely enter the uterine cavity with minimum trauma but have an internal diameter that can comfortably contain the embryo. The catheter also needs to be long enough so that the operator can safely negotiate the passage of the catheter into the vagina, through the cervix and into the uterine cavity whilst essentially operating with their hands in close proximity to, but not inside the vagina.

Embryos are loaded into the more flexible inner catheter between two small volumes of culture medium. The inner catheter is attached to a small syringe which is used by the embryologist to suck up the embryo from the dish in which it is grown and into the tip of the catheter. The inner catheter is then threaded through the outer catheter making sure not to dislodge the syringe. The inner catheter normally protrudes one or two centimetres beyond the external catheter.

The assembled inner and outer sheaths together with the syringe are then handed to the operator who has placed a speculum into the vagina to optimize the view of the cervix. Some operators will remove superficial mucous from the cervical canal before threading the catheter safely and non-traumatically through the cervix. The tip of the catheter is then approximated to within one centimetre of the uterine fundus and once the operator is confident of its position, the embryo is gently expelled by pressure on the plunger of the syringe. The catheter is then swiftly but gently removed from the uterine cavity and handed back to the embryologist who then checks that the embryo has been safely expelled. This technique is known as the single or one step method of embryo transfer. Some operators prefer a two-step technique where the outer sheath of the transfer catheter is placed into the uterine cavity first and then the inner tube containing the embryo is threaded as a second stage into the outer sheath, the theory being to minimise trauma although neither technique has been shown to be superior in terms of outcome.

In a small but significant number of cases, the embryo transfer may be complicated by difficulty negotiating the cervix. For example, the cervical canal may be tight or even stenosed following previous surgery. In such cases, either a more rigid catheter can be used although this may add an additional risk of trauma to the cervix and poorer outcomes; or more commonly, an obturator or stylet is inserted into the outer sheath to confirm more rigidity to the catheter. Once the outer sheath is in situ, the obturator or stylet can be removed to allow the flexible inner sheath containing the embryo to be threaded through the outer sheath and into the uterine cavity with its tip protruding.

More recently, small modifications to the tips of catheters have been incorporated to facilitate the passage of the catheter into the uterus with varying degrees of success. However, a recent innovation has unequivocally improved outcomes to embryo transfer. The incorporation of ultrasonically visible air bubbles into the catheter and around the plastic tip has enabled the catheter to be visible ultrasonically during the process of embryo transfer. This allows the more accurate placement of the tip of the catheter at one centimetre from the uterine fundus before expulsion of the embryo. This in turn optimises the outcome and reduces the risk of the catheter tip being inadvertently placed against the uterine fundus which can cause additional unwanted trauma.

Although technically relatively simple, the art of embryo transfer is difficult to perfect. It is therefore essential that embryo transfer catheters are easy to use, are of high quality and are atraumatic. There also should be ultrasonically visible with the incorporation of a tailor-made obturator or stylet should the need arise.

26.7 Laboratory Process

Following fertilisation check, zygotes are cultured in individual microdrops in standard or timelapse culture. Patients are contacted following fertilisation assessment.

26.7.1 Standard Incubation

DND is used, embryos are assessed for ET on the day of transfer. If there is a low number of embryos (such that selection will not be required), or there is a history of poor or anomalous development, additional observations may be justified. There is insufficient data or evidence to confirm whether an early cleavage stage transfer is preferable to a blastocyst transfer – in such cases, an individualised plan should be made with the patient. Some patients will prefer to know whether the embryos have the capacity to reach the blastocyst stage, accepting the risk of not having an ET. Others will prefer to have an early embryo transfer regardless. Embryologists should consider previous treatment outcomes, and alongside the clinician, give a recommendation, which should be documented in the patient records.

26.7.2 CareMaps

Patients can be given updates from regular assessments made during annotation but, as the algorithms are applied prior to transfer, current standard practice is to contact them at fertilization and then prior to transfer on the day of ET.

On the day of ET, contact the patient to update on development, the embryos for ET may be selected at this time and the agreed number for transfer placed into the designated dish. The degree of fragmentation, morphology of the embryo (shape and form of the blastomeres and their cytoplasm) and time lapse annotation information if available should be considered when assessing the embryo quality and grading.

Day 4 ET: Embryos are observed approximately 96 hours post insemination, documenting cell number and grade, compaction if present. Morula grade 1 where all cells are included should be chosen for transfer over Morula grade 2 when no cavitating blastocyst are present. One/two most advanced and/or best quality day 4 embryo(s) for transfer are selected.

CareMaps has shown that embryos with earlier initiation of blastulation have the highest live birth potential. This time point may not be transferrable to standard incubation but performing the day 4 check later in the day will increase the chances of observing early cavitation and may help in identifying the most suitable embryo for transfer.

Day 5 ET: On day 5, stages of blastocyst development are documented. One/two most advanced blastocysts for transfer based on development and quality are selected. If there are no blastocysts on day 5 of culture, the ET may be performed on day 6. Care fertility wide results (internal data) show equivalence between day 4 and 5 ET.

26.7.3 Embryo Transfer Preparation

See Video 26.1 (Access the videos at www.routledge.com/9781032216577) and Figure 26.1.

Video 26.1 An Embryo Transfer Procedure Performed at CARE Nottingham

1. When the patient arrives to theatre, a patient identity check is carried out with the theatre team (nurse and practitioner) and the embryologist.
2. Electronic witnessing (or equivalent) is used to read the barcoded wristband/photo ID card and the barcode on the culture dish containing the embryos for transfer.
3. Move the ET dish into the mini-incubator within the flowhood (it must stay here for as long as possible before loading is instructed) and the ET medium tube to the tube warmer.
4. Open the catheter (once the practitioner has instructed), syringe and ET medium tube.
5. Move the ET dish under the microscope, ensure it is fully focused and remove the lid.
6. Without touching the outside of the sterile gloves, carefully put them on. (Powder free gloves can be used without washing).
7. Take care not to touch the medium or the tip of the catheter with gloves.
8. Connect the sterile 1ml syringe to the end of the inner catheter.
9. Aspirate medium from the tube into the syringe.
10. Tap the syringe until the medium falls to the top of the syringe barrel and all air bubbles have been removed.
11. Slowly push the medium out, keeping the syringe vertical until all the air bubbles have been expelled.
12. Push out the remaining medium until the top of the plunger reaches no less than 0.1ml marking on the syringe.

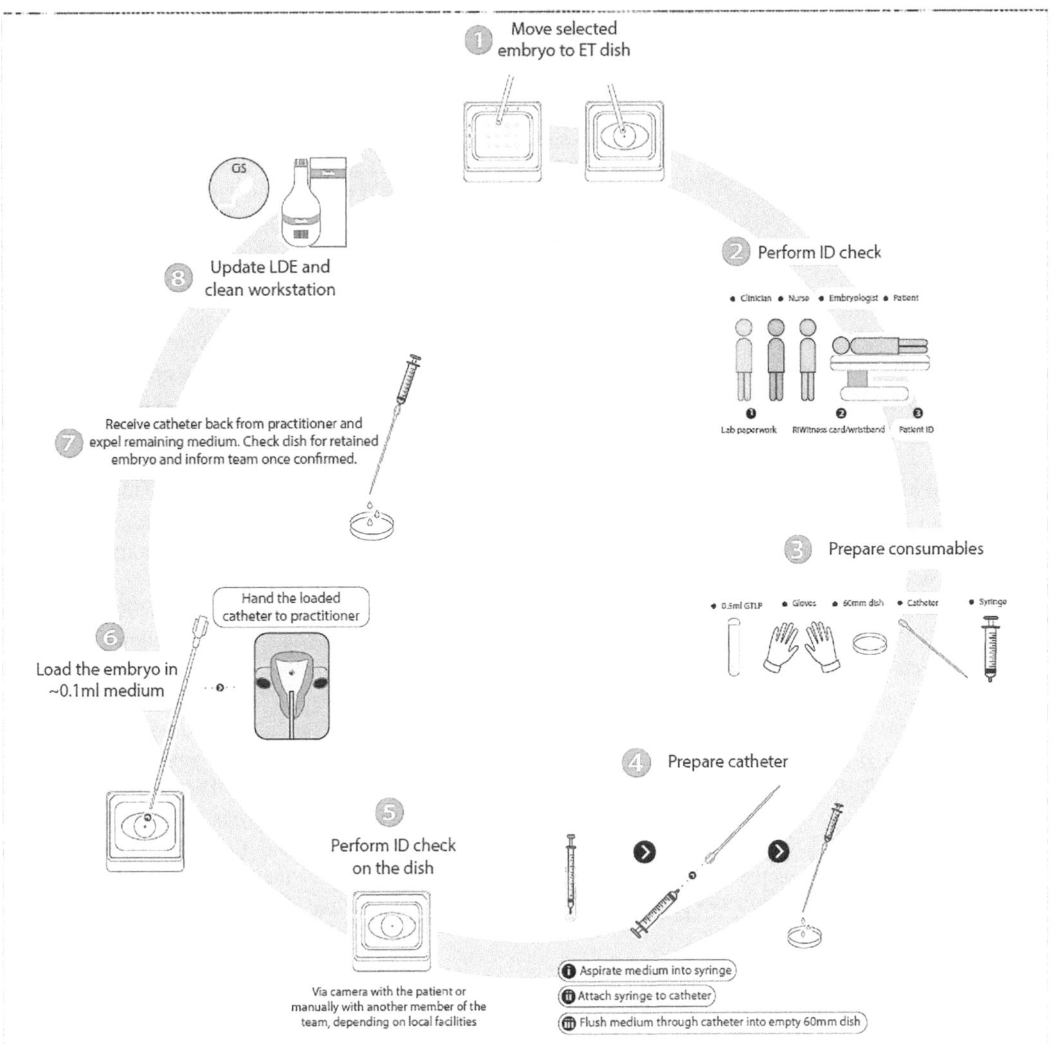

FIGURE 26.1 Embryo transfer.

13. Hold the catheter 2 or 3 inches from the end. Push out any air that may be at the end of the catheter when the tip is placed in the microdrop containing the embryos.
14. Aspirate the embryos, until they are about 1cm from the end of the catheter tube and clearly visible.
15. Check under the microscope that the embryo transfer dish is empty before taking the catheter to the practitioner.
16. Hand the loaded catheter to the practitioner and inject 10–20ul when the catheter is in place and the practitioner has confirmed or the practitioner may expel the contents of the catheter themselves.
17. The practitioner will hand the catheter back. Push out the remaining medium into a clean culture dish and examine. Inform the clinician that the embryos have been delivered successfully or whether an embryo has returned in the catheter.
18. Perform a check of the culture dish to ensure the embryos for transfer are not present.
19. If an embryo(s) has returned in the catheter reload and return to clinician.

26.7.4 Hyaluronan Enriched Media

Hyaluronan enriched media can also be used successfully as a media during embryo transfer. Hyaluronan is a macromolecule that is naturally occurring on the plasma membrane of embryos and endometrial cells, with levels peaking around the time of window of implantation. The addition of high levels of hyaluronan in the transfer medium has been shown to improve implantation. This is thought to mediated by promoting diffusion of the transfer medium into the more viscous uterine secretion, and improving cell adhesion which play an important role in the attachment of the embryo to the endometrium (**16**).

In conclusion, a successful embryo transfer requires knowledge of selecting the correct embryo, the medium for transfer, the timing of the procedure to be synchronised with the readiness of the endometrium and the experience to be able to troubleshoot and react promptly to problems that may occur during the procedure.

REFERENCES

1. Johnson MH. A short history of *in vitro* fertilization (IVF). *Int J Dev Biol.* 2019;63:83–92.
2. Elder K, Johnson MH. The Oldham notebooks: an analysis of the development of IVF 1969–1978. II The treatment cycles and their outcomes. *Reprod BioMed Soc.* 2015;1:9–18.
3. Elder K, Johnson MH. The Oldham notebooks: an analysis of the development of IVF 1969–1979. I. Introduction, materials and methods. *Reprod BioMed Soc.* 2015;1:3–8.
4. Edwards RG, Steptoe PC. Control of human ovulation, fertilization and implantation. *Proc Roy Soc Med.* 1974;67:932–936.
5. Edwards RG, Steptoe PC, Purdy JM. Establishing full-term human pregnancies using cleaving embryos grown in vitro. *Br J Obstet Gynaecol.* 1980;87:737–756.
6. Kellam L, Kasraie J. In: Homburg R, Balan A, Casper R, editors. *50 Big Debates in Reproductive Medicine.* Cambridge, UK: Cambridge University Press; 2021. pp. 151–155.
7. Wei D, Liu J-Y, Sun Y, et al. Frozen versus fresh single blastocyst transfer in ovulatory women: a multicentre, randomised controlled trial. *Lancet.* 2019;393:1310–1318
8. Roque M, Haahr T, Geber S, et al. Fresh versus elective frozen embryo transfer in IVF/ICSI cycles: a systematic review and meta-analysis of reproductive outcomes. *Hum Reprod Update.* 2019;25:2–14.
9. Zaat T, Zagers M, Mol F, et al. Fresh versus frozen embryo transfers in assisted reproduction. *Cochrane Database Syst Rev.* 2021 Feb 4;2(2):CD011184.
10. Campbell A, Fishel S, Duffy S, et al. Embryo selection model defined using morphokinetic data from human embryos to predict implantation and live birth. *Fertil Steril.* 2013;100(3):s502.
11. Campbell A, Fishel S, Bowman N, et al. Retrospective analysis of outcomes after IVF using an aneuploidy risk model derived from time-lapse imaging without PGS. *RBMO.* 2013;27(2):140–146.
12. Letterie G, MacDonald A. Artificial intelligence in in vitro fertilization. *Fertil Steril.* 2020;114:1026–1031.
13. Strowitzki T, Germeyer A, Popovici R, et al. The human endometrium as a fertility-determining factor. *Hum Reprod Update.* 2006;12(5):617–630.
14. Mizrachi Y, Horowitz E, Ganer Herman H, et al. Should women receive luteal support following natural cycle frozen embryo transfer? A systematic review and meta-analysis. 2021. *Hum Reprod Update.* 2021 Jun 22;27(4):643–650.
15. Liu Z, Liu X, Wang M, et al. The clinical efficacy of personalized embryo transfer guided by the endometrial receptivity array/analysis on IVF/ICSI outcomes: a systematic review and meta-analysis. *Front Physiol.* 2022;13.
16. Heymann D, Vidal L, Or Y, et al. Hyaluronic acid in embryo transfer media for assisted reproductive technologies. *Cochrane Database Syst Rev.* 2020;9(9):CD007421.

27

Data and Patient Management in the IVF Laboratory

Rebecca Oakley and Louise Best

27.1 Introduction

Since its inception, the growth of the IVF sector has largely coincided with the digital revolution, and has seen clinics transition from paper records – clinical notes used at consultation, and laboratory records which may have been a single line in a book – to masses of electronic data about every aspect of a patient's journey. A combination of demographic details, consultation notes, consent forms, test results, laboratory records, email communication, and outcome records means that the amount of data a clinic holds about their patients is ever-growing and, in many cases, almost exclusively digital. This chapter will therefore explore our need to manage data, both in terms of how to use it and how to secure it, and discuss how to future-proof clinics in a world of inevitable further digitisation.

27.1.1 The Past

Historically, each fertility patient would have a physical file, into which would be added all paper notes relating to their investigations and treatments. The specifics of the information collected was largely dependent on the individual clinic and what they deemed useful to know regarding their patients. In the 1980s, the UK authorities were considering how to better protect an individual's data and their right to privacy, and, concurrently, beginning to consider how to regulate the emerging IVF sector. The introduction of the Data Protection Act in 1984 and the subsequent Human Fertilisation and Embryology Act in 1990 meant that, in order to standardise care across the country, each clinic had to ensure they were gathering and submitting the same sorts of data about their patients, as well as ensuring that this information was stored and handled securely in accordance with the new privacy laws. Therefore, as the amount of information that clinics collected increased, so grew their need for efficient filing systems (and the associated storage space) so that staff could easily locate a patient's notes as and when needed, and ensure they were managed securely and properly.

27.1.2 The Present

In more recent years – and a trend which has been exacerbated by the coronavirus pandemic in 2020 – clinics have been moving towards becoming paper-light, or even paper-free, whereby nearly every step of a patient's fertility journey is enhanced by specialist technology that ultimately contributes to improved patient care. Overall, digitisation in the IVF sector renders a clinic more flexible, more competitive, more efficient, and improves the level of patient care. This is broadly achieved by:

- **Increasing efficiency** – searching for physical records can be time-consuming as well as frustrating for staff members. Removing the need to search for physical documents can therefore make staff members more productive.
- **Improving resilience** – storing data digitally can mean that should the worst happen and a building is damaged by fire or flood, records are not destroyed. Similarly, files cannot be misplaced if they are stored digitally, meaning that no patient data is lost. Data back up systems must be robust.
- **Improving collaboration** – records can be shared easily between different locations, allowing for joint working and faster decision-making, as well as allowing some staff to work from home, which can improve quality of life.
- **Space saving** – the need for numerous filing cabinets is reduced. Existing hard copies of documents can be scanned and shredded, freeing up physical clinic space.

Despite a move to a more digital way of working that will be described later in this chapter, many records in an IVF laboratory are still handwritten, often used in combination with printed paperwork and digital records. This relies on an accurate recollection of events, as well as decipherable handwriting, in order to document parts of a patient treatment cycle. This steadfast reliance on handwritten paperwork can be attributed to the fact that it is often the quickest way to record events as, incontrovertibly, many events in the laboratory especially are time-critical in nature, and may not take place at a work area where a tablet or computer is readily accessible. It is often quicker to document conversations between an embryologist and patient on a paper record and enter onto the computer later. Adequate and timely access to a computer is essential, but not always provided. Patient paperwork can therefore be much more convenient in a busy laboratory than a computer or a tablet. However, it is inevitable that the advantages of using handwritten notes over technology will be short-lived as digital systems imminently become faster, more convenient, and a seamless part of the laboratory.

DOI: 10.1201/9781003269502-27

27.1.3 The (Near) Future

Improvements in technology not only have the potential to improve efficiency in the laboratory, but also to enhance the patient experience. For example, there are currently apps already available that, with the use of at-home testing kits, help women to track basal body temperature, cycle symptoms, and ovulation, used either with the intent of planning timed intercourse or as a method of contraception. With an increase in wearable technology, smart watches may eventually be able to detect blood pressure and basal body temperature to provide an all-encompassing fertility app with no separate kits or testing required. For men, there are semen analysis apps that provide users with mini clip-on microscopes that attach to a phone camera, with the intent of providing patients a basic idea of their fertility potential. Furthermore, patients can also access at-home, mail-order blood tests that analyse hormone levels to predict ovarian reserve and general fertility well-being. These digital fertility solutions are typically sourced from companies independent of a specialist fertility clinic, and thus can face some criticism for placing a burden on the NHS, as patients subsequently make appointments with their GP to discuss their results. This, of course, does have value if it means that they can be referred for further investigations more quickly, but in a majority of cases these patients would likely go on to conceive naturally in due time and do not actually need medical intervention. Once this at-home technology is more robust and reliable, it may conceivably form part of a patient's journey through an IVF clinic, as it could:

- Reduce waiting times, as without a need for in-clinic testing more patients could begin their journey sooner;
- Increase patient satisfaction, as they would not have to attend the clinic so often;
- Render a treatment more personalised, as tests could be run more often or even continuously in the case of wearable technology.

As exciting as this sounds, careful consideration must be given to legal obligations towards patient data before recommending third-party technology as a supportive tool, as many apps and websites that, for example, help patients to log their menstrual cycle, can treat the data they collect as generic personal data, rather than health data, the latter of which is afforded special protection under the new General Data Protection Regulation (2016). The distinction between personal and health data can seem ambiguous – for example, if a patient stops reporting their menstrual data to an app, does it mean that they have stopped using it, or does it inadvertently reveal that they are pregnant? Any clinics wanting to invest in use of such technology must therefore proceed with caution in this regard.

Many clinics already offer a portal-style service where a patient can manage their appointments and documents, but as app technology develops, patients may soon be able to manage every aspect of their fertility journey in one place – for example, using the same clinic app for video appointments with staff, for reminder notifications to take the right drugs at the right times, and even for viewing their live embryo development in laboratory time-lapse incubators. While a digital laboratory itself may seem rather futuristic, a more digital patient experience through the clinic in general does not seem far off. This chapter therefore explores the digitisation that has already occurred in the IVF sector and how this has been used to the benefit of patients and staff.

27.2 Digitisation in the IVF Clinic

27.2.1 Information Databases

An IVF clinic must have all computers and other devices connected to the same intranet network, allowing for immediate and secure sharing of information around the clinic. While general operating documents can be stored on a network drive or in document control applications, patient data should be stored in a specialised IVF database, which allows multiple, permitted users to access and edit information concurrently. These databases can either be outsourced from a multitude of different companies offering such software, or created in-house. Outsourced software is usually robust and easy-to-use, but is generic, thus not specific or tailorable to each clinic's unique way of working. Software created in-house can be personalised to a clinic's workflow, but on the other hand requires large amounts of IT time and skill, with input from different specialisms, constant improvement work, and frequent updates as the software develops.

In general, IVF databases must be accessible and easy-to-use for all staff members. However, access should be restricted to certain areas of the database based on staff members' position and need to edit certain types of information. For example, embryologists generally do not need to be able to generate an invoice, but they may need to see if a bill has been paid. Similarly, nurses may need to see if a patient has embryos in storage, but would not need to input or edit this information. Staff with the highest level of responsibility should have the widest access and the ability to edit things that others cannot. Restricting access in this way ensures a higher level of data security, as well as ensuring that staff do not inadvertently interfere with a patient's profile or view information that is not needed for their role. Further to this, databases must have the ability to track staff activity, as well as track any changes that have been made to a patient's file.

It is important for clinics to use specialised IVF databases as the software must perform a multitude of functions that only apply to fertility clinics. Ideal fertility database software should give clinics the ability to:

- **Create an electronic file for each individual patient**, and link them to their partner if applicable.
- **Input demographic details for each patient**, and automatically pull any data from an online registration form they may have completed themselves to avoid any transcription errors by administrative staff. When the patient arrives in the clinic they would provide ID and further details, which can be manually added to their digital file.
- **Upload relevant documents to a patient's file** (for example, a scanned copy of their physical notes).

This may require direct links to scanners in the clinic to provide a seamless and time-saving upload.

- **Generate auto-labelled documents from a patient's file** (for example, an embryo freeze sheet, or a letter to be sent). This is time-saving, as the patient details do not need to be written by hand or typed, again eliminating the risk of any transcription errors. This feature may link directly to printers in the clinic.
- **Manage pharmacy and drug management,** where prescribed drugs can be recorded in a patient's file.
- **Input blood results, scan details and clinical outcomes.**
- **Manage donor matching facilities.**
- **Input all laboratory and clinical events** with witnessing details and timestamps. Some clinics may choose to have linked software that is more app-like for use on tablets, to encourage 'live' data entry (performed as soon as possible after the procedure is finished, and by the person who performed it).
- **Input cryostorage information**, as well as have the ability to manage cryopreserved stock, and to monitor sample expiry dates in a bring-forward system.
- **Link to electronic witnessing software,** so that electronic witnessing events are automatically linked to a patient's file.
- **Link to traceability software**, so that batch details of prescribed drugs and of products used in the laboratory/theatre are automatically recorded for each patient.
- **Generate statistics** to allow relevant staff to study cycle data to allow for calculation of KPIs and success rates, and for audit purposes.
- **Manage diaries** and appointments of various staff members and clinic departments.
- **Link to billing and invoicing systems.**
- **Allow for the ability to send messages** between departments to cut down on phone calls and emails.
- **Link to the relevant national register (e.g., HFEA in the UK) cycle reporting system** so that the required reporting forms auto-populate, and automatically send.
- **Create checklists prior to treatment** to ensure that each department has performed the correct checks to allow a treatment cycle to go ahead.

Clinics should also ensure that they maintain a back-up of the database that is updated at frequent intervals, as loss of the entire database would be catastrophic for a clinic. There should also be periodical audits of the collected information to ensure that no data is missing from the system, which would ultimately lead to inaccurate statistics. In a similar way, clinics must make sure they are chasing outcomes from patients and ensuring that these are entered into the system.

27.2.2 Consents

Historically, patients completed paper consent forms (both clinic and regulatory consents), signed by hand. This system relied on clinics giving each patient the correct combination of forms applicable to their treatment, as well as consistent and complete counselling ahead of the signing. This may sound simple, however, due to the complexity of the law surrounding fertility treatment, there are many unique and rare scenarios that can arise and an in-depth knowledge of which consent forms apply to each of these scenarios is required. As such, either due to lack of staff training, or simple human error, patients were on occasion not given the correct consent forms, which has in some cases resulted in legal action against the clinic in question. Also, patients may return their consent forms, but may have failed to tick certain boxes, complete certain sections or sign and correctly date in all the required places. Physical consent forms can go missing, so despite being once completed by a patient, the forms cannot be located.

There are three major problems therefore with physical consent forms: the wrong consents being given by staff; consents completed incorrectly by patients; and forms that are mislaid. Technology has therefore made huge leaps with ensuring consent is informed, complete, and in place. A digital system has the potential to automatically generate which consent forms are needed based on the entered treatment plan and the patient's circumstances. Patients can then use the digital platform to receive and electronically sign the forms – having to first watch a video about each consent form, and complete a short assessment at the end of each module before being allowed to complete it, ensuring informed consent. These videos can be watched at their own leisure, and repeatedly, rather than having an overwhelming consent session in-clinic. Patients can then arrive at their next appointment informed and prepared without taking up staff time in the clinic to go through consents. Forms are auto-populated with the patient's details, and patients have to ensure every section is completed before the consent can be marked as complete and valid. The form can then link back to the information database – for example the number of years a patient has chosen to store their embryos can be added directly into the cryo-management database without a need for staff to transcribe this information, reducing human error. Digital consent platforms also offer more security as patients need login details linked to their email address and phone number, reducing the risk of forged signatures.

27.2.3 The Laboratory

27.2.3.1 Embryology and Andrology

In the IVF laboratory, the vast majority of procedures are still performed manually, as they require high levels of dexterity, coordination and decision-making on a microscopic level that technology has not yet managed to replicate. However, there are many digital tools already used to assist the embryologist – for example, most clinics now use algorithms linked to time-lapse incubators that give embryos a score based on their patterns and timings of divisions, giving some degree of prediction of implantation. This aids in deciding which embryos to transfer or cryopreserve. In order to generate an algorithm score, time-lapse footage must be annotated with the key developmental timepoints of each embryo. This time-lapse footage consists of an amalgamation of images of each embryo taken every few minutes and through multiple focal planes, meaning that for each patient there can be thousands of image files generated across six days of embryo culture. Other advances in the laboratory include the use of computer-assisted semen analysis (CASA), and artificially-intelligent analysis of oocyte images to predict likelihood of a live birth. Considering that clinics can treat thousands of patients each year, new advancements in technology are therefore responsible for generating vast amounts of digital data. Clinics must not only consider how to physically handle this quantity of data (for example, ensuring that the servers are large enough to cope), but also ensure that the data is safe and appropriately managed.

27.2.3.2 Electronic Witnessing

Since 2002, witnessing has been mandatory in UK IVF laboratories to ensure traceability of gametes from egg collection to embryo transfer. Only in recent years have clinics begun to move away from performing witnessing with two laboratory staff both reading patient labels together, and towards electronic witnessing systems. A typical IVF clinic will perform hundreds of checks each month, generating hundreds of chances of human error, such as check omission, involuntary automaticity, and non-contemporaneous checks. The advantages of electronic witnessing are therefore numerous, as it:

- Eliminates the chance of human error.
- Frees up time for staff as they no longer have to witness each other's procedures, minimising stress and interruptions.
- Reduces the need for staff to be present in the laboratory, allowing lone-working.
- Links to batch control – cross-referencing patient cycle witnessing points and material batches, for traceability purposes.
- Supports audit activity and gives more information about an event – timestamps and staff logins demonstrate who did what, where and when, without relying on staff remembering to record these events manually. Useful information can also be gained regarding how long a procedure has taken from start to finish.
- Offers the possibility of linking to cryostorage systems, so that samples can be tracked to a physical location in the storage tanks, removing the need for physical audits and ensuring that samples can always be located in case of transcription errors on paperwork.

Electronic witnessing systems largely fall into two categories: those that use barcodes, and those that use radio-frequency identification (RFID) technology. The former uses barcode readers located in the workstation, whereby each dish or tube has a stick-on barcode label that can be scanned and 'matched' together. Conversely, RFID systems have each dish or tube tagged with a self-adhesive RFID chip that is detected by readers built-in to the work area. See Table 27.1.

TABLE 27.1

Advantages and Disadvantages of Electronic Witnessing Systems

SYSTEM	ADVANTAGES	DISADVANTAGES
BARCODE	Installation into a laboratory is easy and non-disruptive.	Users must remember to match dishes at each step, there are no prompts to remember to do this.
	The necessary hand-held devices that scan barcodes are visible to the patient at egg collection and semen production checks, which can make them feel reassured that the traceability of their samples is taken extremely seriously.	Samples need to be moved within the work area to be scanned and checked, which can be disruptive and may mean that samples are out of the incubator for a longer period.
	Some barcode readers can store photographs of the scanned labels, which can be reassuring to staff and patients retrospectively investigating a cycle that the correct matches were performed.	Two samples from different patients could be in the same work area undetected. If the user does not use the reader and witness the samples correctly, a mismatch could occur.
RFID	Users cannot forget to use the electronic witnessing system. If an unassigned dish is removed from the work area, an alarm will sound alerting the user that they have forgotten to assign the dish.	Installation of an active electronic witnessing system is expensive and disruptive to the laboratory, as the RFID-detecting work stations need to be installed and validated
	Samples do not need to be removed from the work area to be checked, as they are automatically detected. The user quickly presses a button to assign a new dish	
	If two samples from different patients are in the same work area, the system will automatically detect the non-compatible RFID tags and alert the user with a loud alarm.	

27.2.3.3 Facility Monitoring

Considering management of the laboratory itself, monitoring systems are essential to identify changes in critical gas and temperature levels. In a modern clinic, wireless probes can be linked to any essential equipment (incubators, fridges, freezers, storage dewars) that feed into a digital monitoring system. This independent monitoring system records the set parameters continuously. These records are backed up and stored as a record of lab equipment compliance. These systems have the advantage of alerting the embryology team if there is any deviance from the set parameters. During working hours this can be checked, and acknowledged, in person. Out of hours the system sends a text message, or automated call, meaning an embryologist may have to attend the clinic, or remotely access the system. These alarm events are then recorded and saved.

27.2.4 Cyber Security

27.2.4.1 Communication

It is necessary for clinics to send communications to external sources – for example sending emails to other doctors involved in a patient's care, to third party companies like couriers and test providers, and of course, to the patient themselves. In order to adhere correctly to data protection laws, it is critical to not include identifying information in any emails – for example, only including a patient's initials and clinic number – and to ensure that all attached documents are encrypted, in case of interception or of sending an email to an incorrect source. Clinics must take any breach of confidentiality very seriously and report it as an incident to the HFEA.

27.2.4.2 Cyber Attacks

In the past, it was of vital importance to a clinic to secure its premises in order to ensure that patient information could not fall into the wrong hands. Although these physical threats still exist, businesses are more likely than ever to be targeted digitally. This is most likely to arise in the form of a cyber-attack, in which hackers gain access to a clinic's IT infrastructure and install ransomware to render the network unusable, demanding a ransom sum in exchange for decrypting the system. The risk of the patient's confidentiality being breached is the highest concern of a clinic. They should invest in IT security, as well as ensuring the systems are robust enough to be able to recover from the aftermath of an attack, which will involve highly trained expert staff.

27.2.4.3 Off-Site Access

As previously discussed, clinics are progressing towards becoming paper-free, which has enabled some staff to be able to work from home. Staff may also need to access patient records from a remote satellite facility. Digitisation means more and more remote devices must be connected to the network, and therefore to patient records. The greater the number of devices, the higher the chances of loss or theft, and of malicious access to the system. Staff are therefore encouraged to use passwords that are complex, changed regularly, and not used for any other personal purposes. Furthermore, clinics must balance the benefits of being paper-free with resilience planning for how to maintain a normal service if the system stops functioning, and access cannot be gained. All clinics should have a business continuity plan in place in case of the IT network being inaccessible, whether because of an act of cyber-crime, network maintenance, or a general problem in the system.

Clinics should consider how they would be able to go about their day-to-day business if they suddenly lost all access to network, including, for example:

- How would they know which patients were attending for appointments, and when?
- How would they be able to access patient consent forms and blood results, which are critical checks before a patient can proceed with their treatment?
- How would they be able to distinguish between fertilised and non-fertilised embryos in a culture dish, if the laboratory record was not accessible?

27.2.5 Quality Management

27.2.5.1 Incident Reporting

As the amount of patient data stored in a clinic grows exponentially, a robust quality management system is more valuable than ever. Unsurprisingly, technology also has a role to play in this regard. Clinics can use incident reporting software to

- Help manage incidents and complaints.
- Keep a clear record of incidents in one, accessible place.
- Ensure that incident reports are managed in a timely fashion as the software can have deadlines and dates applied to it.
- Alert staff members when incidents have occurred in order to promote group learning.
- Monitor any trends in incidents that suggest training is required, or processes need to be altered.

27.2.5.2 Document Management

Document management can be managed through use of specialised software. It is extremely important that all staff are using the most recent version of policy and paperwork. A searchable document system holds these latest versions, tracks changes and notifies of review dates. It is possible to have an audit trail of who has viewed a document and when. Managing documents digitally therefore helps compliance with the HFEA regulations, as all historic and current versions of documents are reviewed, stored, and classified all in one, easily-accessible place.

27.3 Conclusion

The benefits of digitisation in the IVF laboratory are numerous: reducing human error; reducing subjectivity; decreasing the workload of staff; reducing costs for clinics and patients alike; making clinics more environmentally-friendly as they move away from paper; improving the patient experience; and accurately monitoring success rates. However, advancing technology comes at a cost, not only monetarily, but most notably of how to deal with vast and exponentially-increasing amounts of data and the potential consequences should the data not be dealt with appropriately. It is imperative therefore that this data is properly managed, analysed, and secured. It could also be argued that digitisation presents a risk of staff members becoming de-skilled, over-reliant on technology, and complacent. However, with the right security protection in place, and appropriate training for all involved, it is hoped that these risks can be mitigated, leaving clinics and patients alike to reap the benefits associated with the modern era of fertility treatments.

28

Genomics and Genetic Counselling: Considerations and Challenges with IVF Patients

Karen Sage and Valerie Shaikly

28.1 Introduction

The quest for understanding the underlying molecular basis of many diseases has driven innovation in genetics and genomic technologies. These advances have had a direct effect on reproductive options and are increasingly becoming a significant part of patient care for those seeking assisted reproduction treatment (ART). As genetics becomes part of mainstream routine medicine, genetic specialists and counsellors are called upon to participate in multi-disciplinary teams providing guidance on various aspects of a patient's fertility journey.

Enquiries featuring genetics within the context of ART are an important aspect of clinical discussions. It is essential patients fully understand their available options; the implications for genetic testing including the provision of support for individuals, couples and families as part of their treatment management. This information, often complex, needs to be provided within the context of regulatory and ethical frameworks supporting individual autonomy.

This chapter highlights where genetics questions may occur during ART with points to consider when guiding individuals on genetic and genomic testing for a range of complex conditions and scenarios. Reproductive clinicians and scientists should ensure that any testing strategies offered, are relevant to an individual's specific needs and provide safe and effective patient care. It is important to understand limitations of scope of practice and work in partnership with the multidisciplinary team, including developing relationships with clinical geneticists, genetic counsellors and specialist genetic laboratory clinical scientists.

28.1.1 Genetics and Genomics: An Overview

Genetics is described as the study of hereditary factors and covers the classic types of inheritance: autosomal dominant, autosomal recessive, gender-linked inheritance for changes on the X chromosome mainly, and mitochondrial inheritance patterns.

Genetics focuses on the study of a single gene and the product of that gene (a protein) and how an alteration on the gene affects the protein's functionality. By sequencing a single gene, mutations in the DNA sequence can be classified according to the impact the change is observed to have on the health of an individual. For example, understanding that benign changes which can be tolerated and have no effect on health whilst other changes are deleterious (pathogenic) and are associated with specific genetic disease.

Genomics is a study of gene structure and function. This can include the entire genetic code or multiple genes to understand how these work together. Genomics therefore has application to recognize genetic causes of complex diseases and syndromes.

Generation Genome: In 2016, the Department of Health and Social Care published the chief medical officer's annual report entitled Generation Genome. The report takes a detailed look at genomics and explores how this is currently used in our healthcare systems and how to unlock the potential for further improvement for patients[1] (see Figure 28.1).

Technological innovation has driven genomics forward in recent years. It is now possible to sequence entire sections of the genome and deploy bioinformatics to rapidly elucidate disease-causing mutations. There has been an increase in the development of "gene panels" which analyse a number of genes simultaneously, allowing quicker diagnosis of genetic conditions and in turn, identify carriers of inherited conditions thereby helping many families with treatment and reproductive options.

Examples of diagnostic panels are those currently used for many inherited conditions such as the retinopathies investigating genetic eye disease, cancer genetics and the growing field of inherited cardiac conditions. Genomics also translates to the field of pharmacogenomics that uses precision medicine to tailor medical treatment to how an individual's DNA impacts drug response – the concept of personalised genomic medicine (see Figure 28.2).

28.1.2 Genetic Counselling

Genetic counselling provides information about how inherited conditions might affect an individual, a couple and their wider family. A genetic counsellor or other genetic healthcare professionals are trained to review personal and family health history, gathering key information to help guide genetic testing

Genetic counselling *before* genetic testing can help individuals make informed decisions prior to undertaking genetic testing. Specifically understanding the possible results of genetic investigations and the implications for an individual and the extended family. Genetic counselling *after* a genetic

DOI: 10.1201/9781003269502-28

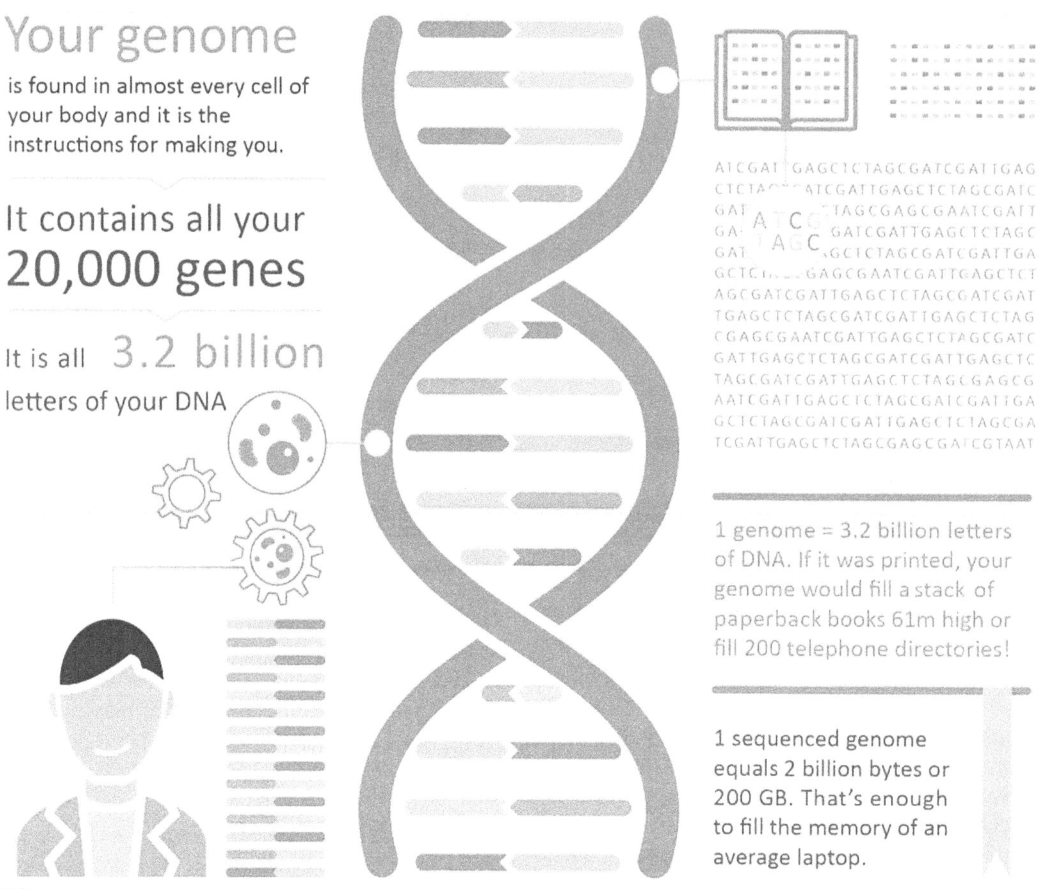

FIGURE 28.1 About your genome (from **1** under Open Government licence).

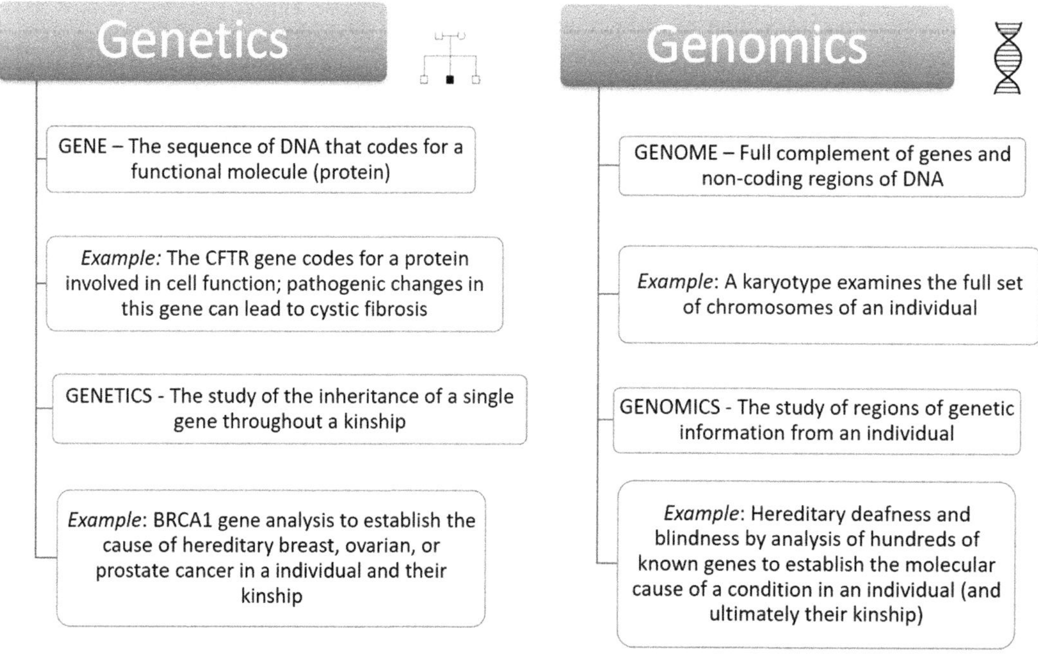

FIGURE 28.2 Overview comparison of genetics vs. genomics (adapted from Health Education England).

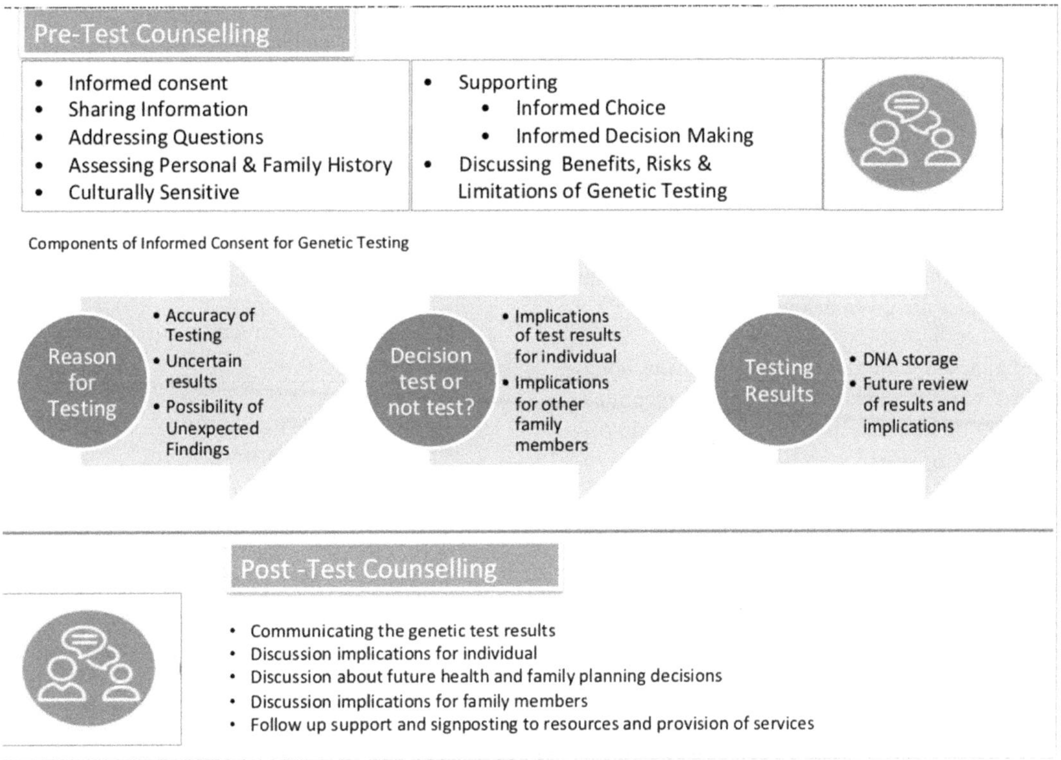

Pre-Test Counselling

- Informed consent
- Sharing Information
- Addressing Questions
- Assessing Personal & Family History
- Culturally Sensitive

- Supporting
  - Informed Choice
  - Informed Decision Making
- Discussing Benefits, Risks & Limitations of Genetic Testing

Components of Informed Consent for Genetic Testing

Reason for Testing
- Accuracy of Testing
- Uncertain results
- Possibility of Unexpected Findings

Decision test or not test?
- Implications of test results for individual
- Implications for other family members

Testing Results
- DNA storage
- Future review of results and implications

Post -Test Counselling

- Communicating the genetic test results
- Discussion implications for individual
- Discussion about future health and family planning decisions
- Discussion implications for family members
- Follow up support and signposting to resources and provision of services

FIGURE 28.3 Key Components of pre-test and post-test genetic counselling pathway.

test can help understand the results and available treatment options. This is simply illustrated in Figure 28.3.

Genetic counselling and genetic discussions can be beneficial for personal health management especially if an individual develops symptoms of a condition, or have a family history of a condition, or if there are concerns for a child that has difficulties that are thought to be genetic in origin. In assisted conception there are many different points where genetic counselling for an individual and couple may be offered.

The following is a list of possible engagement points for genetic counselling in ART.

1. Before pregnancy to understand concerns for genetic factors that might affect fertility, or the health of a child including:
   - Genetic conditions known to run in the family
   - History of fertility problems, recurrent miscarriages, or stillbirth
   - Previous pregnancy or child affected by a birth anomaly or genetic condition
   - Genetic testing options for assisted conception treatment at a fertility clinic
2. During a pregnancy to understand prenatal tests that may be offered and their results including:

   Non-invasive prenatal investigations
   - Early pregnancy screening results with ultrasound anomaly scan findings.
   - Non-invasive prenatal tests (NIPT) for aneuploidy and chromosome micro-deletions and micro-duplications.
   - NIPD bespoke tests for diagnosing a pregnancy at risk of a serious genetic condition.

   Invasive Prenatal investigations
   - Chorionic Villus Sampling (CVS) from 11 weeks of pregnancy
   - Amniocentesis from 15 weeks of pregnancy for aneuploidy and for known or suspected genetic risks.
   - Screening recommended for conditions where there is known familial risk, for example, cystic fibrosis, sickle cell anaemia and other recessive conditions where there is a potential risk.
   - Diagnostic testing for a serious genetic condition, known or suspected
3. Post pregnancy
   - Products of conception following a miscarriage
   - Investigations following investigations into the cause of a symptoms in a child without family history, which is diagnosed as genetic
   - In the event of an adverse outcome following a donor conceived conception – often investigations can take significant time to complete so genetic counselling can provide support for patient(s) during and post investigation.

28.2 Genetic Causes of Infertility

In addition to considerations of genetic disease, genetic causes of infertility are often encountered in the ART setting. Many clinics may offer a treatment pathway for a genetic cause of infertility, it is important that a person understands the results of their specific investigations and the impact this might have on their chances of treatment success, risk for any children they may have, and the risks for their wider family if applicable. Some examples are given below.

- Males diagnosed with azoospermia or severe oligospermia Y chromosome deletions may be identified. Sperm may be available for ICSI and all male offspring will be affected.[2]
- Females diagnosed with premature ovarian failure, a karyotype may show a sex chromosome imbalance. The implications of the chromosome imbalance on health and reproduction can be complex and is not always the same for individuals with the same type of imbalance.
- Males with azoospermia testing of the CFTR gene that is responsible for Cystic fibrosis and CFTR-related conditions can be screened[3]. Females with premature ovarian failure and a family history of premature ovarian failure the FMR1 gene responsible for fragile X can be tested[4]. The implications of findings in CFTR and FMR1 can be complex and will depend on the specific gene alterations reported, but genetic counselling for the individual and the partners and extended family are important prior to and following testing.

A finding from genetic testing can come as shock to the patient(s) who may find it helpful to understand what their specific genetic difference is, what it means to for their health, their fertility journey and risks if any for a pregnancy or child. Support via referral or within the multidisciplinary team should be available to access this information so that patient(s) can make informed decisions and reproductive scientists can provide ongoing support for their treatment pathway.

The nature of a patient(s) fertility history can indicate a genetic cause of infertility and guide a specific genetic test, it should be considered that genetic testing for infertility or for the purposes of donation can also give rise to incidental findings for which an individual requires specialist genetic support. The recommendations for some tests frequently requested in the ART setting are listed below:

Chromosome analysis (karyotype) is recommended for the following indications:

- A couple has 2 or more miscarriages (chance of balanced chromosome rearrangement.
- Severe male factor infertility, defined as azoospermia or severe oligozoospermia.
- First degree relative diagnosed with chromosomal abnormality
- Personal history of stillbirth or fetus affected with congenital abnormality, where the chromosomal investigation of the fetus has not been performed.
- Egg and sperm donors (recommended according to current professional guidelines for screening gamete donors).
- Patient presenting with unexplained infertility have an increased chance of a chromosome abnormality over that of the general population (1%)[4]

Cystic Fibrosis carrier screening is recommended for the following indications:

- Severe male factor infertility, defined as azoospermia or severe oligozoospermia.[3]
- The patient or partner has a family history of CF or a family member is a known carrier (refer for genetic counselling).
- Egg and sperm donor carrier screening (up to 1/25 chance of at alteration in the gene associated with CF in the general Northern European population).[4]

Fragile X pre-mutation testing recommended for the following indications:

- Risk of isolated or familial Fragile X in a patient diagnosed with Premature Ovarian Failure (defined as menopause before 40 years) with 2% isolated and 14% familial risk of Fragile X.[5]
- Family history of unexplained delayed cognitive ability or autism, particularly in young boys.

28.3 Options Available to Individuals Wishing to Reduce Risk of Passing a Genetic Condition to their Child

Figure 28.4 shows the options that patients consider if patients are at risk of passing a genetic condition to a child.

28.4 Preimplantation Genetic Testing

PGT-M and PGT-SR is regarded as diagnostic and intended for patients with a single gene alterations or chromosome rearrangements associated with a risk for a child Patients may also consider the option of additional aneuploidy screening for chromosome balance of the embryos. Genetic counselling to understand the likelihood of success for a treatment pathway is an essential aspect of understanding this treatment option.

Although testing options may be available it should be noted that embryo testing for IVF patients with a known genetic risk is an option and not a default position. For some people embryo testing may not be an option they wish to consider. This is particularly true for families affected by a genetic condition that can be clinically managed and have a lived experience that they understand. People may have fertility problems and

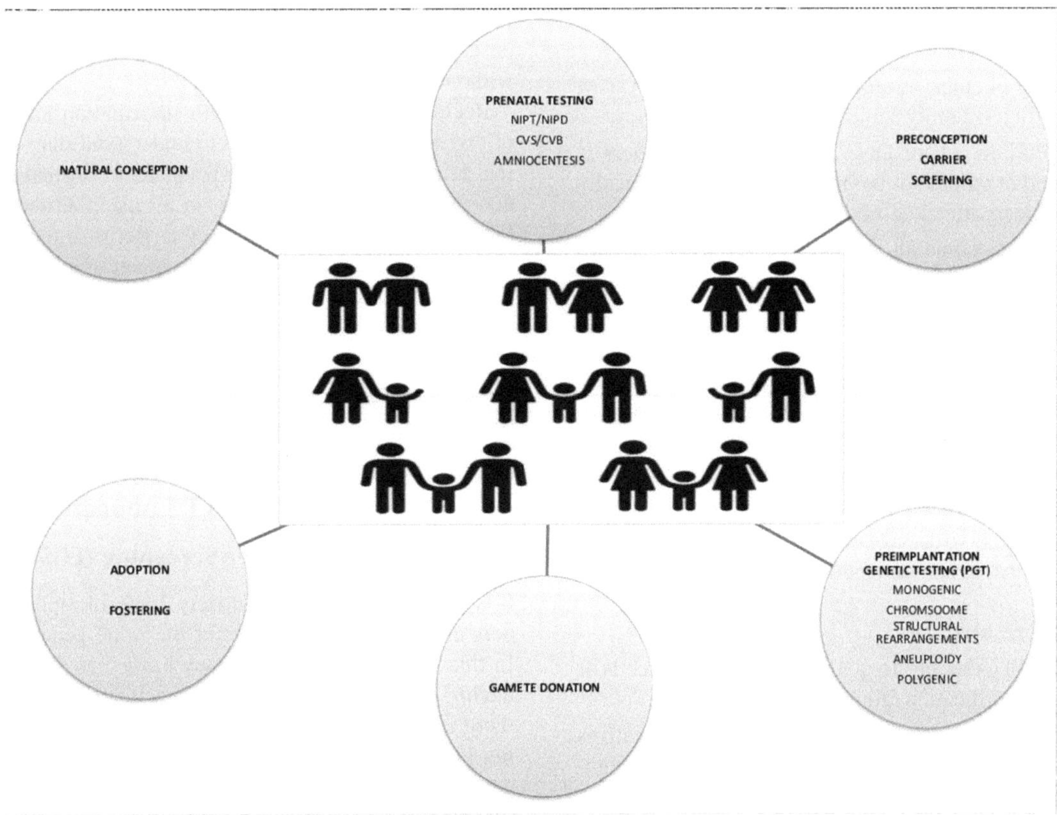

FIGURE 28.4 Overview reproductive options for couples at risk of passing on an inherited condition to their children.

seek assisted conception treatment but not wish to test their embryos. This does not preclude access to ART and treatment can be offered on the understanding of the risk and patient choice. Conditions can be unique to the family and should be reviewed case-by-case basis with MDT agreement for treatment. Genetic counselling can provide additional support in these circumstances. Some clinics may implement a clinic specific consent or genetic acknowledgment documenting discussion, risk, referencing genetic information.

Discussions for risk assessment often involve options for prenatal testing. This is an area that is changing rapidly with the increasing use of non-invasive testing methods which may be available if an assay has been or can be developed for the specific single gene disorders Chorionic villus sampling from 11 weeks of pregnancy is an early invasive option with amniocentesis from 15 weeks offered as gold standard fetal testing.

Gamete donation is an option for patients who may wish to reduce the risk of passing on a genetic condition, or for those who may require gamete donation for treating infertility. Some individuals will consider adoption and fostering or make the decision to remain childless following genetic counselling.

Reproductive scientists and clinicians working within a service offering preimplantation genetic testing through biopsied tissue samples need to be aware of the testing risks, benefits and limitations to assist with patient queries. Often the genetic testing laboratory receiving the biopsied embryo samples are able to provide in-house genetic counselling for patients discussing the potential outcomes of testing prior to giving informed consent.

The reporting for the genetic status of an embryo can vary between laboratories based on the underlying technology, their cut off limits for reporting and the laboratory descriptors. Working closely with clinical scientists at the laboratories providing testing on embryo biopsies is key to understanding what a test result means, so this can be explained to the patient in order to have autonomy in decisions for prioritising embryos for transfer post testing. Transport of embryos between laboratories in the UK and internationally highlights the need for diligence in this aspect of a clinical scientist role. Furthermore, patients may have been able to access embryo testing in other countries, that would not be licensed or accredited the UK. An example of this is the reporting of gender for social reasons in PGT which is currently illegal in the UK under the Human Fertilisation and Embryology Act (HFEA) 2008.

28.5 General Considerations for Clinical Scientists Supporting Patients in PGT Treatment Pathways

Pre-test considerations

- Is the condition licensed for PGT-M testing by the regulatory body in the country (for example the HFEA in the UK)?
- For PGT-M test development, are suitable DNA samples are available from the egg and sperm provider

and reference sample (affected family member, child or pregnancy)?

- Number of embryos required to set phase for PGT-M reporting, if family samples are unavailable?
- For PGT-M where DNA from family members is limited or would not be informative, is it technically possible to offer a de-novo test development?
- For chromosome alterations, is the size of the predicted imbalance(s) detectable within the limits of laboratory detection capability?

Embryology

- Not all eggs fertilise or develop to blastocyst stage embryos suitable for biopsy.
- Embryos will need to be cryopreserved pending test results – associated risks of vitrification and thawing.
- Risk for embryo damage via biopsy, any long term implications that have been reported for biopsied embryos.

Genetic test results

- No result either due to quality of the biopsied cells or DNA amplification failure.
- Accuracy and risk for misdiagnosis false negatives and positives (most laboratories and clinics recommend prenatal testing after PGT).
- Sometimes no embryos are unavailable for transfer after test results are received.
- Mosaic results, is a clinical policy for transfer.

Embryo transfer

- Biopsied embryo cannot be transferred with non-biopsied embryos in the UK.
- Implantation Failure – embryos identified as unaffected (with respect to PGT-M) or balanced (with respect to PGT-SR) with a euploid PGT-A result may not implant or may miscarry.
- Miscarriage risk is a possibility following any embryo transfer.

28.6 Gamete Donation

Gamete donors are clinically reviewed for the possibility of hereditary conditions that may be revealed through a thorough family history review covering 2–3 generations. The decision to accept into the donor programs is based on the information the individual is able to share. Increasingly donors are screened for a fixed number of autosomal recessive. The genes included in the screening panels range from 3 to more than 500 genes, with the most frequently used panels offering screening for 300 conditions. The genes included in the panels can have varying carrier frequencies in different populations and therefore the risks vary for a potential child of a recipient of positively screened donors. In addition, some of the genes can have a mild ffect on the carriers, for example the gene LDLR in carrier form may predispose an individual to adult-onset cardiac disease in their 50s–60s, earlier than individuals without changes in this gene.

Recipients need support with information about the level of screening a donor has had to understand that 'genetic testing' referenced in a donor banks patient information can vary and importantly, does not screen for all inherited conditions. Where a donor is identified as a carrier of a recessive condition, and vials are available for recipient use a genetic discussion to understand what this means in terms of risk for a child and options for counter screening should be offered.

28.7 Other Considerations for Genetics/Genomics for Clinical Scientists Working in the ART Laboratory

28.7.1 Extended Carrier Screening (ECS)

It is estimated that approximately 2–5% of reproductive partners are found to be carriers of the same genetic condition[6]. In this situation every pregnancy has a 1 in 4 or 25% risk of having a baby with a recessive genetic condition even when there is no previous family history. Extended carrier screening identifies known disease-causing changes in a number of genes and can test for hundreds of different recessive conditions simultaneously. This testing is available from commercial providers using different underlying technologies and includes various combinations of genes. It is important that the carrier test selected meets the need of the individual at the time it is taken and that results from the testing are discussed prior to providing a sample, to give informed consent. Single gene carrier screening or extended carrier screening may be offered by a clinic or a patient(s) may source screening outside of the clinic through accredited testing laboratories and share test results to inform a treatment pathway.

28.7.2 Direct-to-Consumer Testing for Carrier Screening

Patients may share direct to consumer genetic test results with the laboratory team to demonstrate that they have been tested for a particular condition and are not carriers. Many direct-to-consumer tests are not clinically validated and this should be confirmed in a clinical setting. This type of testing can be of limited utility in that the analysis may focus only on one or two known disease-causing variants on a gene, which would fail to report the many other possible disease causing variants in a single gene. For example, there are more than a thousand variants in the BRCA1 and BRCA2 genes associated with an increased risk for certain cancers, but 23andMe's BRCA1 and BRCA2 (Selected Variants) Genetic Health Risk report looks at just three (3) of these variants, that are most commonly found in people with Ashkenazi Jewish ancestry.

For individuals who find out they have one of these three variants, which can significantly increase their risk for cancer, this information can be extremely impactful when shared with their providers. But for other individuals who do not carry one of these variants, it is essential that they understand that they may still have a variant not tested, especially if there is a family history of cancer. Home DNA test kits usually do not account for family history, environment, and lifestyle, which can also influence overall risk.

28.7.2.1 Direct-to-Consumer Testing Effect on Donor Anonymity

If an individual undertakes a home DNA kit to find out more about their ancestry it is now possible to select an option to search for family members by % shared DNA as shown in Figure 28.5.

Information relates to markers on one specific chromosome and this can be shared to give clues to side of the family. Contact may then be available to potential family members who are on the same ancestry test registry. Social media and Google ™ profiles can then be used to potentially identify a donor if the individual searching is donor conceived. This information is usually given to recipients and donors via implications counselling or the clinic team, however it is likely that as clinical scientists this topic will arise as part of patient communication.

28.8 Futures

The application of genomic technologies to ART is likely to increase as evidenced by the extensive research into a number of potential promising treatments. The use of whole genome sequencing may become available for embryo biopsies, which could increase the potential for simultaneously testing a number of mono-allelic disease-specific genes with aneuploidy screening. This technology could also generate incidental findings that potentially impact a child and the wider family with associated ethical and governance considerations.

28.8.1 Polygenic Risks Scores (PRS)

Many common complex conditions prevalent in some families are considered to be life-style related and referred to as multi-factorial. This means the onset of these, usually adult conditions, are a result of a combination of genetic predisposition based on family history, environment and social lifestyle choices. Advances in technology allow genetic scientists to interrogate the whole genome and subject the resulting big data set to bioinformatics. Combining the results of data gathered from multiple genes it is possible to produce an estimate of an individual's chance of developing multi-factorial disease – this is the polygenic risk score. This is complex area of genomic research as there are multiple aspects of genetic variants that scientists do not fully understand. Consequently, a PRS may play a role in the estimation of risk but the other factors (environment and lifestyle) may have a greater impact.

Applying this technique to genomic data derived from embryo biopsies could be used to rank and select embryos for reduced risk for multifactorial conditions such as diabetes and coronary heart disease. In the USA, testing of embryos and applying PRS has recently become available and has been subject to much social and ethical debate.[7, 8]

Although this is currently offered by a number of international centres, the clinical utility of application for a small number of genetically similar embryos is disputed. Moreover, European professional bodies hold the position that use of this technology should not be supported in clinical practice. There are ethical concerns that traits such as height and academic achievement could be included in embryo ranking. Guidelines for ethical consequences of generating this additional genetic information have yet to catch up with these technologies. While there may be patient-led demand, future research on the impact of these techniques is required, especially where there is a risk of a trait rather than a confirmed diagnosis.

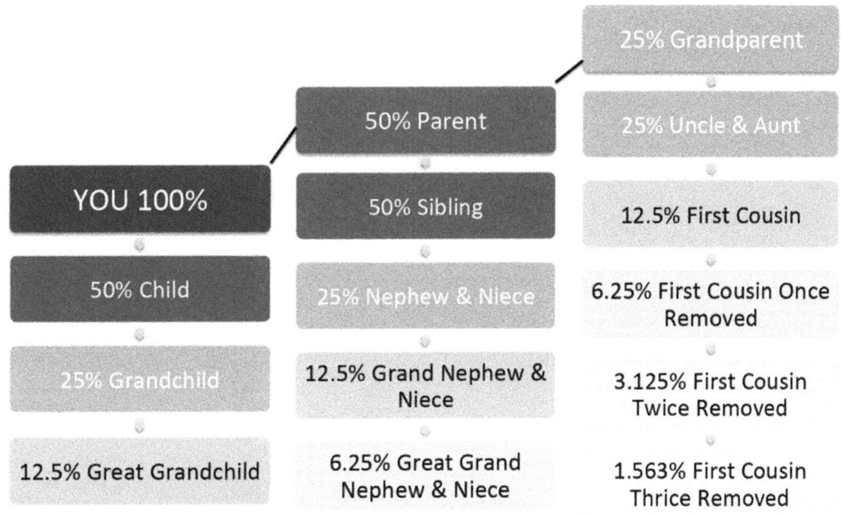

FIGURE 28.5 Discovery of close relatives by % of DNA shared in DNA ancestry databases.

28.8.2 Non-Invasive Preimplantation Genetic Testing of Embryos

Non-invasive PGT, is when embryo cell-free and mitochondrial DNA secreted into culture medium is tested to determine the chromosome balance of an embryo. The reliability of the methodologies currently available has not yet been demonstrated to be as efficacious as biopsied embryo samples, despite some uptake in other countries using laboratory specific protocols.

28.8.3 Metabolomics and Proteomics

Other genomic applications have been investigated in the ART setting involve examining the metabolomic differences in spent culture media in relation to implantation potential. RNA sequencing of granulosa cells to determine oocyte quality, is another area of investigation, although to date these techniques are novel not demonstrated sufficient sensitivity for clinical application.

28.8.4 Genome Editing

On the horizon are genome editing technologies which could replace the need for PGT for genetic conditions. To date, off-target effects have been observed in the research setting. It is anticipated that in the future, as editing techniques and systems improve, an international framework for governance would be required to consider ethical values and principles.

The role of a clinical scientist in ART is likely to include understanding new genomic technologies, their benefits and limitations, how to advise and counsel patients for available treatment options and the interpretation of results for their treatment plans.

SOURCES OF INFORMATION

Genomics Health Education England: www.genomicseducation.hee.nhs.uk

www.genomicseducation.hee.nhs.uk/genomics-in-healthcare/#specialism

National Institute of Health and Care Excellence (NICE)

www.nice.org.uk/guidance/cg156/

Genetic Alliance

https://geneticalliance.org.uk/

Donor Conception Network

www.dcnetwork.org

Bionews

www.bionews.org.uk

American College of Medical Genetics and Genomics

www.acmg.net/ACMG/Medical-Genetics-Practice-Resources/Practice-Guidelines.aspx

The American College of Obstetricians and Gynecologists (ACOG)

www.acog.org/

REFERENCES

1. Annual Report of the Chief Medical Officer 2016: Generation Genome. Published 4 July 2017, Updated 2019. Accessed at: https://assets.publishing.service.gov.uk/government/uploads/system/uploads/attachment_data/file/631043/CMO_annual_report_generation_genome.pdf.
2. Bayer S, Alper M, Penzias A. *The Boston IVF Handbook of Infertility: A Practical Guide for Practitioners Who Care for Infertile Couples.* 4th edition, CRC Press, Boca Raton, 2017.
3. Brennan ML, Schrijver I. Cystic Fibrosis A Review of Associated Phenotypes, Use of Molecular Diagnostic Approaches, Genetic Characteristics, Progress, and Dilemmas. *J Mol Diagn.* 2016,18(1)3–14.
4. Nussbaum R, McInnes R, Huntington F, eds. *Thompson and Thompson's Genetics in Medicine.* 8th edition, Elsevier, Philadelphia, PA, 2015.
5. National Fragile X Foundation. Accessed at: https://fragilex.org/understanding-fragile-x/fxpoi-primary-ovarian-insufficiency/.
6. Gregg AR, Aarabi M, Klugman S, et al. Screening for Autosomal Recessive and X-Linked Conditions During Pregnancy and Preconception: A Practice Resource of the American College of Medical Genetics and Genomics (ACMG). *Genet Med.* 2021,23(10)1793–1806.
7. Gallegos E. Progress Education Trust. *Bionews*, 1130. Accessed at: www.progress.org.uk/no-evidence-for-using-polygenic-risk-scores-in-embryo-selection/.
8. ESHRE. Position Statement of Polygenic Risk Scores. Accessed at: www.eshre.eu/Guidelines-and-Legal/Position-statements/PRS.

29

Third Party Reproduction

Selina Wilkinson and Louise Kellam

29.1 Introduction

The rapid emergence of various IVF technologies now goes beyond two people reproducing biologically (**1**). Third party reproduction refers to the involvement of another individual to help people become the intended parents in the process of reproduction, either through gamete donation or gestational surrogacy.

Third party reproduction provokes different reactions in different cultures and the structure of the traditional family has dramatically transformed, from predominately being married heterosexual couples to single or same sex couples who reproduce by utilising gamete donation or surrogacy. In essence, assisted reproductive technologies have helped remove the stigma of infertility (**1**). It also provides an opportunity for couples or individuals to make their dream of having a child a reality. It is often the final route for those unable to produce or use their own eggs or sperm, for any reason, or for those that require a surrogate to carry their child.

There are many social, ethical, regulatory and legal aspects that can make the donation options available complex, especially surrogacy arrangements which can be controversial and subject to psychosocial scrutiny (**2**). IVF clinics are developing and expanding their donation services so that they can support patients in this area and provide competitive treatment options to anyone requiring donation. What was once seen as a narrow, complicated route is now more accessible with new options and choices. The goal for all involved; from fertility professionals to gamete providers and patients, is to enable the process to move forward as smoothly as possible and result in individuals achieving their goals of parenthood.

29.2 Management of Donation in IVF Clinics in the UK

Historically, donation has commonly been managed by individual clinics with practice and systems varying immensely. Donation has been a niche and specialised area of ART and has usually been managed by either a trained individual or a small team working alongside other aspects of the daily running of the clinic. The size of the team is dependent on the size of the clinic, services offered, case complexity, levels of staff expertise, training available, distribution of clinical caseload, and additional responsibilities.

Covering an effective service has its challenges because of the speciality, especially considering unpredictable staff turnover, annual leave and sickness. Training can be a logistical barrier for a large clinic group where specially trained staff are distributed across different clinics. Care Fertility have found that centralising the donation management (such as consultation, screening and consent) has been an effective way of dealing with this challenge. A dedicated team of specially trained nurses/midwifes, scientists, health care assistants and administrators work together across multiple locations to ensure the best outcomes and experiences for all patients in third party reproduction.

Donation services across the world vary dramatically due to the regulatory framework, laws and availability of donors or surrogates. This chapter is focused on the UK landscape primarily.

29.3 HFEA (Human Fertilisation and Embryology Authority) Regulatory Requirements and Clinic Policy for Donation and Surrogacy

There are specific mandatory requirements that are set out in the HF&E Act and HFEA Code of Practice that must be complied with when recruiting donors or managing surrogacy arrangements; including donor screening, donor consent, use and storage of donor gametes (**3**).

Fertility clinics have their own standard operating procedures and policies, which will ultimately be based on regulatory requirements, but also on evidence-based research, risk considerations, operation and business factors.

All donors are registered with the HFEA and the law requires clinics to inform the HFEA when a donated gamete is used in treatment including the identity of the gamete (egg or sperm) providers, the identity of any person who has an embryo transfer or intrauterine insemination and the outcome of the treatment cycles.

29.4 Gamete Donation

In the UK, donors can be anonymous or known to the recipient. Known donors are generally a close relative or friend of the recipient. Both types of donors must meet the same selection criteria based on clinic policy and HFEA regulatory requirements. Recruitment of enough altruistic donors to meet the increasing demand for third party reproduction remains a challenge.

DOI: 10.1201/9781003269502-29

Social media and other advertising avenues are often used to highlight the need for altruistic donation. Potential donors contact the clinic voluntarily to take part in the programme. Donors are selected based on eligibility criteria such as age and clinical history and are compensated for expenses incurred when making their donation.

Donors can find out the number, sex of the baby, and year of birth of any children conceived from their donation. They can't find out the identity of the children unless a donor-conceived child contacts them after they have reached 18 years of age.

29.5 Embryo Donation

Patients who have had IVF treatment may decide to generously donate super nummary embryos that they no longer wish to use, for the treatment of others. Both egg and sperm providers are screened as donors in accordance with the regulatory requirements. As the original intention was not to donate, the patients may not have been screened for infectious disease at the time of embryo creation and are therefore screened retrospectively. The fact that embryos have a "special status" may permit the donation, although risks are always mitigated.

29.6 Donor Expenses

Donating gametes and embryos in the UK is voluntary and unpaid and donors may be compensated only in line with relevant HFEA Directions. Clinics may offer benefits in kind, in the form of reduced-price or free licensed services (for example, fertility treatment or storage) or quicker access to those services, in return for providing eggs or sperm for the treatment of others (**3**).

Elsewhere in the world there are contrasting practices. In the US, for example, donations can be sold and donors may be paid. This variation is largely determined by ethical and social frameworks linked to fertility treatment provision in that country (**4**).

29.7 Anonymity for Donors

From the age of 16, children born as a result of fertility treatment in the UK have the right to ask the HFEA whether they were born as a result of fertility treatment. When a donor-conceived child reaches age 16, they can ask the HFEA for non-identifying information of their donor such as ethnicity, year and country of birth and a physical description. They may also find out if they are related to someone they plan to marry, enter into a civil partnership or intend to have a relationship with.

At 18, a donor-conceived child can ask the HFEA for the donor's name, date of birth, the town or district where they were born, and their last known postal address as well other identifying information the donor supplied at the time of their donation.

In some countries, like Spain, donors remain anonymous, however, whatever the requirements of local legislation, it is getting more difficult to guarantee anonymity due to the volume of genetic information available to individuals (**5**).

DNA testing and matching services (like those used by people tracing their ancestry) have increased significantly over the last few years. Because of the way DNA matching and tracing services work, the donor or the donor-conceived person themselves doesn't necessarily need to be signed up to such a service for a genetic link, or possibly even their identity, to be revealed if a close family member uses the service. It is important that new donors and recipients are made aware of this prior to donation or treatment.

29.8 Donor Screening, Including Intended Parents in a Surrogacy Arrangement

The screening of donors is comprehensive and is designed to protect the recipients of donor sperm, oocytes and embryos from acquiring infection and donor-conceived people from being born with an infection or serious heritable disorder from the donor (**6**).

Intended parents providing gametes for the creation of embryos that will be transferred to a surrogate must also undergo the same screening as donors as set out in HFEA code of practice. This is also the case for any embryos or gametes imported into the UK for use in donation treatments. Mandatory screening requirements are laid out in the HFEA Code of Practice 9th edition (**3**).

The UK donor screening requirements are complex and can be challenging for clinics to manage as donors move through various stages of the pathway.

29.9 Family Limit

In the UK, the eggs or sperm of a single donor can be used to create up to ten families (not including their own), but the donor has an option to restrict the number of families to fewer than ten if they wish to. However, this does not stop the donor donating in other countries and creating more families through sperm donation.

The legislation regarding family limits differs for other countries, for example, Norway changed their legislation in 2020, stipulating a maximum of 6 families per donor. A US Cryobank; one of the largest sperm banks in the world, supplies donor sperm to the UK and permits 25–30 families per donor worldwide. The HFEA can only record the number families created in the UK as a result of donation.

29.10 Matching Donors and Recipients

Depending on donor availability, a clinic or donor bank may provide the details of all available donors to the potential recipient and invite them to select a donor for treatment. If there are too few donors, the recipient may be asked what donor characteristics were important to them so that they may be offered a suitable donor by the clinic when one becomes available.

In the UK, all non-identifying information about the donor is made available to the recipient prior to use, and not held back until a pregnancy or birth is confirmed. The type of information includes; ethnicity, physical description, medical history, age, country of birth, family background, hobbies, and interests. If the donor has written one, a personal description and goodwill message to any potential children will also be available. Clinics are not expected to match the ethnic background or blood group of the recipient to that of the donor.

If treatment using a donor gamete is successful, and results in a live birth, the recipient may wish to use the same donor in future treatment. In these situations, clinics or banks will aim to match with a 'sibling-donor' where possible. This is more likely in sperm donation where stocks from each donor are more likely to be available.

29.11 Carrier Screening

Expanded carrier screening (ECS) involves identifying the presence or the absence of many gene variants which might be associated with different conditions of varying severity and predictability. Gamete donors may be screening for over 500 more frequent and severe hereditary recessive diseases to reduce the risk of a donor-conceived child inheriting one of the diseases. This technology replaces the routine traditional ethnicity, or family history-based screening.

In the UK there are currently no national guidelines or standardised screening panels specific to ECS, yet much debate on whether gamete donors should undergo ECS. Currently the HFEA does not require UK fertility clinics to carry out ECS and gamete donors are not required to have had this screening.

Although ECS can mitigate risk of a child inheriting certain conditions, its introduction could mean an overall decline in the number of donors available (**7**). In the US, ECS is becoming commonplace for sperm donors with many donors known to have a positive carrier status and available for use in large sperm banks. For UK recipients considering donors that are known carriers for a condition, Care Fertility provides access to genetic counselling services to ensure that the implications are understood, risks explained, and their own testing offered, prior to any decision-making.

29.12 Egg Donation

The first pregnancy resulting from egg donation was reported in 1984. Since then, egg donation has grown markedly across the globe, with an increase of 49% of treatment cycles in the UK since 2011 (**8, 9**).

Egg donor recruitment involves a significant amount of investment for a clinic, in terms of the costs, risks and staff involved in the processes. On average it costs over £2000 to support a donor from initial enquiry through to egg collection. Of course, not all donors respond as expected, based on specific indicators and therefore egg performance is unpredictable with no guarantee of outcome.

Although egg donors are selected to be young and healthy, most will generally respond well to ovarian stimulation, but because the stimulation is a biological process, and many donors are having treatment for the first time, it is difficult to predict how a donor will respond, which is why more clinics are freezing eggs and creating egg banks, rather than set up a fresh match – which can be challenging to synchronise and can delay treatment if things don't go as predicted.

Historically fresh donation has been the preferred option as eggs have been more difficult to freeze successfully than sperm, however with a breakthrough in laboratory cryopreservation processes; vitrification is now used to allow eggs to be frozen and thawed successfully whilst reducing the risk of them being damaged during the process. This method freezes eggs rapidly at -196ºC using liquid nitrogen and is so effective that over 85% of eggs survive the freeze-thaw process (**10**).

29.13 Egg Sharing

Occasionally, fertile women having their own treatment also offer to share half of the eggs that are collected in their own treatment cycle, in exchange for treatment benefits in kind. The HFEA decided in 1992 that the egg sharing provided an acceptable, efficient and effective option; with only one woman undergoing ovarian stimulation and retrieval but two hopefully achieving a pregnancy.

Many clinics in the UK offer egg sharing packages, however, over the last few years, there has been a decrease in the number of egg sharers (**9**). This may be in part due to the improved supply of altruistic egg donors that are not seeking treatment, supported by the increasing success of oocyte vitrification. A descriptive cohort study concluded that egg sharing does not compromise live birth chances for the donor or recipient, and advocates egg sharing as a practical option that maximises the precious resource of human oocytes (**11**).

However, egg sharing has been criticised and debated over the years (**12, 13**). Some feel using financial incentives (discounted treatment) to attract someone into proceeding with an option they may not otherwise choose, at a time when they are experiencing infertility themselves – added to the fact that they could fail and have "sharer regret" if the other person succeed, could be utterly devastating. However, for same-sex female couples egg sharing was reported to be considered particularly favourable as they liked the idea of giving back, as they need donor sperm.

Managing egg sharing arrangements within a clinic also has its logistical challenges, with more expertise required to synchronise the donor treatment with the egg recipient and more emotional support required for all parties in the arrangement. There is commonly a minimum of 8 eggs required in order to egg share, which is not known until the day of egg collection and therefore results in uncertainty and increased anxiety for the egg recipient. If the cycle is cancelled cycle, the process starts again with further planning to rematch, which has further cost implications for the clinic.

29.14 Sperm Donation

It was anticipated that the change in the donor anonymity law would affect the recruitment of altruistic sperm donors, however, sperm donor numbers have remained steady since 2005 and have actually grown year on year (**9, 14**). It would be reasonable to presume that there is little financial motivation for altruistic sperm donation given the limited amount of £35 per visit a sperm donor can claim in expenses. Sperm donors have no legal or moral responsibility for any child they help create.

Unlike egg donors, many sperm donors utilised within the UK, are recruited from outside the UK having met UK regulation in order to be imported for use. US derived donor sperm accounts for 49% of international donors imported and registered in the UK (**9**).

Like several other clinic groups, Care Fertility has its own central sperm bank and recruits sperm donors in its individual clinics across the UK. Care also purchases donor sperm from larger dedicated sperm banks outside the UK in order to supplement the demand for those requiring treatment with donor sperm. Recipient waiting times for those using the Care sperm bank, can be up to 6 months depending on donor availability and preferences of donor by the recipient. Obstacles to facilitate an effective recruitment programme, include staffing resources, specialist skills and logistic practicalities, such as drop-in services for donors within its clinics.

Sperm sharing programmes can improve donor sperm supply and, similar to egg sharing, offer a benefit in kind in the form of discounted treatment in return for the donation. The number of sperm sharing arrangements is not recorded by the HFEA and has arguably greater ethical concerns than egg sharing (**15**).

For same-sex male couples sperm sharing can be a favourable option, with the requirement for surrogacy and egg donation themselves, they may feel they are giving something back in response to the help that has been provided to them. About 90% of sperm sharers at Care Fertility currently are same-sex male couples in a surrogacy arrangement.

Patients may source donor sperm independently from their clinic from a donor sperm bank either in the UK or abroad. Sperm can be shipped to their clinic in advance of treatment. For imported donors, the same HFEA requirements of donor recruitment, screening and consent must be met, however allowances of overseas donor expenses differ slightly. UK clinics must ensure that any imported donor has not received compensation which exceeds reasonable expenses, and that loss of earnings payments of no more than £250 (or local equivalent) were paid to the donor for each course of donation. Each import is recorded, and each overseas donor registered by the HFEA, in the same way as UK donors. Laws regarding donor anonymity, consent and storage are the same for imported donors as UK donors.

Successful management of sperm donor recruitment is dependent on the time and investment allocated to the cause and the ability to reach out and support prospective donors wanting to help others. Sperm banks purely specialising in sperm donor recruitment can be very successful and offer no wait for donor sperm selection by its users. One of Europe's largest sperm banks focuses solely on donor sperm recruitment and has a self-matching online platform with donors that meet the UK regulatory requirement. Not surprisingly the Covid pandemic has affected donor sperm recruitment with sperm banks experiencing a temporary reduction in the amount of sperm donors they would normally offer.

29.15 Shared Motherhood/Parenthood

Donor insemination (DI) of sperm is most commonly used by patients with a female partner, accounting for 44% of all DI treatments (**9**). Although, for female same-sex relationships, IVF treatments has increased as shared parenthood has become a popular choice. Shared motherhood, also known as intra-partner egg donation follows the same general pathway as IVF treatment, using donated sperm with the egg provider's partner having the embryo transfer and carrying the pregnancy.

29.16 Egg and Sperm Recipients

Around 2,700 children in the UK are born each year through the help of a donor. The HFEA holds records of all donors and children born since 1991 (**16**). Egg and sperm donor treatment remain a growing area within fertility (see Figure 29.1), and it has provided the opportunity for same-sex couples, those with no partner and those in the older age range to become parents.

Recipients should be encouraged, by their clinic/counsellor to be open with their donor conceived child about their origins. Studies suggest that being open and honest can avoid the

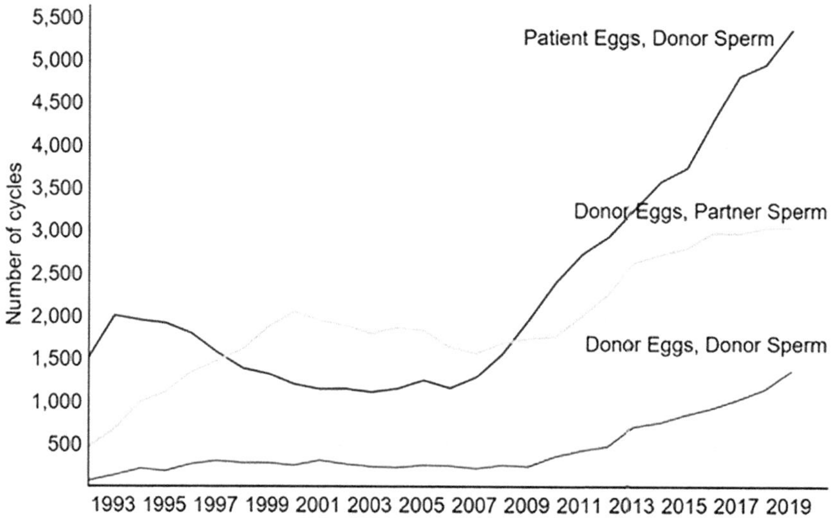

FIGURE 29.1 The number of IVF cycles by egg and sperm shows how the use of donor egg and sperm have increased over the past 30 years (from [**9**] under Open Access licence).

conflict or hurt that can be caused if a child discovers their origins unintentionally or unexpectedly (**17**). The UK laws of the provision of identifiable donor conception information at an earlier stage in the child's life, is currently under review by the HFEA (**18**).

29.17 Egg Recipients

29.17.1 Fresh Donation Treatment

Fresh egg donation involves synchronising the donor's menstrual cycle with that of an egg recipient. For clinics it is more operationally challenging, than frozen donation, as it requires the intervention of a specialised health professional to plan and co-ordinate this synchronisation. Menstrual cycles can be unpredictable for both parties and there is always a risk that donors can potentially pull out of the process during crucial aspects of the treatment. This in turn leaves patients facing uncertainty during what can be a stressful time for the egg recipient.

29.17.2 Frozen Egg Donation Treatment

Using frozen donor eggs instead of fresh donor eggs has a number of advantages for recipients. It is a more natural approach, as preparation for the treatment can be done in synchrony with the patient's own cycle. There doesn't need to be any synchronisation with the donor's cycle, which reduces the chance of hormonal injections and the side effects that accompany them.

Sometimes, fresh donation cycles have to be cancelled at the last minute, if a donor's stimulation doesn't go to plan or pulls out of the process. With frozen eggs, the eggs have already been successfully collected and carefully frozen and therefore there are fewer disruptions for the recipient and more certainty.

The additional freezing and thawing step, associated with frozen donation, slightly reduces the number of eggs which may be available – as some do not survive the freeze-thaw process. It also means that ICSI is required for insemination, due to the mode of preparation of the eggs for the vitrification process (Figure 29.2).

29.18 Surrogacy

In the UK, surrogacy is legal. However, any agreement between parties cannot be enforced by the law. Surrogacy through commercial means, is illegal in the UK and it is an offence for an individual or agency to act on a profit-making basis to organise or facilitate surrogacy for another person (**19**). For this reason, IVF clinics cannot be involved in introducing or identifying surrogates or intended parents.

Surrogacy was often seen as a small aspect of IVF treatments but it has grown immensely in the last 5 years, especially with the law changes in 2019, allowing single people to

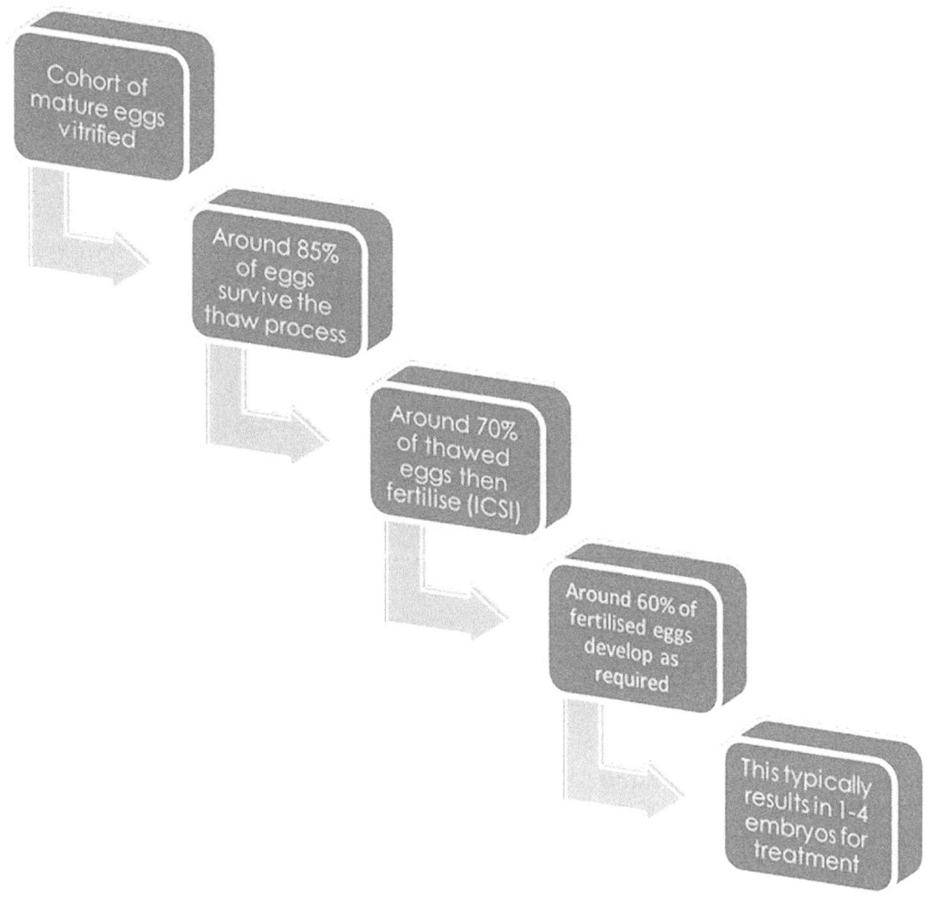

FIGURE 29.2 From mature donor eggs to embryos for transfer. Depicts the cascade commonly observed when working with frozen donor eggs. Values are for illustrative purposes and approximated based on author experience.

proceed with a surrogacy arrangement. Many UK clinics have seen treatments almost doubling year on year and now have a dedicated central team to manage surrogacy.

Surrogacy like other aspects of donation, is a specialised area of expertise with regulatory requirements creating more complex and essential patient workup, so a dedicated team is vital in order to ensure a smooth pathway for patients.

29.19 Legal Parenthood in Surrogacy

In the UK the birth mother of a child is the legal parent. If granted, a parental order transfers the status of the birth mother to the intended parents but the grant of an order is subject to certain legal requirements being met.

29.20 National Health Service (NHS) Funding for Donation Services

NHS funding for fertility varies considerable across the UK, particularly in donation. On average most trusts will offer one funded treatment using donor gametes, but with strict criteria. Surrogacy is rarely funded although there have been sporadic special cases.

Interestingly, NHS funding for donor insemination has increased with the biggest rise being for same-sex female couples (requiring donor sperm), increasing from 25% in 2009 to 44% in 2019 (**9**).

29.21 Fertility Tourism

Couples and single women may decide to seek treatment in a different country for reasons including; cheaper treatment, higher success rates, availability of treatments or to reduce the waiting time for a donor or surrogate. Whilst gamete donation is illegal in a number of countries, for example Germany and Turkey, it is permitted in many. Fertility tourism for surrogacy is driven by legal restrictions or the incentive of lower prices overseas. Popular destinations are those which permit commercial gestational surrogacy, where the cost is relatively low, and which give the intended parents legal rights over the newborn child.

Laws regarding the donor's payments, rights, and responsibilities vary depending on the country. Many people have safe effective treatment abroad but there are risks. It is recommended that the clinic's donor recruitment, health checks, rules of anonymity and limits of donation are all researched by any intended parent prior to making a commitment.

REFERENCES

1. Behjati Ardakani Z, Navabakhsh M, Tremayne S, et al. The impact of third party reproduction on family and kinship. *J Reprod Infertil*. 2021 Jan–Mar;22(1):3–15.
2. ASRM (American Society for Reproductive Medicine). *Third-Party Reproduction: Sperm, Egg, and Embryo Donation and Surrogacy*. 2018. Available from: www.asrm.org/topics/topics-index/third-party-reproduction/
3. HFEA. *Code of Practice*. 9th Edition. London: Human Fertilisation and Embryology Authority; 2021.
4. Samorinha C, De Freitas C, Baía I, et al. Payment to gamete donors: equality, gender equity, or solidarity? *J Assist Reprod Genet*. 2020;37(1):133–140.
5. Harper JC, Kennett D, Reisel D. The end of donor anonymity: how genetic testing is likely to drive anonymous gamete donation out of business. *Hum Reprod*. 2016;31:1135–1140;37(1):133–140.
6. Clarke H, Harrison S, Jansa-Perez M, et al. UK guidelines for the medical and laboratory procurement and use of sperm, oocyte and embryo donors. *Hum Fertil*. 2021;24(1):3–13.
7. Payne MR, Skytte AN, Harper JC. The use of expanded carrier screening of gamete donors. *Hum Reprod*. 2021;36(6):1702–1710.
8. Lutjen P, Trounson A, Leeton J. The establishment and maintenance of pregnancy using in vitro fertilization and embryo donation in a patient with primary ovarian failure. *Nature*. 1984;307:174–175.
9. Human Fertilisation & Embryology Authority. *Trends in Egg and Sperm Donation*. London; 2019. Available from: www.hfea.gov.uk/media/2808/trends-in-egg-and-sperm-donation-final.pdf.
10. Walker Z, Lanes A, Ginsburg E. Oocyte cryopreservation review: outcomes of medical oocyte cryopreservation and planned oocyte cryopreservation. *Reprod Biol Endocrinol*. 2022 Jan 7;20(1):10.
11. Bracewell-Milnes T, Hassain A, Jones BP et al. Does egg-sharing negatively impact on the chance of the donor or recipient achieving a live birth? *Hum Fertil*. 2022;25:1–10.
12. Blyth E. Guidance for egg sharing arrangements: redefining the limits of information-giving in donor assisted conception. *Reprod Biomed Online*. 2001;3:45–47.
13. Blyth E. Subsidized IVF: the development of 'egg sharing' in the United Kingdom. *Hum Reprod*. 2002;17:3254–3259.
14. HFEA. *Rules Around Releasing Donor Information*. London, 2022. Available from: www.hfea.gov.uk/donation/donors/rules-around-releasing-donor-information/.
15. Hodson N. Differences between sperm sharing and egg sharing are morally relevant. *J Med Ethics Published Online*. 2022;49:1.
16. HFEA. *Press Release: The HFEA Respzonds to New Research Showing Link between Frozen-Thawed Embryos and Cancer*. London. Available from: www.hfea.gov.uk/about-us/news-and-press-releases/2022-news-and-press-releases/the-hfea-responds-to-new-research-showing-link-between-frozen-thawed-embryos-and-cancer/#:~:text=About%20the%20HFEA&text=Around%202%2C700%20children%20in%20the,grant%20from%20UK%20central%20government.
17. *HFEA Talk to Your Child About Their Origins*. London: HFEA. Available from: www.hfea.gov.uk/donation/donor-conceived-people-and-their-parents/talk-to-your-child-about-their-origins/
18. LRAG. *HFEA Discussion Paper, Legislative Reform Advisory Group*. London: Human Fertilisation and Embryology Authority; 2022.
19. UK Government. *Surrogacy: Legal Rights of Parents and Surrogates: Overview*. London; 2022. Available from: www.gov.uk/legal-rights-when-using-surrogates-and-donors/print.

30

Add-Ons: Critical Evaluation of Supplementary Treatments

Charlotte Palmer

Experiencing a negative outcome from assisted reproductive interventions can have overwhelming effects on patients and their partners. This can impact on emotional, physical, and psychological wellbeing, in addition to having significant financial implications. Fertility units are constantly evolving their practices in an effort to improve the embryology and subsequent pregnancy outcomes for patients. Many adjunctive treatments have been introduced in addition to standard IVF protocols over recent years. These optional extras are termed 'add-ons'. There is no consensus definition of an 'add-on' but they are generally considered to be a heterogeneous group of additional options for patients to consider in addition to the standard IVF steps depicted in Figure 30.1.

The salient point of an 'add-on' is that the treatment entity is **non-essential**, and can include diagnostic investigations, surgical procedures, medication, supplements, equipment use, laboratory techniques, holistic or alternative therapies. The aim is to increase the likelihood of achieving a pregnancy or reduce the time it takes to conceive and will usually come at an extra financial cost to patients. Availability of add-ons are clinic dependent, with geographical and provider-specific variations between what is offered to patients. Not all add-ons that are integrated into clinical practice have convincing evidence of clinical effectiveness, and this causes controversies amongst the fertility and wider medical and scientific community.

In 2018 the HFEA launched the first ever national fertility patient survey within the UK (**1**). This applied to any patients who had undergone treatment within the preceding five years and gave them the opportunity to give feedback on their experiences. This revealed that 74% of patients had at least one type of add-on included in their treatment in the preceding two years. Information about add-ons is increasingly available online and many patients have strong views or requests for particular treatments, even before they have had an initial consultation.

In 2019 the HFEA released a consensus statement from eleven affiliated societies and colleges regarding treatment add-ons (**2**). This set principles for ensuring patients have consistent, evidence-based treatment and gives guidance for 'responsible innovation' (Box 30.1).

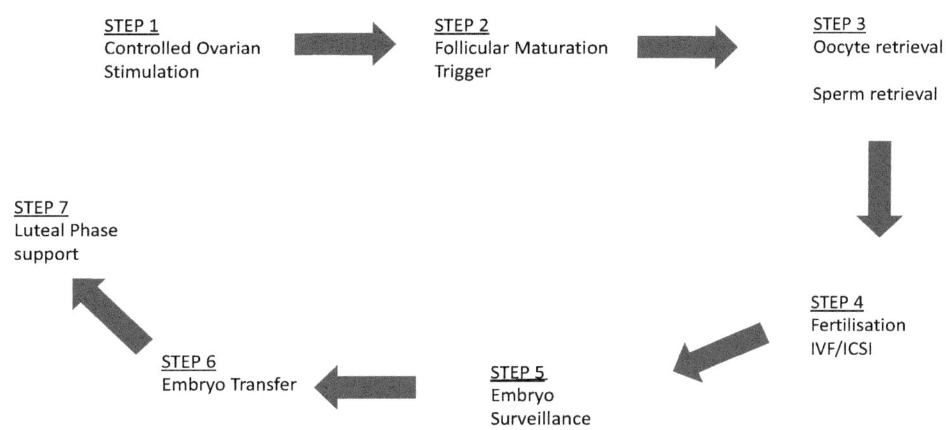

FIGURE 30.1 Conventional fertility cycle.

DOI: 10.1201/9781003269502-30

BOX 30.1 EXTRACTS FROM THE CONSENSUS STATEMENT REGARDING RESPONSIBLE INNOVATION (2)

'Practitioners have a duty of care to patients, which should separate pressure from patients and commercial interests from their best practice advice.

We believe that culture change is required if the potential benefits of new treatments are to be offered responsibly. It's time to have an open and honest conversation about treatment add-ons. This consensus statement sets out the principles of responsible innovation which we believe should guide professionals in the UK.'

1. **Clinics should only offer treatment add-ons under the following conditions:**
   a) ≥1 high quality study to demonstrate the add-on is safe and effective. The clinic must continue to monitor local success rates and long-term data with adequate incident reporting if concerns are raised about safety and effectiveness.
   b) If there is limited or conflicting evidence about an add-on, the clinic must be open about their data to add to the evidence-base for the add-on.
   c) If there is no evidence to support the safety and efficacy, add-ons should only be offered in a research setting approved by a research ethics committee.
2. **Clinics must provide patients with up-to-date information about the evidence base supporting the use of any treatment add-on they offer.**
3. **Patients must be clearly informed of the experimental nature of any treatment add-on which is offered where there is no robust evidence for safety or effectiveness.**
4. **Patients should not be charged extra to take part in research.**

In April 2022, the HFEA released an updated report of key findings from a national patient survey collected in 2021 (**3**).

This demonstrated that 65% of patients had used a treatment add-on with the most common being acupuncture (33%) followed by time-lapse imaging. It also revealed that **treatment option availability**, was the fourth most key factor for patients choosing a clinic location.

CLASSIFYING CLINICAL EFFECTIVENESS OF ADD-ONS

A subcommittee of the HFEA, the Scientific and Clinical Advances Advisory Committee (SCAAC), meets annually together with independent expert reviewers, to evaluate the quality of evidence and research available on treatment add-ons. A rigorous process of evaluation specifically focuses on the availability of multi centre, peer-reviewed, double blinded randomised controlled trials (RCTs), widely accepted as the highest quality study design. To convey these evaluations, a patient centred 'traffic light' classification system has been developed with the aim of simplifying scientific evidence (**2**):

- Green for more than one high quality RCT showing the procedure is effective at improving the chances of having a baby for most fertility patients
- Amber for conflicting evidence from RCTs: the evidence is not conclusive and the add-on should not be recommended for routine use
- Red for no evidence from RCTs

Whilst this is transparent in terms of classifying RCT evidence, it negates evidence that is collected from other study designs such as cross-sectional studies, cohort studies or case-control series. The exclusion of these alternative study designs is based on the presumption that they are less reliable in drawing conclusions about treatment effectiveness and contain more bias.

More recently, this classification system has been challenged, with the view that other sources of evidence should be included for informing patients of their reproductive choices (**4**). There is a further caveat paragraph included with the traffic light classification:

'For specific patient groups there may be reasons for the use of a treatment add-on other than improving your chances of having a baby. In these situations, it may be appropriate for you to be offered a treatment add-on as part of your treatment and not in a research setting.'

Table 30.1 lists the commonly available add-ons; more details on specific widely offered add-ons and their scientific basis is included in the subsequent sections.

TABLE 30.1

The More Common Add-Ons Currently Available with Assisted Conception

IVF Add on	Description
Time lapse imaging systems (TLS)	Time lapse systems are incubators with integrated digital cameras to allow for continuous monitoring of embryos as they develop in culture media. Images are taken frequently at specific time intervals, allowing the embryo to be studied in minute detail without being disturbed. Some fertility units also utilise software or algorithms using data from the TLS that can assist in assessment of embryo quality and selection.
Hyaluronate enriched medium	This is a transfer medium containing hyaluronan (HA). The addition of HA is thought to improve the chances of implantation by improving contact and adherence of the embryo to the endometrium.
Endometrial injury 'scratch'	The endometrium is intentionally 'injured' or 'scratched' using a pipelle device prior to commencing a standard IVF treatment cycle. The theory is that this triggers an immunological reaction at the site of the injury which makes it more receptive to an embryo implanting.
Preimplantation genetic diagnosis (PGD)	In PGD embryos carrying a specific genetic mutation (PGM) or chromosomal translocation are identified and not transferred. Testing involves taking a biopsy from an embryo and performing genetic tests in a laboratory. Patients require adequate genetic counselling and pedigree/inheritance analysis prior to organising these specific tests.
Pre-implantation genetic testing for Aneuploidy (PGT-A)	An embryologist performs a biopsy on appropriate quality embryos. This tissue sample is then genetically analysed for chromosome number with normal 'euploid' embryos being preferentially selected for transfer back to the endometrium for implantation. Aneuploid embryos have an abnormal number of chromosomes and must be discarded or used for research/training.
Artificial egg activation	Calcium ionophores are a type of substance that increases concentration of calcium ions when applied to an egg, which in turn activates the egg so that fertilisation can occur.
Intrauterine administration of hCG	Administering natural or synthetic hCG into the uterus prior to embryo transfer. There are currently variable doses and times of administration as well as different recommended stages of embryo transfer in which this administration is effective (cleavage stage v blastocyst)
Intrauterine culture	Intrauterine culture allows the early stages of embryo development to occur within the uterus. The fertilised eggs are collected and placed in an intrauterine culture device and inserted into the uterus. The device stays in place for several hours during the initial stages of embryo development. When the device is removed, the embryos are put in an incubator until they are ready to be transferred back to the uterus or frozen for future transfer.
Intracytoplasmic morphologic sperm injection (IMSI)	Intracytoplasmic morphologic sperm injection (IMSI) is a laboratory technique whereby ultra-high magnifications are used to identify the morphological appearances of sperm. It is a technology based on ICSI however the higher magnifications allow elucidation of more detail. This is especially useful for identifying defects in the sperm head which would not otherwise be visualised under lower magnifications. Once sperm are selected, the process is the same as ICSI in which the sperm is injected into the oocyte.
Advanced sperm selection	Advanced sperm selection techniques are thought to improve the chance that structurally intact and mature sperm with high DNA integrity are selected for fertilisation. Different selection strategies include selecting based on surface charge, ability to bind hyaluronic acid, sperm apoptosis and sperm birefringence.
Assisted hatching	Assisted hatching is a laboratory technique in which the zona pellucida is thinned or an opening is made in it. This can be achieved chemically, mechanically, via laser or with electric pulses (piezo technology). It is thought that breaching this membrane can aid implantation.
Reproductive immunology tests	There are various treatments in this category of add-on that aims to suppress the patient's immune system and therefore favour implantation and a sustained pregnancy. Treatments include administration of steroids, intravenous immunoglobulins, TNF-alpha blocking agents, intralipid infusions.
Sperm DNA damage tests	There are various tests that look at the DNA integrity of sperm. This is a non-invasive add-on performed on the semen sample provided. The background behind these tests is that during sperm cell maturation DNA is susceptible to strand breakage or fragmentation and this could cause failed IVF cycles or miscarriage.
Endometrial receptivity analysis (ERA)	This is a diagnostic test that determines each woman's unique personalised embryo transfer timing therefore synchronising the embryo transfer with the individualised window of implantation. An endometrial biopsy is taken in a mock embryo transfer cycle.
Microbiome testing	Evaluating the endometrial microbiome can recommend the best probiotic treatment to balance the endometrial flora. If low levels of lactobacilli are found this could reduce the chances of pregnancy.
Screening for chronic endometritis	Screening for chronic endometritis can detect bacteria causing chronic endometritis and recommend specific antibiotics and probiotics fir successful treatment,

Note: This is by no means an exhaustive list as research and development is fast paced, with new add-ons being introduced and popularity of interventions changing on a regular basis.

30.1 Time Lapse Imaging Systems (TLS)

Assessment of embryo development is a vital step in any IVF cycle. Traditionally this was achieved by embryologists removing embryos from the incubator on a daily basis. In more recent years, the development of time lapse imaging systems (TLS) has allowed for more frequent review of embryo development without the physical removal from its stabilised environment. TLS are essentially incubators with in-built digital cameras and their proposed advantage is the ability to detect minute changes and detail that may not have otherwise been identified with traditional review (**5**), together with preventing repeated disturbance.

TLS have the ability to capture images of embryos every 5 minutes over a period of 6 days. This generates thousands of images per embryo and provides specific timings of when a developmental milestone is reached (morphokinetics). Using the TLS data from successful live births, many researchers have developed embryo selection algorithms (ESAs) to score or grade the embryos (**6**).

Despite the wealth of data TLS can provide for embryological assessment, a recent Cochrane review concluded that there is insufficient evidence of differences in live birth, ongoing pregnancy, miscarriage, or clinical pregnancy to choose between TLS, with or without ESAs, and conventional incubation (**7**). Despite these conclusions, TLS remain very popular as demonstrated in the recent patient survey.

30.2 Hyaluronate Enriched Medium

Hyaluronic acid is a natural compound found in the body that acts as a binding and protective agent (**8**). During implantation, there are higher concentrations of hyaluronan present, along with increased expression of its receptors in embryos (**9**). Murine studies in the early 1990's showed improved implantation rates when culture media were enriched with hyaluronic acid (**9**). It has also been suggested that Hyaluronan promotes decidualisation of the endometrium and better mimics the intrauterine environment (**10**).

In 2020 Cochrane published a systematic review comparing embryo transfer media containing functional concentrations of adherence compounds, to media with no or low adherence compound concentrations. It concluded that there was moderate quality evidence to suggest that these adherence compounds improved clinical pregnancy and live birth rates (**11**). Criticisms of this review (**5**) have highlighted that it only included studies with patients up to the age of 35, when in fact such formulations of culture media have greatest benefit in poorer prognosis patients including raised maternal age, previous failed cycles and with poor quality embryos (**12, 13**).

30.3 Assisted Hatching (AH)

The aim of assisted hatching (AH) is to artificially disrupt the zona pellucida (ZP) of the fertilised egg or blastocyst and thereby help initiate the developmental steps leading to implantation. This is a laboratory technique that is sometimes used in IVF or ICSI and involves thinning or incising this membrane to enable 'hatching' of the embryo from its protective coat. It is proposed that failure of ZP rupture after blastocyst expansion, is a possible contributory factor to failed implantation.

Zona Pellucida thickness appears to be influenced by a variety of factors including maternal age, smoking status, the cause of infertility and hormone profile (Raised FSH). Studies have also reported a correlation between increased zona thickness and decreased implantation rates (**14, 15**). Various theories as to how AH improves embryo implantation have been suggested:

- AH may overcome ZP hardening caused by IVF, cell culture or cryopreservation
- AH may lead to implantation occurring one day earlier than unhatched embryos
- AH could enhance hormonal and metabolite exchange and thereby signal transduction between the endometrium and embryo

There are different methods used to disrupt the ZP including mechanical, chemical and laser. AH techniques will also distinguish whether the ZP has remained un-breached (thinning), fully breached (hole made) or has been completely removed. Box 30.2 lists some of the different techniques and extent of ZP disruption utilised for AH.

BOX 30.2 EXAMPLES OF AH TECHNIQUES

- Chemical drilling of ZP with acidic Tyrode's medium
- ZP thinning using acidic Tyrode's medium
- Mechanical piercing of the ZP with a microneedle – partial zona dissection (PZD)
- Mechanical expansion of the ZP with injected hydrostatic pressure
- Carving a hole in the ZP with piezoelectric pulses
- Lazer assisted ZP drilling

An update to a previously conducted Cochrane systematic review (**16**), still reports uncertainties regarding the clinical effectiveness of this add-on. There may be a slightly increased chance of clinical pregnancy with AH, but this is unclear due to the quality of the evidence available (poor). These potential benefits need to be weighed against the risk of techniques causing injury to embryos, and a potential for an increase in multiple pregnancy. The HFEA and NICE do not recommend AH.

30.4 Artificial Oocyte Activation (AOA)

This is a laboratory intervention in which calcium ionophores are added to the culture medium of oocytes to facilitate activation and subsequent fertilisation.

In 1995 this add-on gained further momentum when a study reported that treating oocytes with calcium ionophore after failed ICSI, led to improved fertilisation rates compared to a control solvent (**17**). Subsequent studies have continued to demonstrate the benefit of AOA after ICSI particularly when previous cycles have had suboptimal fertilisation rates (**5**).

Data remains conflicting regarding whether this improvement in fertilisation rate translates to improved outcomes in terms of live birth rates. Again, the existing quality of evidence is limited by sample size and study design.

Further contention regarding the safety of AOA has previously been questioned with the suggestion that manipulation of gametes may lead to birth defects or pregnancy complications such as intrauterine growth restriction, or preterm delivery with its neonatal siliquae (**18**). However, this has recently been rebuffed in a meta-analysis concluding that AOA did not result in any significant increase in either congenital birth defects or chromosomal anomalies (**19**).

30.5 Pre-Implantation Genetic Testing for Aneuploidy (PGT-A)

Embryonic aneuploidy is the leading cause of poor reproductive outcomes in both natural and assisted conception, and it can lead to recurrent miscarriage and implantation failure (**20**).

PGT-A is a laboratory-based technique developed to examine the number of chromosomes present in embryos. Normal 'euploid' embryos are then preferentially selected for transfer whilst abnormal 'aneuploid' embryos that would be destined for failure, are not used for treatment. Selection of the most competent embryos facilitates single embryo transfer (SET) and reduces the risk of multiple pregnancy (**20**).

There is a third potential result of a PGT-A biopsy and that is a 'mosaic' embryo. Embryos that are mosaic can have different proportions of normal and abnormal cells and the laboratory report usually gives some indication of this. Patients often require further consultation with a genetic counsellor to discuss the levels of mosaicism and what implications this could have in terms of potential congenital defects in any resulting child (if any).

PGT-A was first introduced in the early 1990's and has been the subject of ongoing scientific debate and controversy for decades. The earlier genetic analysis techniques first utilised fluorescent in situ hybridisation (FISH) and these quickly gained popularity and were introduced before the technique was validated for clinical settings (**21**). A systematic review and meta-analysis published in 2011, reported that there were no beneficial results of PGTA (using FISH) with some suggestion it may even be harmful (**22**). However, with advances in technology now incorporating comprehensive chromosome screening (CCS), with next generation sequencing (NGS), and trophectoderm (TE) biopsy, the biopsy technique appears to be less operator-dependent with more consistent reproducibility. More material is often available for analysis and there are lower rates of mosaicism which lead to earlier criticism of cleavage-stage biopsies.

Earlier genetic analysis platforms such as array comparative genomic hybridisation (aCGH), real-time quantitative polymerase chain reaction (qPCR), single nucleotide polymorphisms (SNP) and microarray have been superseded by NGS which is now utilised by all accredited PGT-A providers in the UK (**4**).

Despite the advent of CCS in PGT-A, RCTs have still been presenting inconsistent results regarding the clinical effectiveness and improvement in live birth rate with PGTA (**4**). In order to examine the data for PGTA cycle outcomes within the UK, a recent research group requested data from the HFEA via a freedom of information request (**4**). This included data for cycles between 2016 and 2018 and this retrospective study revealed compelling evidence for PGTA in terms of live births per embryo transferred and per cycle.

30.6 Endometrial Receptivity Analysis (ERA)

Implantation is an intricate process that requires synchronisation between a healthy embryo and a receptive endometrium. Endometrial receptivity denotes a time sensitive window of implantation (WOI) in which endometrial maturation, (orchestrated by complex molecular signalling), allows a blastocyst to attach and invade the endometrial stroma. Whilst the WOI most frequently occurs over a 2-to-3-day timeframe within the luteal phase, for various reasons this time period may be shifted or narrowed in some patients undergoing IVF (**5**).

Identification of gene expression profiles for both receptive and non-receptive endometrium has allowed an 'array' to be developed as an objective molecular dating tool – endometrial receptivity analysis (ERA) (**23**). By profiling the transcriptome of 238 genes that are expressed at various stages of the endometrial cycle, the ERA can accurately and reproducibly identify the receptivity status of endometrial tissue. Using this information, a personalised embryo transfer (pET) time can be recommended specific to the patients' own menstrual cycle so called 'precision medicine'.

In order to perform an ERA, an endometrial biopsy is required which is an invasive test and may be painful for the patient. Albeit small, there are also associated risks of introducing infection or causing intrauterine injury or perforation. These need to be considered and discussed when offering this add on investigation to patients. Whilst personalised medicine and genomics-based tests hold a lot of potential for reproductive care, there still remains conflicting evidence and mixed results that ERA offers a justifiable benefit.

30.7 Future Assessment of Add-ons

When evaluating more commonly used add-ons, there is a reoccurring theme of insufficient, high-quality evidence to support clinical effectiveness.

The HFEA continue to prioritise addressing how treatment add-ons are offered to patients and plan to evolve the current traffic light rating system as part of their strategy with updated ratings to be launched early in 2023 (**24**). The three key elements that are being developed include:

- Evolving the rating scale and presentation of this evidence.

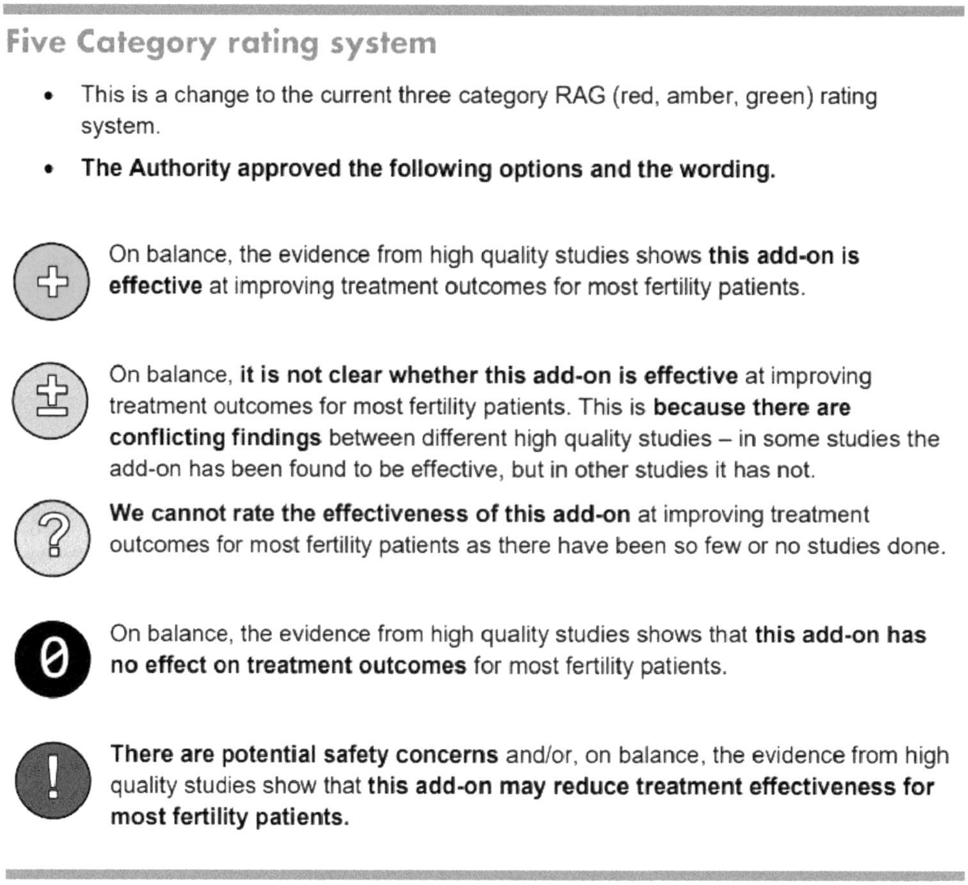

Five Category rating system

- This is a change to the current three category RAG (red, amber, green) rating system.
- **The Authority approved the following options and the wording.**

On balance, the evidence from high quality studies shows **this add-on is effective** at improving treatment outcomes for most fertility patients.

On balance, **it is not clear whether this add-on is effective** at improving treatment outcomes for most fertility patients. This is **because there are conflicting findings** between different high quality studies – in some studies the add-on has been found to be effective, but in other studies it has not.

We cannot rate the effectiveness of this add-on at improving treatment outcomes for most fertility patients as there have been so few or no studies done.

On balance, the evidence from high quality studies shows that **this add-on has no effect on treatment outcomes** for most fertility patients.

There are potential safety concerns and/or, on balance, the evidence from high quality studies show that **this add-on may reduce treatment effectiveness for most fertility patients.**

FIGURE 30.2 Five-category rating system for add-ons to be introduced in 2023 (**24**).

- Incorporating outcomes in addition to live birth rates.
- Determining the evidence base that should be used when rating add-ons.

The HFEA has started a consultation with its stakeholders and agreed a more detailed 5-category rating system which will be introduced for add-ons (Figure 30.2). This is intended to provide patients with an easier understanding of the level of effectiveness or potential safety concerns in relation to specific add-ons.

REFERENCES

1. HFEA. *Pilot National Patient Survey Human Fertilisation and Embryology Authority*. 2018. Available from: www.hfea.gov.uk/media/2702/pilot-national-fertility-survey-2018.pdf.
2. Sanders D, Kasraie J, Lewis S, et al. *The Responsible Use of Treatment Add-Ons in Fertility Services: A Consensus Statement*. Human Fertilisation and Embryology Authority; 2019. Available from: www.hfea.gov.uk/media/2792/treatment-add-ons-consensus-statement-final.pdf.
3. HFEA. *National Patient Survey*. Human Fertilisation and Embryology Authority; 2021. Available from: www.hfea.gov.uk/about-us/publications/research-and-data/national-patient-survey-2021.
4. Sanders KD, Silvestri G, Gordon T, et al. Analysis of IVF live birth outcomes with and without preimplantation genetic testing for aneuploidy (PGT-A): UK Human Fertilisation and Embryology Authority data collection 2016–2018. *J Assist Reprod Genet*. 2021;38:3277–3285.
5. Glatthorn HN, Decherney A. The efficacy of add-ons: selected IVF "add-on" procedures and future directions. *J Assist Reprod Genet*. 2022;39(3):581–589.
6. Barrie A, McDowell G, Troup S. An investigation into the effect of potential confounding patient and treatment parameters on human embryo morphokinetics. *Fertil Steril*. 2021;115(4):1014–1022.
7. Armstrong S, Bhide P, Jordan V, et al. Time-lapse systems for embryo incubation and assessment in assisted reproduction. *Cochrane Database Syst Rev*. 2019;5(5):CD011320.
8. Cochrane. *Special Collection: In Vitro fertilisation – Effectiveness of Add-Ons: Cochrane*. 2021. Available from: www.cochrane.org/news/special-collection-vitro-fertilisation-effectiveness-add-ons.
9. Gardner DK, Rodriegez-Martinez H, Lane M. Fetal development after transfer is increased by replacing protein with the glycosaminoglycan hyaluronan for mouse embryo culture and transfer. *Hum Reprod*. 1999;14(10):2575–2580.
10. Schoolcraft W, Lane M, Stevens J, et al. Increased hyaluronan concentration in the embryo transfer medium results in a significant increase in human embryo implantation rate. *Fertil Steril*. 2002;78:S5.

11. Heymann D, Vidal L, Or Y, et al. Hyaluronic acid in embryo transfer media for assisted reproductive technologies. *Cochrane Database Syst Rev.* 2020;9(9):CD007421.
12. Atkinson B, Woodland E, editors. *Embryo Glue: The Use of Hyaluronan in Embryo Transfer Media. Seminars in Reproductive Medicine.* New York: Thieme, 2021.
13. Hazlett WD, Meyer LR, Nasta TE, et al. Impact of EmbryoGlue as the Embryo Transfer Medium. *Fertil Steril.* 2008;90(1):214–216.
14. Avella MA, Milne KA, Dawood S, et al. Assisted hatching of human embryos for successful implantation. In: Nagy Z, Varghese A, Agrawal A, editors. *In Vitro Fertilization.* Cham: Springer; 2019. Pp. 567–579.
15. Ricardo Loret de Mola J, Garside WT, Bucci J, et al. Analysis of the human zona pellucida during culture: correlation with diagnosis and the preovulatory hormonal environment. *J Assist Reprod Genet.* 1997;14:332–336.
16. Lacey L, Hassan S, Franik S, et al. Assisted hatching on assisted conception (in vitro fertilisation (IVF) and intracytoplasmic sperm injection (ICSI)). *Cochrane Database Syst Rev.* 2021;3(3):CD001894.
17. Tesarik J, Sousa M. More than 90% fertilization rates after intracytoplasmic sperm injection and artificial induction of oocyte activation with calcium ionophore. *Fertil Steril.* 1995;63(2):343–349.
18. Miller N, Biron-Shental T, Sukenik-Halevy R, et al. Oocyte activation by calcium ionophore and congenital birth defects: a retrospective cohort study. *Fertil Steril.* 2016;106(3):590–596. E2.
19. Long R, Wang M, Yang QY, et al. Risk of birth defects in children conceived by artificial oocyte activation and intracytoplasmic sperm injection: a meta-analysis. *Reprod Biol Endocrinol.* 2020;18(1):1–9.
20. L'Heveder A, Jones BP, Naja R, et al. Pre-implantation genetic testing for aneuploidy: the past, present and future. *Obstet Gynecol.* 2020;22(4):293–304.
21. Scott RT, Jr, Upham KM, Forman EJ, et al. Blastocyst biopsy with comprehensive chromosome screening and fresh embryo transfer significantly increases in vitro fertilization implantation and delivery rates: a randomized controlled trial. *Fertil Steril.* 2013;100(3):697–703.
22. Mastenbroek S, Twisk M, Van Der Veen F, et al. Preimplantation genetic screening: a systematic review and meta-analysis of RCTs. *Hum Reprod Update.* 2011; 17(4):454–466.
23. Tan J, Kan A, Hitkari J, et al. The role of the endometrial receptivity array (ERA) in patients who have failed euploid embryo transfers. *J Assist Reprod Genet.* 2018;35:683–692.
24. SCAAC. *Scientific Clinical Advisory Committee (SCAAC) Meeting Papers.* HFEA; 2022. Available from: www.hfea.gov.uk/media/ebobgcmd/2022-10-03-scaac-meeting-papers.pdf.

31

Cryobiology and Cryopreservation of Oocytes and Embryos

Louise Best

31.1 History of Gamete and Embryo Cryopreservation

Cryopreservation of gametes and embryos in human IVF has transformed the options available to patients, as well as maximising the potential from a single oocyte retrieval by the long-term storage of surplus embryos. Cryopreservation is the use of very low temperatures to store cells, tissues or organs to preserve their viability by stopping all biological activity. As human biological systems lack efficient internal defence mechanisms against chilling injuries, it is of the utmost importance to supply adequate external support, in terms of cryoprotectant additives, appropriate cooling/warming rates, and suitable long-term storage (**1**). The combination of these elements has been constantly modified and refined for more than 50 years. Early attempts at freezing human biological cells used spermatozoa, due to their availability, small size, and their motility acting as a simple marker of viability. Successful cryopreservation of fertilised mouse embryos was first reported by Whittingham et al. in 1972 (**2**). This was achieved by slow freezing at a predicted, controlled rate and seeding the storage device containing the cells to induce crystal formation at an exact temperature. The first human pregnancy from a frozen eight-cell embryo was in 1983, in Australia, using similar methods. The first pregnancy from a vitrified blastocyst was reported by Yokota et al. in 2000 (**3**).

The use of vitrification for oocytes and embryos was a major development for cryopreservation in IVF. It dramatically increases post-survival rates, when compared to slow freezing, and has significantly improved clinical outcomes. Vitrification, derived from the Latin word vitreum which means "glass," involves the rapid cooling of a liquid to avoid the formation of the destructive crystals within the cells.

The Human Fertilisation and Embryology Authority (HFEA) in the UK reported that frozen embryo transfers increased by 86% from 2014–2019 (**4**). Frozen embryo transfers made up 41% of all IVF cycles in 2019.

31.2 Principles of Cryobiology

Vitrification achieves minimization of crystal formation within the cytoplasm of cells, which is the main cause of injury challenging its viability. This success is based on two basic elements: Firstly, before cooling, gametes/embryos are placed in

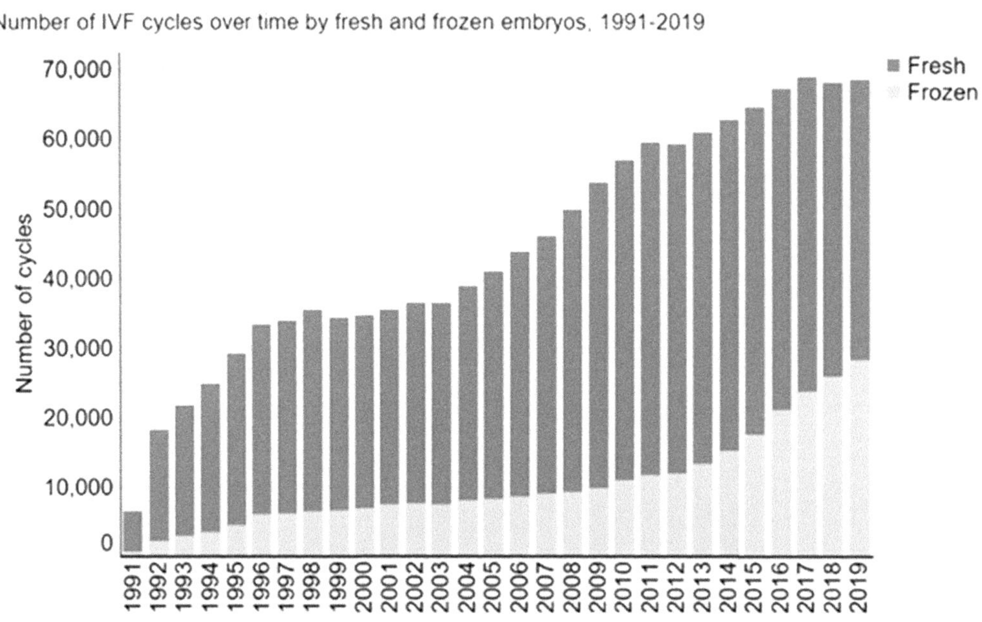

FIGURE 31.1 Number of IVF cycles levelling off, while frozen embryo transfers increase (from [**4**]with permission).

DOI: 10.1201/9781003269502-31

the appropriate cryoprotectant which causes dehydration, and then enter the cells osmotically replacing water, and secondly, by the use of sufficiently high cooling and warming rates between the culture temperature of 37°C and liquid nitrogen's temperature of −196°C. Therefore, the solution and intracellular environment do not form crystals but solidify acquiring a composition similar to that of glass (**5**). The balance between cryoprotectant concentrations and rapid cooling rates dramatically decreased the time required for cryopreservation in the IVF laboratory. As such, vitrification is a highly skilled process that requires a good deal of training.

The steps involved in vitrification and warming protocols are: a) Exposure of oocytes/embryos to progressively higher concentrations of cryoprotectants to cause dehydration, b) loading of oocyte/embryos on a carrier of choice in the smallest volume required, c) rapid freezing-vitrifying, d) storage at -196°C, e) warming by exposure to gradually lower concentration of cryoprotectants aiming towards rehydration and washing in order to remove cryoprotectant material and restore the physiological environment. Part of the success of vitrification is the loading of the oocytes/embryos on to the carrier in a minimal volume (0.5–2μl) which facilitates the rapid cooling rates and even higher warming rates.

Studies show that warming rates may be more important than those of cooling as achieving warming rates of 42,000°C/min ensures a fast passage from the harmful temperature zone which is responsible for the chilling injury and affects the meiotic spindle and cytoplasmic lipid droplets (**6**).

The choice of carrier can also have an effect on the success of the oocyte or embryo. They are largely divided into "open" and "closed" devices. "Open" vitrification devices (such as Cryotec (Cryotech), Cryolock (Irvine Scientific), McGill Cryoleaf (Medicult), Vitri-Inga (Ingamed)) allow direct contact of the oocytes with liquid nitrogen (LN2) and usually provide very high cooling (20,000°C/min) rates. Conversely, closed devices (such as CryoTip, High-Security Vitrification straw (Irvine Scientific), Cryopette (Cooper Surgical), Rapid-I (Vitrolife), VitriSafe (Nextclinics), and MicroSecure (**7**)) may not be able to reach this cooling rate, but they have the advantage that samples can be stored completely isolated from the external environment (**8**). As liquid nitrogen is not routinely sterilised, the direct contact with the samples on an 'open' device has the theoretical risk of potential contamination during the freezing event, or the potential cross-contamination between samples in a liquid storage system. Although the benefits of employing the 'open' versus the 'closed system may outweigh the negligible risk of contamination, it has been reported that the cooling rate obtained with closed devices generates a comparable survival rate if the warming rate is sufficiently high (**9**), or better for oocyte vitrification (**10**).

31.3 Cryoprotectants Used in Cryomedia

Cryoprotectants are constituents used to protect biological material from damage during the freezing and thawing process. Cryoprotective effects of glycerol were discovered accidentally by Polge et al. in 1949 (**11**). Cryoprotectants are divided into two groups: intracellular (such as DMSO, glycerol and propylene glycol) and extracellular (such as sucrose, trehalose, polyvinyl pyrrolidone, ficoll, hydroxyethyl starch and dextran) (**12**). Their modes of action are lowering of the freezing point of the solution, preventing intracellular ice formation, as well as protecting the cell membrane from the drastic changes occurring during the transition between fluid and solid states. Cryoprotectants may, however, be toxic to the cells, therefore over the years a relentless search for less toxic and efficient cryoprotectants ensued as well as for protocols combining several cryoprotectants in order to reduce individual solute concentration and the associated cell toxicity. Non-permeating cryoprotectants are generally higher molecular weight polymers and mimic the dehydration mechanism of penetrating cryoprotectants but remain outside of the cell.

Sucrose and trehalose are the most commonly used non-penetrating cryoprotective agents (CPAs) during vitrification and warming of oocytes and embryos. It has been reported that the inclusion of 0.5 M of either sucrose or trehalose in the vitrification solution improved the percentage of viable oocytes post-warming in sheep as compared to those vitrified in sugar-free solutions (**13**).

Permeating cryoprotectants (e.g., glycerol, propane diol, dimethyl sulphoxide or ethylene glycol) cross the cell membrane through an osmotic gradient displacing water. These agents act to reduce ice crystallization and reduce cell dehydration but are toxic at higher concentrations. More specifically, in vitrification, their role is to completely inhibit ice formation. Permeating cryoprotectants also stabilize intracellular solutes which otherwise would be lethal in a hyperosmotic state. The rate of dehydration is dependent on the controlled working temperature promoting slower or faster dehydration (**14**).

31.4 Oocyte Cryopreservation

Oocytes at metaphase II are the most vulnerable and challenging of the reproductive cells to cryopreserve. This is due to their relatively large size, high water content and the presence of the meiotic spindle. Oocyte freezing may be of benefit to any person who wishes to preserve their fertility for medical or nonmedical reasons, following thorough counselling regarding success rates. Oocytes are cryopreserved almost exclusively at the metaphase II stage, although there may be some circumstances when immature eggs are frozen.

Reasons why eggs may be vitrified:

1. For non-medical/social reasons women may wish to freeze their eggs to delay having children until a more appropriate time in their lives. This is because the efficiency of getting pregnant declines with age and the risk of miscarriage and certain abnormalities (such as Down's syndrome) increase with age. The age of the person when the eggs are replaced (as embryos) is almost irrelevant; it is the age of the person when the egg was removed and preserved that counts the most. Therefore, people who may not want to conceive until their later 30s/early 40s, may consider using eggs from their own "egg bank" of eggs preserved when they were much younger. The

chance of conception in a single cycle with eggs of a 30-year-old person is estimated to be up to 50%, compared with 15% with eggs of a 40-year-old.

2. People suffering from endometriosis, a progressive disease that can impair ovarian function.
3. Cancer: the common treatments for cancer – chemotherapy and radiotherapy – can have the common side effect of damaging the ovaries which may affect a person's future fertility. Unfortunately, for many cancer sufferers the need to quickly commence with cancer treatment does not allow sufficient time to set up a treatment cycle, stimulate the ovaries and collect eggs; as this could delay cancer treatment for 2–6 weeks. There may also be extra risks (for example in people with breast cancer) whose cancer may be sensitive to the high hormone (oestrogen) levels produced when stimulating drugs are given. However, following advice from a person's cancer specialist an attempt at egg freezing in selected cases could be considered where the timing of cancer treatment is less critical and hormone issues are not relevant.
4. Other medical reasons, for example a family history of premature ovarian failure.
5. Eggs may also be frozen if more eggs than sperm are available in an ICSI treatment cycle, or if the couple have ethical concerns about the creation of surplus embryos (e.g., do not want more than two eggs inseminated when larger numbers of eggs are available).

Effective freezing programmes also allows storing of donor eggs in order to provide a bank for recipients to have instant access to, without having to wait to be matched with a donor.

The process of vitrification clearly has some degree of negative effect on the oocyte physiology: the membrane permeability; the hardening of zona pellucida; cytoplasmic and cytoskeletal damage, and depolymerization of the meiotic spindle (**15**). The procedure is carried out at room temperature or 37°C to attempt to reduce the effects of the increased cryoprotectant concentrations, however by exposing oocytes to temperatures below 37°C leads to rapid depolymerisation of the meiotic spindle. This beta-tubulin depolymerisation is completely reversible following 2 hours of incubation post warming, forming morphologically normal metaphases with properly aligned chromatin (**16**).

Since the birth of the first baby following vitrification of oocytes in 1999 (**17**), technology and protocols have refined and improved, leading to much more consistent survival, fertilisation, and pregnancy results. As with embryo cryopreservation there are several vitrification kits available on the market. An evaluation should be made before choosing one as some result in inconsistent survival rates following thawing and others require extensive training. All the kits will contain varying combinations and concentrations of cryoprotectants, but all involve a period of equilibration in a first solution (modified for oocyte cryopreservation with some commercial kits) followed by a fast washing in high concentration cryoprotectant, before plunging into liquid nitrogen, or a supercooled holding device.

The skill involved in successful vitrification comes from the movement, or lack of disturbance, within the medias; the control of transfer between the solutions; the strict adherence to timings within the solutions; and the minimizing of media that the oocytes or embryo is loaded in on the device. Minimizing the volume of the vitrification solution containing oocytes or embryos not only offers the benefit of increasing both cooling and warming rates, but also decreases the chance of ice crystal nucleation/formation in the small sample (**18**).

31.5 Embryo Cryopreservation

Embryo cryopreservation facilitates the maximum potential of every oocyte retrieval. This has been particularly pertinent since the advent of blastocyst culture. In addition to this, time-lapse technology has allowed for algorithms to give a prediction a predictive value to the competence of those stored blastocysts. As such, although less blastocysts than embryos maybe cryopreserved following a treatment cycle, they have a higher, and more understood implantation potential, and gives way to an increase in the trend for freeze all cycles, with no fresh transfer. A freeze- all policy has been shown to significantly increase outcomes for patients who have low progesterone levels, or impaired endometrial receptivity (ER) (**19**). Growing evidence in the literature shows that controlled ovarian stimulation (COS), with its supraphysiologic hormonal levels, may decrease ER (**20**). Moreover, endometrial development can be controlled more precisely during its priming for frozen-thawed embryo transfer (FET) vs. for COS. With the freeze-all policy, the entire cohort of embryos is cryopreserved, and the FET is performed later in a natural cycle, or in a cycle with hormonal replacement for endometrial priming.

Kuwayama's method of vitrification is considered the gold standard in terms of successful outcomes from blastocyst vitrification (**18**). Vitrification of 6328 human blastocysts resulted in 90% survival, and the 5659 transferred blastocysts resulted in 53% clinical pregnancies and 45% live births/transfer. This was using the Cryotop technology.

An added element with regards to vitrifying blastocysts over oocytes, is assessment of the grade as well as the stage. The first issue is which (morphological) type of blastocysts can be selected for vitrification. This question is crucial, as it is well accepted that blastocyst morphology, classified by the degree of expansion and appearance of the inner cell mass (ICM) and trophectoderm (TE), is positively associated with implantation rate (IR) and live birth rate (LBR) after fresh and frozen embryo transfer (**21**). Because of the correlation between morphology and LBR, blastocyst vitrification is generally restricted to embryos with expansion scores of 3–5 on Day 5 and an ICM or TE with minimum Grade B ideally according to the Gardner score (**22**).

The second issue is how to proceed with delayed Day 5 embryos presenting as early blastocysts or with delayed blastulation at the stage of morulae or compacting embryos on Day 5. Embryos frequently reach the blastocyst stage only on Day 6. Reasons for this phenomenon might involve cytoplasmic immaturity of oocytes, chromosomal abnormalities in blastomeres and suboptimal culture conditions that might result in prolonged intermitotic periods and therefore delayed development of the embryo (**23**). Blastocysts are routinely cryopreserved on day 5, 6 or even day 7 post- oocyte retrieval. However, to avoid asynchrony between the stage of the blastocyst and the window of implantation of the endometrium, all blastocysts are warmed and replaced on day 5 of progesterone exposure in an FET cycle.

31.6 Developments in Cryopreservation Materials and Methods

31.6.1 Automated Vitrification

An automated vitrification system, the Gavi®, has been developed by Genea Biomedx in Australia. It automates and standardises the exposure time to cryoprotectants and cooling/warming rates. Potential benefits maybe improved clinical outcomes due to standardisation and the reduced timeframe required for embryologists to achieve high survival rates consistently, when compared to manual systems. Disadvantages would be the deskilling of embryologists to manually vitrify embryos.

The first livebirth reported using warmed oocytes, that had been vitrified using the automated GAVI™, was reported in 2021 (**24**). Fifteen donor oocytes were collected and after cumulus removal, fourteen metaphase II oocytes were identified. They were vitrified 40 hours post hCG using GAVI™ as previously described by Roy and colleagues (**25**). Prior to loading the oocytes into the pod, gametes were cultured for 5 minutes in VitBase in an ungassed incubator. In the meantime, the media vials and the cartridges containing the tips and seals used by GAVI™ were loaded. Finally, the oocytes were loaded individually or in pairs in each pod and pods were loaded into the GAVI™ system. Oocyte vitrification program was initiated and once it had finished, pods were submerged directly into liquid nitrogen. All 14 were warmed for a recipient couple. Seven survived and fertilised following ICSI, resulting in 3 blastocysts that were biopsies and were conventionally vitrified. Two resulted in euploid genetic testing results. One of these was warmed, replaced and resulted in a live birth.

31.6.2 Artificial Intelligence (AI)

AI is being introduced into many aspects of healthcare. It may also help improve IVF success because it provides more sophisticated and faster, standardised ways of analysing big data, including images. AI can be used to assess the quality and potential of eggs before freezing. One such egg AI-assessment product is called VIOLET™ (Figure 31.2) and is more reliable than the expert human eye. VIOLET™ enables the assessment of the probability of each egg reaching the blastocyst stage. Patients are provided with a report that not only includes images of each egg to be frozen, but also predicts the likelihood of them becoming a blastocyst embryo, and a livebirth. This AI technology has been shown to be superior in accuracy to trained senior embryologists by more than 20%. It rapidly predicts the likelihood of an embryo developing at 63% accuracy and is completely non-invasive (**26**).

31.6.3 In Vitro Maturation

Oocyte preservation can be performed for immature oocytes before or after their in vitro maturation (IVM). Conventionally, prophase I (GV) oocytes have been considered more suitable for preservation than metaphase II (MII) oocytes, since during meiosis arresting at GV, chromatin is protected in the germinal vesicle and the spindle is not formed yet (**27**). However, the possible alteration in the cortical granules' distribution, cytoplasmic organelles, RNA, and proteins may compromise their maturation. IVM involves nuclear and cytoplasmic changes that are necessary for the subsequent proper embryonic development. Peinado showed comparable vitrification survival, maturation, and metaphase plate configuration rates whether oocytes were cryopreserved before or after IVM, suggesting a possible benefit if oocytes were vitrified at GV. Furthermore, extending IVM could increase the number of available oocytes without altering their quality, at least regarding the metaphase plate configuration. Currently, the use of immature oocytes (rescue oocytes) is one of the research fields with the greatest potential to develop and optimize emerging assisted reproduction techniques in humans, especially for younger, or pre-chemotherapy patients. Healthy live births can be achieved

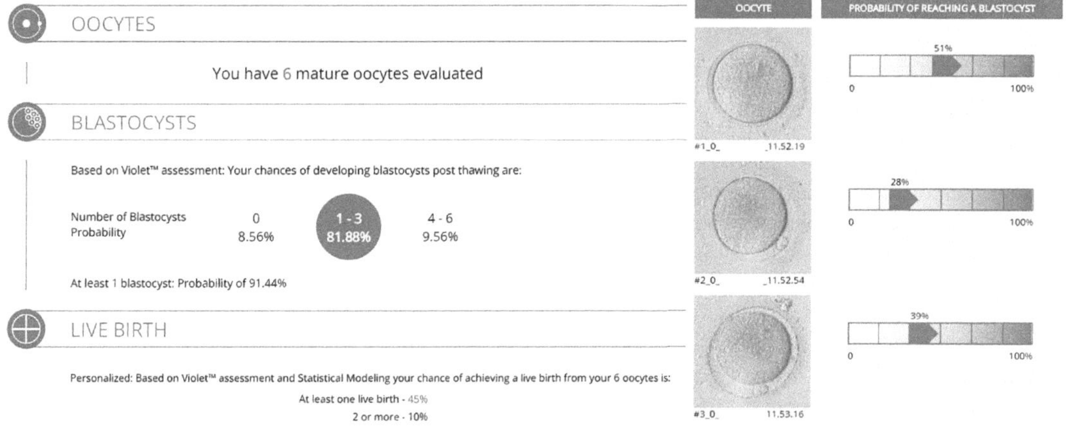

FIGURE 31.2 Sample report using AI (VIOLET™) for egg assessment of development capacity.

from the combination of IVM and vitrification, even if vitrification of in vivo matured oocytes is still more effective (**28**). IVM is explored further in Chapter 32.

31.6.4 Ovarian Tissue Cryopreservation

A small piece of a few millimetres of ovarian cortex contains several thousand primordial follicles. The cryopreservation of ovarian tissue before cancer therapy with re-transplantation after convalescence is increasingly becoming an option for young cancer patients when egg freezing cannot be performed, or in young girls before puberty. The first live birth was reported in Belgium in 2004 (**29**). Ovarian tissue was removed laparoscopically and cryopreserved in 2003. After chemotherapy and 5 years of remission, the thawed tissue was laparoscopically retransplanted into a peritoneal pouch in the ovarian fossa of the right pelvic wall. Three months later, her menopausal symptoms resolved, and she had her first spontaneous menstruation. Six months after re-transplantation, after two normal menstrual cycles, low-dose follicle stimulating hormone (FSH) treatment induced the appearance of a dominant follicle in the tissue graft. Ovulation was then induced with human chorionic gonadotropin (HCG), whereupon the patient conceived naturally. Although there have been over 100 live births worldwide in the last 20 years, and the procedure is no longer considered to be experimental, it is still only carried out at specialist centres that have the expertise in this procedure (**30**).

31.6.5 Re-vitrification/Warm Cycles

Re-vitrification of embryos may be required for a number of reasons: more embryos than required for transfer were stored on the same device; failed transfer following thaw; embryos were thawed and cultured before transfer e.g. a number of 2pn embryos are thawed, cultured to blastocyst and then re-vitrified; or thaw, biopsy for pre-genetic testing and re-freeze event (**31, 32**). Since re-vitrification is not routinely performed, most publications are confined to single case studies. However, studies have suggested that vitrifying and warming embryos twice at blastocyst or at cleavage and then blastocyst stage, can lead to similar reproductive outcomes to embryos vitrified-warmed once, after a single euploid embryo transfer (**33**).

31.7 Management of Gametes and Embryos Cryotanks

The liquid nitrogen cryotank is most commonly used in every reproductive clinic for cryopreservation. These vessels are commonly referred to as dewars, after its inventor, James Dewar (1892). The tanks, or dewars, are essentially a large vacuum container with insulation inside the vacuum chamber, much like an oversized thermos. The working parts are a lid, Styrofoam cork plug that sits inside the neck, the inner chamber that holds the liquid nitrogen, canisters and a "spider" to keep the canisters from moving around. A dewar can hold anywhere between 5 and 500 litres of liquid nitrogen, and 100s to 1000s of specimen, depending on the type of devices used for storage and internal design of the dewar. Some large dewars have liquid nitrogen circulating in the internal walls of the vessel, meaning the samples stored within the dewar are held at -196°C in vapour phase, and are not in direct contact with liquid.

Liquid nitrogen is inert, odourless, colourless, non-corrosive, non-flammable, and achieves temperatures of -196°C (-320°F) in materials that are fully submerged within it. Nitrogen has a boiling point of -195.8°C, and a liquid-to-gas expansion ratio of nitrogen is 1:694 at 20 °C (68°F). As such it requires careful risk management, and specialist training for staff who may be handling it or maintaining the tanks. Risk assessments of liquid nitrogen use need to be carried out around the delivery; the high-volume storage; the dispensing; the handling; and the monitoring and evacuation of the dedicated cryo- storage room. Careless handling of liquid nitrogen, and any objects cooled by it, may result in cold burns. Evaporating nitrogen will reduce the oxygen concentration in the air and can rapidly act as an asphyxiant, especially in confined spaces. Personal protection equipment including specialist gloves and eye protection, should be provided, and low oxygen monitors, connected to alarms and rapid, low level extraction fans, must be present and regular checked.

Failure of a liquid nitrogen Dewar containing patients' gametes and embryos is a devastating loss for the patients affected, as well as a major reputational and financial risk for a company. With this in mind a rolling replacement of tanks should be in place to ensure tanks are not used beyond the manufactures expected lifespan, and daily/weekly monitoring should be in place to detect any early signs of failure. Visual checks daily will detect ice formation on the tank surface, or pooling of water below the tank, as an early sign of vacuum failure. Weekly measuring of the liquid levels, using a ruler, can be plotted to see if liquid evaporation is increasing over time. In the UK the HFEA requires the temperature, or liquid level of any tanks containing patient gametes or embryos, to be constantly monitored, and any deviation from the set limits to trigger an alarm that alerts staff during, and out of work hours, using an auto-dial system. The earlier a problem is detected, and an alarm is communicated, the longer the time is available to respond and act. The inside of a Dewar will remain cold even with low levels of liquid nitrogen but the temperature will rise fast once there are only a few centimetres of liquid nitrogen left at the bottom. Theoretically, temperature probes that are placed closer to the bottom of the Dewar will provide staff very little response time to save the specimen. Monitoring of the levels within a Dewar can be done using probes placed within the tank; by specialist roller base that detects changes in the weight of the Dewar (**34**); or by an infrared thermal monitoring of an entire cryo room (**35**).

A regular audit of all cryopreserved samples should be carried out. Historically, a full physical audit was performed on all cryopreserved samples every two years. This was in line with the HFEA Code of Practice's requirement of a storage review to reconcile clinic records with the material in storage (**36**). However, due to the risk of damaging vitrified samples by unnecessarily exposure to changes in temperature whilst handling them during an audit procedure, and also the time required to audit every sample in storage, a risk assessment can be carried out and the full, physical audits replaced with a sporadic, sampling QA/audit procedure. This involves verifying the location of cryopreserved gametes/embryos against the electronic inventory and any paper records. This is carried out in conjunction with the regular thawing events performed in the IVF laboratory. The points at which this physical check of cryo-location is performed are:

- prior to a patient coming for a frozen embryo replacement or prior to frozen gametes being used in a fresh treatment cycle
- at transfer of gametes/embryos into/out of a clinic
- at disposal of gametes/embryos following patient consent

Good cryo-governance as a minimum should provide, and maintain ventilation systems, oxygen monitors, alarms, training, PPE and adequate documentation. Everything possible must be done to mitigate risk to loss or damage of gametes and embryos; injury to the staff using and maintaining the storage vessels; and legal exposure.

31.8 Clinical Frozen Embryo Transfers (FET) Outcomes

Embryo transfers are conventionally carried out on day 2–5 post insemination, following an oocyte retrieval event. The embryo or embryos considered to have the best chance of implantation (based on a selection criteria) are transferred during the fresh cycle. Any remaining, surplus embryos, that are considered to be of a quality suitable to survive the freezing and thawing process, are then frozen for subsequent use. These cryopreserved embryos are thawed and replaced, when required, in a natural cycle, or a hormonally manipulated cycle. With the advances in cryopreservation technology and protocols, success rates from frozen cycles are now comparable with fresh cycles, with live birth rates per embryo transferred of 23% and 21% respectively (**37**).

There have been numerous studies exploring the obstetric and perinatal outcomes resulting from fresh and thawed frozen embryos. Maheshwari et al. in 2016 analyzed 95,911 fresh and 16,521 frozen single embryo transfers using 10 years of HFEA anonymized data and showed there was no significant difference in the risk of preterm delivery (**37**); a lower risk of having a low birth weight, or very low birth weight, baby as a result of a frozen embryo transfer; and there was no difference in the risk of any congenital anomaly (2.2% fresh vs. 2.3% frozen).

The prolonged storage of embryos has been shown to have no effect on FET outcomes. Canosa (2022) carried out a systematic review and meta-analysis on the effect of cryo-storage for greater than 12 months (**38**). Survival rate, miscarriage rate, live birth and major birth malformation rates were similar as those having had short-term storage. However, although cryopreservation is now an established procedure, due to various cryoprotectants and protocols, long-term follow-up studies remain essential.

REFERENCES

1. Lussig B, Maggiulli R, Fabozzi G, et al. A brief history of oocyte cryopreservation: arguments and facts. *Acta Obstet Gynecol Scand.* 2019;98:550–558.
2. Whittingham DG, Leibo SP, Mazur P. Survival of mouse embryos frozen to -196 degrees and -269 degrees C. *Science.* 1972 Oct 27;178(4059):411–414.
3. Yokota Y, Sato S, Yokota M, et al. Successful pregnancy following blastocyst vitrification: case report. *Hum Reprod.* 2000;15(8):1802–1803.
4. *HFEA Fertility Treatment 2019: Trends and Figures.* London; 2019. Available from: www.hfea.gov.uk/about-us/publications/research-and-data/fertility-treatment-2019-trends-and-figures/#Section4.
5. Rall WF, Fahy GM. Ice-free cryopreservation of mouse embryos at -196 degrees C by vitrification. *Nature.* 985;313(6003):573–575.
6. Mazur P, Seki S. Survival of mouse oocytes after being cooled in a vitrification solution to -196 degrees C at 95 degrees to 70,000 degrees C/min and warmed at 610 degrees to 118,000 degrees C/min: a new paradigm for cryopreservation by vitrification. *Cryobiology.* 2011;62(1):1–7.
7. Gallardo M, Saenz J, Risco R. Human oocytes and zygotes are ready for ultra-fast vitrification after 2 minutes of exposure to standard CPA solutions. *Sci Rep.* 2019;9(1):1–9.
8. Porcu E, Tranquillo ML, Notarangelo L. et al. High-security closed devices are efficient and safe to protect human oocytes from potential risk of viral contamination during vitrification and storage especially in the COVID-19 pandemic. *J Assist Reprod Genet.* 2021;38:681–688.
9. Doyle JO, Richter KS, Lim J, et al. Successful elective and medically indicated oocyte vitrification and warming for autologous in vitro fertilization, with predicted birth probabilities for fertility preservation according to number of cryopreserved oocytes and age at retrieval. *Fertil Steril.* 2016;105(2):459–466. e2.
10. Pujol A, Zamora MJ, Obradors A, et al. Comparison of two different oocyte vitrification methods: a prospective, paired study on the same genetic background and stimulation protocol. *Hum Reprod.* 2019;34(6):989–997.
11. Polge C, Smith AU, Parkes AS. Revival of spermatozoa after vitrification and dehydration at low temperatures. *Nature.* 1949 Oct 15;164(4172):666.
12. Szeptycki J, Bentov Y. Cryopreservation of embryos and gametes: past, present, and future. In: Marco-Jiménez F, Akdemir H, editors. *Cryopreservation in Eukaryotes [Internet].* London: IntechOpen; 2016 [cited 2022 May 23].
13. Fakhrildin MB, Al-Moussawi RHA. Effect of two types and two concentrations of cryoprotectants on ovine oocytes morphology and viability post-vitrification. *Iraqi J Embryos Infertil Res.* 2013;3:38–44.
14. Vincent C, Garnier V, Heyman Y, et al. Solvent effects on cytoskeletal organization and in-vivo survival after freezing of rabbit oocytes. *J Reprod Fertil.* 1989 Nov;87(2):809–820.
15. Larman MG, Minasi MG, Rienzi L, et al. Maintenance of the meiotic spindle during vitrification in human and mouse oocytes. *Reprod Biomed Online.* 2007 Dec;15(6):692–700.
16. Gomes CM, Silva CA, Acevedo N, et al. Influence of vitrification on mouse metaphase II oocyte spindle dynamics and chromatin alignment. *Fertil Steril.* 2008;90(Suppl. 4):1396–1404j.

17. Kuleshova L, Gianaroli L, Magli C, et al. Birth following vitrification of a small number of human oocytes: case report. *Hum Reprod.* 1999;14(12):3077–3079.
18. Kuywayama M. Highly efficient vitrification for cryopreservation of human oocytes and embryos: the Cryotop method. *Theriogenology.* 2007;67(1):73–80.
19. Roque M, Valle M, Guimarães F, et al. Freeze-all policy: fresh vs. frozen-thawed embryo transfer. *Fertil Steril.* 2015;103(5):1190–1193.
20. Shapiro B, Daneshmand ST, Garner FC, et al. Clinical rationale for cryopreservation of entire embryo cohorts in lieu of fresh transfer. *Fertil Steril.* 2014;102(1):3–9.
21. Van den Abbeel E, Balaban B, Ziebe S, et al. Association between blastocyst morphology and outcome of single-blastocyst transfer. *Reprod Biomed Online.* 2013;27:353–361.
22. Gardner DK, Lane M, Stevens J, et al. Blastocyst score affects implantation and pregnancy outcome: towards a single blastocyst transfer. *Fertil Steril.* 2000;73:1155–1158.
23. Campbell A, Fishel S, Bowman N, et al. Retrospective analysis of outcomes after IVF using an aneuploidy risk model derived from time-lapse imaging without PGS. *Reprod Biomed Online.* 2013;27:140–146.
24. Brunetti XO, Cawood S, Gaunt M, et al. The first livebirth using warmed oocytes by a semi-automated vitrification procedure. *J Reprod Infertil.* 2021;22(1):70–72.
25. Roy T, Brandi S, Tappe N, et al. Embryo vitrification using a novel semi-automated closed system yields in vitro outcomes equivalent to the manual Cryotop method. *Hum Reprod.* 2014;29(11):2431–2438.
26. Peschansky C, Patel S, Amir J, et al. Picture perfect? Determining the clinical utilization of artificial intelligence in oocyte cryopreservation. *Fertil Steril.* 2021;116(3):e157.
27. Peinado I, Moya I, Sáez-Espinosa P, et al. Impact of maturation and vitrification time of human GV oocytes on the metaphase plate configuration. *Int J Mol Sci.* 2021;22:1125.
28. Khalili MA, Shahedi A, Ashourzadeh S, et al. Vitrification of human immature oocytes before and after in vitro maturation: a review. *J Assist Reprod Genet.* 2017;34:1413–1426.
29. Donnez L, Dolmans MM, Demylle D, et al. Livebirth after orthotopic transplantation of cryopreserved ovarian tissue. *Lancet.* 2004;364(9443):1405–1410.
30. Marin L, Bedoschi G, Kawahara T, et al. History, evolution and current state of ovarian tissue auto-transplantation with cryopreserved tissue: a successful translational research journey from 1999 to 2020. *Reprod Sci.* 2020;27(4):955–962.
31. Taylor TH, Patrick JL, Gitlin SA, et al. Outcomes of blastocysts biopsied and vitrified once versus those cryopreserved twice for euploid blastocyst transfer. *Reprod Biomed Online.* 2014 Jul;29(1):59–64.
32. De Vos A, Van Landuyt L, De Rycke M, et al. Multiple vitrification-warming and biopsy procedures on human embryos: clinical outcome and neonatal follow-up of children. *Hum Reprod.* 2020 Nov;35(11):2488–2496.
33. Theodorou E, Jones BP, Cardenas Armas DF, et al. Live birth rate following a euploid blastocyst transfer is not affected by double vitrification and warming at cleavage or blastocyst stage. *J Assist Reprod Genet.* 2022;39:987–993.
34. Mora F, Maalouf W, Selley M, et al. The use of cryokinetic variables to ensure correct functioning of liquid nitrogen dewars. *Fertility.* 2023;112:96.
35. Cryosentinel. *Thermographic Cryogenic Storage Monitoring.* 2023: Available from: https://cryosentinel.com/.
36. *HFEA Fertility Treatment 2017: Trends and Figures.* London. Available from: www.hfea.gov.uk/media/3189/fertility-treatment-2017-trends-and-figures.pdf.
37. Maheshwari A, Amalraj Raja E, Bhattacharya S. Obstetric and perinatal outcomes after either fresh or thawed frozen embryo transfer: an analysis of 112,432 singleton pregnancies recorded in the Human Fertilisation and Embryology Authority anonymized dataset. *Fertil Steril.* 2016;106(7):1703–1708.
38. Canosa S, Cimadomo D, Conforti A, et al. The effect of extended cryo-storage following vitrification on embryo competence: a systematic review and meta-analysis. *J Assist Reprod Genet.* 2022;39:873–882.

32

In Vitro Maturation (IVM) and Artificial Oocyte Activation (AOA)

Walid E. Maalouf and Juan Hernandez-Medrano

In vitro maturation (IVM) is the process in which oocytes are retrieved from antral follicles at the germinal vesicle stage, then matured in vitro to allow those to reach the metaphase II (MII) stage (**1**). IVM procedure has the potential to avoid supraphysiological levels of steroids, minimising the risk of ovarian hyperstimulation syndrome (OHSS) (**2**), to salvage immature oocytes for IVF or ICSI after standard stimulation (**3**), to mature oocytes for fertility preservation in women about to undergo cancer treatment (**4**) or patients with oestrogen-sensitive cancer (**5**), and to provide a cost-effective alternative to high cost stimulated cycles (**6**). OHSS is associated with polycystic ovary syndrome (PCOS), which is a common reproductive disorder (**7**). On the other hand, artificial oocyte activation (AOA) is a recent alternative that assist mature eggs activation following fertilisation failure after an IVF or ICSI procedure. Oocyte activation deficiency (OAD) has been directly correlated with a deficiency of the sperm activating factor PLCζ caused by poor sperm maturation or function (**8**). Both interventions can be beneficial to both clinics and patients as they offer alternative clinical treatment options to patients that either would be able to go through a conventional IVF cycle, or due to the inability of the used protocols to generate mature or fertilised eggs and embryos.

32.1 In Vitro Maturation

IVM-IVF is a useful alternative for patients who are higher responders for ovarian stimulation (**9**), with the first live birth from this procedure reported in 1991 (**10**), and more than 5,000 babies born globally to date (**11**). Although a recent a randomised controlled trial (RCT) reported live birth rates (LBR) and cumulative ongoing pregnancy rates (CLBR) similar to conventional ovarian stimulation patients (**12**), it has not been adopted widely due to the low efficiency of current protocols to reproducibly generate competent mature MII eggs (**11**). In recent years, a number of important developments have been made to improve the efficiency of clinical IVM.

Although IVM is defined as a procedure that does not require ovarian stimulation, the method has been modified to include minimal stimulation with gonadotropins or human Chorionic Gonadotropins (hCG) trigger (**13**). This method, also referred to as truncated IVF, include rescue IVM used by some clinics following an oocyte pickup of patients who did not fully respond to the stimulation protocols (**14**). Whether natural or mild stimulation is used, oocyte aspiration will be more difficult due to the smaller size of the follicles aspirated, and which can be as small as 3mm antral follicles (**15**). Therefore, a more rigid, shorter bevel (**16**), and larger gauge aspiration needles were suggested for this type of work (**17**). A smaller gauge needle has been recommended to reduce bleeding and pain in women who are only lightly sedated during oocyte aspiration (**18, 19**). However, the pressure pump will need to be adjusted to minimise the damage that can be caused to the oocytes by high velocity and fluid flowrate, particularly if different gauge needle sizes are used (**20**). Although flushing the follicles does not necessarily increase the number of oocytes retrieved, it can prevent clot formation and enable easier identification of oocytes (**21**).

Once collected GVs or metaphase I (MI) oocytes can be *in vitro* cultured for maturation to the MII stage (Figure 32.1). IVM media can be commercially available (**22**), or formulated based using blastocyst media as the base (**23**). FSH is essential for the *in vivo* development of pre-ovulatory follicles (**24**), and it is added as a standard supplement in IVM media (**23**). hCG can be considered as another supplement, particularly in patients who have not been primed with hCG. Although they have been reported to improve oocyte IVM (**25**), LH and hCG do not necessarily improve the maturation or developmental potential of oocytes (**26**). On the other hand, epidermal-growth factor (EGF) has been reported to have a positive role directly on the oocyte during IVM, as improved outcomes were reported when used with cumulus intact or cumulus denuded oocytes (**27**). Follicular fluid (FF) has been suggested as a protein supplement, however, human serum albumin (HSA) has been used successfully as an alternative (**28, 29**). It has also been suggested to supplement the media with oestradiol (E2) in the absence of FF (**30**). On the other hand, heat inactivated maternal serum has been reported to produce superior results in IVM (**31, 32**), which indicates that additional factors other than serum play essential roles in IVM. Additional factors that are considered for cytoplasmic and nuclear maturation of the oocytes include insulin or insulin-growth factor (IGF) (**33**), and transferrin and selenium as trace elements with antioxidant properties (**23**).

Other developments in IVM include the use of a biphasic two-steps culture protocol, with an initial incubation of 24 hours to synchronise the nuclear and cytoplasmic maturation with a pharmacological agent such as cAMPs analogues or C-type natriuretic peptide (CNP) to delay the germinal vesical breakdown, followed by further 30 hours in IVM media containing EGF-lie factors such as amphiregulin for improved outcomes (**34**). The length of the maturation process will be dependent on the clinical protocol used prior to aspiration of the oocytes, and the oocytes are usually asynchronous during

DOI: 10.1201/9781003269502-32

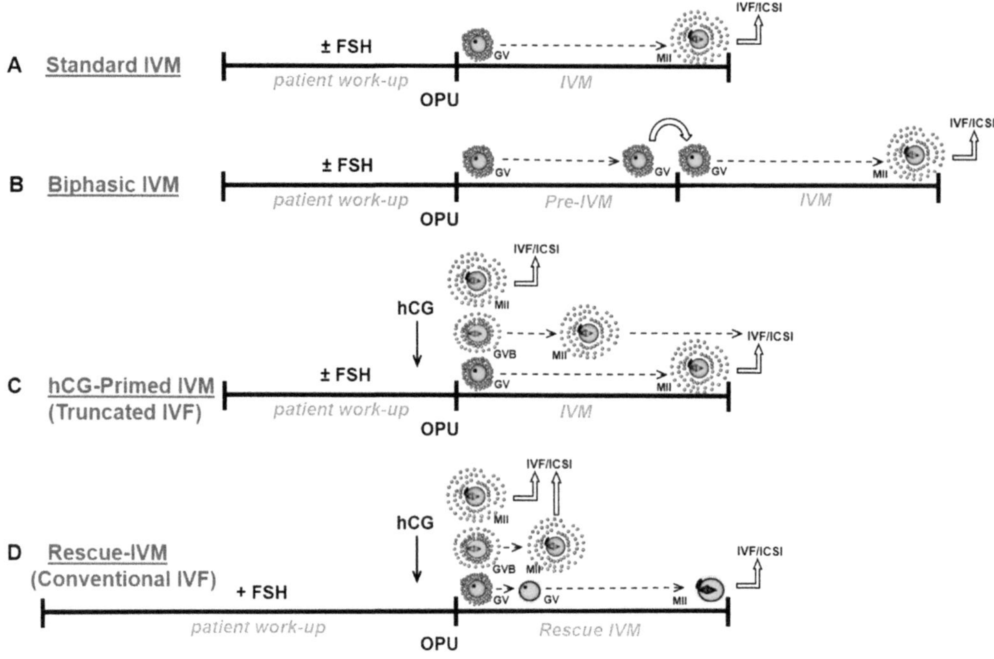

FIGURE 32.1 Various treatment protocols that are collectively referred to as in vitro maturation (IVM) in the clinical literature (from [**40**] under Creative Commons licence).

maturation (**35**). As the insemination of aged oocytes will impede on its competence to develop into blastocysts (**36**), a shorter IVM protocol of 28 hours have been tested with good outcomes on maturation, fertilisation and pregnancies (**37**). A 28-hour procedure also fits better with clinic operations during working hours. Better fertilisation rates were also reported using ICSI instead of IVF (**38**), although others reported no differences (**39**). However, as ICSI requires the removal of the cumulus cells, it offers an advantage over IVF as it allows the embryologists to identify the maturation stage of the oocytes.

The optimal protocol will depend on standard operating procedures, practicalities, technical skills and local or national regulations that may or may not allow certain supplements to be added to a standard culture media. Although published protocols differ and the data is relatively small, a systematic review including 7 quantitative studies on pregnancy outcome and children's development after IVM-IVF appear to be reassuring as the outcomes measured are no different than conventional IVF (**41**), irrespective of whether an ovulation trigger was used in IVM cycles or not.

32.2 Artificial Oocyte Activation

At fertilisation, the sperm contacts the zona pellucida, and the proteolytic enzymes following the acrosome reaction help the sperm burrows its way through the layers to reach the oocyte membrane. Sperm fuses sideways on the equatorial segment to the plasma membrane of the egg on the microvilli. The sperm nucleus breaks up, and goes into the cytoplasm of the oocyte with PLCζ. Sperm PLCζ is a 70kda mammalian protein activated by posttranslational modifications (**42**), and it is responsible for the hydrolysis of phosphatidylinositol 4,5-bisphosphate (PIP2) to inositol 1,4,5-trisphosphate (IP3) and diacylglycerol (DAG). IP3 then binds to specific receptors of the endoplasmic reticulum that induce further Ca+2 release, resulting in oocyte activation (**43–45**). Through a positive feedback mechanism, the Ca+2 release leads to increased PLCζ activity, which, in turn, stimulates a further increase of both Ca+2 and IP3, oscillating the release of calcium. Triggered by calcium output and oscillations, cortical granules are released through the process of exocytosis of ovastacin, plus zinc, which causes the zona pellucida (ZP) to harden and stop any additional sperm from attaching to the ZP (**46**).

The control of nuclear maturation in the oocyte is intrinsically linked to the levels of two cytoplasmic protein kinases, MPF (maturation promoting factor) and MAPK (mitogen activated protein kinase). MPF is a cyclin dependent protein kinase, and its activity is controlled by cyclin B1 and phosphorylation of CDC2 at T14 and Y15 (REF?). MAPK is another kinase that requires phosphorylation on threonine and tyrosine residues to become active (**47**). Activation of the oocyte by the release of calcium at fertilisation also leads to the release of calmodulin-dependent kinase II (CaMKII) and E3 ubiquitin ligase. CaMKII inhibits the cytostatic-static factor (CSF), the most downstream factor in the MAPK pathway, also inactivating cyclin B2 by poly-ubiquitination (**48**), both processes leading to the release of the egg from meiotic arrest at MII.

Once the oocyte is fertilised and activated, it then completes meiosis from the MII stage. Female and male pronuclei formation take place upon Ca+2 oscillations, which continue independently of pronuclear formation (**49**), and the whole process takes around 4–6 hours in humans (**50**). Onset of cell cycle mitosis starts after syngamy of the pronuclei. All the aforementioned events are triggered by the calcium increase in the cytoplasm of the egg as the main stimulus (**51**). The same process of fertilisation is reproduced with IVF and ICSI as PLCζ

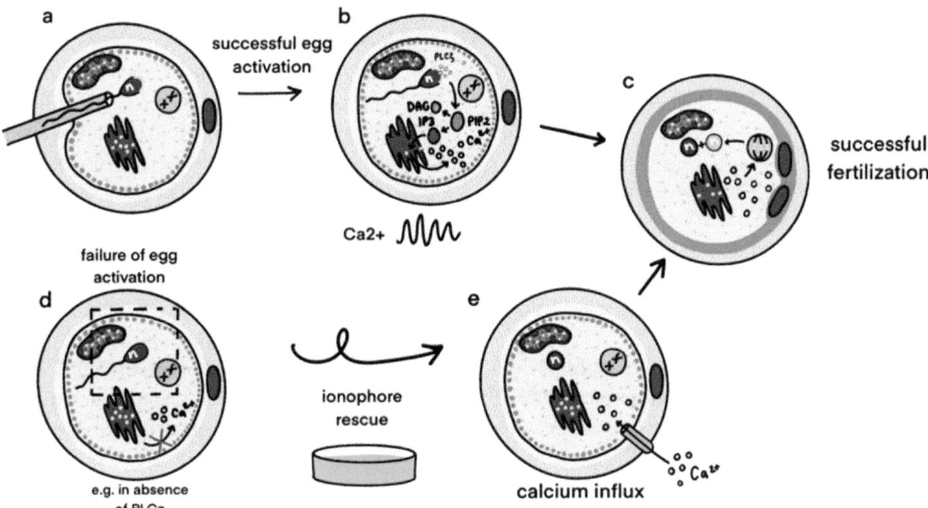

FIGURE 32.2 Artificial oocyte activation (AOA) and the release of calcium, leading to a successful activation (from [**66**] with permission).

is introduced into the egg with the sperm. ICSI has a very good success rates, but total fertilisation failures (TFF) are reported between 1 and 5% of the times (**52–54**). Fertilisation failure per oocyte after ICSI is close 30% actually if TFF included with all other failed fertilised eggs within individual procedures (**55**). Failed fertilisation can be due to either oocyte activation failure or defective sperm decondensation. However, up to 70% of the times, oocyte activation failure seems to be the main reason for the failed fertilisation (**56, 57**) in human studies, and a significant number of those are likely due to the lack or short supply of PLCzeta introduced with the sperm head (**58**).

Oocyte activation can be a problem in those ICSI cases because it is difficult to measure PLCζ when sperm is injected into the egg. However, it is relatively easy to overcome or investigate the lack of activation by using oocyte activators such as calcium ionophore A23187, strontium, ionomycin, or reagents containing similar compounds (**47, 59**). In fact, AOA involves a short incubation of oocytes in calcium ionophore (Figure 32.2) or equivalent activating factor for a short period of 15–20 minutes under oil, followed by two consecutive washes and standard culture thereafter (**60**). This procedure is proposed to cause a significant transient release of calcium from cellular stores, which is different to the frequent multiple spikes calcium release that happen normally, which could be one of the reasons why it is not as effective for activation in mouse or human eggs (**48, 61**). It is suggested that repeated consecutive use of ionophore to mimic what sperm induced calcium release or injecting calcium concurrently might be a better strategy to mimic multiple calcium spikes (**8, 62, 63**). Alternative AOA methods have also been tested including electro-activation (**64**), and mechanical activation through a modified ICSI procedure (**65**), with various relative success rates.

As with maturation age of the eggs *in vitro*, AOA for rescue is typically carried out many hours after hCG trigger and oocyte pick-up. Optimal fertilisation potential is obtained between 37 and 41 hours post-hCG (**67**). Oocyte's sensitivity to PLCζ continues beyond 60 hours after hCG trigger (**68**). However, this sensitivity is reduced as observed by low fertilisation and implantation rates. The low fertilisation rate can be explained by increased chromosomal aberrations that may also correlate with the age of the oocyte at the time of fertilisation (**69**). Systematic reviews of 14 studies reported significant improvement in fertilisation rates, as well as clinical outcomes including live birth rates (**70, 71**). However, it was also reported that there is a risk of increased developmental aberrations and epigenetic related malformations (**72**). The ongoing concerns remain due to lack of standardisation of the procedure (**59**). Although it has potential clinical application for some failed ICSI cases, due to the limited published evidence on the clinical benefits to patients and long terms safety, AOA is classified under the yellow rating by the HFEA (**73**).

32.3 Conclusion

IVM and AOA remain promising intervention technologies that can be beneficial to both clinics and patients as they offer alternative clinical treatment options to patients that either would be able to go through a conventional IVF cycle, or due to the inability of the used protocols to generate mature or fertilised eggs and embryos respectively. Standardisation, science and safety data also remain a priority due to the limited knowledge we have regarding mechanisms involved in the processes.

REFERENCES

1. Chian R-C, Uzelac PS, Nargund G. In vitro maturation of human immature oocytes for fertility preservation. *Fertil Steril*. 2013;99(5):1173–1181.
2. Nargund G, Datta AK, Campbell S, et al. The case for mild stimulation for IVF: ISMAAR recommendations. *Reprod Biomed Online*. 2022;45(6):1133–1144.
3. Mikkelsen AL, Smith SD, Lindenberg S. In-vitro maturation of human oocytes from regularly menstruating women may be successful without follicle stimulating hormone priming. *Hum Reprod*. 1999;14(7):1847–1851.

4. Chang EM, Song HS, Lee DR, et al. In vitro maturation of human oocytes: its role in infertility treatment and new possibilities. *Clin Exp Reprod Med.* 2014;41(2):41.
5. Chian R-C, Wang L, Yang Z-Y. Strategies of infertility treatment with human immature oocytes. *Reprod Dev Med.* 2018;2(4):237–248.
6. Rose BI, Laky D, Miller B. The case for in vitro maturation lower cost and more patient friendly. *J Reprod Med.* 2014;59(11–12):571–578.
7. Yadav A, Malhotra N. Polycystic ovarian syndrome: diagnosis and management of related infertility. *Obstet Gynaecol Reprod Med.* 2022;32(9):197–207.
8. Swann K. The role of Ca2+ in oocyte activation during in vitro fertilization: insights into potential therapies for rescuing failed fertilization. *Biochimica et Biophysica Acta (BBA)-Mol Cell Res.* 2018;1865(11):1830–1837.
9. Lim J-H, Yang S-H, Xu Y, et al. Selection of patients for natural cycle in vitro fertilization combined with in vitro maturation of immature oocytes. *Fertil Steril.* 2009;91(4):1050–1055.
10. Cha KY, Koo JJ, Ko JJ, et al. Pregnancy after in vitro fertilization of human follicular oocytes collected from nonstimulated cycles, their culture in vitro and their transfer in a donor oocyte program. *Fertil Steril.* 1991;55(1):109–113.
11. De Vos M, Smitz J, Thompson JG, et al. The definition of IVM is clear – variations need defining. *Hum Reprod.* 2016;31(11):2411–2415.
12. Vuong LN, Ho VN, Ho TM, et al. In-vitro maturation of oocytes versus conventional IVF in women with infertility and a high antral follicle count: a randomized non-inferiority controlled trial. *Hum Reprod.* 2020;35(11):2537–2547.
13. Lin YH, Hwang JL, Huang LW, et al. Combination of FSH priming and hCG priming for in-vitro maturation of human oocytes. *Hum Reprod.* 2003;18(8):1632–1636.
14. Carles M, Lefranc E, Bosquet D, et al. In vitro maturation of oocytes from stimulated IVF-ICSI cycles using autologous cumulus cell co-culture: a preliminary study. *Morphologie.* 2022;107(356):28–37.
15. Rose B. Approaches to oocyte retrieval for advanced reproductive technology cycles planning to utilize in vitro maturation: a review of the many choices to be made. *J Assist Reprod Genet.* 2014;31(11):1409–1419.
16. Trounson A, Wood C, Kausche A. In vitro maturation and the fertilization and developmental competence of oocytes recovered from untreated polycystic ovarian patients. *Fertil Steril.* 1994;62(2):353–362.
17. Lewin A, Laufer N, Rabinowitz R, et al. Ultrasonically guided oocyte recovery for in vitro fertilization: an improved method. *J In Vitro Fertil Embryo Trans.* 1986;3(6):370–373.
18. Aziz N, Biljan M, Taylor C, et al. Effect of aspirating needle calibre on outcome of in-vitro fertilization. *Hum Reprod.* 1993;8(7):1098–1100.
19. Buisman ETIA, de Bruin JP, Braat DDM, et al. Effect of needle diameter on pain during oocyte retrieval – a randomized controlled trial. *Fertil Steril.* 2021;115(3):683–691.
20. Bols P, Ysebaert M, Van Soom A, et al. Effects of needle tip bevel and aspiration procedure on the morphology and developmental capacity of bovine compact cumulus oocyte complexes. *Theriogenology.* 1997;47(6):1221–1236.
21. Rose B, Laky D. A comparison of the Cook single lumen immature ovum IVM needle to the Steiner-Tan pseudo double lumen flushing needle for oocyte retrieval for IVM. *J Assist Reprod Genet.* 2013;30(6):855–860.
22. Pongsuthirak P, Vutyavanich T. Comparison of medicult and sage media for vitro. *J Fertil.* 2015;3:1.
23. Oktay K, Buyuk E, Rodriguez-Wallberg K, et al. In vitro maturation improves oocyte or embryo cryopreservation outcome in breast cancer patients undergoing ovarian stimulation for fertility preservation. *Reprod Biomed Online.* 2010;20(5):634–638.
24. Macklon NS, Fauser BC. Follicle-stimulating hormone and advanced follicle development in the human. *Arch Med Res.* 2001;32(6):595–600.
25. Hreinsson J, Rosenlund B, Fridén B, et al. Recombinant LH is equally effective as recombinant hCG in promoting oocyte maturation in a clinical in-vitro maturation programme: a randomized study. *Hum Reprod.* 2003;18(10):2131–2136.
26. Ge H-S, Huang X-F, Zhang W, et al. Exposure to human chorionic gonadotropin during in vitro maturation does not improve the maturation rate and developmental potential of immature oocytes from patients with polycystic ovary syndrome. *Fertil Steril.* 2008;89(1):98–103.
27. Goud P, Goud A, Qian C, et al. In-vitro maturation of human germinal vesicle stage oocytes: role of cumulus cells and epidermal growth factor in the culture medium. *Hum Reprod.* 1998;13(6):1638–1644.
28. Jee BC, Han SH, Moon JH, et al. Influence of well defined protein source on in vitro maturation of human oocyte: human follicular fluid versus human serum albumin. *Fertil Steril.* 2008;89(2):348–352.
29. Choi MH, Lee SH, Kim HO, et al. Comparison of assisted reproductive technology outcomes in infertile women with polycystic ovary syndrome: in vitro maturation, GnRH agonist, and GnRH antagonist cycles. *Clin Exp Reprod Med.* 2012;39(4):166–171.
30. Guler A, Poulin N, Mermillod P, et al. Effect of growth factors, EGF and IGF-I, and estradiol on in vitro maturation of sheep oocytes. *Theriogenology.* 2000;54(2):209–218.
31. Mikkelsen AL, Høst E, Blaabjerg J, et al. Maternal serum supplementation in culture medium benefits maturation of immature human oocytes. *Reprod Biomed Online.* 2001;3(2):112–116.
32. Chang EM, Han JE, Seok HH, et al. Insulin resistance does not affect early embryo development but lowers implantation rate in in vitro maturation – in vitro fertilization – embryo transfer cycle. *Clin Endocrinol.* 2013;79(1):93–99.
33. Gómez E, Tarín JJ, Pellicer A. Oocyte maturation in humans: the role of gonadotropins and growth factors. *Fertil Steril.* 1993;60(1):40–46.
34. Sanchez F, Le AH, Ho VN, et al. Biphasic in vitro maturation (CAPA-IVM) specifically improves the developmental capacity of oocytes from small antral follicles. *J Assist Reprod Genet.* 2019;36(10):2135–2144.
35. Combelles C, Cekleniak N, Racowsky C, et al. Assessment of nuclear and cytoplasmic maturation in in-vitro matured human oocytes. *Hum Reprod.* 2002;17(4):1006–1016.
36. Barnes FL, Crombie A, Gardner DK, et al. Blastocyst development and birth after in-vitro maturation of human primary oocytes, intracytoplasmic sperm injection and assisted hatching. *Hum Reprod.* 1995;10(12):3243–3247.
37. Smith SD, Mikkelsen A-L, Lindenberg S. Development of human oocytes matured in vitro for 28 or 36 hours. *Fertil Steril.* 2000;73(3):541–544.

38. Hwang J-L, Lin Y-H, Tsai Y-L. In vitro maturation and fertilization of immature oocytes: a comparative study of fertilization techniques. *J Assist Reprod Genet.* 2000;17(1):39–43.
39. Walls M, Junk S, Ryan J, et al. IVF versus ICSI for the fertilization of in-vitro matured human oocytes. *Reprod Biomed Online.* 2012;25(6):603–607.
40. De Vos M, Grynberg M, Ho TM, et al. Perspectives on the development and future of oocyte IVM in clinical practice. *J Assist Reprod Genet.* 2021;38(6):1265–1280.
41. Strowitzki T, Bruckner T, Roesner S. Maternal and neonatal outcome and children's development after medically assisted reproduction with in-vitro matured oocytes – a systematic review and meta-analysis. *Hum Reprod Update.* 2021;27(3):460–473.
42. Swann K, Saunders C, Rogers N, et al. editors. PLCζ (zeta): a sperm protein that triggers Ca2+ oscillations and egg activation in mammals. *Semin Cell Dev Biol.* 2006;17(2):264–273.
43. Machaty Z. Signal transduction in mammalian oocytes during fertilization. *Cell Tissue Res.* 2016;363(1):169–183.
44. Machaty Z, Miller AR, Zhang L. Egg activation at fertilization. *Vertebr Dev.* 2017;1–47.
45. Yeste M, Jones C, Amdani SN, et al. Oocyte activation and fertilisation: crucial contributors from the sperm and oocyte. *Signal-Mediat Cont Cell Div.* 2017;213–239.
46. Yanagimachi R. Sperm – egg fusion. In: *Current Topics in Membranes and Transport, vol. 32.* Academic Press; 1988. pp. 3–43.
47. Maalouf W, Lee J-H, Campbell K. Effects of caffeine, cumulus cell removal and aging on polyspermy and embryo development on in vitro matured and fertilized ovine oocytes. *Theriogenology.* 2009;71(7):1083–1092.
48. Miyazaki S, Ito M. Calcium signals for egg activation in mammals. *J Pharmacol Sci.* 2006;100(5):545–552.
49. Kono T, Obata Y, Yoshimzu T, et al. Epigenetic modifications during oocyte growth correlates with extended parthenogenetic development in the mouse. *Nat Genet.* 1996;13(1):91–94.
50. Nagy Z, Liu J, Joris H, et al. Time-course of oocyte activation, pronucleus formation and cleavage in human oocytes fertilized by intracytoplasmic sperm injection. *Hum Reprod.* 1994;9(9):1743–1748.
51. Taylor C, Lawrence Y, Kingsland C, et al. Fertilization and early embryology: oscillations in intracellular free calcium induced by spermatozoa in human oocytes at fertilization. *Hum Reprod.* 1993;8(12):2174–2179.
52. Sun B, Yeh J. Calcium oscillatory patterns and oocyte activation during fertilization: a possible mechanism for total fertilization failure (TFF) in human in vitro fertilization? *Reprod Sci.* 2021;28(3):639–648.
53. Shinar S, Almog B, Levin I, et al. Total fertilization failure in intra-cytoplasmic sperm injection cycles – classification and management. *Gynecol Endocrinol.* 2014;30(8):593–596.
54. Farhi J, Cohen K, Mizrachi Y, et al. Should ICSI be implemented during IVF to all advanced-age patients with non-male factor subfertility? *Reprod Biol Endocrinol.* 2019;17(1):1–5.
55. Neri QV, Lee B, Rosenwaks Z, et al. Understanding fertilization through intracytoplasmic sperm injection (ICSI). *Cell Calcium.* 2014;55(1):24–37.
56. Ferrer-Buitrago M, Bonte D, De Sutter P, et al. Single Ca2+ transients vs oscillatory Ca2+ signaling for assisted oocyte activation: limitations and benefits. *Reproduction.* 2018;155(2):R105–R119.
57. Rubino P, Viganò P, Luddi A, et al. The ICSI procedure from past to future: a systematic review of the more controversial aspects. *Hum Reprod Update.* 2016;22(2):194–227.
58. Kashir J, Jones C, Mounce G, et al. Variance in total levels of phospholipase C zeta (PLC-ζ) in human sperm may limit the applicability of quantitative immunofluorescent analysis as a diagnostic indicator of oocyte activation capability. *Fertil Steril.* 2013;99(1):107–117. e3.
59. Ebner T, Montag M. Artificial oocyte activation: evidence for clinical readiness. *Reprod Biomed Online.* 2016;32(3):271–273.
60. Ebner T, Köster M, Shebl O, et al. Application of a ready-to-use calcium ionophore increases rates of fertilization and pregnancy in severe male factor infertility. *Fertil Steril.* 2012;98(6):1432–1437.
61. Sanders JR, Swann K. Molecular triggers of egg activation at fertilization in mammals. *Reproduction.* 2016;152(2).
62. Ozil J-P, Swann K. Stimulation of repetitive calcium transients in mouse eggs. *J Physiol.* 1995;483(2):331–346.
63. Shebl O, Reiter E, Enengl S, et al. Double ionophore application in cases with previous failed/low fertilization or poor embryo development. *Reprod Biomed Online.* 2022;44(5):829–837.
64. Mansour R, Fahmy I, Tawab NA, et al. Electrical activation of oocytes after intracytoplasmic sperm injection: a controlled randomized study. *Fertil Steril.* 2009;91(1):133–139.
65. Tesarik J, Rienzi L, Ubaldi F, et al. Use of a modified intracytoplasmic sperm injection technique to overcome sperm-borne and oocyte-borne oocyte activation failures. *Fertil Steril.* 2002;78(3):619–624.
66. Curnow EC, Vannucci B, Muller CH, et al. Successful live birth outcome following assisted activation of failed fertilized oocytes. *Reprod Sci.* 2023;1–5.
67. Dozortsev D, Nagy P, Abdelmassih S, et al. The optimal time for intracytoplasmic sperm injection in the human is from 37 to 41 hours after administration of human chorionic gonadotropin. *Fertil Steril.* 2004;82(6):1492–1496.
68. Nagy ZP, Staessen C, Liu J, et al. Prospective, auto-controlled study on reinsemination of failed-fertilized oocytes by intracytoplasmic sperm injection. *Fertil Steril.* 1995;64(6):1130–1135.
69. Badenas J, Santalo J, Calafell J, et al. Effect of the degree of maturation of mouse oocytes at fertilization: a source of chromosome imbalance. *Gamete Res.* 1989;24(2):205–218.
70. Sfontouris IA, Nastri CO, Lima ML, et al. Artificial oocyte activation to improve reproductive outcomes in women with previous fertilization failure: a systematic review and meta-analysis of RCTs. *Hum Reprod.* 2015;30(8):1831–1841.
71. Murugesu S, Saso S, Jones BP, et al. Does the use of calcium ionophore during artificial oocyte activation demonstrate an effect on pregnancy rate? A meta-analysis. *Fertil Steril.* 2017;108(3):468–482. e3.
72. Anifandis G, Michopoulos A, Daponte A, et al. Artificial oocyte activation: physiological, pathophysiological and ethical aspects. *Syst Biol Reprod Med.* 2019;65(1):3–11.
73. HFEA. *Treatment Add-Ons With Limited Evidence Online.* HFEA; 2022. Available from: www.hfea.gov.uk/treatments/treatment-add-ons/.

33

ICSI: Micromanipulation Setup, Consumables, and Operational Procedure

Louise Best

33.1 History of ICSI

Intracytoplasmic sperm injection (ICSI) is the procedure by which a single sperm cell is injected directly into the cytoplasm of an oocyte. It may also be used where eggs cannot easily be penetrated by sperm as in the case of warmed vitrified oocytes. It is the first-line choice of treatment for couples with severe male factor infertility. ICSI bypasses the zona pellucida and the acrosome reaction.

Since the inception of IVF for couples where there were sub-optimal sperm parameters this increased the chances of poor fertilisation or complete failure to fertilise. Different techniques were trialled in order to improve the outcome for these patients. Increasing the insemination concentration; use of multi-layer density gradients to selectively prepare the sperm; and improvement of motility using enhancers such as pentoxifylline, however the improvement using these techniques were limited for severe oligo-asthenozoospermia or complete teratozoospermia (**1**). To overcome the zona binding needed during IVF investigators aimed to increase the fertilisation by completely removing the cumulus cells, drilling holes in the zona using acidified Tyrode's solution or partially opening the zona (partial zona dissection PZD). These techniques increased the rates of polyploidy, and increased oocyte damage rate. The PZD technique involved shrinking the oocyte ooplasm by exposure to sucrose and this gave rise to another micromanipulation technique called subzonal insemination (SUZI) (**2**). In this technique up to 3 spermatozoa were brought with an injection pipette through the ZP and deposited into the perivitelline space of a metaphase-II oocyte. Overall pregnancy rate remained low, ranging from 2.9% to 16.3% (**3**).

Microinjection of a spermatozoon directly into the ooplasm of human oocytes was attempted in 11 patients as early as 1987 (**1**). Extensive work was carried out to improve the pre-existing micromanipulators i.e. refining of the injection and holding pipettes, delivery of a constant pressure through a 5 μm diameter micro-needle, as well as standardization of intracytoplasmic sperm injection dishes The first report of human pregnancies using this technique was in 1992 (**4**). Since then, this technique has been adopted world-wide. In their most recent publication, the International Committee for Monitoring Assisted Reproductive Technologies (ICMART) reported that ICSI was utilized in 69.3% cases (**5**). ICSI is being increasingly utilized even in the presence of normal semen parameters. The US national trend for use of ICSI rose from 59.5% in 2019 for cases with unknown infertility factor, and to 74.7% for those cases with male factor diagnosis (**6**). Some clinics use exclusively ICSI for all cases.

33.2 Indications for ICSI

ICSI is most commonly the recommended treatment for male factor infertility:

- Oligozoospermia – fewer than 15million sperm/ml
- Asthenozoospermia or asthenospermia – less than or equal to 32% total motility
- Teratozoospermia – less than 40% normally shaped spermatozoa
- Use of surgically recovered sperm from the testicles or epididymis because a vasectomy, or a blockage that prevents sperm reaching the ejaculate (azoospermia), caused by disease, injury, or a genetic condition
- Presence of anti-sperm antibodies
- Use of frozen sperm

However, it has more routinely been suggested and used for previous failed or low fertilisation with standard IVF insemination, use of frozen-thawed oocytes or typically recommended when testing for a genetic condition or aneuploidy to minimise contamination with sperm and cumulus cells. There are numerous current indications for ICSI, as well as some potential future applications (Figure 33.1).

33.3 ICSI Procedure

33.3.1 Oocyte Denudation

Oocyte nuclear maturity can only be properly assessed after the removal of the cumulus cells and can be identified by the extrusion of the first polar body (PB) in the perivitelline space, indicating a successful completion of meiosis I and arrest at the metaphase II (MII) stage. Some oocytes remain at either the germinal vesicle (GV) or metaphase I (MI) stages. The proportion of MII oocytes retrieved can be affected by follicle

DOI: 10.1201/9781003269502-33

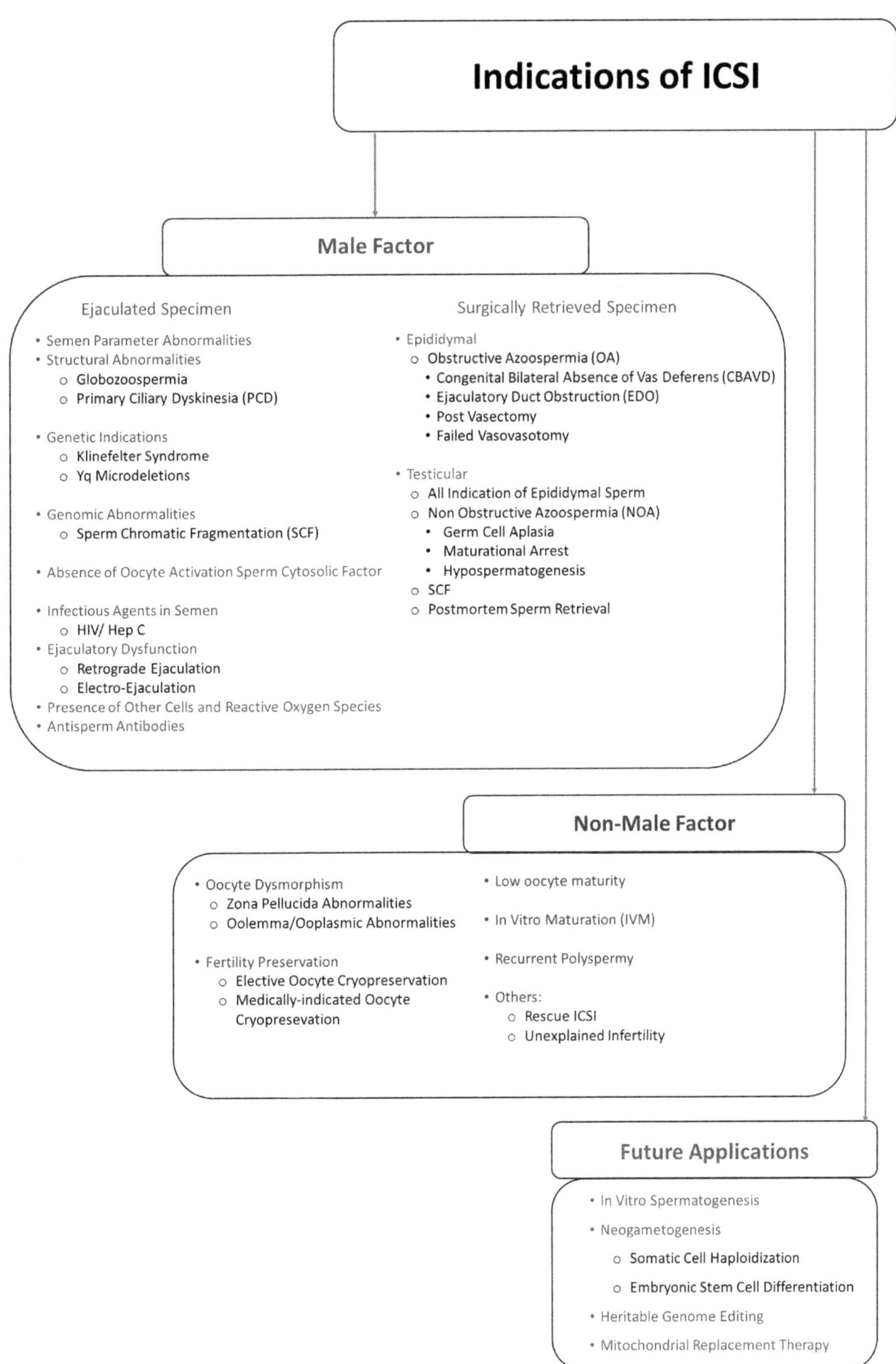

FIGURE 33.1 Indication of ICSI (from [**7**] under open access attribution licence).

size or the ovarian stimulation protocols. Immature oocytes not injected with the majority of the cohort (+/- 40 hours post HCG) are normally discarded.

Denudation of oocytes is a mechanically and chemically stressful procedure for the oocyte. Hyaluronidase is used and although the concentration and processing time varies, it should be kept to the minimum of 40–80 IU/ml and 30–60 seconds respectively (**8**). A pipette of at least 140ul should be used to avoid additional mechanical damage as the oocytes are pipetted up and down within the hyaluronidase until the cumulus and corona cells are removed, before being washed and placed in culture awaiting ICSI.

33.3.2 Dish Preparation

ICSI dishes are commercially available. These are designed to maintain optimal temperature with a true flat bottom that lies flush with the heated place on the ICSI rig. They have low profile edges to allow the angles needles to more easily access a larger area of the dish. They have super polished base for increased optical clarity. These are on top of all the non-toxic mouse embryo assay (MEA) tested requirements of all other IVF culture dishes.

Standard practice dictates the progression of the sperm is slowed using high viscosity polyvinylpyrrolidone (PVP) to ensure better morphological evaluation. This is done by creating a 10–20ul drop of PVP to the ICSI dish, under oil, and adding 1–2ul of the prepared sperm. An alternative to PVP is the use of a semi viscous medium containing hyaluronan. Like PVP, hyaluronan also slows down the movement but by binding the hyaluronic acid which mimics the natural selection of sperm with high DNA integrity by the zona pellucida. Those sperm that have fully matured and have developed receptors for hyaluronan will bind with the hyaluronan and come to a stop. The sperm that have stopped progressing, but their tails are still beating are selected for injection.

Drops of medium are prepared for the oocytes within the ICSI dish under oil. The options for the media, the oocytes are exposed to during ICSI, are buffered and nonbuffered media. Buffered media (e.g., with HEPES or MOPS) maintains the pH for the oocytes during the time that the oocytes are out of the gassed-incubated environment. The non buffered media may be less stressful for the oocytes but puts a time pressure on to the practitioner.

The layout of the ICSI dish must allow the quick and easy movement and orientation between the sperm drop and the oocyte drop. If a high number of oocytes require injecting, two or more injection dishes should be prepared, keeping one warm while the other is being used.

33.3.3 Sperm Selection and Immobilisation

The selection of ideal spermatozoa before ICSI could help to optimize the outcome of the treatment. Occasionally there will be little choice in sperm to select for injection, in which case those showing some degree of movement should be selective chosen. Where there is a good number of progressively motile sperm, a sperm showing a good morphology should be selected.

The most common method of immobilising the sperm is the crushing of the sperm tail against the bottom of the dish using the injection pipette. However, some studies have described the use of a laser as an alternative (**9**). The 'break' should aim to be made midway along the length of the tail, and should create an obvious crook or kink. The sperm should then be aspirated up the injection pipette tail first, and so that it can be moved freely up and down the pipette.

33.3.4 Sperm Injection

ICSI ideally is performed within 2 hours of cumulus removal, but timings are discussed later. The holding and injection needles are set up so they are parallel with the bottom of the dish and equilibrated with medium.

Using gentle suction from the holding pipette, rotate the oocyte in order to hold it with its polar body at approximately 12 or 6 o'clock. Bring the injection pipette into focus. Ensure the oolemma and injection pipette are in focus so that the injection needle enters the centre of the oocyte when injection takes place. Approach the zona from the 3 to 9 o'clock position (depending on which side the injection needle is); this ensures that you will enter the oocyte in the centre. Position the sperm at the needle tip and push the needle into the cytoplasm in one straight, controlled push (Figures 33.2 and 33.3). To ensure that the oolemma is broken before injecting the sperm, aspirate to draw the membrane back into the needle and await the cytoplasmic rush. Gently release the aspirated cytoplasm and

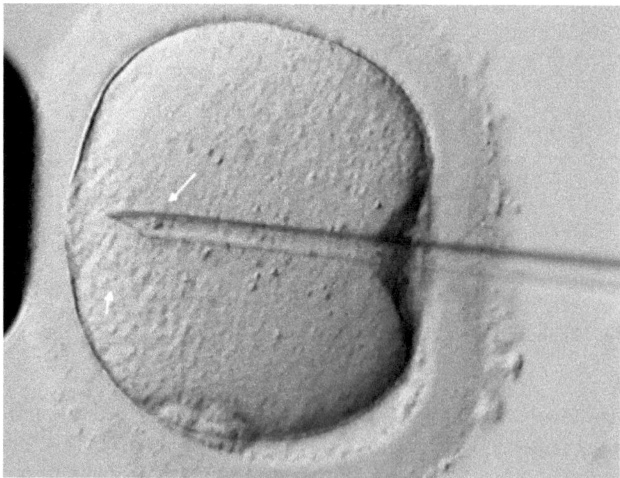

FIGURE 33.2 Culmination of the injection phase. The glass pipette is located close to the opposite membrane region (9 o'clock position) of the oocyte. The first polar body at the 6 o'clock position is out of focus. The large arrow indicates the spermatozoon. The small arrow indicates the area bearing highly polarized mitochondria.

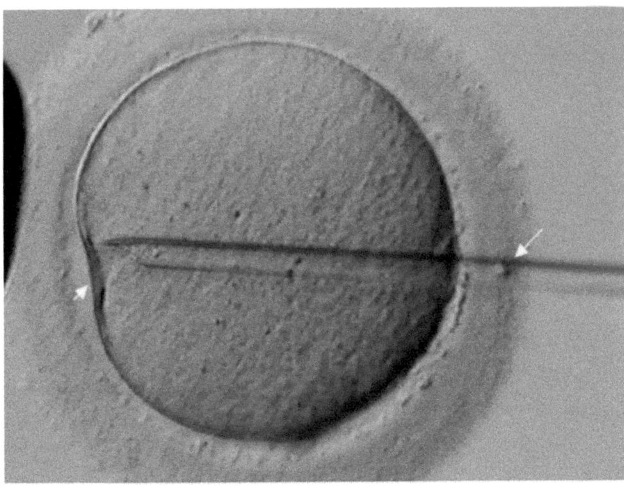

FIGURE 33.3 Culmination of the aspiration phase. During aspiration, the opposite membrane responds with a slight invagination (small arrow). The large arrow indicates the spermatozoon.

the sperm into the ooplasm. Slowly withdraw the needle. Take care not to vibrate or cause the needle to be moved in any other axis than the horizontal plane as this can irreparably damage the oolemma causing lysis. Aim to spend no longer than 2 minutes per oocyte during the ICSI procedure or longer than 15 minutes per dish.

33.4 Developments in ICSI

33.4.1 Artificial Oocyte Activation (AOA)

AOA involves increasing the free intracellular calcium immediately after ICSI using calcium ionophore or equivalent, to mimic the cell signalling that occurs at the point of egg-sperm fusion. In mammalian oocytes, an intracellular calcium rise is the signal responsible for the resumption of meiosis and the beginning of embryo development, thus playing an important role during fertilization (**10**). Sperm contain a specific phospholipase C isoform, PLC-zeta, that is present at a sufficient concentration to induce calcium spiking in the egg (**11**).

Despite there being no product available which is certified as a medical device for IVF clinical use, AOA process was accepted for use by the HFEA in 2012 as a process for carrying out the licensed activity 'Processing Gametes'. Studies have shown that AOA may have a beneficial effect for patients who have had previous failure of fertilisation, or less than 30% fertilisation in previous ICSI cycles (**12**).

In addition, men who repeatedly face failed fertilisation include those with globozoospermia, a rare disorder characterized by round-headed, acrosomeless sperm cells. Several successful pregnancies have occurred after ICSI was used in combination with AOA (**13**). This would suggest that besides the inability to interact with the female gamete due to an abnormal acrosome, globozoospermic sperm may have additional defects that affect their fertilisation capacity. A study by Kuentz et al. (2013) found that the fertilisation rates with AOA are restored to normal when compared with conventional ICSI, in a cohort of globozoospermic patients (**14**). On the other hand, Borges et al. (2009) studied the effects of AOA on ICSI cycles using surgically retrieved sperm (**15**). For patients undergoing TESA, it was reported that AOA did not improve ICSI outcomes. However, for cases in which they injected sperm retrieved from the epididymis, an increased rate of fertilisation and high-quality embryos was observed. The safety of AOA in a clinical setting remains to be assessed. Studies of children resulting from the calcium ionophore method for AOA have no reports of anomalies (**16**). However, as always, patients should be carefully counselled before AOA use. AOA is discussed further in Chapter 32.

33.4.2 Modified ICSI (mICSI)

mICSI is a mechanical means of oocyte activation characterised by aspiration close to the opposite membrane (a region which has high numbers of mitochondria with a high mitochondrial membrane potential), which is followed by central deposition of the sperm. This supplies, theoretically, more energy to the place where the sperm was injected.

Ebner et al. (2004) reported that the oocyte activation defect could be overcome by this simple modification of the micromanipulation technique with no need to use chemical agents such as calcium ionophore (**17**). This method was prospectively applied to the ICSI cycles of patients with a history of failed fertilisation in previous ICSI cycles. Previously there were no 2PN zygotes out of the 70 oocytes injected using conventional ICSI. After mICSI, however, there was an adequate fertilisation rate of 53.6% and a pregnancy rate of 33.3%. In patients without previous failed fertilisation, no improvement in fertilisation rate, blastocyst formation, implantation or clinical pregnancy could be seen.

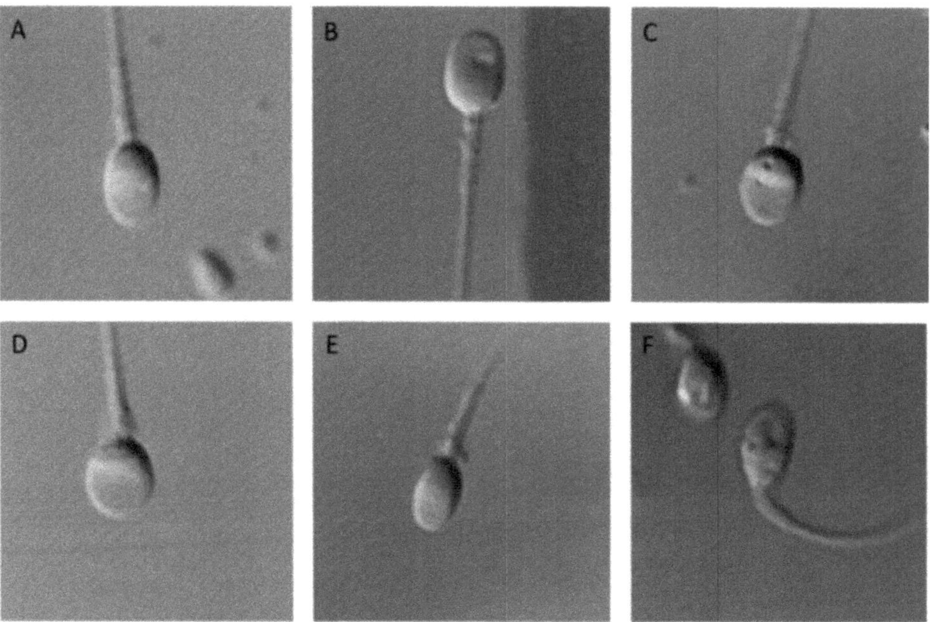

FIGURE 33.4 Sperm head morphology at 6000x magnification. A) Normal morphology. B) Large acrosomal vacuole. C) Equatorial and post-acrosomal vacuoles. D) Wide head. E) Narrow head. F) Highly vacuolated head (from [**19**] under open access attribution licence).

33.4.2.1 Artificial Sperm Activation (ASA)

In cases where ejaculates or surgically recovered sperm contains 100% immotile sperms, ASA can be performed using media containing compounds such as theophylline or caffeine. Motility can be observed after 10 minutes of incubation in the solution, with an effect lasting up to one hour. A study in 2019 showed that although fertilisation rate of oocytes is lower in cases needing ASA, there were similar utilisation of embryos with a control group, and the clinical, obstetric and perinatal outcome was not affected (**18**).

33.4.2.2 MSOME/IMSI

Motile sperm organelle morphology examination (MSOME) is performed in real-time using an inverted light microscope equipped with high-power Nomarski optics (**19**), and was introduced by Bartoov et al. in 2001 (**20**). This requires digital imaging software on a standard ICSI set up to achieve magnification up to 6300×. MSOME enables the detection of subtle sperm organellar malformations in motile spermatozoa. Using this technique together with a micromanipulation system led to a procedure known as intracytoplasmic morphologically selected sperm injection (IMSI). When the spermatozoa with normal morphology and motility selected for ICSI are detected under a magnification of ×400, in IMSI the motile spermatozoa are selected under magnification up to 6300× (Figure 33.4).

Both these modified ICSI techniques require specialised software, objectives and training, and in some studies specialised glass bottomed dishes were used. The additional time required to select the sperm for injection needs to be balanced with the optimal insemination window for the oocytes. A study evaluating the utility of MSOME and IMSI concluded MSOME may be useful for evaluating unexplained infertility, and IMSI can be recommended for men with <2% normal spermatozoa at MSOME (**19**). However, a Cochrane review on 2018 had shown no evidence of increased live birth or miscarriage rates compared to standard ICSI (**21**). Although not at present currently commercially available, further improvement in sperm selection may be achieved in the future, by using AI to select the single highest quality sperm in real-time.

33.4.3 Physiological Intracytoplasmic Sperm Injection (PICSI)

PICSI is a technique used to select sperm to use in ICSI treatment. It involves placing sperm with hyaluronic acid (HA), a natural compound the cumulus surrounding oocytes. Immature sperm do not have the ability to bind to HA, therefore, sperm that can bind to HA are selected for use in treatment. A PICSI dish is commercially available with hyaluronan drops which are hydrated prior to adding the sperm preparation. A systematic review showed no statistically significant difference between the PICSI and the ICSI techniques, for any of the studied outcome measures (**22**), although many studies were under powered, and it was therefore suggested that more information was required.

33.4.3.1 Piezo-ICSI

Piezo-ICSI uses small axial mechanical pulses (Piezo-pulses) to lower stress to the cytoskeleton during zona pellucida and oolemma breakage. A piezo-electric effect (crystal deformation in response to an externally applied voltage) propels a microcapillary forward in a precise and rapid movement that allows the membrane to be penetrated (**23**). The procedure includes specialized Piezo actuators, microcapillaries, and filling medium to transfer mechanical pulses to the cell membranes. The Piezo technique itself was established for animal

ICSI to reduce oocyte damage following conventional ICSI (**24**). Hiraoka and Kitamura working in Japan should an increase in survival and fertilisation rates of Piezo-ICSI injected human oocytes when compared with conventional ICSI, however, the technology has not yet been widely adopted (**25**).

33.5 Factors Affecting Success Rates of ICSI Procedure

There are many factors that impact the outcome of IVF treatments, however the use of ICSI adds some additional complexity that can be mitigated by an experienced practitioner. The sperm immobilisation, oolemma breakage and sperm deposition are the critical components, with other factors adding marginal gains.

33.5.1 Polar Body Positioning

The first polar body is assumed to be associated with the location of the meiotic spindle. Disruption of the spindle can lead to rearrangement of chromosomes in the cytoplasm and may contribute to aneuploidy after fertilization (**26**). To reduce this potential damage the polar body should be positioned at 6 or 12 o'clock, and the injection of the spermatozoa at 3 or 9 o'clock. The orientation of the PB did not significantly affect the proportion of oocytes that failed to survive injection, or the proportion scored as having either zero, one, two or three pronuclei. Stoddart and Fleming (2000) showed the proportion of normally fertilized zygotes that cleaved was not significantly different between the two groups, nor was the proportion of embryos classified as either grade 1, 2 or 3 (**27**). However, the proportion of grade 4 embryos (the poorest grade) was significantly lower in the 12 o'clock, compared to the 6 o'clock group. Most importantly, there was no significant difference between the two groups in the proportion of patients having a positive clinical pregnancy test, nor in either the implantation rate or the mean number of fetal hearts detected per patient presenting with a clinical pregnancy.

Precise identification of the spindle location can be achieved using a polarization microscope. Studies have shown that the spindle is not always adjacent to the polar body (**28**). A meta-analysis to investigate the influence of meiotic spindle visualization in human oocytes on ICSI outcome showed significantly increased fertilisation, cleavage stage embryo quality and blastulation rate when the spindle was visualised prior to ICSI, however, there was no difference observed in the clinical pregnancy or implantation rates (**29**).

33.5.2 Timing of Denudation and Injection, Including IVM and Rescue ICSI

The timing of denudation and injection are largely governed by the lab workflow and staffing levels in the lab. However, as with IVF, the insemination should be carried out as close to the 40-hour post HCG as possible. Studies have shown increased fertilisation rates can be achieved if oocytes are left for at least 1h from oocyte collection before cumulus removal, and ICSI must occur within 2h from cumulus removal (**30**). Studies where the injection of spermatozoon was carried out 9–11h and up to 11h after oocyte retrieval, the result was very poor embryo quality and lower pregnancy rates (**31**). Although there is no universal agreement on denudation and injection timing, most studies suggest that injection should be performed as soon after denudation as possible.

There are occasions where there are no oocytes are at Metaphase II following denudation. In these cases, it is reasonable to keep observing these oocytes for late maturation. Some of these oocytes may mature later on the day of oocyte retrieval, or overnight. In vitro maturation (IVM) of immature oocytes that are injected on the day following oocyte retrieval have been shown to fertilise and go on to achieve Euploid blastocysts (**32**), but it is not part of normal practice in a regular IVF lab. IVM is discussed in Chapter 32.

The term 'Rescue ICSI' may be used to refer to the injection of spermatozoa on day 1 following complete failed fertilisation of previously inseminated oocytes. This was first described by Nagy in 1993 who showed a fertilisation rate of 38% of such oocytes (**33**). However, this practice is currently forbidden by the HFEA Code of practice in the UK.

33.5.3 Troubleshooting

Reasons for ICSI oocyte failure to fertilise, or degeneration, may be due to one or more of these factors: practitioner technique, gamete quality or equipment and consumables. Each ICSI practitioner should be subject to monitoring via pertinent KPIs. The ESHRE Vienna consensus (2017) suggest these should be normal fertilization rate (2pn), oocyte degeneration rate, poor fertilization rate and failed fertilisation rate (**34**). The benchmark for the 2PN rate is >65% including only patients below 40 years of age with at least three oocytes collected. The ICSI damage rate or oocyte degeneration rate target value ranges from 0 to 10%, respectively. This includes oocyte damage observed at three time points during the ICSI process: from the start at stripping, during ICSI, or at the fertilization assess. Oocyte damage that occurs during the ICSI process may not always be seen until fertilisation check. Poor fertilization rate is defined as the proportion of cycles in which <25% of the injected oocytes are fertilized. The Vienna consensus suggests a benchmark value from 0 to 15%. Poor fertilization rate can give an indication of operator competence and reflect gamete quality. In the cases of failed fertilisation rates, meaning all of the oocytes injected failed to fertilise,

Major causes of damage

- Touching the opposing membrane with the injection needle; do not push the injection needle much further than half way.
- Injection of mineral oil; care must be taken when aspirating sperm from the edge of the microdrop.
- Excessive vibration or movement.

Causes of fertilisation failure

- Sperm tail not sufficiently broken.
- Oocyte membrane not penetrated.
- Sperm deposited in vacuoles.
- Excess medium transferred with sperm.

33.6 Risks, Success Rates and Long-Term Health of Offspring

ICSI carries slightly more risks than standalone IVF insemination due to the risk that eggs maybe damaged when they are stripped of cumulus, and when they are injected. Studies have concluded that both IVF and ICSI could pose a risk factor for both mother and baby (**35**), form pregnancy complications such as pre-eclampsia, growth retardation, and prematurity as well as higher rate of congenital malformations, developmental abnormalities and a higher risk of increased aberrations in imprinting patterns due to the possible transmission to progeny from ICSI of chromosomal alterations leading to all the above (**36**). However, an equal number of studies negate any correlation and emphasize that any association could very well be attributed to the increased risk for health problems present in couples undergoing IVF/ICSI cycles and not the actual techniques themselves (**37**). The follow-up studies on children from ICSI have shown that the procedure is safe and the slightly higher incidence of neonatal malformations or de novo gonosomal abnormalities are related to the genetics of the infertile couples (**38**). A meta-analysis in 2004 concluded that the ICSI procedure did not represent a significant risk of major birth defects in addition to the risks involved in standard IVF (**39**).

REFERENCES

1. Rosenwaks Z, Pereira N. The pioneering of intracytoplasmic sperm injection: historical perspectives. *Reproduction*. 2017;154:6.
2. Ng SC, Bongso A, Ratnam SS, et al. Pregnancy after transfer of sperm under zona. *Lancet*. 1988;2:790.
3. Palermo G, Joris H, Devroey P, et al. Induction of acrosome reaction in human spermatozoa used for subzonal insemination. *Hum Reprod*. 1992;7:248–254.
4. Palermo G, Joris H, Devroey P, et al. Pregnancies after intracytoplasmic injection of single spermatozoon into an oocyte. *Lancet*. 1992;340:17–18.
5. ICMART. *Preliminary World Report*. 2017. Available from: www.icmartivf.org/wp-content/uploads/ICMART-ESHRE-WR2017-Preliminary.pdf.
6. Wong A, Wilson B, Murray M. National trends in the use of ICSI with and without a diagnosis of male infertility. *Fertil Steril*. 2021;116(1):E31–E32.
7. Haddad M, Stewart J, Xie P, et al. Thoughts on the popularity of ICSI. *J Assist Reprod Genet*. 2021;38:101–123.
8. Van de Velde H, Nagy ZP, Joris H, et al. Effects of different hyaluronidase concentrations and mechanical procedures for cumulus cell removal on the outcome of intracytoplasmic sperm injection. *Hum Reprod*. 1997;12(10):2246–2250.
9. Montag M, Rink K, Delacretaz G, et al. Laser-induced immobilization and plasma membrane permeabilization in human spermatozoa. *Hum Reprod*. 2000;15:846–852.
10. Carroll J, Jones KT, Whittingham DG. Ca2þ release and the development of Ca2þ release mechanisms during oocyte maturation: a prelude to fertilization. *Rev Reprod*. 1996;1:137–134.
11. Saunders CM, Larman MG, Parrington J, et al. PLC zeta: a sperm-specific trigger of Ca(2þ) oscillations in eggs and embryo development. *Development*. 2002;129:3533–3544.
12. Montag M, Koster M, Van der Ven K, et al. The benefit of artificial oocyte activation is dependent on the fertilization rate in a previous treatment cycle. *Reprod Biomed Online*. 2012;24:521–526.
13. Nasr-Esfahani MH, Razavi S, Javdan Z, et al. Artificial oocyte activation in severe teratozoospermia undergoing intracytoplasmic sperm injection. *Fertil Steril*. 2008;90(6):2231–2237.
14. Kuentz P, Vanden Meerschaut F, Elinati E, et al. Assisted oocyte activation overcomes fertilization failure in globozoospermic patients regardless of the DPY19L2 status. *Hum Reprod*. 2013;28(4):1054–1061.
15. Borges E, Almeida Ferreira Braga DP, de Sousa Bonetti T, et al. Artificial oocyte activation with calcium ionophore A23187 in intracytoplasmic sperm injection cycles using surgically retrieved spermatoa. *Fertil Steril*. 2009;92(1):131–136.
16. Yamano S, Nakagawa K, Nakasak H. Fertilisation failure and oocyte activation. *J Med Invest*. 2000;47:1–8.
17. Ebner T, Sommergrubber M, Jesacher K, et al. Complete oocyte activation failure after ICSI can be overcome by a modified injection technique. *Hum Reprod*. 2004;(19):1837–1841.
18. Sandi-Monroy NL, Musanovic S, Zhu D, et al. Use of dimethylxanthine theophylline (SpermMobil ®) does not affect clinical, obstetric or perinatal outcomes. *Arch Gynecol Obstet*. 2019;300(5):1435–1443.
19. Asali A, Miller N, Pasternak Y, et al. The possibility of integrating motile sperm organelle morphology examination (MSOME) with intracytoplasmic morphologically-selected sperm injection (IMSI) when treating couples with unexplained infertility. *PLoS One*. 2020;15:e0232156.
20. Bartoov B, Berkovitz A, Eltes F, et al. Real-time fine morphology of motile human sperm cells is associated with IVF-ICSI outcome. *J Androl*. 2002;23:1–8.
21. Farquhar C, Marjoribanks J. Ultra-high magnification sperm injection (IMSI) has no evidence of increased live birth or miscarriage rates compared to standard ICSI. "Assisted reproductive technology: an overview of Cochrane reviews". *Cochrane Database Syst Rev*. 2018;(8):CD010537.
22. Avalos-Durán G, Cañedo-Del Ángel A, Rivero-Murillo J, et al. Physiological ICSI (PICSI) vs. conventional ICSI in couples with male factor: a systematic review. *JBRA Assist Reprod*. 2018;22(2):139–147.
23. Costa-Borges N, Mestres N, Vanrell I, et al. Intracytoplasmic sperm injection (ICSI) in the mouse with the Eppendorf PiezoXpert®: how to increase oocyte survival rates after injection. Eppendorf Application Note I No. 395.
24. Kimura Y, Yanagimachi R. Intracytoplasmic sperm injection in the mouse. *Biol Reprod*. 1995;52:709–720.
25. Hiraoka K, Kitamura S. Clinical efficiency of Piezo-ICSI using micropipettes with a wall thickness of 0.625 µm. *J Assist Reprod Genet*. 2015;32(12):1827–1833.
26. Pickering SJ, Johnson MH, Braude PR, et al. Cytoskeletal organization in fresh, aged and spontaneously activated human oocytes. *Hum Reprod*. 1988;3:978–989.

27. Stoddart NR, Fleming SD. Orientation of the first polar body of the oocyte at 6 or 12 o'clock during ICSI does not affect clinical outcome. *Hum Reprod*. 2000;15: 1580–1585.
28. Rienzi L, Ubaldi F, Martinez F et al. Relationship between meiotic spindle location with regard to the polar body position and oocyte developmental potential after ICSI. *Hum Reprod*. 2003;18(6):1289–1293.
29. Petersen CG, Oliveira JBA, Mauri AL, et al. Relationship between visualization of meiotic spindle in human oocytes and ICSI outcomes: a meta-analysis. *RMBO*. 2009;18(2):235–243.
30. Hickman C, Campbell A, Fishel S. Optimising the timing between oocyte collection, cumulus removal and insemination by ICSI or IVF. *Fertil Steril*. 2011;96(3):S79.
31. Yanagida K, Yazawa H, Katayose H, et al. Influence of oocyte preincubation time on fertilization after intracytoplasmic sperm injection. *Hum Reprod*. 1998;13(8):2223–2226.
32. Shani AK, Haham LM, Balakier H, et al. What is the developmental potential of mature oocytes derived from rescue in-vitro maturation (RIVM)? *Fert Steril*. 2021;116(3):E178–E179.
33. Nagy ZP, Joris H, Liu J, et al. Intracytoplasmic single sperm injection of 1-day-old unfertilized human oocytes. *Hum Reprod*. 1993;8(12):2180–2184.
34. ESHRE Special Interest Group of Embryology and Alpha Scientistsin Reproductive Medicine. The Vienna consensus: report of an expert meeting on the development of art laboratory performance indicators. *Hum Reprod Open*. 2017;1–17.
35. Simopoulou M, Giannelou P, Bakas P, et al. Making ICSI safer and more effective: a review of the human oocyte and ICSI practice. *In Vivo*. 2016;30(4):387–400.
36. Eroglu A, Layman LC, Role of ART in imprinting disorders. *Semin Reprod Med*. 2012;30:92–104.
37. Wen J, Jiang J, Ding C, et al. Birth defects in children conceived by in vitro fertilization and intracytoplasmic sperm injection: a meta-analysis. *Fertil Steril*. 2012;97:1331–1337, e1331–1334.
38. Palermo GD, Neri QV, Rosenwaks Z. To ICSI or not to ICSI. *Semin Reprod Med*. 2015;33:92–102.
39. Lie RT, Lyngstadaas A, Ørstavik KH, et al. Birth defects in children conceived by ICSI compared with children conceived by other IVF-methods; a meta-analysis. *Int J Epidemiol*. 2005;34:696–701.

34

Embryo Biopsy and Preimplantation Genetic Testing (PGT)

Lucy Jenner and Colleen Lynch

34.1 Introduction

Preimplantation genetic testing (PGT) of embryos is seen by many, especially the general public, as a new and experimental technology. However, the first babies were born over 30 years ago following this treatment and only 12 years after the birth of the first IVF baby (**1**). In fact, Robert Edwards, a pioneer of both IVF and preimplantation testing, performed the first PGT, by sexing of rabbit blastocysts (**2**), ten years prior to the worlds' first IVF birth that would eventually lead to his Nobel prize.

34.2 The Embryo Culture Environment

The first steps in a successful PGT cycle with embryo biopsy are the same as a standard cycle – oocyte retrieval, sperm preparation, insemination, and embryo culture. Whilst there is no need to deviate from standard laboratory practice, it may be sensible to ensure that PGT oocyte retrievals and inseminations are the first to be performed, to maximise the time for blastocyst development. Dependent on clinic protocol and the requirements of the PGT laboratory, it should be possible to inseminate via IVF or intracytoplasmic sperm injection (ICSI).

Many professional guidelines still recommend ICSI as the preferred means of insemination in PGT cases (**3, 4**). Whilst ASRM and SART acknowledge a lack of data supporting this in practice (**4**), ESHRE states ICSI to be the preferable method of insemination for PGT cases in order to minimise the risk of both maternal contamination from residual cumulus cells, and paternal contamination from surplus spermatozoa attached to the zona pellucida (**5**). However, the risk of maternal contamination remains with ICSI, and embryologists should be rigorous when it comes to the removal of cumulus cells at denudation or fertilization check. Additionally, it is questionable how much risk bound spermatozoa present (**6, 7**). Retrospective analyses (**8, 9**) and prospective studies (**10**) report no significant difference between IVF and ICSI PGT patients in terms of aneuploidy rates, contamination rates, and parental origin of aneuploidy or disomy, indicating no additional risk factors stemming from IVF insemination.

While the culture system may not impact directly on aneuploidy rates – though could foreseeably contribute to mosaicism given it is generated during embryonic mitosis – it does impact on embryo metabolism and ultimately implantation and livebirth rates. Poor blastocyst development or quality will negatively impact PGT outcomes by reducing the number of embryos available for testing. Given that blastocyst development is dynamic, embryos within a cohort may be ready to biopsy at different times or on different days. Embryo development could be hindered by repeatedly checking the embryos; the use of time-lapse incubation to monitor development could reduce the interruption of culture. If time-lapse is not available, the laboratory should identify time points each day to check development.

In addition, strategies should be considered to minimise incubator door openings while embryos are removed for biopsy such as having a "handling incubator" to reduce the impact on other patient's dishes, or using multiple chambers across a benchtop incubator, which have much quicker recovery rate in terms of temperature and gas atmosphere (**11**). Further, it may be sensible to split a cohort of embryos across a number of culture dishes. Single embryo culture is necessary from the point of biopsy onwards, for sample identification and the chain of custody leading to results and may also be considered prior to this.

34.3 Embryo Biopsy

Since the introduction of PGT into assisted reproductive medicine there have been exponential improvements and innovations in the field of genetic diagnostics (**1**). Within the embryology laboratory change has also occurred. There has been movement from single cell biopsy approaches (polar body (PB) or blastomere) to multiple cell biopsy (trophectoderm biopsy), enabled by improvements in embryo culture, and from fresh embryo transfer on days 5 or 6 to vitrification and frozen embryo replacement (**12**).

34.3.1 Polar Body Biopsy

This approach benefits from the fact that no essential cellular material is removed for testing, but can only be used for maternally inherited genetic conditions and will not detect post meiotic chromosomal errors. The biggest advantage of PB biopsy is that the ploidy of PB I and II accurately predicts the ploidy of the zygote as shown through ESHRE's ESTEEM trial (**13**). It is often used where there are legal or ethical contraindications to embryo biopsy. For an accurate result both polar bodies must be removed and tested – either sequentially or simultaneously, the advantage of the former being the greater ease in differentiating them. The timing of the removal of the

DOI: 10.1201/9781003269502-34

second PB is important in terms of the completion of anaphase II, complete cleavage from the oocyte (reducing the risk of the presence of spindle remnants in the cytoplasmic bridge and removal of chromatids from the oocyte), and maximising amplification rates (**14**). The process can be labour intensive, especially if the biopsies are performed sequentially, and given that not all oocytes will fertilise.

34.3.2 Cleavage Stage Biopsy

This technique is less labour intensive than PB biopsy as only embryos reaching the requisite cell number, and of sufficient quality, are biopsied. Depending on the PGT technology, it can allow the return of results for fresh embryo transfer at the blastocyst stage. Newer technologies require embryo freezing and clinics are moving towards frozen transfers to optimise outcomes (**15**). The biopsy is normally performed on the morning of day 3 Criteria should be in place for the selection of embryos suitable for biopsy, usually over 5 cells, no multinucleation/anucleation, and low levels of fragmentation. Moves away from cleavage stage biopsy are mainly related to concerns of a possible reduction in implantation potential (**16**) and false positive/negative results relating to mosaicism (**17**). Cleavage stage biopsy can be used to test for maternally and paternally inherited conditions, as well as meiotic and mitotic errors, but may miss some mitotic errors depending on the stage they arise at, or the cell selected for testing. Embryos should be biopsied in individual drops of HEPES- or MOPS- buffered Ca^{2+}/Mg^{2+} free culture media, which disrupts cell-to-cell adhesion and allows the easy removal of a single blastomere. The blastomere selected for biopsy should be of average size and have a visible nucleus. Ideally only a single blastomere should be removed, as the removal of additional cells impacts on the embryo's implantation potential (**18**). The most common practice is to aspirate the chosen blastomere with a biopsy pipette (Figure 34.1). The blastomere may also be removed by extrusion (where the blastomere is squeezed through the opening in the zona by pushing against the exterior of the embryo with the biopsy pipette) or displacement (where media is gently injected into the embryo to displace the blastomere through the zona breach).

34.3.3 Morula Biopsy

Morula biopsy is a more recent approach to embryo biopsy. The theory is that multiple cells can be taken late on day 3 or on day 4, and testing can be performed to allow fresh transfer. On the face of current evidence, fresh transfer, especially if late on day 5 or on day 6, may not provide the best chance of pregnancy for the patient, but is sometimes necessitated by reproductive health tourism, where the patient has travelled to another country for access to the treatment.

The morula is placed into buffered Ca^{2+}/Mg^{2+} free media to de-compact the embryo, making the individual blastomeres visible and reducing cell-cell adhesion. When the individual blastomeres are visible, biopsy can proceed as per cleavage stage, but with multiple cells taken. The embryo will recompact once it is returned to culture. Data is still limited on this

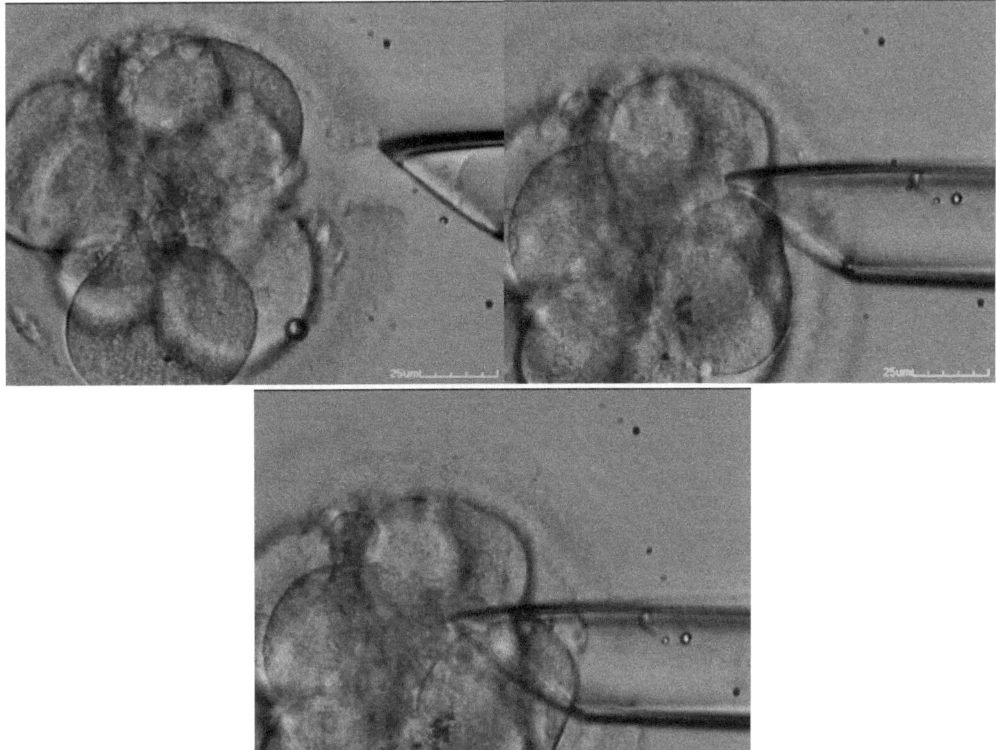

FIGURE 34.1 Blastomere biopsy with selected blastomere and zona breach at around 3 o'clock. With the zona and blastomere on the same plane of focus, the biopsy needle can be inserted through the breach with light suction used to remove the blastomere (courtesy of CARE Fertility).

approach, but early studies and case reports suggest this to be a feasible approach and that embryo development is not affected (**19, 20**).

34.3.4 Trophectoderm Biopsy

Trophectoderm biopsy was first reported in 1990 and clinically applied in 2002 (**21, 22**). It has now become the preferred method of biopsy for all forms of PGT (**23**), enabled by advances in embryo culture techniques which have increased blastulation rates. It confers a number of advantages, the most obvious being that time and resources are not used biopsying and testing embryos that have not reached the blastocyst stage and may not be capable of implantation. This approach can optimise the cost of the procedure, something that is ultimately passed on to the patient (**22**). The biopsy of multiple cells both reduces the risk of test failure and increases diagnostic accuracy (**24**), and at the blastocyst stage, allows certainty that cells are not being taken from part of the embryo that will develop into the foetus, i.e. the inner cell mass (ICM) (**22**). The biopsy of multiple cells also enables reporting of levels of chromosome mosaicism (**25, 26**).

Trophectoderm biopsy can be used for testing in all the same scenarios as cleavage stage and may pick up additional mitotic errors occurring post day 3. Mosaicism still exists at the blastocyst stage, but technologies like next generation sequencing (NGS) allow samples to be categorised as aneuploid, euploid or mosaic. However, this requires limits for each of these categorisations to be set, and assumes that the levels of aneuploidy within the sampled cells is represented in the rest of the embryo. Nonetheless, some clinics are adopting the transfer of mosaic embryos in the absence of the availability of euploids, and achieving livebirths (**27, 28**). These data have enabled the creation of guidelines (**29**) with information for the testing laboratory, the IVF clinic, genetic counsellors and clinical support groups and recommendations for clinicians, including prenatal diagnosis options. While trophectoderm biopsy may initially appear the least labour intensive of the biopsy approaches, blastocysts are biopsied at different times over days 5, 6, and 7, which prolongs the process. They are then vitrified awaiting test results before warming and transfer in a different cycle.

34.3.4.1 Assisted Hatching

Blastocysts can be biopsied once the inner cell mass (ICM) and trophectoderm can be differentiated. In most culture systems, it is not expected that all blastulated embryos will have begun the hatching process *in vitro* concurrently. Although the clinical evidence does not support the use of assisted hatching (AH) in clinical practice to improve live birth rates (**30**), it is generally considered a useful intervention as part of the biopsy process to allow direct access and aspiration and separation of trophectoderm cells. It is common practice to hatch the embryos on day 3 or late on day 4 (when it may be possible to visualise the ICM) to encourage herniation of the trophectoderm and make the biopsy procedure easier on day 5 or 6 (**31**). However, it is also possible to hatch the embryo at the time of biopsy (**32**).

Laser is currently the most widely used method for AH (**5**) being the most standardised, reproducible, and safe (**33, 34**).

34.3.4.2 Blastocyst (Trophectoderm) Biopsy Procedure

The biopsy can be performed using laser or mechanical approaches, or a combination of both. The trophectoderm biopsy most commonly involves assisted hatching via laser on day 3 or day 4, creating a zona breach of 25–30µm. Embryos are cultured to day 5; those with expanded hatching trophectoderm cells are biopsied and the remainder cultured for a further 8–24hrs to be rechecked. A 30µm biopsy pipette is used to aspirate 5–6 trophectoderm cells and, if used, the laser is fired 3–5 times, at a reduced pulse length, a maximum of 3 times to create a weakness between trophectoderm cells at cell junctions. In terms of the biopsy procedure and separation of the trophectoderm cells, two methods encompass the approaches of most groups, and the main differences pertain to when or if hatching is performed, as discussed in the previous section (**5**), and the method of separation of the cells.

34.3.4.2.1 Laser and Stretch

The blastocyst is gently aspirated on the holding pipette with the hatching trophectoderm cells/opening of the zona pellucida opposite from the holding pipette, preferably working in a horizontal line, and with the ICM in clear view. The trophectoderm cells are gently aspirated into the biopsy pipette, holding the embryo securely to create tension. The laser is fired at the thinnest portion of the aspirated cells, directed at cell junctions, until the sample separates (**31, 35**). The biopsy pipette is pulled away from the embryo as the laser is fired, allowing the cells to detach (**23, 31**). This approach has been modified by instead performing hatching at the time of biopsy (**35**) or by using a mixture of laser and mechanical methods to detach the trophectoderm cells (**36**).

34.3.4.2.2 Laser and Flick

The key difference with this approach is that after the trophectoderm cells are gently aspirated into the biopsy pipette, the aspiration pressure is neutralised (Figure 34.2a). The laser may be fired cell junctions along the outside of the opening of the biopsy pipette or the procedure may be performed entirely mechanically. The embryo is then released from the holding pipette. The biopsy pipette is positioned above the holding pipette, ensuring they are on the same plane of focus (Figure 34.2b). The biopsy pipette is moved to the edge of the holding pipette and they are pushed against each other, causing the biopsy pipette to flick across the front of the holding pipette, detaching the trophectoderm sample, which should remain in place in the biopsy pipette (Figure 34.2c) (**36, 37**). See further Videos 1 and 2.

Throughout biopsy and tubing procedures, all embryo movements require an appropriate witness and witness events must be recorded. Manual witnessing will be mandatory for some movements, for example, where more than one embryo is placed in the biopsy dish; in this case we are not simply matching dish to dish or dish to tube, but also that the embryo/sample identifier matches culture drop to culture drop or culture drop to tube.

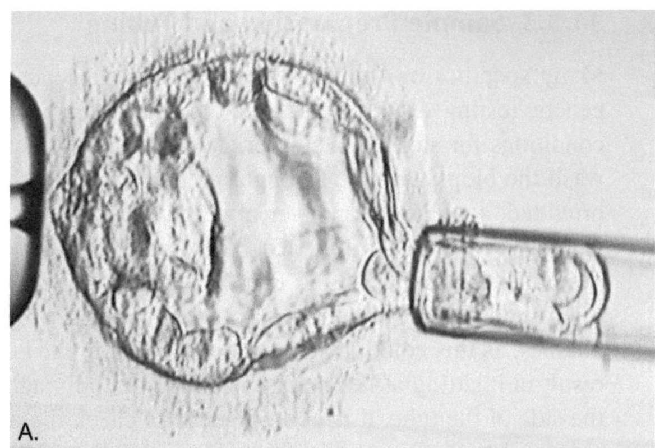

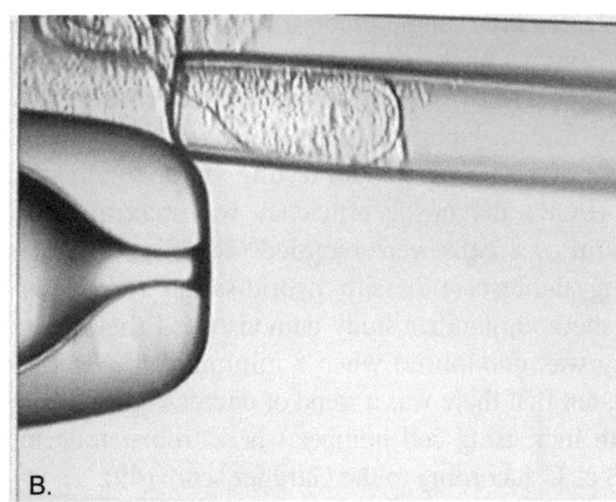

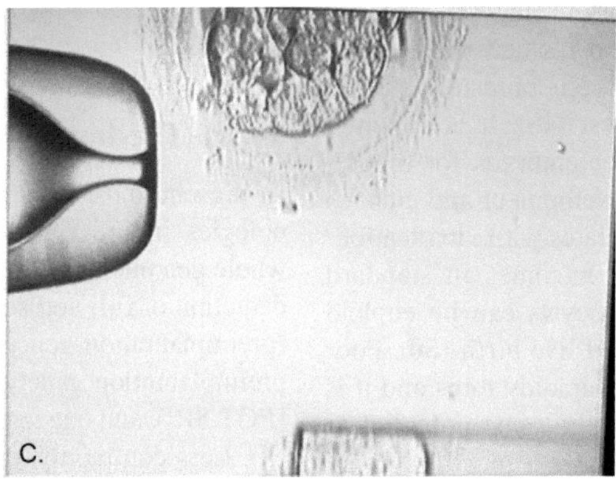

FIGURE 34.2 Biopsy of trophectoderm cells using the laser and flick method. (A) pull cells into the biopsy pipettes, (B) align the edges of the biopsy and holding needles in the same focal place, and (C) slide biopsy needles to cut biopsied cells away from remaining embryo (courtesy of CARE Fertility).

34.3.4.3 Cell Lysis and Damage

Guidance on laser assisted biopsy warns against over-use of the laser as a potential source of cell damage and partial destruction of cellular deoxyribonucleic acid (DNA) (**26**). As with assisted hatching, papers usually reference the make and model of laser use, but much less frequently refer to the pulse length used, the hole size this generates, or the number of times the laser is fired. Kelk et al. (2017) demonstrated no impact to DNA profiles with up to 5 shots of the laser in the range commonly used to perform trophectoderm biopsy (**38**). However, the H1 human embryonic stem cells used may have been more robust than human trophectoderm cells and were not placed under the same stresses i.e. aspiration, stretching, as trophectoderm cells during biopsy. Therefore, it is still possible that stresses on the trophectoderm cells such as increased laser exposure, multiple flicking, scraping on the holding pipette or overstretching could lead to cellular damage that could impact on PGT data, especially where cell lysis is observed. Poor quality samples will lead to lower quality/noisier data that is more difficult to interpret and could lead to overcalling of mosaic changes where data analysis is manual rather than via validated algorithms (**36**). Some groups suggest that using the laser and flick method is recommended (**39**), on the basis that laser and stretch produces more mosaic profiles, but this has not been replicated by all groups investigating the impact of the biopsy method (**40**). Mechanical biopsy via the flicking method on days 5 or 6 (following laser hatching on day 4) has shown similar amplification rates and clinical pregnancy outcomes to blastocysts undergoing biopsy via the "laser and flick", but blastocysts in the latter group demonstrated significantly better survival rates on warming post vitrification (**41**).

34.3.4.4 Blastocyst Quality and Number of Cells Biopsied

When performing biopsy there needs to be a balance between maximising diagnostic accuracy, minimising the failed amplification and "no result" rate and, obviously, impact on the implantation potential of the blastocyst. As such, the number of trophectoderm cells taken at biopsy may be vital, especially given that trophectoderm function is increasingly recognised as vital to implantation and sustained pregnancy (**42, 43**). Where chromosome mosaicism is reported, cell number is also vital in terms of this being a meaningful measure, and as such a minimum sample size of 5 cells has previously been recommended (**26**). If we accept that cell loss through cryopreservation (**44**) and removal of more than a single blastomere at cleavage stage (**45**) impacts on implantation, it is logical to assume that removing too high a number of cells relative to the total number of cells within the trophectoderm could impact on continued development and implantation.

Neal et al. reported biopsies with the highest relative DNA content – estimated at 15–20 cells – were associated with lower live birth rates after single embryo transfer (**46**). Comparing genetic testing technologies requiring different cells numbers has also appeared to show removal of an average of 10 cells negatively affects embryo implantation when compared to an average of 5 cells (**47**). With testing via polymerase chain reaction (PCR), diagnostic efficiency was maximised when a minimum of 8 cells were biopsied (**48**). Similarly, despite employing fluorescent in situ hybridisation (FISH) as the analysis method, another study demonstrated that diagnostic efficiency was maximised when a minimum of 6 cells were biopsied, but that there was a trend of decreasing implantation rates with increasing cell number where trophectoderm was graded B or C according to the Gardner score (**49**).

Factors influencing the "no result rate" post biopsy – a combination of both amplification failure and poor-quality test data – have been demonstrated to include the treating centre, day of biopsy, and number of cells biopsied, but not morphological quality of the blastocyst (**48**). It is common for centres to set selection criteria for embryos for biopsy, basing this on the day and stage of development and embryo morphology, given this normally associates with vitrification/warming survival rates and clinical outcomes in standard cycles. However, poorer quality blastocysts can be euploid and do result in clinical pregnancy and live birth (**50**). Poor quality blastocysts do show higher aneuploidy rates and it is not certain when euploid if they have the same potential as good quality blastocysts, but patients of advanced maternal age particularly benefit from their inclusion in testing. The culture to and biopsy of day 7 embryos has also proved controversial but again, it has been demonstrated that while they have lower euploid rates, they may have similar sustained implantation rates to day 5 and day 6 blastocysts (**51, 52**). Faster and slower growing embryos have been shown to have similar aneuploidy rates (**35**), and so, while it is important that the blastocyst has expanded to the point where the inner cell mass and trophectoderm can be clearly distinguished prior to biopsy, the specific time point at which the biopsy is performed can be left open to include embryos reaching the requisite stage on day 5, 6, or 7.

34.3.4.5 Re-biopsy

With the "no result rate" varying between clinics and testing laboratories, depending on patient circumstance, re-biopsy and re-testing may be requested rather than disposing of the embryo or transferring with unknown genetic status. Given that the in the majority of PGT cycles embryos are vitrified post-biopsy, this requires warming, followed by a second round of trophectoderm biopsy and vitrification. If the embryo proves to be genetically suitable for use, it then must be warmed for a second time. Embryo survival on warming, the return of results, and the genetic status (e.g. euploid vs. aneuploid) has been reported to be similar to first biopsy data (**48**). Similar clinical outcomes have been observed, including gestational age at delivery, and birth weight, as embryos that have only been through one round of biopsy, vitrification, and warming (**53–55**). However, overall numbers of embryos transferred remains relatively very low, and therefore, further data is needed for analysis.

34.3.5 Sample Preparation and Tubing

Many specifics on the tubing procedure will depend on the genetic testing service used; type of buffer, volume of buffer, conditions for storage. However, good standard practise is to wash the biopsy sample through multiple drops of the buffer provided, avoiding carry over of culture media or oil, before placing it in the PCR tube (**5**). The dispensing of the biopsy sample into the PCR tube can be visualised with a stereo microscope during pipetting. Care should be taken not to expel bubbles, as this could displace the sample from the buffer and result in it sitting at the meniscus and potentially adhering to the side of the tube. It is good practice to check the pipette in a drop of buffer post-tubing to confirm that the sample is not retained in the pipette when withdrawing the pipette from the PCR tube (**39**).

34.3.6 Pre-Implantation Genetic Testing

At present, most PGT laboratories employ at least three technologies in order to test embryonic material: One for the whole genome amplification of DNA from the biopsy, one for detection of full and segmental chromosome gains and losses (preimplantation genetic testing for aneuploidy [PGT-A] and preimplantation genetic testing for structural rearrangements [PGT-SR]), and one for detection of monogenic diseases (PGT-M). Less commonly, there is also PGT-P for preimplantation genetic testing for polygenic disorders.

The application of whole genome amplification (WGA) technology means that both PGT-A and PGT-M can be performed on amplified DNA from the original trophectoderm biopsy. WGA is the precursor step to both single nucleotide polymorphism (SNP) arrays and NGS as it enables the production of several micrograms of DNA from a single cell (**56**). It is expected that PGT-M will ultimately also be performed via NGS, with single gene and chromosome information being provided by a single test on one platform.

34.3.7 Adverse Outcomes and Misdiagnosis

A misdiagnosis is generally considered to have occurred when conception occurs, but the foetus or child born does not genetically match the PGT result. The true incidence of misdiagnosis in PGT is difficult to gauge. Many will go undetected if pregnancy or livebirth does not occur, where there are no adverse indications (i.e. unaffected vs. carrier), or where embryos are discarded without confirmatory diagnosis. Conversely, misdiagnosis may be incorrectly presumed in place of a natural conception. The ESHRE PGD consortium aims to collect and publish such data, although not all clinics offering the treatment report to the consortium. Between 1997 and 2010 they have reported 21 misdiagnoses via FISH for PGT and 13 via PCR based approaches for PGT-M. This represents less than a 0.5% risk of misdiagnosis and is almost certainly lower than the actual figure (**57, 58**).

The causes of misdiagnosis can be categorised as human error, technical, or biological. In addition to this the cause may be intrinsic (a known phenomenon or limitation) or extrinsic (introduced to the process) (**59**). Some potential examples are

TABLE 34.1

Summary of Potential Causes of Adverse Incidents in PGT and Preventive Actions (Adapted from [**59**])

Cause of Incident	Error Type	Potential Preventive Action
Natural conception	Human	Patient information and consents state to avoid unprotected intercourse
Mislabelled sample	Human	Robust labelling system
Misidentified samples	Human	Robust witnessing procedures
Misinterpreted report	Human	Identification suitable individuals to communicate results and appropriate training and witnessing
Transfer of incorrect embryo	Human	Robust witnessing procedures
Use of incorrect reagents	Human	Appropriate training and
Haploid cells	Intrinsic/biological	Use of linked markers or SNP array
Polyploid cells	Intrinsic/biological	Use of linked markers or SNP array
Chromosomal mosaicism	Intrinsic/biological	Biopsy of multiple cells
Test failure	Extrinsic/technical	Pre-clinical validation. Whole genome amplification allows repeat testing
Maternal contamination	Extrinsic/technical	Removal of all cumulus cells prior to biopsy
Paternal contamination	Extrinsic/technical	Use of ICSI to prevent extraneous bound sperm
Operator contamination	Extrinsic/technical	Appropriate training, personal protective equipment a lab model rules
Allele drop out	Intrinsic/technical	Multiple cell biopsy. Multiple linked markers
Incorrect setting of genetic phase	Human	Appropriate training and competency
Uniparental disomy	Intrinsic/biological	Use of linked markers or SNP arrays

outlined in Table 34.1 along with possible preventive action. Further to the cause of a misdiagnosis it is important to identify the specific root cause to implement effective corrective action to prevent recurrence. For example, human errors may result from inadequate training, inadequate staff levels, or a failure of the standard operating procedure to fully or correctly describe the procedure.

Quality management is an essential part of PGT. Identification and analysis of the likelihood and seriousness of risk and the implementation of preventive action is a necessity given the potential level of severity of adverse incidents in this field. Robust staff training and competency assessment and confirmatory diagnosis of non-transferred embryos are vital parts of the embryology aspect of PGT programmes.

Videos

34.1 "Flick" Biopsy with Laser (Access the videos at www.routledge.com/9781032216577)

34.2 "Flick" Biopsy without Laser (Access the videos at www.routledge.com/9781032216577)

REFERENCES

1. Handyside AH, Kontogianni EH, Hardy K, et al. Pregnancies from biopsied human preimplantation embryos sexed by Y-specific DNA amplification. *Nature.* 1990;344(6268):768–7670.
2. Edwards RG, Gardner RL. Sexing of live rabbit blastocysts. *Nature.* 1967;214(5088):576–577.
3. Kokkali G, Traeger-Synodinos J, Vrettou C, et al. Blastocyst biopsy versus cleavage stage biopsy and blastocyst transfer for preimplantation genetic diagnosis of β-thalassaemia: a pilot study. *Hum Reprod.* 2007;22(5):1443–1449.
4. ASRM T. Intracytoplasmic sperm injection (ICSI) for non-male factor infertility: a committee opinion. *Fertil Steril.* 2012;98(6):1395–1399.
5. Kokkali G, Coticchio G, Bronet F, et al. ESHRE PGT consortium and SIG embryology good practice recommendations for polar body and embryo biopsy for PGT. *Hum Reprod Open.* 2020;2020(3):hoaa020.
6. Patassini C, Garolla A, Bottacin A, et al. Molecular karyotyping of human single sperm by array-comparative genomic hybridization. *PLoS One.* 2013;8(4):e60922.
7. Lynch C, Armstrong E, Charitou M, et al. Investigation of the risk of paternal cell contamination in PGT and the necessity of intracytoplasmic sperm injection. *Hum Fertil.* 2022:1–6.
8. Feldman B, Aizer A, Brengauz M, et al. Pre-implantation genetic diagnosis – should we use ICSI for all? *J Assist Reprod Genet.* 2017;34(9):1179–1183.
9. Palmerola KL, Vitez SF, Amrane S, et al. Minimizing mosaicism: assessing the impact of fertilization method on rate of mosaicism after next-generation sequencing (NGS) preimplantation genetic testing for aneuploidy (PGT-A). *J Assist Reprod Genet.* 2019;36(1):153–157.
10. De Munck N, El Khatib I, Abdala A, et al. Intracytoplasmic sperm injection is not superior to conventional IVF in couples with non-male factor infertility and preimplantation genetic testing for aneuploidies (PGT-A). *Hum Reprod.* 2020;35(2):317–327.
11. Swain JE. Decisions for the IVF laboratory: comparative analysis of embryo culture incubators. *Reprod Biomed Online.* 2014;28(5):535–547.
12. Coll L, Parriego M, Boada M, et al. Transition from blastomere to trophectoderm biopsy: comparing two preimplantation genetic testing for aneuploidies strategies. *Zygote.* 2018;26(3):191–198.

13. Geraedts J, Montag M, Magli MC, et al. Polar body array CGH for prediction of the status of the corresponding oocyte. Part I: clinical results. *Hum Reprod.* 2011;26(11): 3173–3180.
14. Magli MC, Montag M, Köster M, et al. Polar body array CGH for prediction of the status of the corresponding oocyte. Part II: technical aspects. *Hum Reprod.* 2011;26(11):3181–3185.
15. Coates A, Kung A, Mounts E, et al. Optimal euploid embryo transfer strategy, fresh versus frozen, after preimplantation genetic screening with next generation sequencing: a randomized controlled trial. *Fertil Steril.* 2017;107(3):723–730. e3.
16. Scott RT, Jr, Upham KM, Forman EJ, et al. Cleavage-stage biopsy significantly impairs human embryonic implantation potential while blastocyst biopsy does not: a randomized and paired clinical trial. *Fertili Steril.* 2013;100(3):624–630.
17. Baart EB, Martini E, van den Berg I, et al. Preimplantation genetic screening reveals a high incidence of aneuploidy and mosaicism in embryos from young women undergoing IVF. *Hum Reprod.* 2006;21(1):223–233.
18. Goossens V, De Rycke M, De Vos A, et al. Diagnostic efficiency, embryonic development and clinical outcome after the biopsy of one or two blastomeres for preimplantation genetic diagnosis. *Hum Reprod.* 2008;23(3):481–492.
19. Zakharova EE, Zaletova VV, Krivokharchenko AS. Biopsy of human morula-stage embryos: outcome of 215 IVF/ICSI cycles with PGS. *PLoS One.* 2014;9(9):e106433.
20. Orvieto R, Feldman B, Wiesel M, et al. Is day-4 morula biopsy a feasible alternative for preimplantation genetic testing? *PLoS One.* 2020;15(9):e0238599.
21. Dokras A, Sargent I, Ross C, et al. Trophectoderm biopsy in human blastocysts. *Hum Reprod.* 1990;5(7):821–825.
22. De Boer K, McArthur S, Murray C, et al. O-54. First live birth following blastocyst biopsy and PGD analysis. *Reprod Biomed Online.* 2002(4):35.
23. Van Montfoort A, Carvalho F, Coonen E, et al. ESHRE PGT consortium data collection XIX-XX: PGT analyses from 2016 to 2017. *Hum Reprod.* 2021;3.
24. Forman EJ, Hong KH, Treff NR, et al. Comprehensive chromosome screening and embryo selection: moving toward single euploid blastocyst transfer. *Semin Reprod Med.* 2012;30(3):236–242.
25. Mamas T, Gordon A, Brown A, et al. Detection of aneuploidy by array comparative genomic hybridization using cell lines to mimic a mosaic trophectoderm biopsy. *Fertil Steril.* 2012;97(4):943–947.
26. Cram D, Leigh D, Handyside A, et al. PGDIS position statement on the transfer of mosaic embryos. *Reprod Biomed Online.* 2019;39:e1–e4.
27. Greco E, Minasi MG, Fiorentino F. Healthy babies after intrauterine transfer of mosaic aneuploid blastocysts. *N Engl J Med.* 2015;373(21):2089–2090.
28. Munné S, Grifo J, Wells D. Mosaicism: "survival of the fittest" versus "no embryo left behind". *Fertil Steril.* 2016;105(5):1146–1149.
29. Leigh D, Cram DS, Rechitsky S, et al. PGDIS position statement on the transfer of mosaic embryos. *Reprod BioMed Online.* 2022;45(1):19–25.
30. Lacey L, Hassan S, Franik S, et al. Assisted hatching on assisted conception (in vitro fertilisation (IVF) and intracytoplasmic sperm injection (ICSI)). *Cochrane Database Syst Rev.* 2021;3(3):CD001894.
31. McArthur SJ, Leigh D, Marshall JT, et al. Pregnancies and live births after trophectoderm biopsy and preimplantation genetic testing of human blastocysts. *Fertil Steril.* 2005;84(6):1628–1636.
32. Capalbo A, Romanelli V, Cimadomo D, et al. Implementing PGD/PGD-A in IVF clinics: considerations for the best laboratory approach and management. *J Assist Reprod Genet.* 2016;33(10):1279–1286.
33. Kanyó K, Konc J, Solti L, et al. Assisted reproductive research: laser assisted hatching and spindle detection (spindle view technique). *Acta Vet Hung.* 2004;52(1):113–123.
34. Taylor TH, Gilchrist JW, Hallowell SV, et al. The effects of different laser pulse lengths on the embryo biopsy procedure and embryo development to the blastocyst stage. *J Assist Reprod Genet.* 2010;27(11):663–667.
35. Capalbo A, Rienzi L, Cimadomo D, et al. Correlation between standard blastocyst morphology, euploidy and implantation: an observational study in two centers involving 956 screened blastocysts. *Hum Reprod.* 2014;29(6):1173–1181.
36. Whitney JB, Anderson RE, Garner F, et al. Aneuploidy rates are associated with the blasotcyst biopsy technique. *Reprod Biomed Online.* 2018;36:e12–e13.
37. Mizobe Y, Kuwatsuru Y, Kuroki Y, et al. The effects of differences in trophectoderm biopsy techniques and the number of cells collected for biopsy on next-generation sequencing results. *Reprod Med Biol.* 2022;21(1):e12463.
38. Kelk D, Sawarkar S, Liu Y, et al. Does laser assisted biopsy introduce mosaic or chaotic changes to biopsied cells? *Fertil Steril.* 2017;108(3):e88.
39. Aoyama N, Kato K. Trophectoderm biopsy for preimplantation genetic test and technical tips: a review. *Reprod Med Biol.* 2020;19(3):222–231.
40. Benavent M, Escriba M, Miret C, et al. Evaluation of the impact of the pulling and flicking trophectoderm biopsy procedures on the integrity of the biopsied cells and their correlation to PGT-A results. *Fertil Steril.* 2019;112(3):e242.
41. Armstrong E, Campbell A, Castro I, et al. Should we be more lenient when selecting blastocysts for PGT-A? *Reprod Biomed Online.* 2022;45:e40–e41.
42. Honnma H, Baba T, Sasaki M, et al. Trophectoderm morphology significantly affects the rates of ongoing pregnancy and miscarriage in frozen-thawed single-blastocyst transfer cycle in vitro fertilization. *Fertil Steril.* 2012;98(2):361–367.
43. Ahlström A, Westin C, Reismer E, et al. Trophectoderm morphology: an important parameter for predicting live birth after single blastocyst transfer. *Hum Reprod.* 2011;26(12):3289–3296.
44. El-Toukhy T, Khalaf Y, Al-Darazi K, et al. Effect of blastomere loss on the outcome of frozen embryo replacement cycles. *Fertil Steril.* 2003;79(5):1106–1111.
45. De Vos A, Staessen C, De Rycke M, et al. Impact of cleavage-stage embryo biopsy in view of PGD on human blastocyst implantation: a prospective cohort of single embryo transfers. *Hum Reprod.* 2009;24(12):2988–2996.
46. Neal SA, Franasiak JM, Forman EJ, et al. High relative deoxyribonucleic acid content of trophectoderm biopsy adversely affects pregnancy outcomes. *Fertil Steril.* 2017;107(3):731–736.e1.
47. Guzman L, Nuñez D, López R, et al. The number of biopsied trophectoderm cells may affect pregnancy outcomes. *J Assist Reprod Genet.* 2019;36(1):145–151.

48. Cimadomo D, Rienzi L, Romanelli V, et al. Inconclusive chromosomal assessment after blastocyst biopsy: prevalence, causative factors and outcomes after re-biopsy and re-vitrification. A multicenter experience. *Hum Reprod.* 2018;33(10):1839–1846.
49. Zhang S, Luo K, Cheng D, et al. Number of biopsied trophectoderm cells is likely to affect the implantation potential of blastocysts with poor trophectoderm quality. *Fertil Steril.* 2016;105(5):1222–1227.e4.
50. Cimadomo D, Soscia D, Vaiarelli A, et al. Looking past the appearance: a comprehensive description of the clinical contribution of poor-quality blastocysts to increase live birth rates during cycles with aneuploidy testing. *Hum Reprod.* 2019;34(7):1206–1214.
51. Tiegs A, Sun L, Patounakis G, et al. Worth the wait? Day 7 blastocysts have lower euploidy rates but similar sustained implantation rates as day 5 and day 6 blastocysts. *Hum Reprod.* 2019;34(9):1632–1639.
52. Hernandez-Nieto C, Lee JA, Slifkin R, et al. What is the reproductive potential of day 7 euploid embryos? *Hum Reprod.* 2019;34(9):1697–1706.
53. Zhang S, Tan K, Gong F, et al. Blastocysts can be rebiopsied for preimplantation genetic diagnosis and screening. *Fertil Steril.* 2014;102(6):1641–1645.
54. Neal SA, Morin SJ, Tiegs AW, et al. Repeat biopsy for preimplantation genetic screening (PGS) reanalysis does not adversely impact obstetrical outcomes. *Fertil Steril.* 2018;109(3):e41.
55. Neal SA, Sun L, Jalas C, et al. When next-generation sequencing-based preimplantation genetic testing for aneuploidy (PGT-A) yields an inconclusive report: diagnostic results and clinical outcomes after re biopsy. *J Assist Reprod Genet.* 2019;36(10):2103–2109.
56. Zheng Y-M, Wang N, Li L, et al. Whole genome amplification in preimplantation genetic diagnosis. *J Zhejiang Univ Sci B.* 2011;12(1):1–11.
57. De Rycke M, Belva F, Goossens V, et al. ESHRE PGD Consortium data collection XIII: cycles from January to December 2010 with pregnancy follow-up to October 2011. *Hum Reprod.* 2015;30(8):1763–1789.
58. Moutou C, Goossens V, Coonen E, et al. ESHRE PGD consortium data collection XII: cycles from January to December 2009 with pregnancy follow-up to October 2010. *Hum Reprod.* 2014;29(5):880–903.
59. Wilton L, Thornhill A, Traeger-Synodinos J, et al. The causes of misdiagnosis and adverse outcomes in PGD. *Hum Reprod.* 2009;24(5):1221–1228.

35

Computer Assisted Sperm Analysis (CASA)

Walid E. Maalouf and Mathew Tomlinson

35.1 Introduction

Infertility is a disease of the reproductive system, and it is defined by the failure to achieve a successful pregnancy after 12 months of regular sexual intercourse (**1**). It is one of the major health issues affecting up to 12% of couples of reproductive age globally (**2**), with the male factor accounting for about 50% of the cases (**3**), and an increasing trend of male factor worldwide due to a mixture of biological, behavioral, environmental and sociological factors (**4, 5**). Male factors must therefore be excluded so a s semen analysis is part of the essential workup in the evaluation of the subfertile couple? In fact, the American Urological Association (AUA) strongly recommends an initial evaluation of male fertility should include a reproductive history, also include one or more semen analyses (**6**).

However, semen analysis is labor intensive, subjective, and often poorly reproducible, and reference values used by the World Health Organisation are at best only weakly predictive of fertility. Subjectivity associated especially with motility and morphology can often lead to clinical confusion, misdiagnosis and inappropriate or delayed infertility treatment. This has led to the development of a battery of advanced sperm function tests looking at live-dead sperm (**7**), and sperm chromatin, oxidative stress and DNA damage (**8–11**), and computer assisted sperm analysis (CASA) systems that can automate, or at least, semi-automate semen analysis (**12, 13**) and remove a degree of subjectivity and uncertainty from the diagnosis. Conventional CASA systems include three main components, an upright microscope, a camera and a computer and monitor powered by an appropriate software to capture a series of images of the sperm that can be tracked within the field of view of the attached camera. Sperm detection and tracking still depends largely on image quality provided by phase contrast microscopy but providing the system is properly calibrated and non-sperm cells are excluded from the analysis, sperm concentration and motility can be provided with a high degree of accuracy and precision. Moreover, motility is provided with a degree of objectivity with measurements based on individual sperm swimming speed and units of microns per second. This is in contrast to the totally subjective nature of manual motility estimates which cannot be labelled as a 'measure' and cannot be validated. In addition the benefit of automation offers other significant advantages over manual assessment as more sperm can be analyzed and then tracked in a relatively shorter time and if required an increased number of cells can be counted and provide overall improved accuracy and reliability in reporting. Increasing the number of sperm cells evaluated manually is difficult to justify in terms of the impact on staffing and cost of providing a diagnosis. (**12**). Although CASA has a clear role to play in diagnostic semen analysis, other potentially equally important applications are in the provision of quantitative motility and reliable sperm concentration assessments for therapeutic andrology, including: sperm preparation for ART, fertility preservation and in the processing (pre and post thaw) of donor sperm for treatments such as IUI or IVF.

35.2 Principles of CASA Operation

Conventional CASA systems should be programmed to operate using the definitions and reference values of the WHO laboratory manual for the examination and processing of human semen (**14**). That said, in the past 10–12 years, the WHO has recently changed its guidance on motility grading, moving from 4 to 3 grades in 2010 but then completely reversing this decision 10 years later. Although most CASA systems retained the 4-grade system knowing that grade 1 and 2 (rapid and slow progression) could simply be added together, it is important that any system can take account of updated guidance. More importantly, CASA is able to assess sperm swimming speed in microns per second which enables classification of motility in a quantitative approach. The pre-examination procedures up to sample liquefaction are identical. In manual sperm assessment, 2 separate slide preparations are required, one wet preparation slide for assessing sperm motility, then another sperm sample is diluted with a fixative to assess sperm concentration in an improved Neubauer ruling or alternative haemocytometer chamber (**15**). The haemocytometer has a grid with known dimensions including depth, which allows the calculation of the volume and ultimately the concentration of the sample being analyzed. The CASA operates on a similar basis, in that providing the area under the microscope is known and the slide is of a fixed-depth (often 20 micron), then providing the system is able to correctly identify the object (sperm) in a given volume of fluid, then a simple calculation will provide an output in millions per ml (Figure 35.1).

However, the main difference is that only one slide is prepared for both sperm concentration and motility, and the outputs are provided simultaneously, and often in less than 1 minute. Typically used slides have a depth of either 10 or 20 microns, but choice is often a compromise, since the aim is to create only a monolayer of sperm but at the same time permit full sperm tail rotation. This is why the WHO recommend a 10 microlitre drop of sample under a square 22mm coverslip.

DOI: 10.1201/9781003269502-35

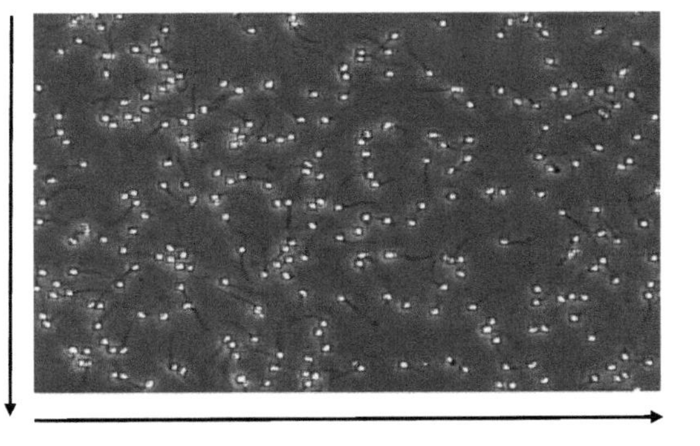

FIGURE 35.1 Typical CASA screenshots showing sperm identification in a pre-defined area/volume.

35.2.1 Count and Concentration

One of the main sources of errors in CASA systems is in their performance to distinguish between immotile spermatozoa, from debris or other cells (**16**). This could be due to the differences in the type of microscopic imaging used such as bright-field or darkfield, the resulting resolution of the objective and camera image, and the algorithm built into the software to define a sperm. The algorithm can use a multitude of physical and biological features to filter out non-sperm objects such as dimension measurements, elongated shape, light refraction, presence of tail. This was a major problem for earlier systems with over-estimated concentration and of course an inflated percentage of 'static' objects a significant issue and for a while led to CASA having a damaged reputation. However, some easy fixes have since become standard features of more modern CASA systems, including: image optimisation, re-setting object size thresholds (gaiting) and more recently field editing which enables the removal of incorrectly identified objects or the re-instatement of missed sperm. Such features have led to improved sperm concentration measurements in terms of parity with the WHO Gold standard haemocytometer and as a result, improved motility.

Error or moreover 'measurement uncertainty' can arise from a number of other sources (**17**), not least those associated with semen as a biological test fluid. All methods of sperm assessment are totally dependent on the assumption of 100% heterogeneity (equal sperm dispersion) throughout the sample. However, we know that hyper viscosity is common and affects mixing/heterogeneity for both manual and CASA analysis alike. Moreover, sperm agglutination and aggregation will always affect accuracy more difficult cases, a representative semen analysis result is almost impossible. In these cases (whether manual or automated), analysis can only be improved by increasing not only the number of sperm evaluated but also the aliquots removed for analysis as well as repeated full testing. The other source of error is the operator due to either methodology of preparing the same sample and filling the chambers, or lack of appropriate validation of their methods on the instrument, which can all compound on performance and reporting.

35.2.2 Motility

The second part of semen analysis is the classification of spermatozoa by their motility into rapid progressive, slow progressive, non-progressive and immotile. A standard glass slide, a 10 microlitre drop of semen and a coverslip are prepared to count the motile spermatozoa. In some laboratories, an eyepiece reticle is used to aid manual assessment of sperm count and motility as it provides a reference of distance travelled by sperm under the field of view. Importantly, yet often overlooked is the need for some form of temperature control when analyzing motility, without which leads to huge inconsistency and variation in results. Motility and velocity are both of course temperature sensitive and sperm behave very differently at relative cool ambient temperature 20–22°C when compared to body temperature. The WHO states that as a minimum temperature should be measured at a consistent temperature. The majority of laboratories rightly address this at a more physiological temperature of 36–37°C achieved using a warm microscope stage. The CASA system will be capturing a series of frames, track the movement of the sperm head to calculate motion kinematic measurements (Figure 35.2, Table 35.1), and use that information to estimate motility accordingly (**18**).

Sperm kinematic parameters (described in Table 35.2) have been used as an adjunct to traditional % motility or motility grades in an attempt to better provide quantitative measures

TABLE 35.1
Short Description and Function of Different Variables (Compiled from [**19**])

CASA Variables	Description and Function
ALH	Amplitude of Lateral Head displacement is calculated as the maximum value of the lateral oscillation of the sperm head from average path line.
MAD	Mean Angular Displacement is calculated as the average time of angle rotation of the sperm head on the curvilinear path.
VAP	Average Path Velocity is average path line of the sperm head from all the frame positions, divided by the elapsed time.
VCL	Curvi-Linear Velocity measured by adding the straight lines distance between the sperm head positions of each frame, then dividing by the elapsed time.
VSL	Straight-Line Velocity measured as the distance travelled between first position and last position of sperm head, divided by the elapsed time.

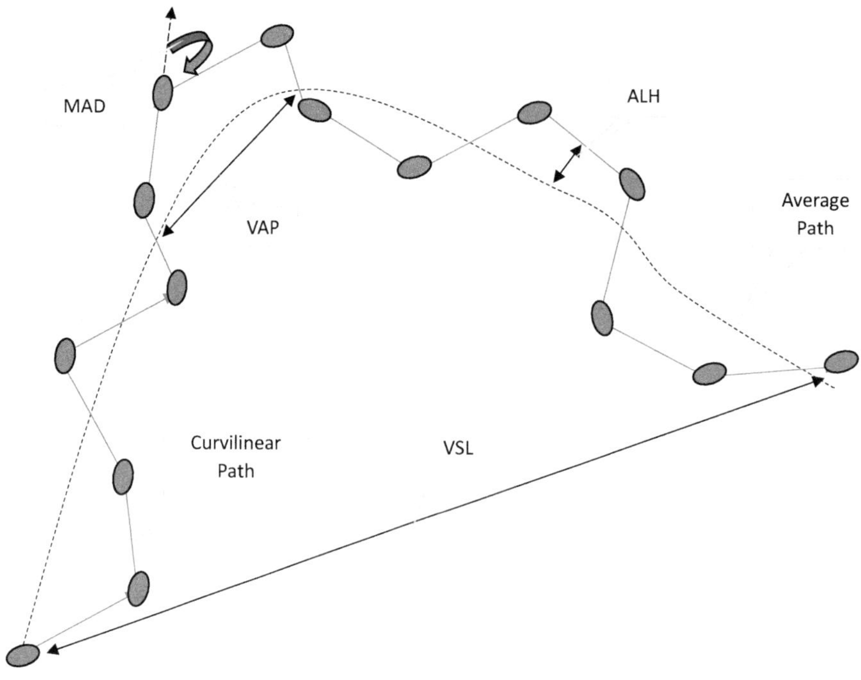

FIGURE 35.2 Different variables measured by CASA systems (with permission from [**19**]).

TABLE 35.2

Summary of Sperm Kinetic Parameters Attempting to Provide an Adjunct to Traditional Motility Percent (from [**20**] with Permission)

Publication	Setting (natural or assisted conception	CASA system track length, frame rate, temperature	No significance	Significant predictors
Barratt et al. (1993) (**21**)	Natural	HTM 0.8, 25, 37	VSL, LIN, STR, BCF	VAP, VCL
Sukcharoen et al. (1996) (**22**)	IVF	HTM 0.8, 25, 37	VSL, LIN, STR, BCF, VAP, VCL	None
Larsen et al. (2000) (**23**)	Natural	CRISMAS 2.6, 25	ALH, WOB, LIN	VCL, VAP, BCF
Hirano et al. (2001) (**24**)	IVF	HTM, no other detail	ALH, BCF, STR NS	VCL, VAP (swim-up)
Garrett et al. (2003) (**25**)	Natural	HTM, 0.5, 60, 37	VCL, VAP, LIN, STR, ALH, BCF	VSL, % progression
Shibhara et al. (2004) (**26**)	IUI		ALH, LIN, BCF	VSL, VAP, VCL
DeGeyter et al. (1998) (**27**)	IVF	HTM 0.8, 25, 37	LIN, BCF	VCL, VAP, VSL, ALH
Jedrzejczak et al. (2005) (**28**)	IVF	no detail	BCF,	VSL, ALH, VCL
Andersen et al. (2002) (**29**)	Natural TTP	HTM 0.8, 25, 37		None
Freour et al. (2009) (**30**)	DIUI	unknown	VAP, VL, VSL, LIN, ALH, STR	% motile, motile concentration
Tan et al. (2014) (**31**)	IUI	HTM no other details	VAP, VL, VSL, LIN, ALH, STR	Total motile sperm concentration

as opposed to the more subjective estimates provided by manual analysis. Although they have been useful in determining behavioral characteristics in a particular environment, for example in describing and defining sperm hyperactivation, there is no consensus on their influence on male fertility. From many studies over the past 30 years, it is very clear that some form of velocity measurement (whether VSL, VCL or VAP) adds to the clinical value of the motility assessment (**20**).

If the sperm heads are all counted and tracked correctly between frames, then an algorithm can be optimized and used to apply the WHO definitions of motility grading (**15**):

A. Rapidly progressive sperm are those moving ≥ 25µm/s (or half the tail length).
B. Slow progressive sperm are those moving between 5 and 25µm/s.

C. Non-Progressive motile sperm are those sperm with active sperm movement (eg twitching), or moving at a speed under 5µm/s.
D. Immotile sperm are those with no recorded activity movements in the tail.

This is an exercise that is almost impossible to perform manually, a fact borne out by EQA (external quality assessment) reports over the past 25 years. CASA offers the ability to grade sperm for speed based on the specified definition for A, whereas manual analysis (which can take several minutes) almost always leads to over-estimation of the motile fraction. CASA algorithms suffer similar source of errors to manual analysis depending on the concentration of sample. Depending on the system, deviations at high concentrations have been reported in a number of CASA validation studies (**12, 32, 33**), and a dilution of samples to lower the concentration below this threshold is recommended to obtain accurate and reproducible results (**14**).

Of course, any inaccuracies associated with sperm concentration will have consequences for subsequent sperm tracking and motility analysis. On the opposite end, for oligozoospermic and azoospermic samples, the counting chamber and the number of fields required to work out an accurate reporting become practically difficult and statistically low accuracy to report a reliable concentration based on low number of spermatozoa included in the count, similarly to the level of error reported in the manual assessment (**34**). Again, a number of validation reports have been published on low accuracy of CASA results at low concentration (**34–36**). However, it should be noted that at very low sperm concentration, all methods lose accuracy and precision, since errors associated with sampling and homogeneity are simply exacerbated. A manual assessment method will offer better speed, accuracy and precision when reporting low sperm concentration samples of under 2 M/ml over current CASA systems (**15, 19**). Overall, the haemocytometer requires around 10 minutes to prepare and for sperm to settle before counting manually 200 sperm on each side of the chamber. In the meantime, two wet preparations of semen sample under a coverslip are prepared for a repeated motility assessment of another 200 spermatozoa. A total of 15–20 minutes is estimated to complete both concentration and motility, which is a time that is significantly reduced using a CASA instrument down to 1–3 minutes depending on the type of instrument, concentration range, and number of repeats required to report.

35.2.3 Quality Control

Quality control can be conducted in a similar manner to manual assessment on a number of commercial CASA systems. Internally, a number quality control samples with known target mean and range can be purchased to check if the instrument is calculating accurately the number of cells in the sample (**37**). Similarly, pre-recorded videos of known motility samples can be used to check the CASA's performance in classifying motility. If manual methods are validated through external quality assurance programmes in a laboratory, then the CASA can be always checked against manual methods using patient samples and using QA sample materials (**38**). One caveat to this and

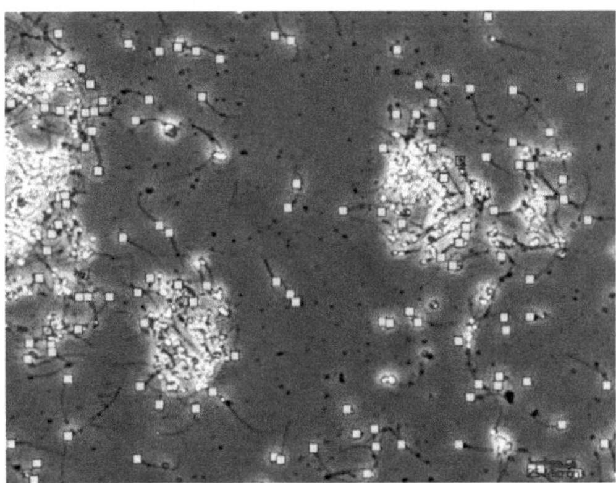

FIGURE 35.3 Agglutination/aggregation renders homogenisation of the sperm suspension and hence accurate assessment of sperm number almost impossible. Depending on the CASA model, the algorithm (identifying head centre or head area) will find sperm detection very difficult.

word of warning is in the use of formalin fixed-pooled semen samples as QC material. As years of EQA results have shown, such samples are prone to significant aggregation, which significantly hampers 'homogenisation' and makes reliable/reproducible analysis almost impossible (**17**). Laboratories considering providing their own Stock QC material should therefore consider using cryopreserved material as a superior alternative (see Figure 35.3).

A Shrewhart type of plot to monitor the mean values of repeated analyses of internal QC result measurements and the standard deviations (**38**), and Westgard QC rules can be applied to warn operators when QC fails and a rectifying action is needed (**37**). Assessing reproducibility of CASA measures are at distinct advantage over manual methods since automation removes any operator bias that is inherent to manual counts and motility. Prior knowledge of the previous answer will always influence the operator, especially with regard to motility which is clearly more subjective.

Similar methods can be used to check inter- and intra- operator variabilities in sample preparation and analysis methods. Additionally, a Bland-Altman and scatter plot graphs were used to plot the difference between CASA and manual measurements and calculate the limits of agreement between the two counts (**12, 38**). These are ideal approaches for demonstrating the 'interchangeability' of methods.

35.2.4 Morphology

A number of commercial CASA systems have the ability to analyse sperm morphology including sperm head, midpiece and most of the tail defects (**39**). Additional sources of error can compromise the automated morphology assessment including level of illumination, focus on sample using 100x oil immersion, and the quality of smear and stain used (**40, 41**). In terms of the pre-defined criteria for describing the 'normal' sperm, the accuracy and precision of the method can be over 90% if proper control measures are in place (**39, 42, 43**), which can make such computerised systems acceptable, or even superior, than experienced operators for routine diagnostic applications. The one major weakness with CASA morphology which it has in common with manual methods is in the uncertainty surrounding current definitions of 'normal'. Similarly to QC for concentration and motility, fixed morphology slides can be purchased and analysed to verify correct operations of the instrument (**14, 38, 39**).

35.2.5 CASA in IVF

In addition to semen analysis for diagnostic purposes, CASA has the potential to improve workflow in the IVF laboratory (**44**). Patients typically repeat semen analysis during consultation at the IVF clinic after referral by the general practitioner, then have another two semen analyses at day of OPU, one before and one after oocyte pick-up. In addition, semen analyses are carried before and after sperm freezing and storage for fertility preservation. CASA can be useful in providing trained staff with a high-number sperm motility categorization quickly and with less analytical variance than manual assessment (**45**), and increase objectivity in predicting IVF fertilization rates (**24, 45**). In addition, if the kinetic movements of the sperm are measured correctly, the proportion of hyperactivated sperm sub-population in the analysed sample can be calculated in washed or prepared sample for IVF (**46**). This can be done by applying an algorithm that defines the typical sperm hyperactive sperm movement, and a threshold to work out the proportion of hyperactive spermatozoa (**47, 48**).

35.3 Conclusion

CASA remains a promising tool, particularly with improved quality of imaging and AI applications. Training operators remain the main barrier for wider implementation due to higher complexity of a number of systems in operation or validation. Better efficiency, accuracy, specificity and sensitivity are achievable if the CASA system is set-up correctly and validated regularly.

REFERENCES

1. WHO. *ICD-11 for Mortality and Morbidity Statistics*. 11th Edition. Geneva: WHO; 2022.
2. Vander Borght M, Wyns C. Fertility and infertility: definition and epidemiology. *Clin Biochem*. 2018;62:2–10.
3. Mascarenhas MN, Flaxman SR, Boerma T, et al. National, regional, and global trends in infertility prevalence since 1990: a systematic analysis of 277 health surveys. *PLoS Med*. 2012;9(12):e1001356.
4. Kumar N, Singh AK. Trends of male factor infertility, an important cause of infertility: a review of literature. *J Hum Reprod Sci*. 2015;8(4):191.
5. Okonofua FE, Ntoimo LFC, Omonkhua A, et al. Causes and risk factors for male infertility: a scoping review of published studies. *Int J Gen Med*. 2022;5985–5997.
6. Schlegel PN, Sigman M, Collura B, et al. Diagnosis and treatment of infertility in men: AUA/ASRM guideline part I. *J Urol*. 2021;205(1):36–43.
7. Blom E. A one-minute live-dead sperm stain by means of eosin-nigrosin. *Fertil Steril*. 1950;1:176–177.
8. Check J, Graziano V, Cohen R, et al. Effect of an abnormal sperm chromatin structural assay (SCSA) on pregnancy outcome following (IVF) with ICSI in previous IVF failures. *Arch Androl*. 2005;51(2):121–124.
9. Spanò M, Bonde JP, Hjøllund HI, et al. Sperm chromatin damage impairs human fertility. *Fertil Steril*. 2000;73(1):43–50.
10. Larson-Cook KL, Brannian JD, Hansen KA, et al. Relationship between the outcomes of assisted reproductive techniques and sperm DNA fragmentation as measured by the sperm chromatin structure assay. *Fertil Steril*. 2003;80(4):895–902.
11. Saleh RA, Agarwal A, Nada EA, et al. Negative effects of increased sperm DNA damage in relation to seminal oxidative stress in men with idiopathic and male factor infertility. *Fertil Steril*. 2003;79:1597–1605.
12. Tomlinson MJ, Pooley K, Simpson T, et al. Validation of a novel computer-assisted sperm analysis (CASA) system using multitarget-tracking algorithms. *Fertil Steril*. 2010;93(6):1911–1920.
13. Mortimer D, Aitken R, Mortimer S, et al. Workshop report: clinical CASA – the quest for consensus. *Reprod Fertil Dev*. 1995;7(4):951–959.
14. WHO. Advanced examinations. In: WHO, editor. *WHO Laboratory Manual for the Examination and Processing of Human Semen*. 6th Edition. Geneva: WHO; 2021. pp. 139–160.
15. WHO. Basic examination. In: WHO, editor. *WHO Laboratory Manual for the Examination and Processing of Human Semen*. 6th Edition. Geneva: WHO; 2021. pp. 9–82.
16. Finelli R, Leisegang K, Tumallapalli S, et al. The validity and reliability of computer-aided semen analyzers in performing semen analysis: a systematic review. *Transl Androl Urol*. 2021;10(7):3069.
17. Tomlinson M. Uncertainty of measurement and clinical value of semen analysis: has standardisation through professional guidelines helped or hindered progress? *Andrology*. 2016;4(5):763–770.
18. Serres C, Feneux D, Jouannet P, et al. Influence of the flagellar wave development and propagation on the human sperm movement in seminal plasma. *Gamete Res*. 1984;9(2):183–195.
19. WHO. Optional procedures. In: WHO, editor. *WHO Laboratory Manual for the Examination and Processing of Human Semen*. 5th Edition. Geneva: WHO; 2010. pp. 115–141.
20. Tomlinson MJ, Naeem A. CASA in the medical laboratory: CASA in diagnostic andrology and assisted conception. *Reprod Fertil Dev*. 2018;30(6):850–859.
21. Barratt CLR, Tomlinson MJ, Cooke ID. Prognostic significance of computerized motility analysis for in vivo fertility. *Fertil Steril*. 1993;60(3):520–525.
22. Sukcharoen N, Keith J, Irvine DS, et al. Prediction of the in-vitro fertilization (IVF) potential of human spermatozoa using sperm function tests: the effect of the delay between testing and IVF. *Hum Reprod*. 1996;11(5):1030–1034.
23. Larsen L, Scheike T, Jensen TK, et al. Computer-assisted semen analysis parameters as predictors for fertility of men from the general population. *Hum Reprod*. 2000;15(7):1562–1567.

24. Hirano Y, Shibahara H, Obara H, et al. Andrology: relationships between sperm motility characteristics assessed by the computer-aided sperm analysis (CASA) and fertilization rates in vitro. *J Assist Reprod Genet.* 2001;18:215–220.
25. Garrett C, Liu D, Clarke G, et al. Automated semen analysis: 'zona pellucida preferred' sperm morphometry and straight-line velocity are related to pregnancy rate in subfertile couples. *Hum Reprod.* 2003;18(8):1643–1649.
26. Shibahara H, Obara H, Ayustawati, et al. Prediction of pregnancy by intrauterine insemination using CASA estimates and strict criteria in patients with male factor infertility. *Int J Androl.* 2004;27(2):63–68.
27. De Geyter C, De Geyter M, Koppers B, et al. Diagnostic accuracy of computer-assisted sperm motion analysis. *Hum Reprod.* 1998;13(9):2512–2520.
28. Jędrzejczak P, Rzepczyńska I, Taszarek-Hauke G, et al. Effect of sperm subpopulation's kinetics on human fertilization in vitro. *Arch Androl.* 2005;51(3):185–193.
29. Andersen A, Ziebe S, Jørgensen N, et al. Time to pregnancy in relation to semen quality assessed by CASA before and after sperm separation. *Hum Reprod.* 2002;17(1):173–177.
30. Freour T, Jean M, Mirallie S, et al. Predictive value of CASA parameters in IUI with frozen donor sperm. *Int J Androl.* 2009;32(5):498–504.
31. Tan O, Ha T, Carr BR, et al. Predictive value of postwashed total progressively motile sperm count using CASA estimates in 6871 non-donor intrauterine insemination cycles. *J Assist Reprod Genet.* 2014;31:1147–1153.
32. Agarwal A, Selvam MKP, Ambar RF. Validation of LensHooke® X1 PRO and computer-assisted semen analyzer compared with laboratory-based manual semen analysis. *World J Mens Health.* 2021;39(3):496.
33. Schubert B, Badiou M, Force A. Computer-aided sperm analysis, the new key player in routine sperm assessment. *Andrologia.* 2019;51(10):e13417.
34. Davis R, Katz D. Operational standards for CASA instruments. *J Androl.* 1993;14(5):385–394.
35. Vantman D, Koukoulis G, Dennison L, et al. Computer-assisted semen analysis: evaluation of method and assessment of the influence of sperm concentration on linear velocity determination. *Fertil Steril.* 1988;49(3):510–515.
36. Togni G, Gallicciotti G, Coccia P, et al. Computer-aided semen analysis: sperm concentration assessment by the Strömberg-Mika system. *Andrologia.* 1995;27(1):55–65.
37. Vernon DD, Johnson JE, Houwing AM, et al. Accu-Beads as a quality control measure for manual and automated methods of measuring sperm concentration – an observational study. *J Assist Reprod Genet.* 2014;31:25–33.
38. WHO. Quality assurance and quality control. In: WHO, editor. *WHO Laboratory Manual for the Examination and Processing of Human Semen.* 6th Edition. Geneva: WHO; 2021. pp. 185–210.
39. Coetzee K, Kruger TF, Lombard CJ, et al. Assessment of interlaboratory and intralaboratory sperm morphology readings with the use of a Hamilton Thorne Research integrated visual optical system semen analyzer. *Fertil Steril.* 1999;71(1):80–84.
40. Lacquet F, Kruger T, Du Toit T, et al. Slide preparation and staining procedures for reliable results using computerized morphology. *Arch Androl.* 1996;36(2):133–138.
41. Menkveld R, Lacquet F, Kruger T, et al. Effects of different staining and washing procedures on the results of human sperm morphology evaluation by manual and computerised methods. *Andrologia.* 1997;29(1):1–7.
42. Garrett C, Baker HG. A new fully automated system for the morphometric analysis of human sperm heads. *Fertil Steril.* 1995;63(6):1306–1317.
43. Kruger TF, du Toit TC, Franken DR, et al. Sperm morphology: assessing the agreement between the manual method (strict criteria) and the sperm morphology analyzer IVOS. *Fertil Steril.* 1995;63(1):134–141.
44. Timvere T, Gregaoire R, editors. *Computer Aided Semen Analysis (CASA) in Therapeutic Semen Analysis Improves Embryologist Efficiency and Accuracy.* Poster/presentation at Fertility. Belfast, ARCS; 2023.
45. Dearing C, Jayasena C, Lindsay K. Can the sperm class analyser (SCA) CASA-Mot system for human sperm motility analysis reduce imprecision and operator subjectivity and improve semen analysis? *Human Fertil.* 2021;24(3):208–218.
46. Mortimer D, Mortimer ST. Computer-aided sperm analysis (CASA) of sperm motility and hyperactivation. *Spermatogenesis: Methods Protoc.* 2013:77–87.
47. Mortimer ST. Minimum sperm trajectory length for reliable determination of the fractal dimension. *Reprod Fertil Dev.* 1998;10(6):465–470.
48. Katz MJ, George EB. Fractals and the analysis of growth paths. *Bull Math Biol.* 1985;47(2):273–286.

36

Time-Lapse Embryo Culture Systems and Morphokinetics in Clinical Embryology: A Brief Overview on the Evolution of Embryo Scoring System

Rachel Smith and Walid E. Maalouf

Traditional microscopic examination of the developing embryos at specific intervals, typically the morning up to every day of pre-implantation embryo culture, allows the embryologists to carry out a basic embryo grading for the purpose of selection or de-selection of embryos. The correlation between the observed morphological parameters and developmental potential have been extensively reported in the literature. For embryos up to the cleavage stage, the number and evenness of blastomeres as well as level of fragmentation are most commonly used as markers of embryo viability. Whereas for the blastocyst stage embryos, the level of expansion, inner cell mass and trophectoderm quality are the superseding markers of quality. Additional markers that have been used include pronuclear morphology, polar body alignment and appearance, appearance of cytoplasm and zona pellucida, early cleavage, blastomere number and symmetry, multinucleation and degree of fragmentation (**1–5**).

A number of grading systems use an alphanumeric grading system based on morphological features at the time observed, with different grades reflecting the quality of the embryo and its predictive ability to result in a successful clinical outcome (**6–8**). Whilst those scoring systems are based on a single observation at day 3 or day 5 of embryo development in vitro, a cumulative embryo scoring system based on multiple observations of morphology at different stages of embryo development including the cumulus egg complex at the time of egg retrieval have also been described previously (**9**). Multiple observation points to score embryo development have been reported to provide a superior alternative to a single point assessment of development, but in order to reduce both the workload and stress to the embryos resulting from taking them out of the incubators frequently, the Alpha Scientists in Reproductive Medicine and ESHRE Special Interest Group of Embryology, in 2011, developed a set of consensus points to locate optimal stages for morphological assessment (**10**). However, each standard morphological assessment exposes the embryos to sub-optimal conditions as a result of the physical removal of embryos from the incubator system. This exposes the embryos to environmental fluctuations including fluctuations in temperature, gaseous environment, pH, VOCs and additional handling risk. In addition, basic embryo grading must rely on five to six observations that introduce the risk of assessment variability between embryologists (**11, 12**).

36.1 Description of a Time-Lapse System (TLS)

In a laboratory context, a time-lapse system (TLS) refers to several approaches for time-lapse imaging of a biological sample. A number of those approaches were developed in a research environment and include equipping a microscope with a chamber to hold the material and a camera for recording changes over time; those have been described in the literature (**13–15**). In a clinical IVF setting, two broad categories of TL systems have been introduced, one that you can place inside existing boxed incubators such as the Eeva™ (**16**) and the Primo Vision™ systems (**17**). The other category includes the fully integrated TL systems which feature the incubator, imaging camera and a computer interphase (**16**); those are becoming the gold standard in the IVF laboratory.

As the first type of TL systems does not offer a stable culture environment due to culture in a box incubator, which following door openings has a large change in environmental condition. This is particularly problematic when more than a single patient or imaging unit is used within the incubator (**17**). The rest of the description of TL systems will focus therefore on the integrated type of TLS. There are many commercially available TL systems, with various integrated technologies, leading to a variety of capabilities and capacity which may have practical considerations to the laboratory when deciding on a suitable system.

In no particular order, one of the main considerations is the size of the machine when placed on the laboratory bench. Integrated TL instruments vary from 53 cm to 96 cm in width. At the same time, the capacity of those systems in terms of the number of patient slides that can run per single instrument will vary from 6 to 15 patient slides, and based on the number of wells in the custom-made slides for TLS, the total number of embryos that can run in one instrument at full capacity can vary between 72 and 240 embryos (**18**). Some TL manufacturers allow multiple capacity instruments to run on the same platform which can be useful from an operational perspective

DOI: 10.1201/9781003269502-36

to add instruments with a capacity that will be proportional to the workload required.

The second consideration is the quality of the incubator, type of gas required, gas consumption, humidity option, recovery, and monitoring. TL incubators will either have their own gas mixer to allow changing the setpoints desired for CO2 and O2, or work using a premixed gas source only. Consumption can vary from 0.5 up to 10 Litres/hour, and this can depend on type of gas used and the rate the system recirculates the gas environment. In addition, the design will affect recovery which can vary between from under 3 minutes to under 15 minutes with a 30 seconds door opening (**18**). Internal air filtration and purification are also key factors with some TL incubators allowing UV purification from biological VOCs, and HEPA and carbon activated filtration. Most instruments allow the validation of the gas levels and temperature inside the incubation chamber, and most will allow the connection to an external monitoring system to alert for failure. Certain TL instruments allow the option to humidify the incubation environment, but other manufacturers have designed their TL embryo culture dishes with volumes of media and oil that allow minimal evaporation for the duration of in vitro embryo culture (**19**).

The image quality is another key consideration as this will be the image the embryologist or the software will analyse and save as part of the patient files. The specifications can vary from the type of illumination, but a short exposure time and short frequency with a red LED light is usually preferred (**20, 21**). The quality of the time-lapse sequence generated is dependent on the camera and objective lens used in the system, and the time between acquisitions which can vary from 5 to 15 minutes, and the number of focal planes used varies from 3 to 11 (**18**). Those time-lapse videos are the basis of morphokinetic analyses, algorithms of embryo (de-)selection and AI developments for automatic annotations or embryo grading (**22**).

The setup will require a separate computer and network terminal with appropriate software to monitor the embryos growing in a TLS in real time. The software should allow the review of the time-lapse videos, with the ability to annotate the developmental characteristics of the developing embryo, and then to apply algorithms for embryo ranking or selection (**22, 23**). Additionally, there are final considerations regarding the installation, training and support provided by the manufacturer that can facilitate the integration of the time-lapse into the standard operating procedure, and also the ability of the instruments to communicate with other 3rd party software such as electronic medical records (EMRs) (**18**).

We have examined the array of timelapse devices that can be introduced into the laboratory, in this section of the chapter we examine morphokinetics, the dynamic change of the embryo over time and the potential benefits of identifying these kinetic markers to aid selection of a single embryo with the 'best' implantation potential. Morphokinetics used in conjunction with time-lapse incubation (TLI) has the benefit of providing in depth information on the embryo, non-invasively, without disturbing the environmental conditions of culture. Standard incubation (SI), is still the more commonly used method of culture for gametes and embryos prior to a fate decision of either transfer, cryopreservation or discard.

Standard incubation is considered a lower cost option to TLI as the equipment necessary for continuous image capture of the developing embryo is considered expensive and is not an option for all laboratories. SI requires the embryo to be removed from the incubator at specific time points to assess the stage and quality of the embryo. These static observations involve handling the dishes outside of the incubator on a stereo microscope, the timing of the assessment is laboratory specific. Evidence on the value of information gathered from a sequence of static observations during embryo culture, weighted against the need to remove the embryo from the incubator, disturbing the environmental conditions, has been seen to offer little advantage, with many laboratories choosing to provide undisturbed culture in SI with the fate on the embryo being determined from one observation on the day of transfer (**24**). The assessment of embryo competence for implantation is largely performed using defined morphological grading systems, at the cleavage stage, this is determined by the number of cells, presence of fragmentation and uniformity of the cell size for blastocyst assessment the scoring system considers the inner cell mass (ICM) and trophectoderm (TE) quality along with the degree of expansion, with the most widely used grading system defined by Gardner and Schoolcraft (**25**). These morphological classifications are subject to operator subjectivity (**26, 27**), and only loosely correlate to embryo viability. Can time-lapse culture improve our understanding of embryo development and in turn improve the patient experience by identifying the embryo with the highest propensity for live birth outcome with greater certainty than existing methodologies?

Selecting the best embryo for transfer from a cohort of available embryos does not impact the cumulative pregnancy rate, but may help to reduce the time to live birth outcome. This in turn reduces the financial burden and emotional stress of repeated treatments by minimising the number of interventions needed. The identification of the 'single' best embryo also reduces the need to replace multiple embryos in one cycle with the elevated risk of multiple pregnancy and the risks associated with an increase in perinatal morbidity and mortality and increased maternal morbidity (**28**). Time-lapse imaging allows for the capture of images at regular intervals (5–15mins) providing over 5000 images in the course of embryo culture over 5 days in an undisturbed environment. To benefit embryo selection these images can be annotated for known morphokinetic parameters which have been identified to infer information on embryo competence (**10**).

Morphokinetics refers to the identification of dynamic changes in the developing embryo over time, these changes can be transient in nature so are therefore only observed in combination with time-lapse culture. These morphokinetic variables are defined by Ciray et al. 2014 (**29**), to ensure consistency of the nomenclature and implementation of agreed practices for identification of these key dynamic events within laboratories. The process of determining theses key events is performed by reviewing the timelapse images or video, manually or using the device software to document the key events from the oocyte through fertilisation to the developing embryo prior to a decision on the fate to transfer, cryopreserve or discard.

36.2 Oocyte Morphology

Although a systematic review highlighted that no morphological features were unanimously evaluated to have prognostic value for further developmental competence of oocytes (**30**), the lack of any dysmorphism is normally considered a prerequisite for a good quality oocyte. The main inclusions regularly annotated are the presence of smooth endoplasmic reticulum (SERc) or vacuoles within the cytoplasm. In early studies the presence of SERc in the oocyte had lower IVF success rates, as well as increased obstetrical complications and neonatal outcomes. More recent studies have questioned the degree of these reported negative outcomes from SER oocytes, if any at all. Currently many IVF labs either deselect SER oocytes to their last priority embryo (if it had led to a blastocyst) or ignore it as a prognostic variable.

36.3 Fertilisation Assessment

Following insemination, the earliest sign of potential fertilisation is the appearance of the second polar body (tPB2) in addition to the time of presentation a further annotation of the orientation of the second polar body in relation to the first polar body has been linked to implantation success (**31**). Appearance of the pronuclei is transient and the pronuclei number can occasionally change over time so time-lapse imagery can offer a reassurance for this critical assessment. For ICSI fertilisation the use of TLI over SI has been shown to potentially increase the number of available embryos, Barrie et al. (**32**) revealed 11% of normally fertilised oocytes (n3000) would have been assessed within the study cohort as unfertilised if cultured in standard incubation and assessed at the recommended time of 17+/- hours post insemination (hpi).

36.4 Early Embryo Development

From the identification of normal fertilisation numerous defined changes are expected to occur within the developing embryo, the pronuclei fade (tPNf) and the first cell division occurs and continues as the cells replicate and divide into 2 daughter cells (t2-t8). Each annotation is identified as the first image when the 2 cells become discrete entities. From these timed events cell cycles can be determined, the time taken to complete a cell cycle is related to embryo competence (**33**) for example CC3 the time for division from 3 cell to 5 cell is calculated as t5-t3 (see Figure 36.1 for examples). Synchronisation could be considered a simpler alternative to cell cycles as they account for the completion of a synchronised event, i.e. 2 cell to 4 cell and 4 cell to 8 cell. These are recorded as S2 and S3, where S2 is the time from 3cell to 4cell and S3 is the time from 5 cell to 8 cell. Syngamy or pronuclei fading (tPNf) is often used instead of time of insemination to allow the comparison of IVF and ICSI by removing the time taken for the sperm to enter the egg in IVF but this will also act to eliminate any prognostic information in delays from t0 to completing the first cell cleavage.

These early cleavage morphokinetic variables can provide valuable information on the embryo's potential to become a blastocyst, historically early cleavage at 22–24hpi was considered a prognosticator for implantation potential when a cleavage transfer was the only option available. Recently Campbell et al. 2022 (**34**) determined the value of single morphokinetic variables and their ability to predict blastulation, embryo utilisation and live birth outcome, in a large study of over 31,000 embryos, tPNf and t2 were reliable markers of prediction for achieving full blastocyst with an AUC of 0.63 and 0.65 respectively.

Anomalies within the early stages of division are well documented and are discussed in more detail in chapter 40, these

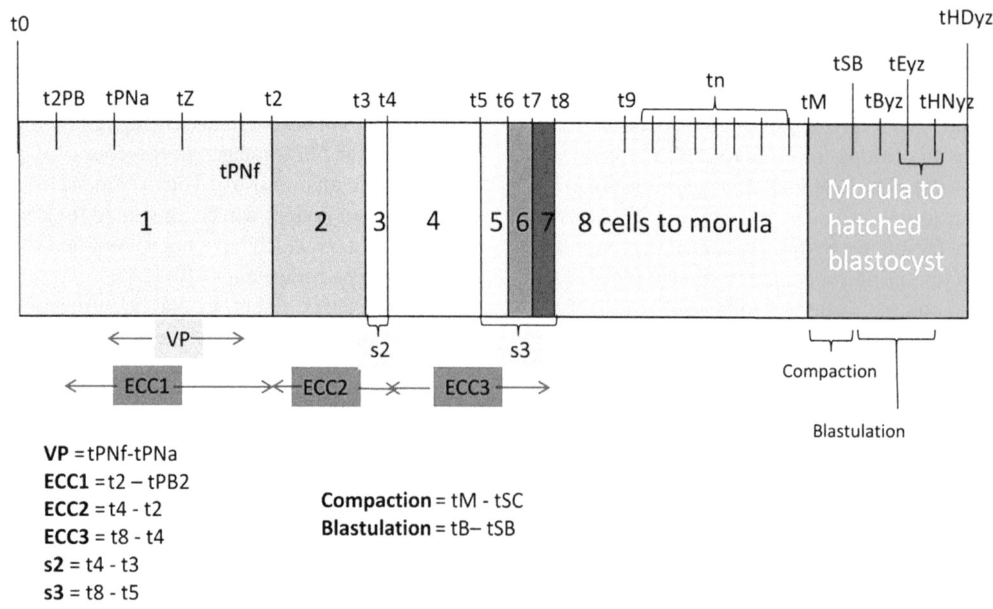

FIGURE 36.1 Definitions for the morphokinetic variables that are monitored during preimplantation embryo development (from [**29**] with permission).

include multi nucleation, multichotomous division, 4 cell planar and merged cells or reverse cleavage. These irregular cell divisions are often linked to poor embryo development and often result in failure of the embryo to become a blastocyst. Observance of these irregularities highlight to the operator the potential for lower implantation potential if no other blastulating embryo is available for replacement. Outcomes have been achieved from replacement of these embryos once they achieve appropriate development after 5 days of culture (**35, 36**), therefore, it is considered acceptable to replace or cryopreserve any embryos that result in a blastocyst following one of these irregular events in their early development. In most cases these embryos are more likely to arrest and therefore result in failure to achieve a viable blastocyst.

Early markers of development predictive of implantation, hold importance to reduce the time in culture without compromise to embryo selection as a blastocyst has greater implantation potential compared to a cleavage embryo but with the increased evidence of altered gene expression and epigenetic inheritance linked to prolonged embryo culture a cleavage transfer may reduce these risks (**37**).

36.5 Compaction to Blastulation

Prolific cell division leads to compaction, where the cell-to-cell adhesion increases until the cell boundaries are undetectable at full compaction at the morula stage. The determination of these events is difficult to pin point as the changes are more subtle in nature and therefore often overlooked when considering static observations. TLI allows for closer observation of compaction and time of morula with both being linked in multiple studies of improved outcomes for euploid embryos (**38**), and prediction of euploidy with prolonged or late compaction linked to detrimental embryo development (**38–40**). These findings are hard to collaborate as these timings although defined are hard to annotate and therefore open to subjectivity. At compaction time lapse imaging allows documentation of a number of physical characteristics of the morula including extruded versus excluded cells. Coticchio et al. proposed that exclusion prior to compaction and extrusion during compaction require further study to consider possible mechanisms of correction (**41**). Other visual markers are the appearance of late onset or spontaneous vacuoles which, depending on size and timing, have been linked to reduced blastocyst formation and poor-quality blastocysts (**42**), and a lower chance of live birth outcome (**43, 44**).

Blastulation follows full compaction, the first appearance of the blastocoel cavity or time to start blastulation is a key morphokinetic variable predictive of implantation, utilised for risk classification for ploidy status (**18, 23**) and the precursor to full blastulation. Embryos with early appearance of the blastocoel cavity <95hpi have been shown to have a significantly higher implantation rate when compared to embryos with a longer time frame of >96hpi (**45**). Using tSB as a sole predictor is reflected in an analysis by Campbell et al. (**12**) individual morphokinetic variables were consider for prediction of live birth, tSB was the strongest predictive variable from 12 assessed with t0 as time of insemination. The strength of this variable could be related to the ease of annotation, the first appearance of the cavity is less subjective than other late-stage markers such as time to morula or time to full blastocyst. Full blastocyst is determined when the blastocoelic cavity expands to the point prior to the thinning of the zona and is often used to collate the duration of blastulation (tB-tSB) as an important indicator of embryo viability when used in a in house developed algorithm was more predictive than morphology alone to determine live birth outcome (**24**). Further events within blastocyst development would otherwise be unseen without TL technology with cytoplasmic strings and blastocyst collapse (**25**) linked to embryo competence with lots of scope for investigation to understand the mechanisms of embryo development that would otherwise be undetected.

Determination of optimal timings for all cell cycle durations and key morphokinetic timings are dependent on multiple factors, from chromosomal and genetic competence and specific laboratory conditions and protocols. Different patient and culture environments can therefore have a profound effect on the timing of key events making reproducibility of findings from studies difficult to replicate, limiting the transference of findings, there is an urgent need for collation of large, diverse, quality annotated image derived data sets to be widely available to drive reproducibility.

36.5.1 What to Annotate

Table 36.1 shows a selection of the types of events that can be observed and documented and the rationale for including the assessment, but it is not an exhaustive list. The decision on what to annotate will largely depend on the experience of the annotators, time to complete and the value to the user for either assessment of embryo potential for implantation for selection or to develop in house derived embryo selection models or in the pursuit of research for future evaluation.

36.6 Quality Assured Manual Annotations

Manual annotation is well defined (**29**), but can still be open to inter observer variation. A study by Sundvall et al. 2013 (**37**) investigated inter practitioner variation and showed consistency across time lapse annotations was high between operators, this is dependent on appropriate training and continuous monitoring to ensure quality is assured. These results indicate that annotations may be less subjective than routine morphology-based embryo grading as a marker of competence which is known to be less than optimal (**4**). Regular assessment can be performed in the laboratory with all annotators reviewing the same 3–5 embryos and comparing the intra-class correlation coefficient (ICC) between the predicted timed events. For large groups of clinics reviewing the same embryos may not be possible but there are a number of cloud-based systems for quality assurance for example ART compass or NEQAS, consideration of the quality of annotations is imperative if they are being used to determine the embryos fate or to rank viability within an embryo selection model

TABLE 36.1

Annotations

Parameter	Value of description	Sample image	Evidence for annotation
t0	Time of insemination - Day 0		Documented to access hours since insemination (HPI)
tPB2	Time of extrusion of the second polar body		Size, time of appearance (**19**) and the position of the second PB compared to the first polar body and fertilisation events linked to embryo quality
Polar body (PB) extrusion	Position of second PB in relation to the first (e.g. adjacent or non-adjacent – see inset image)	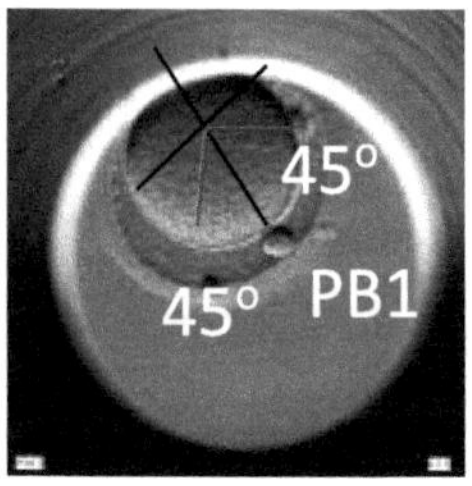 45° 45° PB1	Zhang et al. (**26**) 'PB2 angle can be used for prediction of implantation success'
tPNa	Time of PN appearance Day1		Asynchronous appearance of the pronuclei and relative movement of the pronuclei in the cytoplasm (**28**)
Pronuclei Number	0PN 1PN 2PN 3PN (inset image) =/>4PN	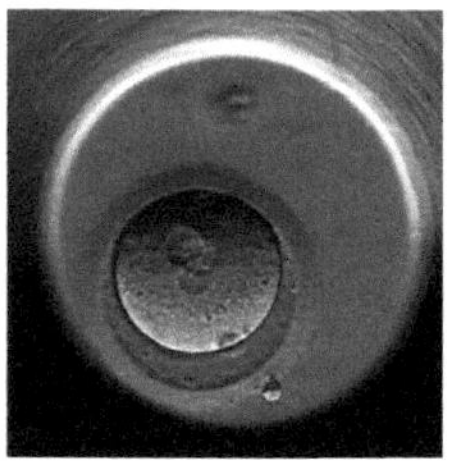	Pronuclei morphology can be considered including nuclear precursor bodies patterns and score currently, no link to live birth outcome (**27**). Correct identification of fertilisation prior to syngamy. Barrie et al. 2021 (**10**) using TLI prevented 11% of oocytes being categorised as unfertilised as syngamy had occurred prior to 17hpi
tPNf	Time to pronuclei fading (see image of tPNf in two consecutive time-lapse images)	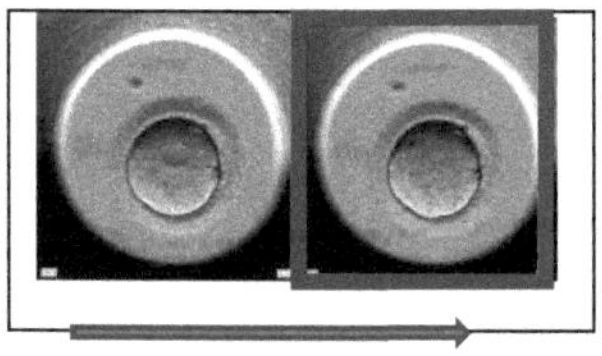	Alignment of ICSI and IVF using tpnf as start of development if wish to compare morphokinetic values by irradicating time taken for sperm to enter the oocyte. Predictive of blastocyst formation when used as a sole morphokinetic variable Campbell et all 2022 (**12**)
t2, t3 and t4	Time to each defined cell cleavage (Inset image: 2cell, correct t2 in green)	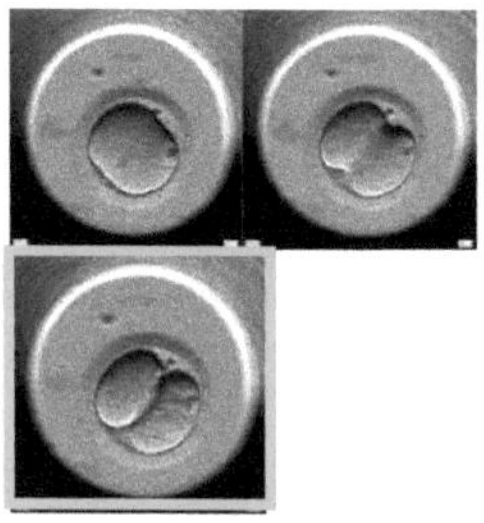	Success or failure to reach the blastocyst stage has been linked to early cleavage development and is likely inherited from the oocyte. (**15**) Various predictive algorithms have linked the timing of early cleavage markers to implantation potential (**29**).
4 cell orientation	Tetrahedral (TET) or non-tetrahedral (nTET): Marks divisional orientation of cells from 2/3 cell to 4 cell	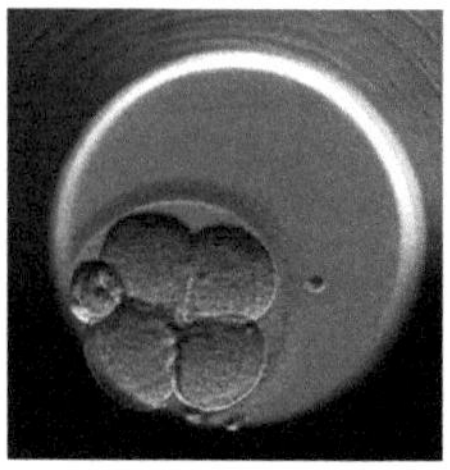	Desai et al. 2019 (**30**) nTET significantly fewer developed into 'top' grade embryos. Effect on clinical outcomes is unclear (**30, 31, 32**).

TABLE 36.1 ***(Continued)***

Annotations

Parameter	Value of description	Sample image	Evidence for annotation
t5-t9	Time to cell division of discrete cells until compaction precludes observance of divisions.		t5 was highlighted by Meseguer et al. 2011 as a pivotal variable for ranking embryo potential (**33**).
Direct cleavage	Single cell divides from one to three daughter cells directly	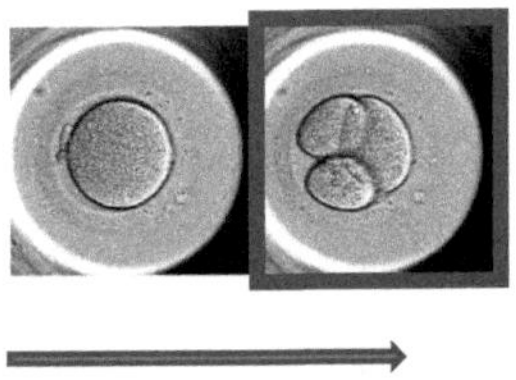	Observance of this anomaly is linked to reduced implantation potential (**34**).
tSc	The first frame in which evidence of compaction is present	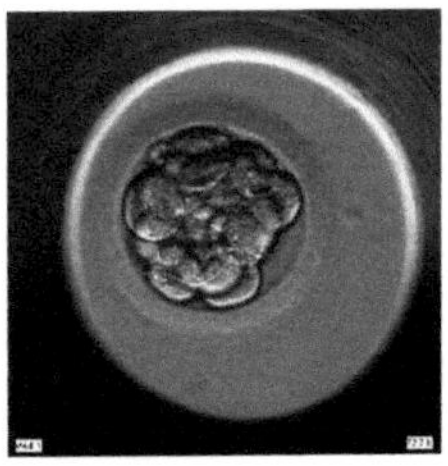	Kramer et al. identified a correlation between duration of compaction and euploidy prediction (**17**).
tM	Time of completion of compaction. Compaction can include all cells or be partial where cells are excluded.	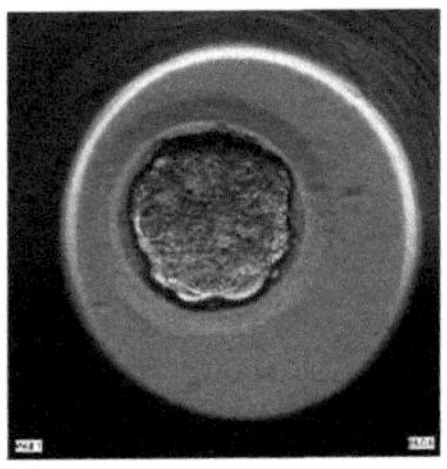	Rienzi et al. (**16**) lots to be learnt from the morula as an important precursor to the blastocyst with cell differentiation with tM >=80 hpi linked to live birth outcome.
Morula Morphology	M1 inclusion of all cells (see tM previous image) M2- partial inclusion		Morula grade linked to outcome with morula 1 highly correlate to clinical pregnancy. Boardman et al. (**35**).
Morula exclusion of cells	Exclusion/extrusion documentation as a % of the entire cell volume.		Coticchio et al. (**19**), consider exclusion or extrusion and possible corrective mechanisms linked to outcome.
tsb	Time of the first appearance of the blastocoel cavity	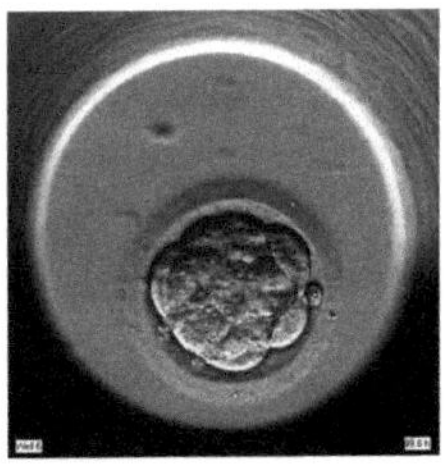	Highly predictive variable for implantation and livebirth outcome, as a sole predictor or within an algorithmic model (**12, 23**), also linked to risk classification of ploidy status. and ploidy prediction Campbell 2013 (**18**).
tB	Full blastocyst marked at the time prior to the first thinning of the zona pellucida	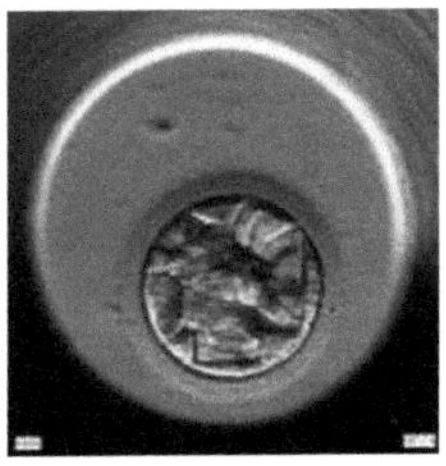	Blastocoel collapse as a measure of competence with further links to cavity diameter as an accurate measure of expansion (**25**). For thawed embryos there are links to improved clinical outcome when re-expansion is seen within a defined time prior to transfer.

(Continued)

TABLE 36.1 *(Continued)*

Annotations

Parameter	Value of description	Sample image	Evidence for annotation
tEXB	Time to expanded blastocyst; when the blastocyst had increased in diameter by more than 30% and the zona pellucida started to thin by about 50%		Expansion and collapse are considered a strong predictor of implantation potential (**25**).
tHB	Time to hatching blastocyst, when trophectoderm herniation through the zona pellucida was first observed		Hatching also a predictive variable for potential improved outcome when comparing non hatched to hatched blastocyst (**36**).

36.7 Automated Annotations

The time taken to manually annotate an individual embryo in culture to day 5 could take an experienced practitioner, on average 5–10 mins over 5 days of culture. This could account for a 1–2 of hours of laboratory time when applied to a cohort of embryos and average patient numbers per week. Factoring in quality assurance that is required to ensure all practitioners are able to robustly assess morphokinetic variables there has been an increase in supporting software to provide auto annotations. Fully automated systems using artificial intelligence with deep learning to derive annotation points by training convolutional neural networks (CNN) to determine morphokinetic variables using large data sets of quality assured manual annotations. These systems can predict annotations with accuracy with the promise of speed, reproducibility and consistency and the removal of subjectivity. They can be implemented regardless of the TLI experience, but similar to any introduction should be validated before implementation. With more reproducible outcomes they could provide improvement to prediction when used in conjunction with selection algorithms.

36.8 Use and Development of Prediction Algorithms

Understanding the morphokinetic differences between embryos and links to embryo viability paired with a quality assured annotation program naturally leads to the development or use of embryo prediction algorithms.

An in-house model has the benefit of being built on annotations derived from your specific patients and laboratory environment, these factors are known to impact the transference of predictive models between laboratories, any model will be 'tailored' and more clinically relevant to your patients and working practices (**10**). Commercially available models avoid this issue by drawing outcomes and annotations from various clinics, sampling a more diverse population and laboratory practices. This has the effect of potentially diluting the prediction to allow for a more transferrable model. These models will provide an instantaneous ranking system and often come integrated within the instrument (KID score day 5, Embryoscope, Vitrolife (**38**)). Models incorporating AI are now coming onto the commercial market which incorporate all of the previously described benefits of automatic morphokinetic assessment with embryo selection to determine prediction related to embryo viability.

The question of what the model needs to achieve will determine the design, the outcome measure is largely decided by the data available, data with an outcome of whether an embryo became a blastocyst or not, is more prevalent than the gold standard outcome measure of live birth. Models can predict blastulation, fetal heart (FH), livebirth outcome or ploidy status. When using FH or LB outcomes, remember these factors are affected by variables other than just embryo competence including endometrial quality, transfer techniques, practitioner competence and maternal factors to establish a pregnancy. Once the outcome measure has been determined ensure the suitability of the data set by considering the quality and size of the data to ensure accurate prediction with limited overfitting. Whether developing an in-house model, replicating a published model or using a commercially available model the prediction of the model must be validated on your own data prior to use to ensure the ranking of embryos is expected against clinical outcomes.

36.9 Benefits of Morphokinetics and TL Culture for the Patient

There is no doubt that TLC has deepened our knowledge of embryo development through the identification of discrete morphokinetic markers which would otherwise be undetected in SI. There are obvious benefits of undisturbed embryo culture and efficiencies within the laboratory, capturing fertilisation and identifying the time of biopsy through real time monitoring of hatching, but how does this technology improve patient outcomes. A recent Cochrane review by Armstrong et al. (**39**) reviewed 8 RCT's (n 2303) their findings concluding that there was insufficient evidence to conclude an improvement in live birth outcomes or reduction in miscarriage when comparing timelapse culture to standard incubation with morphological assessment for embryo selection. Earlier meta-analysis, Pribensky et al. (**40**), reviewed the outcomes of 5 RCT's (n1637) and revealed that the application of time-lapse monitoring was associated with a significantly higher ongoing clinical pregnancy rate (51.0% versus 39.9%), with a pooled odds ratio of 1.542 ($P < 0.001$, reduced early pregnancy loss and increased live birth outcomes when compared to embryo selection using a static morphological observation. Further evidence is therefore required to answer this question definitively, but it is evident that this technology has the potential to improve our understanding of the embryo and reduce the time to clinical pregnancy. Morphokinetics in relation to ploidy status is still a much-debated area and remains unclear, many studies reveal morphokinetic markers linked to increased incidence of aneuploidy but these findings to date have not been reproducible and further studies are required to understand the link of known events in the pre implantation embryo and chromosomal competency.

36.10 Conclusion

Images generated by time lapse are being exposed to the power of artificial intelligence, with convolutional neural networks and deep learning neural networks, it is now possible to unlock features within the embryo image, beyond the interpretation of the human eye, linked to outcomes of clinical pregnancy, live birth or ploidy status to train a model to determine the potential of an embryo to implant. These AI models have the potential to be reproducible, non-invasive and time saving with minimal cost for equipment as they are largely cloud based with the caveat that they may not be easily interpretable and should be built on large, diverse data sets to ensure accuracy. These technologies are not solely being used for embryo selection but have the potential to revolutionise the clinical application of reproductive technology and are discussed in length in the final chapter of this book. Timelapse technology is becoming more widely used in clinics and as artificial intelligence uses imagery there are potential avenues to explore further avenues to improve our understanding of the embryo with this technology. From the oocyte to the hatching blastocyst more secrets can be revealed, to further improve the patient experience, enlighten our understanding and drive quality in our laboratories.

REFERENCES

1. Rienzi L, Ubaldi F, Iacobelli M, et al. Significance of morphological attributes of the early embryo. *Reprod Biomed Online*. 2005;10(5):669–681.
2. Johansson M, Hardarson T, Lundin K. There is a cutoff limit in diameter between a blastomere and a small anucleate fragment. *J Assist Reprod Genet*. 2003;20(8):309–313.
3. Hardarson T, Hanson C, Sjogren A, et al. Human embryos with unevenly sized blastomeres have lower pregnancy and implantation rates: indications for aneuploidy and multinucleation. *Hum Reprod*. 2001;16(2):313–318.
4. Pickering SJ, Taylor A, Johnson MH, et al. An analysis of multinucleated blastomere formation in human embryos. *Hum Reprod*. 1995;10(7):1912–1922.
5. Cummins JM, Breen TM, Harrison KL, et al. A formula for scoring human embryo growth rates in in vitro fertilization: its value in predicting pregnancy and in comparison with visual estimates of embryo quality. *J In Vitro Fert Embryo Transf.* 1986;3(5):284–295.
6. Racowsky C, Vernon M, Mayer J, et al. Standardization of grading embryo morphology. *J Assist Reprod Genet*. 2010;27(8):437–439.
7. ACE/NEQAS. *The ACE/NEQAS Embryo Grading Scheme is Changing Online: Gamete Expert*. 2017. Available from: https://gamete-expert.com/userfiles/file/New%20UK%20NEQAS%20embryo%20grading%20scheme.pdf.
8. ASEBIR. *ASEBIR Criteria for Morphological Assessment of Oocytes, Early Embryos and Human Blastocysts Online: ASEBIR*. 2015. Available from: https://asebir.com/cuadernos-asebir/criterios-asebir-de-valoracion-morfologica-de-oocitos-embriones-tempranos-y-blastocistos-humanos/.
9. Steer CV, Mills CL, Tan SL, et al. The cumulative embryo score: a predictive embryo scoring technique to select the optimal number of embryos to transfer in an in-vitro fertilization and embryo transfer programme. *Hum Reprod*. 1992;7(1):117–119.
10. ALPHA/ESHRE. The Istanbul consensus workshop on embryo assessment: proceedings of an expert meeting. *Hum Reprod*. 2011;26(6):1270–1283.
11. Sciorio R, Rapalini E, Esteves SC. Air quality in the clinical embryology laboratory: a mini-review. *Ther Adv Reprod Health*. 2021;15:2633494121990684.
12. Campbell A. Clinical aspects of time lapse imaging. In: Campbell A, Fishel S, editors. *Atlas of Time Lapse Embryology*. Florida: CRC Press, Taylor & Francis; 2015. pp. 7–11.
13. Ede DA, Counce SJ. A cinematographic study of the embryology of Drosophila melanogaster. *Wilhelm Roux Arch Entwickl Mech Org*. 1956;148(4):402–415.
14. Blandau RJ, Rumery RE. The attachment cone of the guinea pig blastocyst as observed under time-lapse cinematography. *Fertil Steril*. 1957;8(6):570–585.
15. Taylor AC. Responses of cells to pH changes in the medium. *J Cell Biol*. 1962;15:201–209.
16. Tan L, Shen S, Chen A. Description of time-lapse systems: EevaTM test. In: Meseguer M, editor. *Time-Lapse Microscope in In Vitro Fertilization*. 1st Edition. Cambridge: Cambridge University Press; 2016. pp. 51–76.
17. Pribenszky C. Description of time-lapse systems: Primo VisionTM. In: Meseguer M, editor. *Time-Lapse Microscope*

in In Vitro Fertilization. 1st Edition. Cambridge: Cambridge University Press; 2016. pp. 31–50.
18. Apter S, Ebner T, Freour T, et al. Good practice recommendations for the use of time-lapse technology(dagger). *Hum Reprod Open*. 2020;2020(2):hoaa008.
19. Mestres E, Matia-Algue Q, Villamar A, et al. Characterization and comparison of commercial oils used for human embryo culture. *Hum Reprod*. 2022;37(2):212–225.
20. Li R, Pedersen KS, Liu Y, et al. Effect of red light on the development and quality of mammalian embryos. *J Assist Reprod Genet*. 2014;31(7):795–801.
21. Ottosen LD, Hindkjaer J, Ingerslev J. Light exposure of the ovum and preimplantation embryo during ART procedures. *J Assist Reprod Genet*. 2007;24(2–3):99–103.
22. Campbell A. Time lapse, the cell cycle, distribution of morphokinetic timings, and known implantation data. In: Campbell A, Fishel S, editors. *Atlas of Time Lapse Embryology*. Florida: CRC Press, Taylor & Francis; 2015. pp. 13–18.
23. Tejera A, Basile N, Caiazzo M, et al. Embryo quality (classification and selection). In: Meseguer M, editor. *Time-Lapse Microscope in In Vitro Fertilization*. 1st Edition. Cambridge: Cambridge University Press; 2016. pp. 104–127.
24. Alhelou Y, Mat Adenan NA, Ali J. Embryo culture conditions are significantly improved during uninterrupted incubation: a randomized controlled trial. *Reprod Biol*. 2018;18(1):40–45.
25. Gardner DK, Schoolcraft WB. Culture and transfer of human blastocysts. *Curr Opin Obstet Gynecol*. 1999;11(3):307–311.
26. Adolfsson E, Andershed AN. Morphology vs morphokinetics: a retrospective comparison of inter-observer and intra-observer agreement between embryologists on blastocysts with known implantation outcome. *JBRA Assist Reprod*. 2018;22(3):228–237.
27. Storr A, Venetis CA, Cooke S, et al. Inter-observer and intra-observer agreement between embryologists during selection of a single day 5 embryo for transfer: a multicenter study. *Hum Reprod*. 2017;32(2):307–314.
28. HFEA. *Fertility Treatment Trends and Figures 2014*. London, UK: Human Fertilisation and Embryology Authority; 2014.
29. Ciray HN, Campbell A, Agerholm IE, et al. Proposed guidelines on the nomenclature and annotation of dynamic human embryo monitoring by a time-lapse user group. *Hum Reprod*. 2014;29(12):2650–2660.
30. Rienzi L, Vajta G, Ubaldi F. Predictive value of oocyte morphology in human IVF: a systematic review of the literature. *Hum Reprod Update*. 2011;17(1):34–45.
31. Zhang Q, Guo XM, Li Y. Optimal polar bodies angle for higher subsequent embryo viability: a pilot study. *Fertil Steril*. 2016;105(3):670–675.e2.
32. Barrie A, Smith R, Campbell A, et al. Optimisation of the timing of fertilisation assessment for oocytes cultured in standard incubation: lessons learnt from time-lapse imaging of 78 348 embryos. *Hum Reprod*. 2021;36(11):2840–2847.
33. Herrero J, Tejera A, Albert C, et al. A time to look back: analysis of morphokinetic characteristics of human embryo development. *Fertil Steril*. 2013;100(6):1602–1609.e1–4.
34. Campbell A, Petersen B, Smith R, et al. Prediction of blastulation, embryo utilisation and live birth from single morphological or morphokinetic variables. *Fertil Steril*. 2022(4):e138.
35. Athayde Wirka K, Chen AA, Conaghan J, et al. Atypical embryo phenotypes identified by time-lapse microscopy: high prevalence and association with embryo development. *Fertil Steril*. 2014;101(6):1637–1648.e1–5.
36. Almagor M, Or Y, Fieldust S, et al. Irregular cleavage of early preimplantation human embryos: characteristics of patients and pregnancy outcomes. *J Assist Reprod Genet*. 2015;32(12):1811–1815.
37. Wong CC, Loewke KE, Bossert NL, et al. Non-invasive imaging of human embryos before embryonic genome activation predicts development to the blastocyst stage. *Nat Biotechnol*. 2010;28(10):1115–1121.
38. Campbell A, Fishel S, Bowman N, et al. Modelling a risk classification of aneuploidy in human embryos using non-invasive morphokinetics. *Reprod Biomed Online*. 2013;26(5):477–485.
39. Rienzi L, Cimadomo D, Delgado A, et al. Time of morulation and trophectoderm quality are predictors of a live birth after euploid blastocyst transfer: a multicenter study. *Fertil Steril*. 2019;112(6):1080–1093.e1.
40. Kramer YG, Kofinas JD, Melzer K, et al. Assessing morphokinetic parameters via time lapse microscopy (TLM) to predict euploidy: are aneuploidy risk classification models universal? *J Assist Reprod Genet*. 2014;31(9):1231–1242.
41. Coticchio G, Lagalla C, Sturmey R, et al. The enigmatic morula: mechanisms of development, cell fate determination, self-correction and implications for ART. *Hum Reprod Update*. 2019;25(4):422–438.
42. Ebner T, Moser M, Sommergruber M, et al. Occurrence and developmental consequences of vacuoles throughout preimplantation development. *Fertil Steril*. 2005;83(6):1635–1640.
43. Mayer RB, Shebl O, Oppelt P, et al. Good-quality blastocysts derived from vacuolized morulas show reduced viability. *Fertil Steril*. 2018;109(6):1025–1029.
44. Smith R, Campbell A, Montgomery S, et al. Is the time of appearance of vacuoles critical to live birth outcome? *RBMO*. 2022;45(E19=E20):1.
45. Soukhov E, Karavani G, Szaingurten-Solodkin I, et al. Prediction of embryo implantation rate using a sole parameter of timing of starting blastulation. *Zygote*. 2022;1–8.

37

Abnormal Cleavage, Self-Correction of Aneuploidy and Decision-Making Regarding Embryo Fate

Natalie Davis and Alison Campbell

The introduction of time-lapse imaging to embryology laboratories has allowed the observation and recording of dynamic cellular events during human embryo development. In contrast, static observations, performed either daily or solely at the blastocyst stage observe a snapshot, from which the intervening developmental stages cannot be ascertained. Therefore, as time-lapse imaging has become commonplace within the IVF laboratory over the last 10 years, the knowledge of human embryo developmental patterns has also grown. The normal pathway for embryo development is discussed in Chapter 13, but key aspects of this will also be covered here.

37.1 The Cell Cycle

Chromosomal errors within human embryos result most commonly from errors in maternal meiosis or post-fertilisation mitotic errors. Maternal meiotic errors would result in the oocyte being aneuploid, which unless corrected during second polar body extrusion, would result in all of the cells of the preimplantation embryo containing this aneuploidy. Post fertilisation mitotic errors can occur at any stage but have been widely reported to occur most commonly in the first 3 cell cycles. The majority of these mitotic errors will result in the formation of a mosaic embryo, as whichever cell undergoes the abnormal cleavage event will likely result in one or more aneuploid daughter cells, creating a new aneuploid cell line. The major exception to this is the direct cleavage of the zygote from 1 to 3 cells, which would likely result in all chaotic aneuploid cells due to chromosomes being divided between 3 daughter cells. This chapter focusses on the errors of mitotic division, what we understand about the genetic outcome of these errors and how they impact the developmental potential of the embryo. It is now widely accepted that mosaicism rates are lower at the blastocyst stage than the cleavage stage, which is suggestive of one of more embryo self-correction methods taking place. Current knowledge regarding these mechanisms and their limitations will be discussed as will the requirements for future research.

A cell cycle is a series of events involving cellular and nuclear processes, resulting in the cell's division to two daughter cells. Mitosis consists of nuclear division and cytokinesis and involves several stages; prophase, prometaphase, metaphase, anaphase, and telophase. Interphase precedes these stages and encompasses stages GAP-1 (G1), synthesis (S), and GAP-2 (G2) of what is known as the cell cycle. An association between cell cycle length and embryo viability has been determined, with prolonged or rapid cell cycles associated with DNA repair, cellular rearrangements or failure of an embryo to undergo cell cycle checkpoints. Both potentially compromise embryo development.

For the patient undertaking an IVF cycle, the important issue is how we use all of this information to enable selection of the embryo with the highest chance of viability for transfer and to select which embryos are suitable for cryopreservation. Current perspectives regarding this will be considered.

37.2 Abnormal Patterns of Cell Division

Many of the anomalous patterns of cell division most commonly observed have been analysed and are detailed below:

37.2.1 Direct Cleavage/Multichotomous Mitosis

Multichotomous mitosis (MM) is the term given to a single cell dividing by mitosis resulting in 3 or more daughter cells, each observed to have an identifiable nucleus. It can occur at any stage throughout preimplantation development but is most commonly observed throughout the first 3 cleavage divisions (**1**). It has been shown to occur more frequently after the appearance of multinucleation in the parent cell and in many cases, is followed by reverse cleavage. The occurrence rate of multichotomous mitosis is reported as between 4.4% and 13.7% (**2, 3**). Even with time-lapse imaging, it would be technically challenging to observe this anomaly after the third cell cycle due to the size of the cells and the difficulty in determining the origin of each cell when so many are present, along with the onset of compaction.

When MM occurs during the first cell cycle, the embryo divides directly from 1–3 cells, which is likely to lead to all of the daughter cells having a sub-diploid chromosomal complement, resulting in chaotic aneuploidy. The embryo is highly unlikely to be able to correct this. The Zhan study reported that upon MM occurrence during the first cell cycle, no live births resulted following day 3 embryo transfer (**1**). They also reported that euploidy rates following MM increased from MM during the first cell cycle through to the third and that later stage MM appeared to have a reduced impact on embryo development, likely due to impacting a smaller proportion of

DOI: 10.1201/9781003269502-37

the embryo. Recent studies have suggested a possible mechanism to be the formation of tripolar spindles within diploid cells (**4, 5**). If the chromosomes were then randomly recruited to the axes of the tripolar spindle, this would result in daughter cells with a reduced, chaotic chromosome compliment. Current evidence suggests this may occur due to centrosome anomalies. Although centrosomal components are derived from the sperm during fertilisation, so abnormal centrosome number could lead to this occurrence, it is also considered that dysregulation of centrosome duplication could be a cause. However, the quantitative trait locus spanning PLK4 in the maternal genome has also been implicated as a factor in tripolar mitosis occurrence (**4**).

37.2.2 Rapid Cleavage

Rapid cleavage describes the cleavage of a single cell to 2 daughter cells faster than the 'normal' duration, which has not yet been fully defined for each cell cycle (**6**). This occurrence is most commonly seen during the early cleavage stages, and is most studied when an embryo cleaves from 2 to 3 cells within 5 hours of completion of the first cell cycle. A standard cell cycle would be expected to last between 10 and 12 hours. A further division in less than 5 hours, as it the case with rapid cleavage is thought to be associated with reduced implantation (**3**). It is postulated that there is not time for complete replication of the chromosomes or for DNA repair to occur when two consecutive cytokineses are separated by less than 5 hours. This may then result in aneuploidy through leading to uneven chromosome distribution between the daughter cells. However, it is worth noting that the stage of embryo development at which this occurs could have an impact on its developmental potential. If it occurs during the later cleavage stages, fewer cells and therefore a smaller proportion of the embryo would be involved, potentially resulting in a mosaic embryo.

37.2.3 Reverse Cleavage (RC)/Cell Fusion

Cell fusion is defined as a reduction in the number of cells of an embryo during development due to cells merging or fusing together (**6**). It is separate event to the merging of cells seen at the beginning of compaction prior to morula formation. In order to be classed as 'reverse cleavage' each cell must have a complete membrane around it prior to the fusion, so as not to be confused with failed cytokinesis. This definition also excludes the reabsorption of cellular fragments. As such, each cell should have a visible nucleus during interphase prior to the occurrence of reverse cleavage. Its occurrence rate is reported as in between 6.8% and 10% of embryos (**7, 8**). It is possible for RC to occur more than once within the cleavage stage of the same embryo, with it retaining the ability to reach the blastocyst stage, albeit from a small cohort of embryos (**7**).

In terms of embryo developmental potential, opposing results have been obtained. Hickman et al. showed that embryos exhibiting RC blastulated at a similar rate to those which did not exhibit RC, and also had an equivalent euploid: aneuploid ratio (**7**). However, studies by Lagalla and Desai showed a reduced proportion of embryos reaching the blastocyst stage or being suitable for trophectoderm biopsy following RC (**8, 9**). Liu et al. performed cleavage stage transfers of RC embryos and found no implantation (0/22), suggesting a significant detriment of this occurrence (**10**). A more recent study looking at KID live birth outcomes found that there was no significant difference between the live birth rate of RC and non-RC embryos, if they had reached the start of blastulation prior to transfer (**11**).

A significant association between the use of GnRH antagonist cycles and increased occurrence of RC has been shown when compared to agonist stimulation cycles (**7, 10**), suggestive of an impact of the follicular environment and oocyte development on this occurrence. Reduced progressive sperm motility has also been shown to be associated with increased RC occurrence, as has increased multinucleation by the 4-cell stage (**10**). RC was assumed to be associated with an increase in polyploidy, or aneuploidy, due to the merging of sibling cells, but this association has not been shown. As a result, further work is required to determine how the environment within the ovary and sperm parameters may lead to RC occurrence.

37.2.4 Fragment Generation/Reabsorption

The observation of fragments during the early cleavage stages is widely seen during both conventional and time-lapse embryo observations. These excluded fragments contain cytoplasm, with the presence of chromosomes resulting from malsegregation or exclusion also previously reported. The presence of large fragments was suggested to reduce the implantation rate of the embryo, possibly due to too high a volume of cytoplasm, its associated cellular proteins and mitochondria being removed from individual cells (**12**). Fujimoto et al. reviewed several mechanisms which may lead to fragmentation and found that fragmented embryos often had reduced mitochondrial DNA levels and therefore lower adenosine triphosphate (ATP) content (**13**). Widespread minor fragmentation did not appear to affect the implantation rate. In addition, Hardarson reported the reincorporation of fragments into cells, by an as yet undetermined mechanism, thought to potentially be associated with self-correction (**14**).

37.2.5 Exclusion of Cells from the Morula

During normal embryo development all of the cells produced within the cleavage stage would be incorporated into the morula. However, it is widely recognised using time-lapse observations that cellular exclusion from the morula is a common occurrence. Associated with decreased implantation rates compared to fully compacting morulae, limited research into the content of the excluded cells has been performed. In one study, the cells excluded at the morula stage of 18 blastocysts were analysed by aCGH, along with a trophectoderm biopsy from each blastocyst (**9**). Of the excluded cells corresponding to the euploid blastocysts, 2 were euploid and 5 aneuploid. Six failed to amplify, as may be expected of degenerating DNA, likely to occur if the excluded cell is degrading. They hypothesised that the excluded cells may be excluded because they are aneuploid, and that this may be linked to a self-correction mechanism which will be discussed later in this chapter. In addition, they noted the appearance of cells excluded from

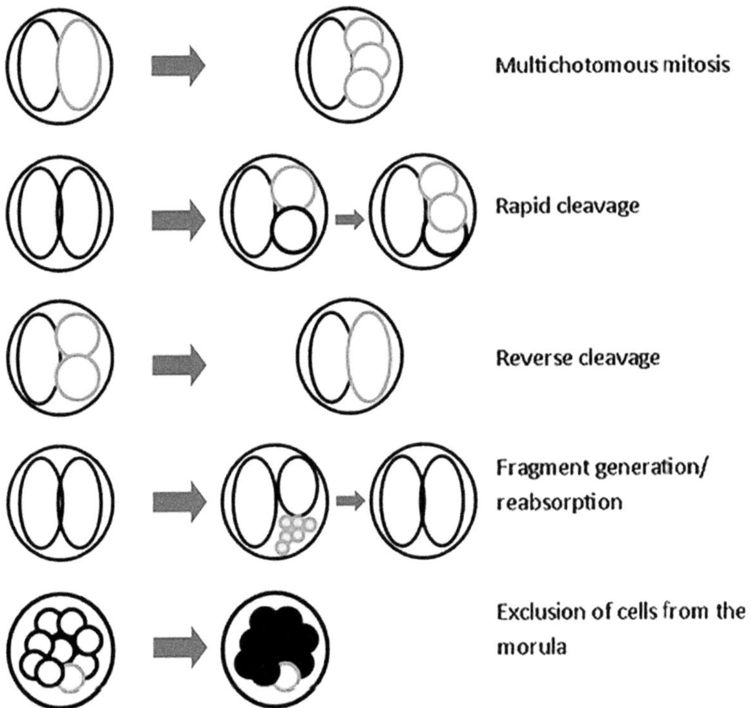

FIGURE 37.1 Examples of cleavage anomalies observed within human embryos.

the morula at a higher rate in embryos which have undergone aberrant cleavage events compared to those which had not (100% vs. 46% respectively).

There is a clear requirement for further studies to fully elucidate the mechanisms by which the cleavage abnormalities detailed previously in this chapter occur and to determine their full effect on embryo developmental potential. Most outcomes do not appear to be so severe as to automatically prevent pregnancy and healthy live birth occurring if they are observed during embryo culture. Where not all cells are implicated in the cleavage abnormality (for example MM from 2–5 cells, where one cell divides normally and the other cell divides to form 3 cells), mosaicism is likely to ensue. Recent evidence reports mosaic embryos as resulting in lower implantation rates and higher miscarriage rates than fully euploid embryos (**15**), but crucially reports link mosaic embryo transfers with healthy live births. However, the first report of mosaic live birth following mosaic embryo transfer was reported in 2020 (**16**). This concept leads to the question of whether some form of embryo 'correction' occurs as development proceeds, allowing a mosaic embryo to correct or exclude these cells, resulting in an embryo with an increased proportion of euploid cells. Several pieces of evidence support this idea. Munné et al. (2005) tested 24 previously aCGH aneuploid embryos, using FISH at on day 12 and found 7 euploid embryos and 11 showing an increase in the proportion of euploid cells (**17**). A further study looked at self-correction between days 3 and 5 of embryo development and noted a 38.1% rate of self-correction in embryos which reached the blastocyst stage, with the rate reducing with declining embryo quality (**18**). Chromosome abnormality levels have also been shown to be lower at day 5 than day 3 (**19**), and mosaic blastocysts cultured to day 12 have been shown to often have euploid outgrowths (**20**), with self-correction a possible mechanism causing this.

Four major methods of self-correction have been propose (**21**). These are described in the following sections.

37.2.5.1 The Embryonic Mortality Model

Mitotic errors can result in the formation of aneuploid cell lines. This self-correction model is the idea that when these aneuploid cell lines account for a small enough proportion of the embryo, the embryo can select against them during development. Where the aneuploid portion of the embryo is too great, embryo development will arrest. Using a mouse embryo model, Bolton et al. used the enzyme reversine to induce the creation of aneuploid cell lines, creating control: reversine cell line chimeras. They created 1:1 control:reversine and 1:3 control:reversine chimeras. Significantly fewer of the implantation sites contained a viable embryo in the 1:3 group than the 1:1 group, suggesting the aneuploid load was too great for the embryo to correct, but that it could be corrected in the 1:1 group (**22**). This model is also supported by a study observing mitotic abnormalities and their development to the blastocyst stage. Lagalla et al. reported that all of the embryos which underwent a cleavage abnormality either arrested or reached the blastocyst stage, but had excluded cells at the morula stage (**9**). They performed aCGH on the resultant blastocysts and excluded cells and found that the proportion of euploid blastocysts was higher than in the control group. All of the excluded cells from aneuploid blastocysts exhibited additional aneuploidies, whilst 5 of the 7 excluded cells from euploid blastocysts which amplified were aneuploid. These results support the idea that the embryo is able to select against cells which are aneuploid to correct itself, but these studies are small, with the key study based on a mouse model. Further work to confirm this and exclude other explanations is required.

37.2.5.2 The Clonal Depletion Model

Related to the embryonic mortality model, this is the idea that aneuploid cells within the embryo undergo apoptosis or reduced propagation compared to euploid cells. In the Bolton study just discussed, they showed that the rate of apoptosis in the inner cell mass of euploid/aneuploid mosaic embryos is higher than in the trophectoderm, resulting in a reduction in the proportion of aneuploid cells in the ICM from 53% at the early blastocyst stage, to 47% at the mature blastocyst stage (**22**). No difference in the proportion was seen in the TE. They used time-lapse imaging to show that this was not due to preferential allocation of aneuploid cells to the TE. Therefore they concluded that it must be due to increased apoptosis of aneuploid ICM cells, which also showed slower cell cycles compared to the euploid cells. Kahraman suggested that these cell lines are lost during implantation (**16**), but this model focuses primarily on the preimplantation basis for this. Lal et al. described that preferential apoptosis of aneuploid cells may occur during preimplantation development, by looking at the cell free DNA content derived from blastocoel fluid, collected after trophectoderm biopsy (**23**). cfDNA results from cellular apoptosis and has been found alongside extracellular vesicles and microRNAs linked to apoptosis in this fluid, from which the conclusion is drawn that cellular apoptosis must occur during the early cleavage stages and potentially also at the blastocyst stage, likely as part of a self-correction mechanism. In addition, through assessing the markers of apoptotic and proliferative activity in euploid, mosaic and aneuploid embryos, an increase in proliferative activity and cell death was seen in mosaic and aneuploid embryos compared to euploid ones. A possible, although as yet unproven reason for this could be that the aneuploid cells proliferate more slowly and apoptose, whilst the euploid cells compensate for this by increasing their proliferative rate (**24**).

Finally, several groups have analysed the presence of proteins associated with cell cycle checkpoints. Aurora B regulates the first mitotic division and allows time for possible self-correction of chromosomal aberrations. Its presence is also required for mitotic arrest deficient 2 (MAD2) expression in the chromatin of embryos, which is a protein required for aneuploidy repair. The effect of in vitro culture and oxidative stress on the cell cycle has also been shown by several groups assessing the presence of cell cycle checkpoints and their associated proteins in aneuploid cells. When Aurora B is inhibited, MAD2 is undetectable and the mosaicism rate increases (**25**). Oxidative stress reduces expression of mitosis promoting factor (MPF) (**26**), and leads to increased aneuploidy. Together, this information suggests reduced propagation of aneuploid cells, as suggested by this model, due to the repair mechanisms taking place and delaying mitosis.

Although this data provides the beginnings of an explanation of how this self-correction model takes places, further work looking at apoptotic markers is required to understand it further.

37.2.5.3 The Trisomic/Monosomic Rescue Model

This model is thought to contribute to a minor proportion of the self-correction seen in embryos. It is the idea that an aneuploid embryo can gain or lose a copy of a chromosome during mitosis, giving it a diploid complement. In some instances, this would result in the embryo containing one copy of the affected chromosome from each parent, making it indistinguishable from an embryo which had undergone normal mitotic division. In other cases, including all cases involving monosomy rescue, it would result in uniparental disomy (UPD), where both copies of the chromosome originate from one parent. A study of UPD in 3401 embryos showed its occurrence is low, at 0.06% (**27**). Correction of paternal origin trisomy is rare, as often an additional centriole will have been inherited with the additional chromosome, impacting spindle formation and normal cell division patterns. As a result, the majority of these rare occurrences derive from maternal trisomies (**28**).

37.3 Preferential Allocation of Aneuploid Cells to the Trophectoderm Model

This model suggests that the ICM is not a conducive environment for aneuploid cell development, which presumably encourages the development of a euploid foetus. Instead, the aneuploid cells are preferentially allocated in the trophectoderm, and later post implantation, in the placenta. A number of groups have attempted to provide evidence of this as a method of self-correction with opposing results. Chuang et al. biopsied 33 human embryos within the ICM, opposite the ICM and near to the ICM, seeing no preferential allocation of aneuploid cells to the trophectoderm (**29**), whilst Taylor et al. tested mural, polar and a mid-area of trophectoderm in between these two, showing a decreasing trend of aneuploidy from the polar to the mid to the mural trophectoderm (**30**). Whilst the rates between the polar and mural trophectoderm were significantly different, this was attributed to biological methods including mosaicism and differences in how embryologists performed the biopsy procedure. The most recent study used single cell genomic data to assess mosaicism across the embryo. They found low-grade mosaicism throughout the embryo, but no statistical difference between the aneuploid cell proportions between the inner cell mass and trophectoderm, with a caveat that the confidence interval was wide, making a modest difference possible (**31**). They have previously shown that in post-implantation embryos there is enrichment of aneuploid cells compared to the lineages derived from the inner cell mass, suggesting that this phenomenon is more common during later developmental stages.

37.4 Self-Correction: Where Are We Now?

Current research is suggestive of the presence of embryo self-correction in a variety of forms, but only a limited subset of these studies relate to human embryos. Research is limited by the number of embryos donated to research and the inability to assess the chromosomal compliment of all cells of an embryo to be used in treatment due to it requiring embryo destruction.

This means that the confirmation of the molecular mechanisms underpinning self-correction and the high quality studies with high embryo numbers required to confirm these are not yet available.

37.5 Decision-Making Regarding Embryo Fate

Embryologists use the information gained during the preimplantation period to determine the fate of each embryo; to transfer, cryopreserve or discard.

As a minimum, without genetic PN assessment alongside PGT-A, an embryo would be assessed twice; once to determine the number of pronuclei present and the second to determine its developmental stage and grade at the point of transfer/cryopreservation. The addition of adjuvant treatments can increase the amount of information available with which to make the decision regarding fate. This includes the use of time lapse imaging, where annotations of specific developmental stage time-points (2c, 5c, tM, tSC etc) can be run through an algorithm such as CAREMaps™ to create a ranking system, where higher scores are associated with a higher chance of live birth. It can also be used for observation of dynamic aberrant cleavage patterns, allowing preferential selection of embryos which have not exhibited this behaviour. In addition the use of preimplantation testing for aneuploidy (PGT-A) or other emerging technologies such as metabolomics, proteomics and artificial intelligence (AI) may play an increasing role in embryo selection in the future. An AI model predicting β-hCG result has already been reported (**32**).

With different methods of embryo selection available, a system of prioritisation is required (Figure 37.2). Due to providing knowledge of the chromosomal content of the tested cells, an available PGT-A result will provide the first selection. An aneuploid embryo will become unavailable for patient use and a euploid, no result, or mosaic embryo may be used for transfer or remain cryopreserved for future use. Embryos which have not undergone PGT, or where more than one euploid embryo is available, will then be assessed using a time-lapse algorithm. Using CARE Maps™ as an example, an embryo with a higher score will be prioritised for transfer over one with a lower score due to the reducing likelihood of live birth with decreasing score. Where embryos return very similar scores, the developmental stage and morphology assessment are used to determine the ranking order of the embryos and thereby which gains the overall highest score (used for transfer) with those reaching a suitable level cryopreserved. As standard, a high-grade embryo which has reached at least the full blastocyst stage would be considered suitable for vitrification.

There are situations where the highest scoring embryo using a time-lapse algorithm may not be selected for transfer, in favour of the next highest scoring embryo. This is rare and the decision should be made by a senior staff member. It would occur in the event the highest scoring embryo was showing signs of degeneration, or if all embryos achieved a lower morphokinetic score and the highest scoring one had a particularly poor morphology, compared to the others. It could also be the case if the embryo had shown repeated cleavage abnormalities such as several rounds multichotomous mitosis and reverse cleavage when another embryo within the cohort had not. However, due to the limited research and lack of definitive outcome data concerning the cleavage abnormalities, and the possibility of self-correction, care should be taken if selecting against an embryo based on these characteristics alone. It may be appropriate to cryopreserve these embryos and transfer an embryo showing normal cleavage stage development, thereby retaining them for future use.

The subjectivity of embryo morphology assessment and time-lapse annotation should also be considered. Embryologists must show proficiency at embryo grading and annotation before being allowed to perform these clinically. In order to retain competency, internal and external quality assurance is performed, including the UK NEQAS scheme for embryo morphology, biannual competency assessment and quarterly IQA exercises, where all embryologists annotate developmental time-points of the same 3 embryos to ensure concordance. This is important to ensure the patient receives the same standard

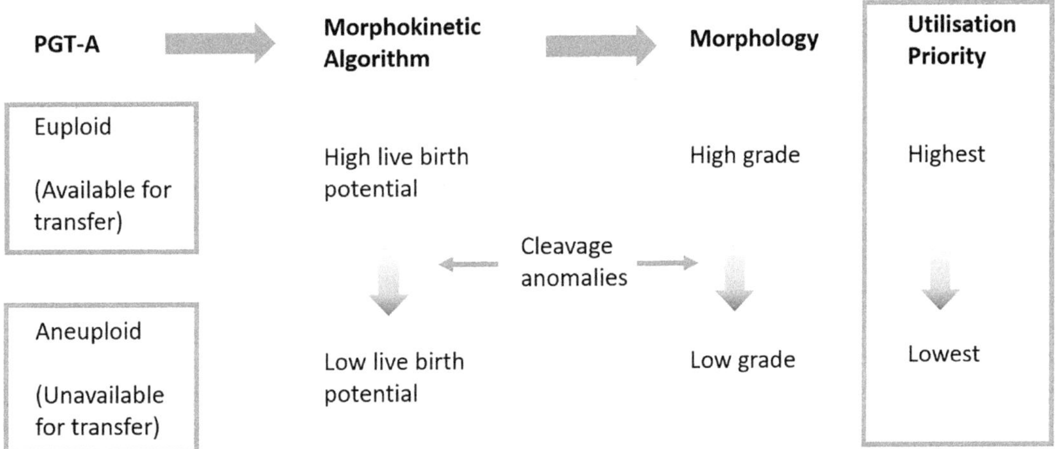

FIGURE 37.2 A hierarchy of embryo selection. When available, PGT-A results are prioritised, then a morphokinetic algorithm and then morphology. Embryologists may also prioritise embryos which have not undergone abnormal cleavage over those which have with a similar morphokinetic score or morphology.

of care whichever embryologist assesses their embryos be it in terms of selection for transfer, or to ensure the morphokinetic score achieved by their embryos is appropriate due to accurate data inputting. Despite this, humans are individual and there will always be small differences which can have a minimal impact on the grading, annotation and embryo selection performed. Currently, AI systems which have undergone machine learning through analysis of existing embryo images are starting to be implemented in IVF laboratories to perform automatic annotation of developmental time-points, making this process more consistent and reducing inter-operator variability.

The scientific assessment of an embryo is not the only factor to be considered when determining an embryo's fate. We must remember that these embryos belong to our patients, whose opinions, beliefs and requests must be respected and followed. In order to do this we must support our patients in gaining an understanding of the process of embryo development and the relevance of the observations we report to them. This process is complicated by the fact that none of the criteria we use give a definitive outcome. For example, the observation of reverse cleavage does not preclude an embryo from leading to live birth, but may reduce its chances. It is now common practice to culture embryos to the blastocyst stage prior to transferring or cryopreserving them, especially when cleavage abnormalities have been observed. An embryo which does not get to that stage is removing itself from the cohort of viable embryos, but one which does may have potential. As discussed previously, how we compare an embryo with a cleavage abnormality but high morphokinetic score to an embryo with a lower morphokinetic score, but with no cleavage abnormalities observed, or an embryo with higher morphology scoring than either of these must be managed carefully. Most importantly, how do we express this to patients and how much of this information should we be sharing with them? Whilst it is important that this information is available to them to understand why a particular embryo has been selected for a particular fate, we must remember that our patients come from all walks of life, and such complex information may be very difficult for them to understand. Add to that that their treatment may also be placing a large financial and emotional burden on them as well and it is not difficult to understand why many patients report feeling stressed and confused by a lack of understanding regarding embryo grading (**33**).

Patients' opinions regarding embryo fate can also vary dramatically. Embryologists are taught to select the embryo(s) believed to have the highest potential for live birth for transfer, with additional embryos considered to have high potential being cryopreserved. Patient opinion does not always follow this pattern. The financial, emotional and personal impact must be considered. For some patients, disposal of a developing embryo, regardless of low grade or slow development is unacceptable. Whilst for some this may be for a religious reason, for others it is the concept of risking disposing a viable embryo, however small the chance of viability may be. In these instances, patients may request the transfer of the embryo which is deemed unsuitable for cryopreservation and have the remainder frozen for future use, thereby utilising a higher proportion of their embryos. Whilst it would always be recommended to transfer the highest grade embryo to give the highest chance of live birth in this cycle and to minimise the need for further medicated cycles, with the associated financial, emotional and physical implications of this, we must respect out patient's wishes. Therefore, as long as the implications of their decision are understood and the realistic chances of live birth associated with their decision explained, reasonable requests should be adhered to.

Although the decision as to which embryos are suitable is usually taken by the embryologist, it is relatively common for a patient to request the cryopreservation of those embryos deemed unsuitable by the embryologist. This presents an ethical dilemma. Whilst we must respect out patient's wishes, the request to cryopreserve an embryo with a low morphokinetic score, combined with low morphological grading must be carefully considered. Whilst a developing embryo can be vitrified, its chances of survival of the procedure will be reduced if it has poor morphology. In addition, if it has a known low morphokinetic score, this would also suggest a reduced potential to reach live birth. A cost benefit analysis would need to be considered and discussed with the patient. The cost associated with freezing, storing, warming and transferring a frozen embryo is high, along with that of any associated medication. A lower grade embryo would have a higher risk of not surviving the warming procedure or post-survival, not achieving a pregnancy, than a higher-grade embryo. As it would be usual practice to use any higher-grade frozen embryos first, these embryos could remain frozen for several years before use, providing hope that may be unsubstantiated. It has been reported that patients feel shocked when they are informed of a low utilisation rate of their embryos (**33**), but this does not necessarily mean we should freeze lower grade embryos to make patients feel better in the short term. It may delay them beginning a further fresh cycle, which with the known decrease in success rates with IVF with increasing maternal age could unfortunately lead to some patients having a worse long-term outcome.

37.6 Conclusion

Overall, time-lapse imaging has allowed the rapid advancement of knowledge relating to how embryo development proceeds. This implications of this for embryo viability are not yet fully understood. Further research is required to determine how embryologists treat morphokinetic observations and cleavage abnormalities to ensure we utilise embryos in the most appropriate way for our patients.

REFERENCES

1. Zhan Q, Ye Z, Clarke R, et al. Direct unequal cleavages: embryo developmental competence, genetic constitution and clinical outcome. *PLoS One*. 2016;11(12):e0166398. doi: 10.1371/journal.pone.0166398.
2. Barrie A, Homburg R, McDowell G, et al. Preliminary investigation of the prevalence and implantation potential of abnormal embryonic phenotypes assessed using time-lapse imaging. *RBM Online*. 2017;34:455–462.
3. Rubio I, Kuhlmann R, Agerholm I, et al. Limited implantation success of direct-cleaved human zygotes: a time-lapse study. *Fertil Steril*. 2012;98:1458–1463.

4. McCoy RC, Newnham LJ, Ottolini CS, et al. Tripolar chromosome segregation drives the association between maternal genotype at variants spanning PLK4 and aneuploidy in human preimplantation embryos. *Hum Mol Gen.* 2018;27(14):2573–2585.
5. Ottolini CS, Kitchen J, Xanthopoulou L, et al. Tripolar mitosis and partitioning of the genome arrests human preimplantation development in vitro. *Sci Rep.* 2017;7(1):9744.
6. Ciray HN, Campbell A, Agerholm IE, et al. Proposed guidelines on the nomenclature and annotation of dynamic human embryo monitoring by a time-lapse user group. *Hum Rep.* 2014;29(12):2650–2660.
7. Hickman CFL, Campbell A, Duffy S, et al. Reverse cleavage: its significance with regards to human embryo morphokinetics, ploidy and stimulation protocol. *Hum Repod.* 2012;27:103–105.
8. Desai N, Goldberg JM, Austin C, et al. Are cleavage anomalies, multinucleation, or specific cell cycle kinetics observed with time-lapse imaging predictive of embryo developmental capacity or ploidy? *Fertil Steril.* 2018;109(4):665–674.
9. Lagalla C, Tarozzi N, Sciajno R, et al. Embryos with morphokinetic abnormalities may develop into euploid blastocysts. *RBM Online.* 2017;34:137–146.
10. Davis N, Smith R, Campbell A, et al. Cell fusion in the preimplantation human embryo is not associated with a significantly decreased live birth rate. *Hum Fertil.* 2020;23.
11. Liu Y, Chapple V, Roberts P, et al. Prevalence, consequence, and significance of reverse cleavage by human embryos viewed with the use of the Embryoscope time-lapse video system. *Fertil Steril.* 2014;102:1295–1300.
12. Alikani M, Cohen J, Tomkin G, et al. Human embryo fragmentation in vitro and its implications for pregnancy and implantation. *Fertil Steril.* 1999;71(5):836–842.
13. Fujimoto VY, Browne RW, Bloom MS, et al. Pathogenesis, developmental consequences, and clinical correlations of human embryo fragmentation. *Fertil Steril.* 2011;95:1197–1204.
14. Hardarson T, Löfman C, Coull G, et al. Internalization of cellular fragments in a human embryo: time-lapse recordings. *RBM Online.* 2002;5(1):36–38.
15. Viotti M, Victo AR, Barnes FL. Using outcome data from one thousand mosaic embryo transfers to formulate an embryo ranking system for clinical use. *Fertil Steril.* 2021;115:1212–1224.
16. Kahraman S, Cetinkaya M, Yuksel B, et al. The birth of a baby with mosaicism resulting from a known mosaic embryo transfer: a case report. *Hum Reprod.* 2020;35(3):727–733.
17. Munné S, Velilla E, Colls P, et al. Self-correction of chromosomally abnormal embryos in culture and implications for stem cell production. *Fertil Steril.* 2005;84(5):1328–1334.
18. Barbash-Hazan S, Frumkin T, Malcov M, et al. Preimplantation aneuploid embryos undergo self-correction in correlation with their developmental potential. *Fertil Steril.* 2009;92:890–896.
19. Harton GL, Munné S, Surrey M, et al. Diminished effect of maternal age on implantation after preimplantation genetic diagnosis with array comparative genomic hybridization. *Fertil Steril.* 2013;100(6):1695–1703.
20. Popovic M, Dhaenens L, Taelman J, et al. Extended in vitro culture of human embryos demonstrates the complex nature of diagnosing chromosomal mosaicism from a single trophectoderm biopsy. *Hum Reprod.* 2019;34(4):758–769.
21. Coticchio G, Barrie A, Lagalla et al. Plasticity of the human preimplantation embryo: developmental dogmas, variations on themes and self-correction. *Hum Reprod Update.* 2021;27(5):848–865.
22. Bolton H, Graham SJL, Van Der Aa N, et al. Mouse model of chromosome mosaicism reveals lineage-specific depletion of aneuploid cells and normal developmental potential. *Nat Commun.* 2016;7:665–666.
23. Lal A, Roudebush W, Chosed RJ. Embryo biopsy can offer more information than just ploidy status. *Front Cell Dev Biol.* 2020;8:78.
24. Victor AR, Tyndall JC, Brake AJ, et al. One hundred mosaic embryos transferred prospectively in a single clinic: exploring when and why they result in healthy pregnancies. *Fertil Steril.* 2019;111:280–293.
25. Li J, Ha S, Li Z, et al. Aurora B prevents aneuploidy via MAD2 during the first mitotic cleavage in oxidatively damaged embryos. *Cell Prolif.* 2019;52(5):e12657.
26. Huang Y, Ha S, Liz, et al. CHK1-CENP B/MAD2 is associated with mild oxidative damage-induced sex chromosome aneuploidy of male mouse embryos during in vitro fertilization. *Free Radic Biol Med.* 2019;137:181–193.
27. Gueye NA, Devkota B, Taylor D, et al. Uniparental disomy in the human blastocyst is exceedingly rare. *Fertil Steril.* 2014;101(1):232–236.
28. Grau N, Escrich L, Galiana Y, et al. Self-correction in tripronucleated human embryos. *Fertil Steril.* 2011;96(4):951–956.
29. Chuang TH, Hsieh JY, Lee MJ, et al. Concordance between different trophectoderm biopsy sites and the inner cell mass of chromosomal composition measured with a next-generation sequencing platform. *Mol Hum Reprod.* 2018;24(12):593–601.
30. Taylor TH, Stankewicz T, Katz SL, et al. Preliminary assessment of aneuploidy rates between the polar, mid and mural trophectoderm. *Zygote.* 2020;28(2):93–96.
31. Starostik MR, Sosina OA, McCoy RC. Single-cell analysis of human embryos reveals diverse patterns of aneuploidy and mosaicism. *Genome Res.* 2020;30:814–825.
32. Chavez-Badiola A, Farias AFS, Mendizabal-Ruiz G, et al. Predicting pregnancy test results after embryo transfer by image feature extraction and analysis using machine learning. *Sci Rep.* 2020;10:4394.
33. Rothwell E, Lamb B, Johnson E, et al. Patient perspectives and experiences with in vitro fertilization and genetic testing options. *Ther Adv Reprod Health.* 2020;14:1–12.

38

Artificial Intelligence Application in the ART Laboratory

Walid E. Maalouf and Rachel Smith

In 1964 President Johnson signed the bill creating the National Commission on Technology, Automation, and Economic Progress in order to reassure citizens that automation is an ally for a stronger future and better security rather than a technology that will just wipe out jobs (**1**). Advances in artificial intelligence (AI) are now leading a new world of automation and augmentation with machines performing at least equally to experienced skilled workforce in a range of activities including physical and those that require cognitive capabilities. In their analysis of potential of automation on the global economy, McKinsey and company summarise the impact of automation on activities that can enable businesses and individuals to perform better by minimising errors, accelerating productivity and achieve competitive advantages. They estimate the pace of automation is determined by the cost of the technology or its deployment (economical), technical feasibility, regulatory or social factors, and the labour market. Either way, people will need to learn to work alongside machines to help achieve the high productivity and survive the change in the activities of the labour force (**2**).

Healthcare services are under severe strain due to shrinkage in workforce exacerbated with mental health and long-lasting symptoms of COVID-19 affecting their performance (**3**). Job strain has been reported to correlate with coping strategies, and negatively associate with work performance and workforce morale (**4, 5**). The constantly changing environment in healthcare and the working conditions becoming increasingly demanding and stressful is a risk factor to the professional's health and safety (**6**), and the patients they look after (**7**). In their study, Portoghese and colleagues conclude that reducing workload will increase the sense of control among workers and reduce the likelihood of burnout (**6**). Therefore, when the strategy of employing more workers is not an option, the introduction of technology to alleviate part of the workload will allow healthcare professionals to spend more time on areas such as direct patient care or to simply provide more flexibility and slack in the system to minimise mistakes particularly in a sector such as fertility services. Paradoxically, if the technology is introduced, without planning it into a strategy of implementation, this can lead to unintended disruption of workflow and workarounds (**7**), which can be potentially harmful to patients (**8, 9**).

AI is a broad term that refers to any algorithm, code, or mixed technology designed to mimic human intelligence, and to display characteristic reasoning and thinking patterns of humans (**10**). AI is gaining traction in every sector, and the field of healthcare is showing remarkable potential for growth, in particular as a result of rapid advancement in medicine, longer life expectancy and growing demand on health services to meet the needs of the patients whilst maintaining the quality expected (**11**). Since the birth of Louise Brown, the first IVF baby (1978), the proportion of IVF babies born currently account for 2–5% of all births, and over 8 million babies born to date (**12**). Significant progress has been made in IVF and the ART laboratory using organic human intelligence, however, problems arise due to variations that can be found in the system, particularly, where human efforts are predominant. With this logarithmic growth of data available in IVF alongside with the increase in computer processing speed, we are in the era where effective AI derived algorithms can be successfully introduced.

Clinical embryologists are spending less time on trial-and-error methods than in the early days, with most of what is used today being commercially available. On the other hand, time dedicated by IVF clinical scientists for each treatment cycle have tripled over time, and with the need to master over 50 different types of procedures to be experienced embryologists (**13**), and this was before accounting for cryopreservation of oocytes and embryos, and time-lapse technology in clinical practice. In 2021, Forbes magazine asked the question: 'Could Artificial Intelligence Be the Future of Fertility Treatment?' where one AI application, to predict the chance of fertilisation was also tested at CARE fertility, and reporting that the technology can give clinical professionals a clearer view on the viability of oocytes and embryos so they can make more informed decisions and ultimately shorten the patient's journey to having a healthy baby (**14**). With clinical success rates remaining relatively low and due to the large number of variables involved, AI has been thought as a promising paradigm shift in IVF to fill in the gaps and manage the IVF patient journey more effectively.

One of the pillars for an effective IVF treatment is to ensure that clinic and laboratory protocols are designed to ensure healthy, high-quality gametes and embryos throughout the IVF journey. However, there are multiple clinical protocols and medications that can be used ahead of oocyte pick-up, and multiple ways to fertilise, culture and select gametes and embryos as part of the treatment. A number of factors therefore contribute to the success or failure of the IVF journey for patients, and therefore there are number of candidate variables for machine learning. The common data that is usually relevant to all patients is the baseline demographic characteristics such as age, BMI, ethnicity, medical history, cause and type of infertility, AMH, AFC, and previous cycle outcome

DOI: 10.1201/9781003269502-38

or complication. A number of baseline characteristics are part of the minimal information needed for medical reporting and any potential generalisation of AI development (**15**). In reproductive medicine, information on the clinical protocol used is expected, and this includes serum hormone levels, ovarian reserve, type of stimulation, dose and duration.

A number of candidates are typically collected and reported following ovarian stimulation for analysis including the number of mature oocytes obtained and OHSS. Concurrently, on the male side, semen analysis including sperm count, concentration, motility and morphology, allow determination of the severity of the male factor. In the laboratory, a number of outcomes are usually obtained such as type of fertilisation and fertilisation rates, fresh or frozen cycle, good quality cleavage stage embryos or blastocysts, morphokinetics if using time-lapse, PGT-A if applicable, number of embryos transferred and cryopreserved, endometrial thickness, any complications or adverse events. Further down, clinical outcomes will include biochemical, ongoing pregnancy, miscarriage, live births, and further detailed information on neonatal outcomes can also be reported if available (**16, 17**).

As more of this data is digitised in electronic medical records (EMRs) (**10**), AI application to automate, improve decision-making or reduce errors in the IVF laboratory have advanced significantly. Apart from data about the patient, hormone measurements and information on consumable used as part of the protocols and procedures, the majority of the candidate variables recorded require an imaging instrument, which is either a trans-vaginal ultrasound machine or a microscope. AI and imaging offer the greatest promise to enhance human performance in medicine. For example, when AI powered imaging diagnostic of cancer pathology is combined with trained pathologists, the accuracy score moved from 92% to 99.5% (**18**). In clinical IVF for example, 3D ultrasound imaging coupled with AI can be used for optimising trigger time, predicting ovarian hyper-response, and improved oocyte retrieval outcome (**19**). In the IVF laboratory, a number of AI applications have been developed for improving semen analysis and sperm viability testing, on oocyte maturity and viability scoring, and more importantly, on embryo selection for transfer, cryopreservation or discard (**20**).

Artificial intelligence-based technology can potentially enhance the accuracy of semen analysis (**21**). Sperm morphology (**22, 23**), sperm DNA fragmentation, viability and hyaluronic binding (**24**), are also additional sperm diagnostic tests that can be analysed with support of deep learning algorithms. Recent developments in the field including combining computer vision and artificial intelligence to create an algorithm that can aid embryologists in selecting the 'best' spermatozoa during an ICSI procedure (**25**). AI was also applied in determining egg quality and probability for successful fertilisation and development to blastocyst to improve egg freezing cycles, information provision and patient expectations (**26–28**). Oocyte imaging and AI was also extended to try and improve the ICSI procedure by identification of the best location to inject the sperm (**29**).

A significant development has been in the area of time-lapse technology and morphokinetics. The advantages of time-lapse have been discussed in chapter 39, but to mention the ability to annotate morphokinetic events of embryo development to help improve embryo selection (**30**). However, the time taken to manually annotate consistently embryos in culture to day 5 could take an experienced practitioner, on average 5–10 mins per embryo over 5 days of culture. This could account for a 1–2 of hours of laboratory time when applied to a cohort of embryos and average patient numbers per week. Factoring in quality assurance that is required to ensure all practitioners are able to robustly assess morphokinetic variables there has been an increase in supporting software to provide auto annotations. Software have been developed to guide the operator to a specific morphokinetic event for a manual confirmation, but still utilising the skills of the manual annotator. Fully automated systems use artificial intelligence with deep learning to derive annotation points by training convolutional neural networks (CNN) to determine morphokinetic variables using large data sets of quality assured manual annotations. These systems can predict annotations with accuracy with the promise of speed, reproducibility and consistency and the removal of subjectivity (**31, 32**). They can be implemented regardless of the TLI experience but similar to any introduction should be validated before implementation. With more reproducible outcomes they could provide improvement to prediction when used in conjunction with selection algorithms.

Images generated by time lapse are being exposed to the power of artificial intelligence, with convolutional neural networks and deep learning neural networks it is possible to unlock features within the embryo image, beyond the interpretation of the human eye, linked to outcomes of clinical pregnancy, live birth or ploidy status to train a model to determine the potential of an embryo to implant. These AI models should be built on large, diverse data sets to ensure accuracy, generalisation, and reproducibility of the algorithms More importantly, they are non-invasive and provide significant time saving as they can circumvent the need to annotate morphokinetic variables are they will be trained to analyse those features and a million plus other datapoints for each embryo. AI powered software that analyses time-lapse videos to predict implantation and live birth have been successfully reported (**33–35**). Other applications of AI and embryo imaging include automatic blastocyst grading (**36–39**), optimisation of criteria for embryo vitrification or biopsy (**40**), best area to perform laser assisted hatching (**36, 41**), and predicting ploidy (**42–45**).

With more digitised data, AI has also found its place in quality control and assurance of the IVF laboratory. Benchmarks and KPIs need to be set and monitored as part of the quality control and management routine of the laboratory (see Chapter 6 on quality control and quality management). In order to obtain finer granularity in the data, data entry into electronic medical records become an essential tool to link or add information such as operators, laboratory monitoring, tools and equipment used, and lot number of consumables. The AI-QM tool can monitor performance of clinicians and embryologists in relation to individual procedure performed, and provide an early warning system in case there is a shift or skew from benchmarks (**46, 47**), instead of waiting for monthly or quarterly manually generated spreadsheets and reports (**48, 49**), which can be time-consuming, inaccurate and subjective. As part of quality management, AI-based tools can be extended to identify embryos based on their morphological features to improve robustness of witnessing, tracking of individual embryos, and minimising risk of mix-up (**50**).

More data availability about the patient and their treatment cycle will also impact AI algorithm developments of other associated tests carried out. In particular, tests that require genetic analysis due to the vast amount of data output from next generation sequencers. This can lead to more objective and accurate calling of mosaics in PGT-A cycles (**51**), and further improving personalised embryo transfer when testing for endometrial receptivity (**52**). In parallel, AI and robotics to standardise a number of ART processes such as ICSI (**29**), vitrification (**53**), and even embryo culture, through developments of microfluidics, and nanoscale microchip devices that can also provide a wealth of data on embryo metabolomics (**54**).

As mentioned earlier in this chapter, the number of specialist procedures that the clinical embryologists are performing has more than tripled over the years, and therefore, managers are having to delegate a number of processes to more junior members of staff such as laboratory technologists. In turn, more junior staff are more likely to be from generation Z and therefore prefer new technologies (**55**), also, this will present a different challenge for their professional development other than the mundane routine laboratory tasks. With EMRs and digitisation, AI is an area of development that will grow very rapidly in the coming years. The main limitation currently is the lack of regulation and heterogeneity in the quality of data used in the development of algorithms, which makes the reliance of the reported outcomes difficult to interpret. Ethics and regulation of AI in IVF, and healthcare in general, will therefore become a pertinent issue in particular in terms of privacy and data governance, technical robustness, standardisation, inclusivity in development and fairness, accountability (**56**). AI will likely to continue to find more ways in supporting clinical embryology by standardising processes, supporting decisions in gamete and embryo selection, reducing number of issues and incorrect treatments, and ultimately, improving clinical outcome.

REFERENCES

1. Frey C, Osborne M. *The Future of Employment.* Oxford Martin Programme; 2013. Available from: www.oxfordmartin.ox.ac.uk/downloads/academic/The_Future_of_Employment.pdf.
2. McKinsey & Company. *A Future that Works.* McKinsey Global Institute; 2017. Available from: www.mckinsey.com/~/media/mckinsey/featured%20insights/Digital%20Disruption/Harnessing%20automation%20for%20a%20future%20that%20works/MGI-A-future-that-works-Executive-summary.ashx.
3. Campbell D. Strain on NHS as tens of thousands of staff suffer long Covid. *The Guardian*; 2021. Available from: www.theguardian.com/society/2021/apr/03/nhs-feels-strain-tens-thousands-staff-long-covid.
4. Wazqar DY, Kerr M, Regan S, et al. An integrative review of the influence of job strain and coping on nurses' work performance: understanding the gaps in oncology nursing research. *Int J Nurs Sci.* 2017;4(4):418–429.
5. Napier J, Clinch M. Job strain and retirement decisions in UK general practice. *Occup Med (Lond).* 2019;69(5): 336–341.
6. Portoghese I, Galletta M, Coppola RC, et al. Burnout and workload among health care workers: the moderating role of job control. *Saf Health Work.* 2014;5(3):152–157.
7. Rathert C, Williams ES, Lawrence ER, et al. Emotional exhaustion and workarounds in acute care: cross sectional tests of a theoretical framework. *Int J Nurs Stud.* 2012;49(8):969–977.
8. Koppel R, Wetterneck T, Telles JL, et al. Workarounds to barcode medication administration systems: their occurrences, causes, and threats to patient safety. *J Am Med Inform Assoc.* 2008;15(4):408–423.
9. Koppel R, Leonard CE, Localio AR, et al. Identifying and quantifying medication errors: evaluation of rapidly discontinued medication orders submitted to a computerized physician order entry system. *J Am Med Inform Assoc.* 2008;15(4):461–465.
10. Davenport T, Kalakota R. The potential for artificial intelligence in healthcare. *Future Healthc J.* 2019;6(2):94–98.
11. Spatharou A, Hieronimus S, Jenkins J. *Transforming Healthcare with AI: The Impact on the Workforce and Organizations.* McKinsey & Company; 2020. Available from: www.mckinsey.com/industries/healthcare-systems-and-services/our-insights/transforming-healthcare-with-ai.
12. ESHRE. *Eight Million IVF Babies Since the Birth of the World's First in 1978 ESHRE.* ESHRE; 2018. Available from: www.focusonreproduction.eu/article/ESHRE-News-GlobalIVF18.
13. Alikani M, Go K, McCaffrey C, et al. Comprehensive evaluation of contemporary assisted reproduction technology laboratory operations to determine staffing levels that promote patient safety and quality care. *Fertil Steril.* 2014;102(5):1345–1349.
14. Broster A. *Could Artificial Intelligence be the Future of Fertility Treatment?* Forbes: Forbes; 2021. Available from: www.forbes.com/sites/alicebroster/2021/01/11/could-artificial-intelligence-be-the-future-of-fertility-treatment/.
15. Hernandez-Boussard T, Bozkurt S, Ioannidis JP, et al. MINIMAR (MINimum Information for Medical AI Reporting): developing reporting standards for artificial intelligence in health care. *J Am Med Inform Assoc.* 2020;27(12):2011–2015.
16. Jayaprakasan K, Pandian D, Hopkisson J, et al. Effect of ethnicity on live birth rates after in vitro fertilisation or intracytoplasmic sperm injection treatment. *BJOG.* 2014;121(3):300–307.
17. Maalouf W, Maalouf W, Campbell B, et al. Effect of ethnicity on live birth rates after in vitro fertilisation/intracytoplasmic sperm injection treatment: analysis of UK national database. *BJOG.* 2017;124(6):904–910.
18. Bejnordi BE, Veta M, Van Diest PJ, et al. Diagnostic assessment of deep learning algorithms for detection of lymph node metastases in women with breast cancer. *JAMA.* 2017;318(22):2199–2210.
19. Liang X, Liang J, Zeng F, et al. Evaluation of oocyte maturity using artificial intelligence quantification of follicle volume biomarker by three-dimensional ultrasound. *Reprod Biomed Online.* 2022;45(6):1197–1206.

20. Dimitriadis I, Zaninovic N, Badiola AC, et al. Artificial intelligence in the embryology laboratory: a review. *Reprod Biomed Online*. 2021;44(3):435–448.
21. Parrella A, Ortega-López L, Briones YG, et al. Enhancing the accuracy of semen analysis with artificial Intelligence-based technology. *Fertil Steril*. 2021;116(3):e189–e190.
22. Thirumalaraju P, Kanakasabapathy MK, Bormann CL, et al. Human sperm morphology analysis using smartphone microscopy and deep learning. *Fertil Steril*. 2019; 112(3):e41.
23. Mirsky SK, Barnea I, Levi M, et al. Automated analysis of individual sperm cells using stain-free interferometric phase microscopy and machine learning. *Cytometry A*. 2017;91(9):893–900.
24. Dimitriadis IL, Bormann C, Kanakasabapathy MK, et al. Automated smartphone-based system for measuring sperm viability, DNA fragmentation, and hyaluronic binding assay score. *PLoS One*. 2019;14(3):e0212562.
25. Mendizabal-Ruiz G, Chavez-Badiola A, Figueroa IA, et al. Computer software (SiD) assisted real-time single sperm selection associated with fertilization and blastocyst formation. *Reprod Biomed Online*. 2022;45(4):703–711.
26. Patel RS, Bachu R, Adikey A, et al. Factors related to physician burnout and its consequences: a review. *Behav Sci*. 2018;8(11).
27. Manna C, Nanni L, Lumini A, et al. Artificial intelligence techniques for embryo and oocyte classification. *Reprod Biomed Online*. 2013;26(1):42–49.
28. Sacha CR, Vagios S, Souter I, et al. Maturity of oocyte cohort impacts blastocyst development as classified by artificial intelligence (AI). *Fertil Steril*. 2021;116(3):e161.
29. Dickinson I, Meyer A, Kelly N, et al. Advancement in the future automation of ICSI: use of deep convolutional neural networks (CNN) to identify precise location to inject sperm in mature human oocytes. *Hum Reprod*. 2020;35.
30. Ciray HN, Campbell A, Agerholm IE, et al. Proposed guidelines on the nomenclature and annotation of dynamic human embryo monitoring by a time-lapse user group. *Hum Reprod*. 2014;29(12):2650–2660.
31. Meseguer M. Workflow efficiency related to iDAScore. The 4th IVF Worldwide Online Congress; Online 2021.
32. Bori L, Meseguer F, Valera MA, et al. The higher the score, the better the clinical outcome: retrospective evaluation of automatic embryo grading as a support tool for embryo selection in IVF laboratories. *Hum Reprod*. 2022;37(6):1148–1160.
33. Ueno S, Berntsen J, Ito M, et al. Pregnancy prediction performance of an annotation-free embryo scoring system on the basis of deep learning after single vitrified-warmed blastocyst transfer: a single-center large cohort retrospective study. *Fertil Steril*. 2021;116(4):1172–1180.
34. Ueno S, Berntsen J, Ito M, et al. Correlation between an annotation-free embryo scoring system based on deep learning and live birth/neonatal outcomes after single vitrified-warmed blastocyst transfer: a single-centre, large-cohort retrospective study. *J Assist Reprod Genet*. 2022;39(9):2089–2099.
35. Tran D, Cooke S, Illingworth PJ, et al. Deep learning as a predictive tool for fetal heart pregnancy following time-lapse incubation and blastocyst transfer. *Hum Reprod*. 2019;34(6):1011–1018.
36. Bormann CL, Thirumalaraju P, Kanakasabapathy MK, et al. Consistency and objectivity of automated embryo assessments using deep neural networks. *Fertil Steril*. 2020;113(4):781–787.e1.
37. Khosravi P, Kazemi E, Zhan Q, et al. Deep learning enables robust assessment and selection of human blastocysts after in vitro fertilization. *NPJ Digit Med*. 2019;2(1):1–9.
38. VerMilyea M, Hall J, Diakiw S, et al. Development of an artificial intelligence-based assessment model for prediction of embryo viability using static images captured by optical light microscopy during IVF. *Hum Reprod*. 2020;35(4):770–784.
39. Thirumalaraju P, Kanakasabapathy MK, Bormann CL, et al. Evaluation of deep convolutional neural networks in classifying human embryo images based on their morphological quality. *Heliyon*. 2021;7(2):e06298.
40. Souter I, Vagios S, Sacha C, et al. Validation of a deep convolutional neural network trained to assess whether an embryo meets criteria for biopsy/cryopreservation using a test set of PGT embryos. *Hum Reprod*. 2020;35:1257–1258.
41. Kelly N, Bormann CL, Dickinson J, et al. Future of automation: use of deep convolutional neural networks (CNN) to identify precise location to perform laser assisted hatching on human cleavage stage embryos. *Fertil Steril*. 2020;114(3):e144.
42. Campbell A, Fishel S, Bowman N, et al. Modelling a risk classification of aneuploidy in human embryos using non-invasive morphokinetics. *Reprod Biomed Online*. 2013;26(5):477–485.
43. Chavez-Badiola A, Flores-Saiffe-Farías A, Mendizabal-Ruiz G, et al. Embryo ranking intelligent classification algorithm (ERICA): artificial intelligence clinical assistant predicting embryo ploidy and implantation. *Reprod Biomed Online*. 2020;41(4):585–593.
44. Meyer A, Dickinson J, Kelly N, et al. Can deep convolutional neural network (CNN) be used as a non-invasive method to replace preimplantation genetic testing for aneuploidy (PGT-A)? *Hum Reprod*. 2020;35:I238–I238.
45. Pennetta F, Lagalla C, Borini A. Embryo morphokinetic characteristics and euploidy. *Curr Opin Obstet Gynecol*. 2018;30(3):185–196.
46. Cherouveim P, Jiang VS, Kanakasabapathy MK, et al. Quality assurance (QA) for monitoring the performance of assisted reproductive technology (ART) staff using artificial intelligence (AI). *J Assist Reprod Genet*. 2022:241–249.
47. Bormann CL, Curchoe CL, Thirumalaraju P, et al. Deep learning early warning system for embryo culture conditions and embryologist performance in the ART laboratory. *J Assist Reprod Genet*. 2021;38(7):1641–1646.
48. Stanger J. Troubleshooting in IVF laboratories. In: Nagy ZP, Varghese AC, Agarwal A, editors. *In Vitro Fertilization*. Switzerland: Springer; 2019. pp. 823–832.
49. Olofsson JI, Banker MR, Sjoblom LP. Quality management systems for your in vitro fertilization clinic's laboratory: why bother? *J Hum Reprod Sci*. 2013;6(1):3.
50. Hammer KC, Jiang VS, Kanakasabapathy MK, et al. Using artificial intelligence to avoid human error in identifying embryos: a retrospective cohort study. *J Assist Reprod Genet*. 2022;39(10):2343–238.
51. Monahan D, Harton G, Griffin D, et al. 2. Clinical comparison of two PGT-A platforms utilizing different

thresholds to determine ploidy status. *Reprod Biomed Online*. 2019;39:e27–e28.

52. Ruiz-Alonso M, Valbuena D, Gomez C, et al. Endometrial receptivity analysis (ERA): data versus opinions. *Hum Reprod Open*. 2021;2021(2):hoab011.
53. Miao S, Jiang Z, Luo J, et al. A robotic system with embedded open microfluidic chip for automatic embryo vitrification. *IEEE Trans Biomed Eng*. 2022;69(12):3562–3571.
54. Gardner DK, Reineck P, Gibson BC, et al. Microfluidics and microanalytics to facilitate quantitative assessment of human embryo physiology. In: Nagy ZP, Varghese AC, Agarwal A, editors. *In Vitro Fertilization*. Switzerland: Springer; 2019. pp. 557–566.
55. Karandish D. *Technology is Critical to Recruit and Retain a Workforce that is Only Getting Younger*. Forbes; 2019. Available from: www.forbes.com/sites/forbestechcouncil/2019/04/09/technology-is-critical-to-recruit-and-retain-a-workforce-that-is-only-getting-younger/.
56. Sounderajah V, McCradden MD, Liu X, et al. Ethics methods are required as part of reporting guidelines for artificial intelligence in healthcare. *Nat Mach Intell*. 2022;4(4):316–317.

Index

Note: Page numbers in *italics* indicate a figure and page numbers in **bold** indicate a table on the corresponding page.

Q

R

S

For Product Safety Concerns and Information please contact our EU representative GPSR@taylorandfrancis.com Taylor & Francis Verlag GmbH, Kaufingerstraße 24, 80331 München, Germany

T - #0306 - 160425 - C74 - 280/210/14 - PB - 9781032216577 - Gloss Lamination